Anesthesia, Intensive Care and Pain in Neonates and Children

Series editor:
Antonino Gullo
Marinella Astuto
Ida Salvo

D1569433

Marinella Astuto • Pablo M. Ingelmo
Editors

Perioperative Medicine in Pediatric Anesthesia

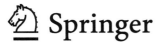 Springer

Editors
Marinella Astuto
UCO di Anestesia e Rianimazione
AO-U Policlinico di Catania
Catania
Italy

Pablo M. Ingelmo
Department of Anesthesia
MUHC Montreal Children's Hospital
McGill University
Montreal, QC
Canada

ISSN 2281-1788   ISSN 2281-1796   (electronic)
Anesthesia, Intensive Care and Pain in Neonates and Children
ISBN 978-3-319-21959-2   ISBN 978-3-319-21960-8   (eBook)
DOI 10.1007/978-3-319-21960-8

Library of Congress Control Number: 2015955168

Springer Cham Heidelberg New York Dordrecht London

Printed on acid-free paper

Springer International Publishing AG Switzerland is part of Springer Science+Business Media
(www.springer.com)

Foreword

For some readers, the title of this book might raise a main question: why a book on perioperative medicine in pediatric anesthesia. The reply is in the understanding that the anesthesia practice has evolved from a limited environment such as the operating room to the whole perisurgical care, starting from the time a patient is referred by the surgical treating team till the time the infant-child has recovered and is back with his own family and community. Therefore, it would make sense that pediatric anesthesiologists apply this concept to their own milieu. The introduction of sophisticated technology in endoscopic surgery and the better understanding of the pathophysiology of neonatal surgical stress emphasize the role of the anesthesiologist as a perioperative physician. For example, there has been an expansion of regional anesthesia applied to pediatric surgery as a result of improved and more reliable imaging techniques together with better training. This has allowed a better quality of analgesia and accelerated recovery. Other examples are the interactions of pediatric anesthesiologists with respiratory physiologists and neuroscientists to better understand the control of breathing and neurobehavioral development, thanks to major development in modern molecular biology and physiology. Also, better monitoring has allowed complex surgeries to be performed on an outpatient basis, and over the years a greater proportion of surgical operations are safely performed on an outpatient basis. Each chapter stresses the scientific principles necessary to understand and manage various situations encountered in pediatric anesthesia from a multidisciplinary point of view.

I commend Drs. Astuto and Ingelmo, both pediatric anesthesiologists in two large pediatric institutions in Italy and Canada, respectively, who have assembled an international group of illustrious experts to dissect the topic of perioperative pediatric medicine and to present the various aspects of pediatric anesthesia care, from preoperative preparation of the child, education of the family and optimization of medical, physical, nutritional and psychological functions, to perioperative management of specific conditions. The last four chapters are dedicated to acute and chronic pain and to the impact of anesthesia and surgery on the infant brain. Overall, these chapters will guide not only the trainee, but also the experienced and seasoned clinicians who are interested in expanding their knowledge on topics of relevant importance.

Francesco Carli, MD, MPhil
Department of Anesthesia
MUHC, Montreal General Hospital, McGill University,
Montreal, QC, Canada

Preface

Perioperative clinical outcomes in procedures involving infants and children have dramatically improved in recent years. Various factors may be responsible for those benefits such as emerging of new technologies, standardized anesthesia protocols, minimally invasive surgeries, improvements in acute postoperative care, and widespread use of perioperative safety standards, to mention just a few.

Traditionally, surgeons coordinate perioperative care of patients undergoing surgery. In some European countries, most of the perioperative care relies on anesthesiologists and pediatricians. Perioperative medicine becomes a multidisciplinary speciality aiming to provide continuum of care with coordinated interventions in the preoperative, intraoperative, and postoperative periods. The collaboration among a variety of doctors and nurses with specific pediatric training in pediatric environments allows the development of multidisciplinary clinical care pathways incorporating multiple evidence-based interventions.

With this book, we aim to provide a comprehensive overview of current practices in pediatric perioperative care. In all sections, from the preoperative care to the consequences of anesthesia and surgery through the perioperative care during surgery and in special clinical conditions, we look for practical answers to the most common questions of pediatric perioperative care.

This book was possible due to the efforts of an exquisite list of anesthesiologists, pediatricians, and surgeons from Europe and North America. This international team of contributors ranges from worldwide experts who had changed the way we care for our patients to young specialists who will lead the future of perioperative medicine. We are truly and deeply grateful for their collaboration and friendship.

There has been a progressive accumulation of good evidence related to perioperative care in the last decade. A long series of well-designed studies now permit an evidence-based approach to pediatric perioperative care. However, translation of research findings and guidelines into clinical practice remains a significant barrier affecting real clinical scenarios. Differences in type of surgeries, ages, interventions, clinical settings, and their interaction justify the need of establishing procedure-specific perioperative programs. Perioperative care is a multidimensional phenomenon, requiring multimodal management plan and strategies. It is evident that not a single specialist is able to provide solutions in all circumstances. Perioperative medicine gives us a unique opportunity to re-imagine the anesthetic-surgical-pediatrician relationship. This partnership should not continue to be experienced as independent entities divided by the operating theater "blood-brain barrier," but as a united team working towards the shared goal of optimal patient trajectory throughout the perioperative process to normality.

Catania, Italy   Marinella Astuto, MD
Montreal, QC, Canada   Pablo Mauricio Ingelmo, MD

Acknowledgments

I would like to express my deep gratitude to Professor Gullo for his patient guidance and enthusiastic encouragement of my work.

I would also like to thank my dear friend Dr. Pablo Ingelmo for his invaluable support throughout the planning and development phases of this book. Finally, I thank all the authors who honored me with their contributions.

Prof. Marinella Astuto M.D.

I wish to thank my wife, Francesca, and my sons, Matteo and Marco, for their patient support. I also wish to thank Prof. Miguel Angel Paladino and Prof. Roberto Fumagalli for their mentorship in shaping my clinical and academic career, and to the KISS group to make it valuable. Finally, this would not be possible without my friends: Walter, Marinella, and Pierre.

Pablo M. Ingelmo M.D.

Contents

1 Perioperative Medicine 1
Gabriele Baldini

Part I Perioperative Care Before Surgery

2 Preoperative Evaluation in Pediatric Anesthesia 11
Giovanni Mangia, Caterina Patti, and Paola Presutti

3 Preoperative Preparation 21
Luciano Bortone, Luca La Colla, and Marinella Astuto

**4 Preoperative Consideration in Common Pathological
and Nonpathological Conditions** 39
Marinella Astuto, Gianpaolo Serafini, Simonetta Baroncini,
Fabio Borrometi, Luciano Bortone, Cristina Ceschin,
Andrea Gentili, Elisabetta Lampugnani, Giovanni Mangia,
Luisa Meneghini, C. Minardi, Giovanni Montobbio,
Francesca Pinzoni, Barbara Rosina, Carlotta Rossi,
Marina Sammartino, Emre Sahillioğlu, Rita Sonzogni,
Valter Sonzogni, Simonetta Tesoro, Costanza Tognon,
Tiziana Tondinelli, Nicola Zadra, and Pablo M. Ingelmo

Part II Perioperative Care During Surgery

5 Perioperative Care in Day Hospital Surgery 55
Simonetta Tesoro and Laura Marchesini

6 Perioperative Care in Remote Locations 75
Maria Sammartino, Fabio Sbaraglia,
and Francesco Antonio Idone

7 Perioperative Care in Paediatric Orthopaedic Surgery 87
A.U. Behr

8 Perioperative Care of the Pediatric Neurosurgical Patient 115
Massimo Lamperti

9   **Pain After Surgical Correction of Congenital Chest Wall Deformities**. 131
Robert Baird and Pablo M. Ingelmo

10   **General Approach to Abdominal and Pelvic Procedures**. 137
Jean-Francois Courval

Part III   Perioperative Care in Special Situations and Conditions

11   **Perioperative Care of Children with a Difficult Airway** 147
Alan Barnett and Thomas Engelhardt

12   **Perioperative Care of Children with Neuromuscular Disease**. 159
Fabrizio Racca and Chiara Robba

13   **Perioperative Care of Children with a Metabolic Disease**. 175
Veyckemans Francis and Scholtes Jean-Louis

14   **Perioperative Care of Children with OSA**. 187
Gianluca Bertolizio and Karen Brown

15   **Perioperative Care of Children with Trauma**. 213
Leonardo Bussolin

16   **Perioperative Care of Children with Cancer**. 229
Navi Virk, B. Senbruna, and Jerrold Lerman

17   **Perioperative Care of Children with Cerebral Palsy and Behavioral Problems** 259
Martin Jöhr and Thomas M. Berger

18   **Perioperative Care of Neonates with Airway Obstruction** 273
Pierre Fiset and Sam J. Daniel

Part IV   Important Techniques for Perioperative Care

19   **Vascular Access in the Perioperative Period** 285
Thierry Pirotte

20   **US-Guided Nerve Targets** 341
Giorgio Ivani and Valeria Mossetti

21   **Noninvasive Hemodynamic and Respiratory Monitoring During the Perioperative Period**. 379
Brian Schloss and Joseph D. Tobias

Part V   Early and Long Term Consequences of Anesthesia and Surgery

22   **Negative Behaviour After Surgery**. 403
Marta Somaini and Pablo M. Ingelmo

23 Acute Pain Management and Prevention 417
Sylvain Tosetti

**24 Long-Term Consequences of Anesthesia (and Surgery)
on the Infant Brain**. 437
Tom Giedsing Hansen

25 Prevention of Chronic Postsurgical Pain 447
Gonzalo Rivera

Index 455

Contributors

Marinella Astuto Anesthesia, Intensive Care, University of Catania, Policlinico Hospital, Catania, Italy

Dipartimento di Anestesia e Rianimazione, Ospedale Universitario Policlinico, Catania, Italy

Robert Baird, MDCM, MSc, FRCSC, FACS Department of Pediatric Surgery, MUHC, Montreal Children's Hospital, McGill University, Montreal, QC, Canada

Gabriele Baldini, MD, MSc Department of Anesthesia, Montreal General Hospital, McGill University Health Center, Montreal, QC, Canada

Alan Barnett Department of Surgery, Radiology, Anaesthesia and Intensive Care, The University of the West Indies, Mona, Jamaica, West Indies

Simonetta Baroncini Dipartimento di Anestesia e Rianimazione Pediatrica, Ospedale S. Orsola-Malpighi, Università di Bologna, Bologna, Italy

A. U. Behr Istituto di Anestesia e Rianimazione, Azienda Ospedaliera Università, Padova, Italy

Thomas M. Berger Neonatal and Pediatric Intensive Care Unit, Children's Hospital, Luzern, Switzerland

Gianluca Bertolizio Department of Anesthesia, Montreal Children's Hospital, McGill University, Montreal, QC, Canada

Fabio Borrometi Servizio di Cure Palliative e Terapia del Dolore, Ospedale Santobono Pausilipon, Napoli, Italy

Luciano Bortone First Service of Anesthesia and Intensive Care, Parma Hospital, Parma, Italy,

Dipartimento di Anestesia e Rianimazione, Azienda Ospedaliera di Parma, Parma, Italy

Karen Brown Department of Anesthesia, Montreal Children's Hospital, McGill University, Montreal, QC, Canada

Leonardo Bussolin Department of Neuroanesthesia and Neurointensive Care, Pediatric Trauma Center, Pediatric Hospital Meyer, Florence, Italy

Cristina Ceschin Servizio di Anestesia e Rianimazione, Dolo Hospital, Mirano, Italy

Jean-Francois Courval Anesthesia Department, Montreal Children's Hospital, Montreal, QC, Canada

Sam J. Daniel, MD, FRCPC Department of Pediatric Surgery and Otolaryngology, Montreal Children's Hospital, MUHC, McGill University, Montreal, QC, Canada

Thomas Engelhardt Department of Anaesthesiology, Royal Aberdeen Children's Hospital, Aberdeen, UK

Pierre Fiset, MD, FRCPC Department of Anesthesia, Montreal Children's Hospital, MUHC, McGill University, Montreal, QC, Canada

Veyckemans Francis, MD Anesthesiology, Cliniques universitaires St Luc, Université Catholique de Louvain, Bruxelles, Belgium

Andrea Gentili Dipartimento di Anestesia e Rianimazione Pediatrica, Ospedale S. Orsola-Malpighi, Università di Bologna, Bologna, Italy

Tom Giedsing Hansen, MD, PhD Department of Anesthesiology and Intensive Care – Pediatric Section, Odense University Hospital, Odense, Denmark

Institute of Clinical Research – Anesthesiology, University of Southern Denmark, Odense, Denmark

Francesco Antonio Idone Department of Anesthesia and Intensive Care, Catholic University of Sacred Heart, Training Hospital "A. Gemelli", Rome, Italy

Pablo M. Ingelmo, MD Department of Anesthesia, Montreal Children's Hospital, MUHC, McGill University, Montreal, QC, Canada

Giorgio Ivani Anesthesiology and Intensive Care, Regina Margherita Children Hospital, Turin, Italy

Scholtes Jean-Louis, MD Anesthesiology, Cliniques universitaires St Luc, Université Catholique de Louvain, Bruxelles, Belgium

Martin Jöhr Pediatric Anesthesia, Department of Anesthesia, Luzerner Kantonsspital, Luzern, Switzerland

Luca La Colla First Service of Anesthesia and Intensive Care, Parma Hospital, Parma, Italy

Massimo Lamperti, MD Anesthesiology Institute, Cleveland Clinic Abu Dhabi (CCAD), Abu Dhabi, United Arab Emirates (UAE)

Elisabetta Lampugnani Dipartimento di Anestesia e Rianimazione, IRCCS Ospedale dei Bambini G. Gaslini, Genova, Italy

Jerrold Lerman, MD, FRCPC, FANZCA University of Rochester, Rochester, NY, USA

Giovanni Mangia Department of Anesthesia, San Camillo Hospital, Rome, Italy

Laura Marchesini, MD Department of Anesthesia, Analgesia and Intensive Care, University of Perugia, Perugia, Italy

Luisa Meneghini Dipartimento di Anestesia e Rianimazione, Università di Padova, Padova, Italy

C. Minardi Dipartimento di Anestesia e Rianimazione, Università di Padova, Padova, Italy

Giovanni Montobbio Dipartimento di Anestesia e Rianimazione, IRCCS Ospedale dei Bambini G. Gaslini, Genova, Italy

Valeria Mossetti Anesthesiology and Intensive Care, Regina Margherita Children Hospital, Turin, Italy

Caterina Patti Surgeon Freelancer, Rome, Italy

Francesca Pinzoni Dipartimento di Anestesia Pediatrica, Ospedali Civili, Brescia, Italy

Thierry Pirotte Department of Anesthesia, Cliniques universitaires Saint-Luc, Université catholique de Louvain – UCL, Brussels, Belgium

Paola Presutti Department of Anesthesia, San Camillo Hospital, Rome, Italy

Fabrizio Racca, MD Anesthesiology and Intensive Care Unit, S.C. Anestesia e Rianimazione Pediatrica Azienda Ospedaliera SS Antonio Biagio e Cesare Arrigo Hospital, Alessandria, Italy

Gonzalo Rivera, MD Department of Anesthesia, Clinica Las Condes, Santiago, Chile

Chronic Pain Service, Department of Anesthesia, The Montreal Children's Hospital, McGill University, Montreal, QC, Canada

Chiara Robba Anesthesiology and Intensive Care Unit, SS Antonio Biagio e Cesare Arrigo Hospital, Alessandria, Italy

Barbara Rosina Dipartimento di Anestesia Pediatrica, Ospedali Civili, Brescia, Italy

Carlotta Rossi Servizio di Anestesia e Rianimazione, Dolo Hospital, Mirano, Italy

Emre Sahillioğlu Department of Anesthesiology and Reanimation, Acibadem University, Istanbul, Turkey

Maria Sammartino Dipartimento di Anestesia e Rianimazione, Ospedale Universitario A. Gemelli, Università Cattolica del Sacro Cuore, Rome, Italy

Department of Anesthesia and Intensive Care, Catholic University of Sacred Heart, Training Hospital "A. Gemelli", Rome, Italy

Fabio Sbaraglia Department of Anesthesia and Intensive Care, Catholic University of Sacred Heart, Training Hospital "A. Gemelli", Rome, Italy

Brian Schloss, MD Department of Anesthesiology and Pain Medicine, Nationwide Children's Hospital, Columbus, OH, USA

Department of Anesthesiology and Pain Medicine, The Ohio State University, Columbus, OH, USA

B. Senbruna, MD University of Rochester, Rochester, NY, USA

Gianpaolo Serafini Anestesia e Rianimazione 1, Fondazione IRCCS Policlinico S. Matteo, Università di Pavia, Pavia, Italy

Marta Somaini, MD Department of Anaesthesia and Intensive Care, Niguarda Ca' Granda Hospital, Milan-Bicocca University, Milan, Italy

Valter Sonzogni Primo Servizio di Anestesia e Rianimazione, Ospedali Riuniti di Bergamo, Bergamo, Italy

Rita Sonzogni Primo Servizio di Anestesia e Rianimazione, Ospedali Riuniti di Bergamo, Bergamo, Italy

Simonetta Tesoro, MD Sezione di Anestesia, Analgesia e Rianimazione, Dipartimento di Medicina Clinica e Sperimentale, Università di Perugia, Perugia, Italy

Department of Anesthesia, Analgesia and Intensive Care, University of Perugia, Perugia, Italy

Joseph D. Tobias, MD Department of Anesthesiology and Pain Medicine, Nationwide Children's Hospital, Columbus, OH, USA

Department of Anesthesiology and Pain Medicine, The Ohio State University, Columbus, OH, USA,

Department of Pediatrics, The Ohio State University, Columbus, OH, USA

Costanza Tognon Dipartimento di Anestesia e Rianimazione, Università di Padova, Padova, Italy

Tiziana Tondinelli Dipartimento di Anestesia, Ospedale S. Camillo, Rome, Italy

Sylvain Tosetti, MD Anaesthesia Department, The Montreal Children's Hospital, Montreal, QC, Canada

Navi Virk, MD University of Rochester, Rochester, NY, USA

Nicola Zadra Dipartimento di Anestesia e Rianimazione, Università di Padova, Padova, Italy

Perioperative Medicine

1

Gabriele Baldini

1.1   What Is Perioperative Medicine?

Perioperative medicine is the practice of medicine that relates to and encompasses all aspects of care provided to patients from the moment surgery is considered the primary treatment to when patients are discharged from the hospital after the operation [1, 2]. It is considered a multidisciplinary speciality that aims to provide continuum of care with coordinated and evidence-based interventions in the preoperative, intraoperative, and postoperative period with the ultimate goals to prevent the occurrence of adverse outcomes, timely diagnose and treat perioperative complications (*timely rescue*) [3], and optimize surgical recovery.

1.2   Patients, Surgery, and Complications

Complications not only delay surgical recovery and increase healthcare costs but can also determine patients' survival [4, 5]. In the last years, significant advancements in surgical care have been achieved. Despite advancements in anesthesia and surgical care have significantly attenuated the stress response associated with surgery, complications still occur in a significant proportion of patients. This demonstrates that the development of postoperative complications mainly depends on the interaction between patient's physiologic reserve and the metabolic and inflammatory response induced by surgery [6]. Consequently, improvement of perioperative care by optimizing patients' physiologic reserve and medical needs, and

G. Baldini, MD, MSc
Department of Anesthesia, Montreal General Hospital,
McGill University Health Center, Montreal, QC, Canada
e-mail: gabriele.baldini@mcgill.ca

© Springer International Publishing Switzerland 2016
M. Astuto, P.M. Ingelmo (eds.), *Perioperative Medicine in Pediatric Anesthesia*,
Anesthesia, Intensive Care and Pain in Neonates and Children,
DOI 10.1007/978-3-319-21960-8_1

minimizing organ dysfunction caused by surgery, might significantly reduce adverse outcomes and further accelerate surgical recovery.

1.3   A Model of Perioperative Medicine: Learning from Enhanced Recovery After Surgery (ERAS) Programs

Traditionally, surgeons coordinate perioperative care of patients undergoing surgery. Enhanced recovery after surgery (ERAS) programs are multidisciplinary clinical care pathways incorporating multiple evidence-based preoperative, intraoperative, and postoperative interventions designed to decrease the surgical stress response, enhance recovery, and improve outcomes (Fig. 1.1). They have been successfully adopted by a variety of surgical specialities, and they have shown to decrease hospital stay and reduce postoperative complications without increasing readmission rates [7]. As consequence, variability in perioperative clinical practice has been reduced, and collaboration among a variety of medical specialities, such as anesthesiologists, surgeons, internists, physiotherapists, and dieticians, increased. For these reasons, ERAS programs can be considered a well-proven clinical model of perioperative care that encompasses many of the perioperative care principles.

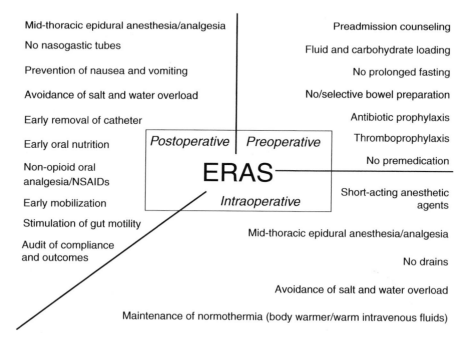

Fig. 1.1 Enhanced recovery after surgery (ERAS) for abdominal surgery: perioperative elements. Published by Varadhan KK et al Crit Care Clin 2010;26:527–47– Fig. 3. Components of ERAS. – Elsevier Inc

ERAS programs have been effectively developed also for pediatric patients [8–12], but further studies are warranted to establish their safety in this population.

1.4 Areas of Perioperative Medicine

1.4.1 Preoperative Phase

1.4.1.1 Preoperative Risk Assessment and Optimization
Patients' comorbidities are one of the main determinants of postoperative complications. In the preoperative period, the aim of perioperative medicine is to assess preoperative risk and optimize functional reserve and preoperative conditions that delay surgical recovery and increase the risk of morbidity and mortality. Ideally, once high-risk patients have been identified, multidisciplinary meeting should discuss the efficacy of alternative treatments to surgery to avoid the occurrence of surgical adverse events without affecting patients' care [13]. If surgery remains the best treatment, preoperative strategies to optimize patients' comorbidities should be adopted to minimize adverse outcomes [13].

1.4.1.2 Pre-habilitation
In the preoperative phase physicians should also take the opportunity to commence lifestyle changes by supporting adolescent or adult patients with smoking and alcohol cessation programs, improve nutritional status and functional capacity. Recovering from surgery takes longer than expected. Even in absence of surgical complications, physiological and functional capacities are reduced by 20–40 % after surgery and take time to return to baseline values. Surprisingly, even following a relatively invasive surgical procedure such as ambulatory laparoscopic cholecystectomy, more than 50 % of patients do not recover to baseline activity levels 1 month after surgery [14]. Pre-habilitation programs aim at improving functional capacity and physiologic reserve before surgery and are becoming popular and effective preoperative strategies to help adult patients recover faster from surgery [15–17]. They include preoperative multimodal interventions such exercise training, nutrition supplement, and relaxation techniques for a period of 3–4 weeks, and they have demonstrated to be more effective than rehabilitation programs intervening only in the postoperative phase [18]. Although pre-habilitation programs enhance functional exercise capacity and reduce hospital stay, it remains unclear if they positively affect clinical outcomes [17].

1.4.2 Intraoperative Phase

Anesthesia care plays a pivotal role to attenuate surgical stress and minimize organ dysfunction associated with surgery. Several intraoperative interventions directly controlled by anesthesiologists [19], such as avoidance of hypothermia and deep anesthesia, glycemic control, optimal fluid management, adequate hemodynamic monitoring, and appropriate analgesia, have shown to improve clinical outcomes and accelerate the early and intermediate phase of surgical recovery [20].

1.4.3 Postoperative Phase

1.4.3.1 Intensity of Postoperative Care

Postoperative care of surgical patients is essential to ensure adequate surgical recovery. Determining the intensity of postoperative care is pivotal as early recognition and treatment of postoperative complications has been shown to significantly reduce surgical mortality [5]. The intensity of postoperative care should be determined considering patient's preoperative risk and the invasiveness of the surgery. Admission to intensive care units or high dependency units should be reserved for high-risk patients or for complicated surgeries.

1.4.3.2 Postoperative Pain Management

Postoperative acute pain management must ensure optimal analgesia, minimizing opioid side effects and facilitating early mobilization. The introduction of acute pain services has facilitated the management of surgical patients with inadequate pain control or with adverse events related to common analgesia techniques. It has also improved patients' satisfaction and accelerated hospital discharge. The use of ultrasound-guided regional analgesia techniques for inpatients and outpatients has increased and successfully improved postoperative pain control. Indeed, also ambulatory patients can be comfortably and safely discharged home with continuous peripheral nerve blocks.

1.4.3.3 Hemodynamic Management and Echocardiography

Perioperative hemodynamic management is essential to guarantee optimal organ perfusion and oxygen delivery. The use of cardiac output monitoring was typically limited in cardiac patients during the intraoperative and postoperative period or for critically ill patients admitted to intensive care units. Recently, the widespread use of perioperative echocardiography and noninvasive cardiac output monitors outside the operating room has gained popularity even in patients undergoing noncardiac surgery. Thanks to these devices physicians can now administer intravenous fluids based on more objective and accurate measures of hypovolemia, facilitating the hemodynamic management of high-risk surgical patients [21] and hemodynamically unstable patients [3]. In the perioperative period, echocardiography can also be utilized as diagnostic tool, for example, to identify preoperative cardiopulmonary conditions that can influence the management of surgical patients.

1.4.3.4 Noncardiac Ultrasound

The use of ultrasound in the perioperative period is gaining popularity also to mange patients without cardiac conditions. For example, ultrasound-guided peripheral nerve blocks are considered standard of care in many institutions; bedsides, ultrasound of the lungs guides physicians to promptly diagnose and treat postoperative

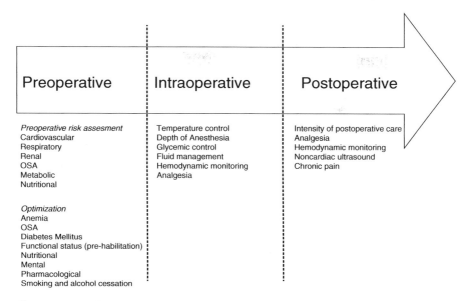

Fig. 1.2 Areas of perioperative medicine

respiratory complications such as pulmonary edema, lung consolidation, pleural effusion, and pneumothorax [22]; ultrasound assessment of the gastric content provides important information about the individual risk of aspiration before the induction of anesthesia [23–26].

1.4.3.5 Chronic Postsurgical Pain

Chronic postsurgical pain (CPSP) can affect a significant proportion of surgical patients even following minor surgical procedures. Although the incidence of CPSP is higher after certain surgeries than others, uncontrolled severe acute surgical pain represents one of the main risk factors associated with the development of CPSP [27]. Identification of patients at higher risk of CPSP, nerve-sparing surgical techniques, and prevention and treatment of acute postoperative pain represent perioperative interventions that must be considered in every surgical patient to decrease the occurrence of this physically, mentally, and socially disabling condition [28].

Figure 1.2 summarized the most important areas of perioperative medicine discussed in this section.

1.5 Perioperative Medicine: A Natural Extension of Anesthesiology?

Anesthesiologists possess extensive perioperative knowledge and skills to be considered the ideal perioperative physician [6]. While many anesthesiologists have already identified themselves as perioperative physicians (some anesthesiology departments have already entitled their departments "Department of Anesthesia and Perioperative Medicine"), others still consider their practice limited to the operating room. This mixed vision can be attributed to several reasons, such as workforce and economic issues, absence of a cohesive and consensus-based perioperative medicine curricula, and lack of a formal and recognized training [1, 2, 29].

Despite these considerations, it is unquestionable that anesthesiologists should start looking beyond the intraoperative period, as they have done in critical care and pain management [6]. Improvements of anesthetic knowledge and advancements in anesthesia care have made the delivery of anesthesia a safer practice. Consequently the need of anesthesiologists in every operating room has started to be considered not essential, and many institutions, especially in the North America, have already tried to replace anesthesiologists with physicians' assistants, certified nurse anesthetists, and other nonphysician figures. If anesthesiologists continue to exclusively practice in the operating room, the speciality of anesthesiology will be at risk of being undervalued, the role of the anesthesiologists underestimated, and perioperative medicine might be practiced by other specialities (e.g., internal medicine, surgery).

However, before being considered a true perioperative speciality, anesthesiology must face important challenges. The residency program should be redesigned by implementing a robust perioperative curriculum that considers the continuum of care and clearly defines the required, basic, intermediate, and advanced competencies that a perioperative physician must have. For this purpose, collaboration with other specialities such as internal medicine, cardiology, and respirology is essential, and it must be intensified during the residency training to improve anesthesiologists' perioperative knowledge. Alternatively, a perioperative fellowship program could be offered to those anesthesiologists who specifically want to support patient's care throughout the entire perioperative period and obtain advance perioperative knowledge and skills [29]. Finally, expanding the horizons of anesthesia beyond the operating theatre will provide strong basic science and clinical knowledge to improve perioperative care.

In conclusion, perioperative medicine aims to provide continuum of care with coordinated and evidence-based interventions in the preoperative, intraoperative, and postoperative period with the ultimate goals to reduce morbidity and mortality and accelerate surgical recovery.

References

1. Rock P (2000) The future of anesthesiology is perioperative medicine. Anesthesiol Clin North America 18(3):495–513, v
2. Carli F (2001) Perioperative medicine. Are the anesthesiologists ready? Minerva Anestesiol 67(4):252–255
3. Yang H (2015) Perioperative medicine: why do we care? Can J Anaesth 62(4):338–344
4. Khuri SF, Henderson WG, DePalma RG, Mosca C, Healey NA, Kumbhani DJ (2005) Participants in the VANSQIP. Determinants of long-term survival after major surgery and the

adverse effect of postoperative complications. Ann Surg 242(3):326–341; discussion 341–323

5. Ghaferi AA, Birkmeyer JD, Dimick JB (2009) Variation in hospital mortality associated with inpatient surgery. N Engl J Med 361(14):1368–1375
6. Grocott MP, Pearse RM (2012) Perioperative medicine: the future of anaesthesia? Br J Anaesth 108(5):723–726
7. Greco M, Capretti G, Beretta L, Gemma M, Pecorelli N, Braga M (2014) Enhanced recovery program in colorectal surgery: a meta-analysis of randomized controlled trials. World J Surg 38(6):1531–1541
8. Howard F, Brown KL, Garside V, Walker I, Elliott MJ (2010) Fast-track paediatric cardiac surgery: the feasibility and benefits of a protocol for uncomplicated cases. Eur J Cardiothorac Surg 37(1):193–196
9. Mattioli G, Palomba L, Avanzini S, Rapuzzi G, Guida E, Costanzo S, Rossi V, Basile A, Tamburini S, Callegari M, DellaRocca M, Disma N, Mameli L, Montobbio G, Jasonni V (2009) Fast-track surgery of the colon in children. J Laparoendosc Adv Surg Tech A 19(Suppl 1):S7–S9
10. Reismann M, Arar M, Hofmann A, Schukfeh N, Ure B (2012) Feasibility of fast-track elements in pediatric surgery. Eur J Pediatr Surg 22(1):40–44
11. Reismann M, Dingemann J, Wolters M, Laupichler B, Suempelmann R, Ure BM (2009) Fast-track concepts in routine pediatric surgery: a prospective study in 436 infants and children. Langenbecks Arch Surg 394(3):529–533
12. Reismann M, von Kampen M, Laupichler B, Suempelmann R, Schmidt AI, Ure BM (2007) Fast-track surgery in infants and children. J Pediatr Surg 42(1):234–238
13. Glance LG, Osler TM, Neuman MD (2014) Redesigning surgical decision making for high-risk patients. N Engl J Med 370(15):1379–1381
14. Feldman LS, Kaneva P, Demyttenaere S, Carli F, Fried GM, Mayo NE (2009) Validation of a physical activity questionnaire (CHAMPS) as an indicator of postoperative recovery after laparoscopic cholecystectomy. Surgery 146(1):31–39
15. Durrand JW, Batterham AM, Danjoux GR (2014) Pre-habilitation. I: aggregation of marginal gains. Anaesthesia 69(5):403–406
16. Corovic A, Griffiths R (2014) Pre-habilitation. II: time for a patient-doctor contract? Anaesthesia 69(5):407–410
17. Carli F, Scheede-Bergdahl C (2015) Prehabilitation to enhance perioperative care. Anesthesiol Clin 33(1):17–33
18. Gillis C, Li C, Lee L, Awasthi R, Augustin B, Gamsa A, Liberman AS, Stein B, Charlebois P, Feldman LS, Carli F (2014) Prehabilitation versus rehabilitation: a randomized control trial in patients undergoing colorectal resection for cancer. Anesthesiology 121(5):937–947
19. Carli F, Baldini G (2011) Fast-track surgery: it is time for the anesthesiologist to get involved! Minerva Anestesiol 77(2):227–230
20. Kehlet H, Wilmore DW (2008) Evidence-based surgical care and the evolution of fast-track surgery. Ann Surg 248(2):189–198
21. Hamilton MA, Cecconi M, Rhodes A (2011) A systematic review and meta-analysis on the use of preemptive hemodynamic intervention to improve postoperative outcomes in moderate and high-risk surgical patients. Anesth Analg 112(6):1392–1402
22. Lichtenstein D, van Hooland S, Elbers P, Malbrain ML (2014) Ten good reasons to practice ultrasound in critical care. Anaesthesiol Intensive Ther 46(5):323–335
23. Perlas A, Chan VW, Lupu CM, Mitsakakis N, Hanbidge A (2009) Ultrasound assessment of gastric content and volume. Anesthesiology 111(1):82–89
24. Bouvet L, Mazoit JX, Chassard D, Allaouchiche B, Boselli E, Benhamou D (2011) Clinical assessment of the ultrasonographic measurement of antral area for estimating preoperative gastric content and volume. Anesthesiology 114(5):1086–1092
25. Bouvet L, Miquel A, Chassard D, Boselli E, Allaouchiche B, Benhamou D (2009) Could a single standardized ultrasonographic measurement of antral area be of interest for assessing gastric contents? A preliminary report. Eur J Anaesthesiol 26(12):1015–1019

26. Perlas A, Davis L, Khan M, Mitsakakis N, Chan VW (2011) Gastric sonography in the fasted surgical patient: a prospective descriptive study. Anesth Analg 113(1):93–97
27. Kehlet H, Jensen TS, Woolf CJ (2006) Persistent postsurgical pain: risk factors and prevention. Lancet 367(9522):1618–1625
28. Gilron I, Kehlet H (2014) Prevention of chronic pain after surgery: new insights for future research and patient care. Can J Anaesth 61(2):101–111
29. Gharapetian A, Chung F, Wong D, Wong J (2015) Perioperative fellowship curricula in anesthesiology: a systematic review. Can J Anaesth 62(4):403–412

Part I

Perioperative Care Before Surgery

Preoperative Evaluation in Pediatric Anesthesia

2

Giovanni Mangia, Caterina Patti, and Paola Presutti

2.1   Introduction

The preoperative assessment is the process of evaluating the patient's clinical condition, aimed to define the risks and eligibility for anesthesia and surgery. The information needed to make decisions comes from the anamnesis, the physical exam, and the complementary test collected by a multidisciplinary team including surgeons, nurses, pediatricians, and anesthetists.

The preoperative evaluation defines the physical status of the child, foresees the surgical and anesthetic risks, prescribes preoperative tests and therapies or special preparation, and provides information regarding the perioperative care. It also helps to make appropriate use of hospital resources and programs the surgical activities based on the clinical characteristic and the risk of the patients.

Although other medical specialists may provide additional information in deciding the eligibility of a patient for anesthesia, the preoperative evaluation is an anesthesiologist's responsibility. Only an anesthesiologist can define the eligibility for anesthesia.

2.2   Operating Risk Stratification

The clinical risk is the probability of a patient presenting "damage or inconvenience caused, even if unintentionally, by the medical care given during the hospitalization period, that causes a prolongation of hospitalization, a health status deterioration or

G. Mangia (✉) • P. Presutti
Department of Anesthesia, San Camillo Hospital, Rome, Italy
e-mail: mangia.giovanni@fastwebnet.it

C. Patti
Surgeon Freelancer, Rome, Italy

© Springer International Publishing Switzerland 2016   11
M. Astuto, P.M. Ingelmo (eds.), *Perioperative Medicine in Pediatric Anesthesia*,
Anesthesia, Intensive Care and Pain in Neonates and Children,
DOI 10.1007/978-3-319-21960-8_2

death" [1]. The negative outcome of a surgery depends on several factors including the patient condition, comorbidity, and the type of surgery (Table 2.1).

The American Society of Anesthesiologist Physical Status classification (ASA-PS) is routinely used for risk prediction [2–4] in the perioperative period. The NARCO-SS score developed by Clavien for adult patients is a risk assessment system that includes both pre- and intraoperative information [5] and has been recently adapted for pediatric population [6, 7]. Additionally, the use of local and regional epidemiological data may contribute to further identify specific risk [8].

The ASA-PS is the most frequently used system to evaluate the preoperative physical status. Five classes can be distinguished: I normal healthy patient, II patient with mild systemic disease, III patient with severe systemic disease that limits activity but not incapacitating, IV patient with incapacitating disease that is a constant threat to life, and V moribund patient not expected to survive 24 hours with or without surgical operation. In the event of an emergency operation, an E is placed after the physical status class. The main advantage of this system is its simplicity. However, its interrater reliability is subjected to an open discussion. [2–4]. Younger age (infants and children with less than 3 years of age) and higher ASA-FS (III to V) were strongly correlated with a higher risk of anesthesia-related cardiac arrest [9–14].

The NARCO is a score risk system based on the preoperative neurological status (N), airway (A), respiratory (R), cardiac activity (C), and other items (O). The total score is supplemented by a score of surgical severity (SS), with the identification of two categories (A and B) according to surgery invasiveness. It is thereby obtained an overall risk score (low, moderate, high, higher) and information on the postoperative care level (day surgery, PACU, PICU). This system shows a more accurate prediction rate of adverse events and care intensification – escalation, morbidity, and mortality – compared with the ASA-PS [5].

Weinberg et al. and Wood et al. studied the predictors of perioperative complications 30 days after surgery [6, 7]. Prematurity, ASA-PS >3, cardiac surgery, neurosurgery, major orthopedic interventions need for intraoperative transfusion of albumin and/or red blood cells, surgery lasting more than two hours, and SpO2 less than 96 % were associated with postoperative complications and reoperations.

Table 2.1 Johns Hopkins surgery risk classification system (JHSRCS)

JHSRCS status	Description	Example
1	Noninvasive procedure, minimal risk	Excision of lesion of the skin
2	Procedures limited in their invasive nature mild risk	Inguinal hernia repair, diagnostic laparoscopy
3	More invasive procedures moderate risk, moderate blood loss	Open abdominal procedures
4	Procedures posing significant risk	Planned postoperative intensive care, open thoracic procedure, intracranial procedure

2.3   Timing and Organization of the Preoperative Evaluation

The timing of the preoperative evaluation could be influenced by the demographic characteristics, the institutional organization, the patient's clinical condition, and the surgical procedure. The organizational system used for the clinical evaluation and preoperative risk stratification and clinical planning varies among institutions and type of intervention [15].

Hospitalization of healthy children for a preoperative evaluation the day before surgery should be considered as improper in most minor elective surgical procedures. A day hospital stay does not reduce costs nor does it save time because the patient should be evaluated again on the day of surgery [16].

The ASA-PS can provide suggestions on the timing of preoperative visit [17]. The ASA Task Force on Preanesthesia Evaluation suggested that for low-risk patients undergoing low grading procedures, preanesthesia could be performed the same day of the surgery [18]. The "one-stop anesthesia" modality is a clinical pathway designed for day surgery procedures (Fig. 2.1). This modality reduces the access to the hospital for day surgery interventions with significant social, psychological, and economic advantages. It is also characterized by a high diagnostic accuracy and a high parents' satisfaction [19–23]. The "one-stop anesthesia" is a modification of the "one-stop surgery" where patients are screened before the procedure by external specialists [24, 25].

The preoperative evaluation of high-risk patients and/or scheduled for major surgery should be performed before the day of surgery [23, 26]. Nurses and the pediatrician have a central role on the screening and preparation of the surgical patient independent of the type of surgery [27–30].

The preoperative risk stratification has organizational consequences including the care settings (in hospital, day of surgery), the postoperative care levels (e.g., PACU, PICU, etc.), and the selection of the institution (hospital vs ambulatory surgery center) [31].

2.4   Medical History and Physical Examination

The preoperative assessment should precede any request of laboratory and instrumental tests. The anamnesis usually takes advantage of questionnaires, submitted to parents, in a "face-to-face" procedure, by phone, online, or compiled at home [32, 33] (Appendix A). As an assessment support, it is also possible to use a specific software, which helps to reduce the amount of preoperative tests [34]. The medical history should provide information of all the present and past medical problems. It should include extensive information of medication intake including natural medicines. Any allergic reaction to food, medications, or other substances (e.g., latex) must be addressed.

When looking for information regarding previous anesthesia experiences, it is extremely important to focus the airway management and respiratory or cardiovascular complications. It is also important to consider the postoperative consequences

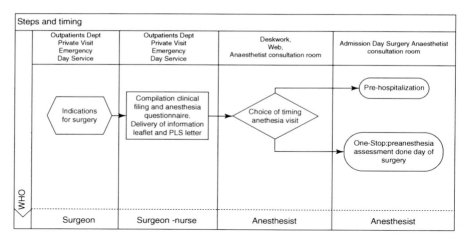

Fig 2.1 Clinical pathways "one-stop anesthesia"

of anesthesia and surgery like nausea and vomiting, pain or unsettled behavior (i.e., emergence delirium) during awakening, and behavioral changes persisting days or weeks after surgery.

The family history should include information of genetically transmitted diseases (malignant hyperthermia, neuromuscular disease, etc.), cases of unexplained deaths, bleeding disorders, passive smoking, or other environmental or social conditions.

The preoperative evaluation can also be an opportunity to observe the parent's behavior and the relations within the family, with indications of the possible preoperative anxiety level.

A thorough assessment of the airway; the cardiovascular, respiratory, and nervous system; and the state of hydration should be performed before any procedure including anesthesia. The physical examination should take into account the awareness of the motor, cognitive, language, and social development of the child [35].

The physical examination may vary according to the age of the patients. The physical examination of infants should be flexible, in order to take advantage of the periods in which the child is quiet or asleep, to auscultate the lungs or heart in the parents' arms. Better collaboration results can be achieved with a pacifier, a smile, a comforting speech, and the use of toys or custom distraction.

Toddlers can be active, curious, or, conversely, shy or less cooperative. Much of the neurological and musculoskeletal assessment may be inferred from the child observation when playing and walking into the visit room. The anxiety reduction can be achieved with a demonstration of the instrument use on the parent or on his reassuring object (e.g., his moppet, favorite toy, etc.).

Providing preschool child's simple explanations of the evaluation phases is always useful. Inviting them to count, explain the colors, talk about a favorite activity, and externalize your approval is all useful strategies during the evaluation.

The school-age children willingly cooperate during the examination. They appreciate the information regarding what you do and why you are doing it.

Teenagers may show concern about their developing body. The choice of performing the physical exam with the parents belongs to the patient.

The body weight and length should be measured and compared with the reference values. During the first 4 years of life, there is a rapid growth rate. The height, with minimal difference between the sexes, increases on average, by 24 cm in the first year of life, by 11 cm in the second year, by 8 cm in the third, and by 7 cm in the fourth. Babies double the birth weight around the 5th months. Their weight triples around the 1st year and quadruples around the 2nd year. From four years old to the beginning of puberty, the growth is more restrained and relatively constant in time. The stature increase is on average 5–6 cm per year in both male and female children. The weight gain per year varies between 1,770 and 2,800 grams [36]. The Pediatric Early Warning Score (PEWS) could be useful in children with abnormal physical examination and/or in emergency situation and may provide additional clinical elements for the evaluation of children undergoing urgent surgical procedures [37].

2.5   Preoperative Tests

Preoperative test and radiological studies should not be requested on a routine basis [16]. The indications for these investigations should be documented and based on the information derived from the medical history and physical exam and/or justified by the proposed surgical procedure.

The American Academy of Pediatrics stated, "preoperative tests should be ordered only when they can provide added value, i.e., when there is a reasonable certainty that they will reveal, or better define the clinical conditions that are relevant to the planned anesthesia and/or may affect the anesthesia or surgical outcome" [38]. Specific tests could be requested for diagnostic purposes (e.g., a cardiac ultrasound for exclusion of unknown congenital heart disease), for therapeutic purposes (e.g., allergy tests to exclude cross allergy conditions), and when it is appropriate to have baseline value (i.e., concentration of Hb in a potentially bleeding operation) [39].The usefulness of routine preoperative laboratory tests for one-day surgery in healthy children was confirmed from some Italian authors since several years [40].

Several national societies produced guidelines and recommendations for the preoperative tests. The National Institute for Health and Clinical Excellence (NICE – UK) suggested to avoid request routine test for patients younger than 16 years ASA1 scheduled for elective surgery grade 1 and 2 [41]. For the Italian Society of Pediatric and Neonatal Anesthesia and Intensive Care (SARNePI), the "systematic prescription of complementary tests in children should be abandoned, and replaced by a selective and rational prescription, based on the patient history and clinical examination" [16]. Those recommendations are based on non-randomized cohort studies with concurrent or historical controls, retrospective case-control studies or case series without control groups. A previous blood test (within 6 months) should only be repeated in case of significant changes on the previous clinical conditions.

There is no justification for the routine examination of hemoglobin and hematocrit before minor surgery, and it should be restricted to potentially bleeding surgical cases [42]. The incidence of anemia in children is rare and occurs more easily in infants younger than 1 year. Moreover, the presence of a certain level of anemia does not affect the decision to proceed with surgery [43, 44].

The determination of blood glucose cannot predict the blood glucose concentration at the time of induction. Numerous studies have actually shown a minimum risk of hypoglycemia in children even after prolonged fasting.

The measurement of plasma electrolytes is not justified in asymptomatic children and should be required only in the presence of vomiting, diarrhea, use of diuretics, or other conditions associated with acid-base modifications [45].

There is consensus on the uselessness of nonselective coagulation screening. This test should be restricted to patients with history of coagulopathy and/or as a baseline measure for procedures with high risk of significant bleeding. The routine request of coagulation tests before ENT surgery or central blocks remains one of the most controversial topics of the perioperative care. Most studies show low sensitivity, specificity, and predictive value of partial thromboplastin activated time, prothrombin time, and thrombin time [46–50]. Moreover, false-positive aPTT prolongation is commonly associated to nonspecific antiphospholipid antibodies often present in children with ENT infections or after vaccination [48, 49]. Standardized questionnaires have shown better sensitivity and negative predictive values than aPTT as coagulation screening before surgery. However, it is difficult to find hemorrhagic signs in small children. The impossibility of obtaining a family history of one or both parents' may compromise the reliability of the questionnaire [51].

Routine request of a preoperative ECG is not recommended in healthy children [52]. The SARNePI recommended the request of a preoperative ECG eventually associated to a cardiac ultrasound in case of pathologic/uncertain heart murmur, suspicion of congenital heart disease, obstructive sleep apnea, severe scoliosis, bronchopulmonary dysplasia (BPD), neuromuscular disease, and in neonates/infants under 6 months of life [16]. The ECG in newborns and infants can detect conduction abnormalities, such as long QT syndrome (LQTS) and the Wolff-Parkinson-White one (WPW) [53]. Investigating maternal factors and fetal factors associated to sudden infant death (smoking, alcohol, intrauterine hypoxia, prone position while asleep, and passive smoke) should be also part of the standard preoperative evaluation. Some congenital heart diseases have asymptomatic evolution during the first weeks after birth [54]. A recent study reveals that up to 30 % of babies and infants with congenital heart disease were discharged from the hospital without diagnosis [55]. Routine physical exam looking for a congenital heart disease between the sixth and eighth week of life is highly recommended.

The chest radiography adds little information to the history taking and to the clinical examination, and its systematic request is not longer justified [56]. A chest radiograph could be indicated after the physical examination and when the medical history supports the need of additional information or in case of chronic lung disease, bronchial pulmonary dysplasia (BPD), severe asthma, neuromuscular disease, severe scoliosis, etc.

Conclusion

The preoperative assessment is the process of evaluating the patient's clinical condition, aimed to define the risks and eligibility for anesthesia and surgery. The preoperative evaluation is mandatory before any diagnostic or therapeutic procedure requiring anesthesia or sedation. The preoperative evaluation should provide the elements to select a shared and individualized perioperative plan.

The prescription of complementary tests in children should be selective and based on the patient history and clinical examination. The preoperative evaluation is an anesthesiologist's responsibility, and only an anesthesiologist can define the eligibility for anesthesia.

2.6   Appendix A

MEDICAL SURVEY QUESTIONNAIRE FOR THE PEDIATRIC ANESTHESIA

GENERALITY

Name and Surname ....…....................Gender: M □ F □, Date of Birth..................…................

Weight.............Height......... Surgery ....…..............Surgeon...

FAMILY HISTORY

Family or relatives related problems during anesthesia : NO □ YES □

If yes, specify type and outcome:

□ allergic reactions, □ fever and/or malignant hyperthermia, □ headache, □ nausea and/or vomit, □ delayed awakening, □ agitated awakening, □ intense pain, □ difficult intubation, □ other...

Familial Severe Allergies NO□, YES□ such as.. ....

Malformation Syndromes   NO□ YES□ such as.............................Rare Diseases NO□ YES□ such as............................

Metabolic Diseases NO□, YES□ such as...................................Coagulopathies NO□ YES□ such as............................

Parents smokers: □ none, □ both, □ mother only, □ father only

MEDICAL HISTORY AIMING TO MAJOR ANAESTHETIC COMPLICATIONS PREVENTION

Certain or suspected episodes of Malignant Hyperthermia or perianaesthetic unexplained deaths in relatives NO □, YES □

Previous anesthesia adverse reaction, suspected of Malignant Hyperthermia in the examinated patient   NO □, YES □

Familiar neuromuscolar diseases and/or personal notes or to be suspected   NO □, YES □

Familiar and/or personal history of Latex Allergy   NO □, YES □

PERSONAL PHYSIOLOGICAL HISTORY

Normal pregnancy: Yes□ No□ If No, specify the problem...

Childbirth: Natural □, □ Indication for Cesarean...

Gestational age <37 weeks (indicate which ....) □, 37-42 weeks □ , > 42 weeks □

Birth weight.............. Problems at Birth NO □ YES□ If yes, specify .... Apgar index......./.......

Neonatal Intensive Care NO □ YES □ If yes specify ....

□ normal psychomotoric development, pathological□.

Regular Growth NO □ YES □. Bowel disorders NO□ YES □.

Date of last menstruation (in adolescent patients) ....

PERSONAL REMOTE PATHOLOGICAL HISTORY

Previous hospital admissions: NO □, YES □. If yes specify: hospitalization age, cause, ward, hospital, Intensive neonatal care hospitalization, Pediatric, DH, Emergency Department visits Hospitalization surgery :

age.................cause......................................…...................ward............................hospital.....…...............

...

age.................cause......................................…...................ward.........................hospital.........…..............

age.................cause......................................…...................ward............................hospital..............…..........

age.................cause......................................…...................ward............................hospital.........…................

Anesthesia problems in previous surgery NO □ YES □ if yes, specify:

References

1. Kohn LT, Corrigan JM, Donaldson MS (2000) To err is human: building a safer health system. National Academy Press, Washington
2. Aplin S, Baines D, DE Lima J (2007) Use of the ASA Physical Status Grading System in pediatric practice. Paediatr Anaesth 17(3):216–222
3. Jacqueline R, Malviya S, Burke C, Reynolds P (2006) An assessment of interrater reliability of the ASA physical status classification in pediatric surgical patients. Paediatr Anaesth 16(9):928–931
4. Burgoyne LL, Smeltzer MP, Pereiras LA, Norris AL, De Armendi AJ (2007) How well do pediatric anesthesiologists agree when assigning ASA physical status classifications to their patients? Paediatr Anaesth: Upper Saddle River, New Jersey 17(10):956–962
5. Udupa AN, Ravindra MN, Chandrika YR, Chandrakala KR, Bindu N, Watcha MF (2015) Comparison of pediatric perioperative risk assessment by ASA physical status and by NARCO-SS (neurological, airway, respiratory, cardiovascular, other-surgical severity) scores. Paediatr Anaesth 25(3):309–316
6. Weinberg AC, Huang L, Jiang H, Tinloy B, Raskas MD, Penna FJ, Freilich DA, Buonfiglio HB, Retik AB, Nguyen HT (2011) Perioperative risk factors for major complications in pediatric surgery: a study in surgical risk assessment for children. J Am Coll Surg 212(5):768–778
7. Wood G, Barayan G, Sanchez DC, Inoue GN, Buchalla CA, Rossini GA, Trevisani LF, Prado RR, Passerotti CC, Nguyen HT (2013) Validation of the pediatric surgical risk assessment scoring system. J Pediatr Surg 48(10):2017–2021
8. Paterson N, Waterhouse P (2011) Risk in pediatric anesthesia. Paediatr Anaesth 21(8):848–857
9. Murat I, Constant I, Maud'huy H (2004) Perioperative anaesthetic morbidity in children: a database of 24,165 anaesthetics over a 30-month period. Paediatr Anaesth 14(2):158–166
10. Jimenez N, Posner KL, Cheney FW, Caplan RA, Lee LA, Domino KB (2007) An update on pediatric anesthesia liability: a closed claims analysis. Anesth Analg 104(1):147–153
11. Morray JP, Geiduschek JM, Ramamoorthy C, Haberkern CM, Hackel A, Caplan RA, Domino KB, Posner K, Cheney FW (2000) Anesthesia-related cardiac arrest in children: initial findings of the Pediatric Perioperative Cardiac Arrest (POCA) Registry. Anesthesiology 93(1):6–14
12. Ramamoorthy C, Haberkern CM, Bhananker SM, Domino KB, Posner KL, Campos JS, Morray JP (2010) Anesthesia-related cardiac arrest in children with heart disease: data from the Pediatric Perioperative Cardiac Arrest (POCA) registry. Anesth Analg 110(5):1376–1382
13. Bhananker SM, Ramamoorthy C, Geiduschek JM, Posner KL, Domino KB, Haberkern CM, Campos JS, Morray JP (2007) Anesthesia-related cardiac arrest in children: update from the Pediatric Perioperative Cardiac Arrest Registry. Anesth Analg 105(2):344–350
14. Flick RP, Sprung J, Harrison TE, Gleich SJ, Schroeder DR, Hanson AC, Buenvenida SL, Warner DO (2007) Perioperative cardiac arrests in children between 1988 and 2005 at a tertiary referral center: a study of 92,881 patients. Anesthesiology 106(2):226–237
15. Varughese AM, Hagerman N, Townsend ME (2013) Using quality improvement methods to optimize resources and maximize productivity in an anesthesia screening and consultation clinic. Paediatr Anaesth 23(7):597–606
16. Serafini G, Ingelmo PM, Astuto M, Baroncini S, Borrometi F, Bortone L, Ceschin C, Gentili A, Lampugnani E, Mangia G, Meneghini L, Minardi C, Montobbio G, Pinzoni F, Rosina B, Rossi C, Sahillioğlu E, Sammartino M, Sonzogni R, Sonzogni V, Tesoro S, Tognon C, Zadra N (2014) Preoperative evaluation in infants and children: recommendations of the Italian Society of Pediatric and Neonatal Anesthesia and Intensive Care (SARNePI). Minerva Anestesiol 80(4):461–469
17. Sgandurra A, Petrini F (1998) Valutazione e selezione dei pazienti. In: Gullo A (ed) Anestesia Clinica. Springer, Milano, pp 49–60
18. American Society of Anesthesiologists Task Force on Preanesthesia Evaluation, Pasternak LR, Arens JF, Caplan RA, Connis RT, Fleisher LA, Flowerdew R, Gold BS, Mayhew JF,

Nickinovich DG, Rice LJ, Roizen MF, Twersky RS (2012) Practice advisory for preanesthesia evaluation: an updated report by the American Society of Anesthesiologists Task Force on Preanesthesia Evaluation. Anesthesiology 116(3):522–538

19. Mangia G, Presutti P, Antonucci A, Bianco F, Bonomo R, Ferrari P (2009) Diagnostic accuracy of anesthesiology evaluation timing: the 'One-Stop Anesthesia' in pediatric day-surgery. Paediatr Anaesth 19(8):764–769

20. Mangia G, Bianco F, Bonomo R, Di Caro E, Frattarelli E, Presutti P (2011) Willingness to pay for one-stop anesthesia in pediatric day surgery. Ital J Pediatr 37:23

21. Twersky R, Frank D, Lerovits A (1990) Timing of preoperative evaluation for surgical outpatients-does it matter? Anesthesiology 73:3A

22. Pasternak LR (2008) Preanesthesia evaluation and testing. In: Beverly KP, Twersky RS (eds) Handbook of ambulatory anesthesia, 2nd edn. Springer, New York, pp 1–23

23. Wittkugel EP, Varughese AM (2006) Pediatric preoperative evaluation – a new paradigm. Int Anesthesiol Clin 44(1):141–158

24. Tagge EP, Hebra A, Overdyk F et al (1999) One-stop surgery: evolving approach to pediatric outpatient surgery. J Pediatr Surg 34:129–132

25. Astuto M, Disma N, Sentina P et al (2003) One-stop surgery in pediatric surgery. Aspect of anesthesia. Minerva Anestesiol 69:137–144

26. Ferrari LR (2004) Preoperative evaluation of pediatric surgical patient with multisystem considerations. Anesth Analg 99:1058–1069

27. Rushforth H, Burge D, Mullee M, Jones S, McDonald H, Glasper EA (2006) Nurse-led paediatric pre operative assessment: an equivalence study. Paediatr Nurs 18(3):23–29

28. Varughese AM, Byczkowski TL, Wittkugel EP, Kotagal U, Dean Kurth C (2006) Impact of a nurse practitioner-assisted preoperative assessment program on quality. Paediatr Anaesth 16(7):723–733

29. Section on Anesthesiology and Pain Medicine (2014) The pediatrician's role in the evaluation and preparation of pediatric patients undergoing anesthesia. Pediatrics 134(3):634–641

30. Wittkugel E, Varughese A (2015) Development of a nurse-assisted preanesthesia evaluation program for pediatric outpatient anesthesia. Paediatr Anaesth 25(7):719–726

31. Mangia G, Bianco F, Ciaschi A, Di Caro E, Frattarelli E, Marrocco GA (2012) De-hospitalization of the pediatric day surgery by means of a freestanding surgery center: pilot study in the Lazio Region. Ital J Pediatr 38:5

32. Brennan LJ (1999) Modern day-case anaesthesia for children. Br J Anaesth 83(1):91–103

33. Patel RI, Hannallah RS (1992) Preoperative screening for pediatric ambulatory surgery: evaluation of a telephone questionnaire method. Anesth Analg 75(2):258–261

34. Flamm M, Fritsch G, Hysek M, Klausner S, Entacher K, Panisch S, Soennichsen AC (2013) Quality improvement in preoperative assessment by implementation of an electronic decision support tool. J Am Med Inform Assoc 20(e1):e91–e96

35. London ML, Ladewig PW, Davidson MC, Ball JW, Bindler RC, Cowen KJ (2014) Maternal & child nursing care, 4th edn. Prentice Hall

36. Bona G, Miniero R (2013) Pediatria pratica. Edizioni Minerva Medica, Torino

37. Solevåg AL, Eggen EH, Schröder J, Nakstad B (2013) Use of a modified pediatric early warning score in a department of pediatric and adolescent medicine. PLoS One 8(8), e72534

38. American Academy of Pediatrics. Section on Anesthesiology (1996) Evaluation and preparation of pediatric patients undergoing anesthesia. Pediatrics 98(3 Pt 1):502–508

39. Patel RI, Hannallah RS (2000) Laboratory tests in children undergoing ambulatory surgery: a review of clinical practice and scientific studies. Ambul Surg 8(4):165–169

40. Meneghini L, Zadra N, Zanette G, Baiocchi M, Giusti F (1988) The usefulness of routine preoperative laboratory tests for one-day surgery in healthy children. Paediatr Anaesth 8(1):11–15

41. National Collaborating Centre Acute Care (2003) Preoperative test, the use of routine preoperative tests for elective surgery. National Institute for Clinical Excellence (NICE), London

42. Olson RP, Stone A, Lubarsky D (2005) The prevalence and significance of low preoperative hemoglobin in ASA 1 or 2 outpatient surgery candidates. Anesth Analg 101(5):1337–1340

43. Hackmann T, Steward DJ, Sheps SB (1991) Anemia in pediatric day-surgery patients: prevalence and detection. Anesthesiology 75(1):27–31
44. Roy WL, Lerman J, McIntyre BG (1991) Is preoperative haemoglobin testing justified in children undergoing minor elective surgery? Can J Anaesth 38(6):700–703
45. Maxwell LG, Deshpande JK, Wetzel RC (1994) Preoperative evaluation of children. Pediatr Clin North Am 41(1):93–110
46. Chee YL, Crawford JC, Watson HG, Greaves M (2008) Guidelines on the assessment of bleeding risk prior to surgery or invasive procedures. British Committee for Standards in Haematology. Br J Haematol 140(5):496–504
47. Samková A, Blatný J, Fiamoli V, Dulíček P, Pařízková E (2012) Significance and causes of abnormal preoperative coagulation test results in children. Haemophilia 18(3):e297–e301
48. Pajot S, Asehnoune K, Le Roux C, Léturgie C, Surbled M, Bazin V, Lejus C (2009) Evaluation of the haemostasis before a central block in children: what is the French anaesthesiologist's attitude? Ann Fr Anesth Reanim 28(1):3–10
49. Chee YL, Greaves M (2003) Role of coagulation testing in predicting bleeding risk. Hematol J 4(6):373–378
50. Scheckenbach K, Bier H, Hoffmann TK, Windfuhr JP, Bas M, Laws HJ, Plettenberg C, Wagenmann M (2008) Risk of hemorrhage after adenoidectomy and tonsillectomy. Value of the preoperative determination of partial thromboplastin time, prothrombin time and platelet count. HNO 56(3):312–320
51. Watson-Williams EJ (1979) Hematologic and hemostatic considerations before surgery. Med Clin North Am 63(6):1165–1189
52. von Walter J, Kroiss K, Höpner P, Russwurm W, Kellermann W, Emmrich P (1998) Preoperative ECG in routine preoperative assessment of children. Anaesthesist 47(5):373–378
53. Quaglini S, Rognoni C, Spazzolini C, Priori SG, Mannarino S, Schwartz PJ (2006) Cost-effectiveness of neonatal ECG screening for the long QT syndrome. Eur Heart J 27(15):1824–1832
54. Knowles R, Griebsch I, Dezateux C, Brown J, Bull C, Wren C (2005) Newborn screening for congenital heart defects: a systematic review and cost-effectiveness analysis. Health Technol Assess 9(44):1–152
55. Wren C, Reinhardt Z, Khawaja K (2008) Twenty-year trends in diagnosis of life-threatening neonatal cardiovascular malformations. Arch Dis Child Fetal Neonatal 93(1):F33–F35
56. Wood RA, Hoekelman RA (1981) Value of the chest X-ray as a screening test for elective surgery in children. Pediatrics 67(4):447–452

Luciano Bortone, Luca La Colla, and Marinella Astuto

3.1 Non-pharmacological Preparation

Preparation of the child and his/her family for anesthesia and surgery should begin when the surgeon sets the date and type of surgery for the child. Pediatricians also have an important role in preparing children and families for anesthesia and surgery. Once it has been ascertained that the child is in good physical condition for surgery, the pediatrician will help the family deal with the surgery in terms of cognitive, emotional, and logistical elements [1].

3.1.1 Preoperative Anxiety

Since more than half of children develop anxiety in the preoperative period, close cooperation between the pediatrician, surgeon, anesthesiologist, nurses, and nonmedical personnel is essential for a positive perioperative experience for the child and his/her family. Preoperative anxiety in children could be assessed by the modified Yale Preoperative Anxiety Scale (mYPAS), containing 27 items grouped into five categories (activity, emotional expressivity, state of arousal, vocalization, and use of parents) [2].

There are two distinct components of anxiety: a transient state anxiety, variable over time and intensity, characterized by a sense of tension, apprehension,

L. Bortone • L. La Colla
First Service of Anesthesia and Intensive Care, Parma Hospital, Parma, Italy

Dipartimento di Anestesia e Rianimazione, Azienda Ospedaliera di Parma, Parma, Italy
e-mail: lbortone@ao.pr.it

M. Astuto (✉)
Anesthesia, Intensive Care, University of Catania, Policlinico Hospital, Catania, Italy

Dipartimento di Anestesia e Rianimazione, Ospedale Universitario Policlinico, Catania, Italy
e-mail: marinella.astuto@gmail.com

© Springer International Publishing Switzerland 2016
M. Astuto, P.M. Ingelmo (eds.), *Perioperative Medicine in Pediatric Anesthesia*,
Anesthesia, Intensive Care and Pain in Neonates and Children,
DOI 10.1007/978-3-319-21960-8_3

nervousness, and worry, and a stable trait anxiety, more or less constant over time, linked to individual differences in the propensity to develop anxiety. The development of preoperative anxiety in children depends on many factors, such as awareness of the disease and the need for surgery, fear of separation from parents, the feeling of lack of control and the unpredictable character of the event that is about to happen, infant temperament, previous experience in a hospital environment, and the emotional state of the parents. Risk factors for the development of preoperative anxiety include being a preschooler, a shy and introverted character, previous surgeries, relationships with health personnel related to previous hospitalizations, the presence of anxious parents, and having participated in preparation programs prior to the intervention [3].

Some children are able to verbalize their fears explicitly; others express them through behavioral changes, such as crying, agitation, tremor, stoppage of play, increased muscle tone, and even real attempts to escape. Preoperative anxiety is associated with increased circulating catecholamines [4].

High levels of preoperative anxiety may adversely affect the postoperative period, with higher incidence of pain as well as short- and long-term behavioral changes such as emergence delirium, enuresis, sleep disorders, nightmares, apathy, eating disorders, and separation anxiety [5]. In clinical practice, one can predict the occurrence of adverse postoperative effects based on the levels of preoperative anxiety. High levels of preoperative anxiety, with a particularly stressful induction of anesthesia and reduced doses of anxiolytics, cause the development of anxiety and behavioral disorders in the postoperative period, even a few months after hospitalization [6].

Low levels of preoperative anxiety are associated with a good postoperative behavioral outcome. It is useful to prevent and treat anxiety in the child and parents through a comprehensive and multidisciplinary approach that accompanies the child and his/her family from the admittance to the hospital until the time of induction of anesthesia. Fundamental moments are represented by preoperative visits by the surgeon and anesthesiologist; preparation for the intervention by psychologists or play specialists; strategies adopted in the operating theater before induction of anesthesia, namely, premedication; and the parental presence in the operating room.

The preoperative visit is a "psychologically" important part of preparation for surgery. Parents express their concern about anesthesia often in the presence of the child; they are more often frightened by the risks related to anesthesia than the surgery. The very detailed description of the proposed anesthetic technique with its potential complications can generate a particularly strong state of anxiety. The data about the emotional state of the parents after a more or less detailed interview with the anesthesiologist are conflicting; some studies report levels of tension, depression, and irritability associated with higher preoperative detailed information, while others conclude that patients and parents informed in detail about the anesthesia and its risks are not more anxious than those less well informed.

As a general rule, it is reasonable to adapt the type of information to the psychological characteristics and the "receptivity" of the patient and the parents. A family looking for comprehensive information will benefit from a detailed anesthetic interview, while parents with negative attitudes toward potentially dangerous situations will react with stress and anxiety to a conversation full of details.

The anesthesiologist must be prepared to deal with parents and children with ideas, life views, and religions differing from their own in order to avoid verbal conflict which could result in an increase in preoperative anxiety for the family. Our goal is to bring the child to surgery as peaceful as possible. The informed consent provides adequate information to parents about the anesthetic procedure and the infrequent possible risks. A good method of requesting consent can help reduce the anxiety of the parents and the child. To say that anesthesia is as risky as traveling by train is different from saying that, although rarely, anesthesia can be fatal.

3.1.2 Preparation for Surgery

Programs destined for pediatric anesthesia preparation aim to reduce the anxiety of children and parents prior to surgery. By using play and games in the hospital, in which the child has full control, they can reduce their fears and teach them tools to deal with otherwise extremely stressful experiences [7].

Over the last 50 years, there have been different patterns of preparation. The "informative" approach was used in the 1960s. It was aimed to encourage emotional expression and to establish a relationship of trust between the medical staff, child, and family. "Modeling" techniques were developed in the 1970s and were based on the ability of the child and his parents to experience anesthesia and surgery through video simulations with dolls. In the 1980s, "coping" techniques included the active involvement of the child and were designed to promote adaptation and the ability to cope with a critical situation. Currently, in pediatric hospitals, that objective is pursued by specialized support staff through a multimodal approach. Play experiences and information on the procedures are explored together with the description of the feelings that the young patient will experience. In addition, the child is given the opportunity to examine and manipulate the instruments that will be used in the operating room.

The development of coping techniques is considered the gold standard of psychological preparation, followed by modeling, play therapy, visiting the operating room, and the distribution of informative material. Compared to other methods (such as modeling and distribution of informative materials), the preparation of the child through coping is associated with lower levels of preoperative anxiety at the day of surgery and at the time of separation from their parents before entering the operating theater [3].

The choice and timing of the preparation program must be based on the age, maturity, and cognitive capacity of the child. Age greater than or equal to 6 years old is an indication to apply the program over five days before the surgical procedure, in order to ensure that the child has time to process the information received and to complete the process of coping. Children over the age of 6 years who underwent psychological preparation one week preoperatively showed decreased levels of anxiety during and immediately after preparation, followed by a reduction in stress during the five days prior to surgery [8]. On the other hand, children aged between

3 and 5 years old gradually acquire the ability to discern fantasy from reality. The skill is not yet present in those younger than three, and therefore, the application of preparation programs based on reality may be useless if not counterproductive by increasing anxiety.

The success of the preoperative preparation can be compromised by past bad experiences of the child in hospital. In this case, the preparation, in addition to not adding any information, could produce an exaggerated emotional response and worsen the anxiety state.

The parents' anxiety influences the psychological condition of their child. Hence, it is optimal that the preparatory projects actively involve the family of the young patient. Watching explanatory movies can reduce preoperative anxiety in parents.

Kain et al. [9] proposed a preparation project focused on the family called "ADVANCE." They demonstrated that this approach reduces the anxiety of both the child and parents before and during induction of anesthesia. Also ADVANCE was proved as effective as midazolam in the management of children undergoing induction and was associated with faster discharge from the recovery room and lower doses of analgesics during the postoperative period. This approach, however, is very costly and requires appropriate health personnel.

Fortier and Kain introduced a new web-based approach for children and their families to impact perioperative pain and anxiety [10].

Music therapy is considered necessary at the time of separation of the child from the parents upon entering the operating theater, while it does not seem useful to reduce anxiety during induction of anesthesia [11].

Recently, new techniques have been tested. Seiden et al. have compared midazolam to a "tablet-based interactive distraction" (TBID) in children aged 2–11 years old. They found that TBID reduced perioperative anxiety, emergence delirium, and time to discharge and increased parental satisfaction in patients undergoing ambulatory surgery [12].

Play specialists in our hospital prepare children before surgery, with a parent present (www.giocamico.it). Aided by two puppets, they teach the children how to use the oximeter, the pressure cuff, the electrocardiogram patches, facemask, and intravenous cannula. The play specialists show pictures of the instruments and provide explanations on what happens in the operating room. They also show the children and their parents how all the people they meet will be dressed upon entering the operating theater. The preparation is offered to all boys and girls aged between 5 and 11 years old, a few days before surgery. For older children, a book with photos and drawings is used. Children are also offered the opportunity to test the diagnostic and therapeutic tools (Fig. 3.1).

Specialists also prepare children who have to undergo painful procedures in sedation analgesia.

Also promising is the preparation of children aged 5–10 years old for MRI. The aim is to reduce the number of MRI done under general anesthesia (Fig. 3.2).

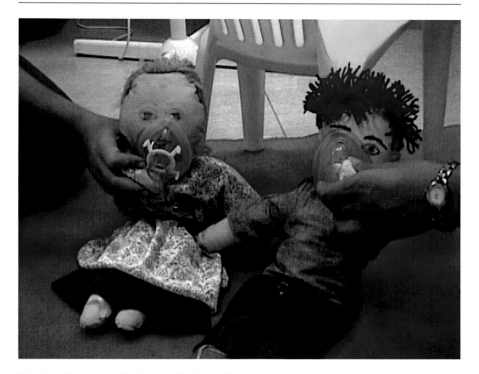

Fig. 3.1 Play preparation for anesthesia by Giocamico

3.1.3   Parental Presence During Induction of Anesthesia (PPIA)

In 1985, an ophthalmic surgeon, Adrian While, wrote in the *British Medical Journal* that he had not been allowed to accompany his 3-year-old daughter to the operating room for induction and argued that parents should be admitted to the operating room to help their child. Gauderer indicated that virtually all parents, given a choice, went into the operating room with their children; only two parents had a fainting spell. Nurses, anesthesiologists, and surgeons were excited about this new approach, which appeared to be safe, simple, and effective [13]. A study by Kain compared PPIA to drug preparation and demonstrated that children who were premedicated had a lesser degree of anxiety at the time of separation before induction compared to the control group and to the PPIA group [14]. In another study, the presence of a parent in the room did not reduce the anxiety of the child who had already received midazolam, while there was a reduction in the anxiety of the parents and their greater satisfaction [15].

Nevertheless, it seems that children aged older than 4 and anxious parents might get some benefit from PPIA [9].

Fig 3.2 Play preparation
for MNR by Giocamico®

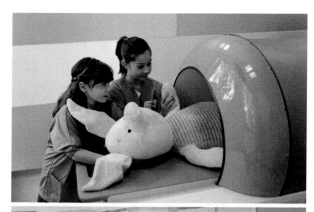

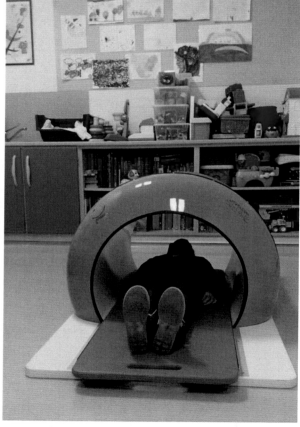

Lerman believes that the presence of the parents is not an undeniable right but rather a therapeutic option to facilitate the induction of anesthesia to be used at the sole discretion of the anesthesiologist [16]. Despite this theory, there is no doubt that some children (such as those with special needs, very anxious, or subjected to multiple hospitalizations) may actually benefit from PPIA, which should ideally be preceded by a preparation program for parents.

In our experience, of over 15 years, we propose that one of the parents accompanies the child into the operating room for induction of anesthesia, excluding pregnant moms, parents with health problems, and anxious parents to whom we explain that their presence could increase the child's anxiety and create problems for the staff. When the parent comes into the room, the preschoolers are normally premedicated with midazolam, while older children can choose, in agreement with the parent, whether or not to have premedication. They can also choose the type of induction of anesthesia, inhalation or intravenous, which helped in the choice by the anesthesiologist. A staff member accompanies the parent in every moment of his stay in the operating room.

Different "side effects" of PPIA have been described in the literature: parents taking their children out of the operating room, parents who faint, and even parents who want the anesthesiologist to discontinue anesthesia and awaken their child. Hence, it is important to select the right parents (excluding, e.g., those who are anxious) and possibly make them undergo a preparation process. In addition, it is important to have a staff member always close to the parent. This member will escort the parent outside the operating room at the end of induction or whenever the child's condition changes and the parents' presence might be distracting or disruptive to the induction of anesthesia.

Hospitalization before surgery and prolonged preoperative fasting represent for the child an additional source of discomfort. At our hospital, young patients can be admitted 1–2 h before surgery. Regarding preoperative fasting, it is necessary to minimize the fasting hours (especially in smaller patients) in accordance with the directions of the American Society of Anesthesiology for healthy pediatric patients undergoing elective surgery (see below). In particular, the reduction in fasting hours is not associated with an increased gastric residual volume, or indirect index of risk of aspiration pneumonia. Furthermore, a less restrictive fasting regimen reduces dehydration, increases hemodynamic stability during anesthesia, facilitates venous vascular access, guarantees glucose homeostasis, reduces irritability in the young patient, and increases the overall satisfaction of the child and parents.

The pain from venipuncture is one of the greatest fears of the hospitalized pediatric patient. The pain generated by venipuncture is classified as moderate to severe. The procedure should be reduced to the absolute minimum, such as preoperative blood tests prescribed only on the basis of anomalies detected in the patient history or by physical examination [17]. The intravenous line needed for the surgery is normally placed after induction of anesthesia when the child is asleep and the veins well dilated. However, if the child prefers an intravenous induction, it is recommended to apply an anesthetic cream over the skin of the most visible veins 40 minutes before the surgery.

3.2   Pharmacological Preparation

The second part of this chapter will briefly review only the most widespread routes of administration of the most common drugs that are currently used for pharmacological preparation of children before surgery.

The goals of premedication in children are the reduction in anxiety, block of autonomic (especially vagal) reflexes, reduction of airway secretions, amnesia, prophylaxis against pulmonary aspiration of gastric contents, facilitation of induction of anesthesia, and possible analgesia and to potentially mitigate the stress response and prevent malignant cardiac arrhythmias [18].

A list, although not necessarily exhaustive, of the main indications for premedication in children includes:

- Children/teenagers who already show a high degree of anxiety
- Children who cannot be separated easily from the parent
- Cases in which the anesthesiologist thinks that PPIA is not of benefit
- Children with previous experience of surgery, perhaps characterized by a negative memory or discomfort
- Children with neurological and behavioral disorders
- Children with comorbidities requiring smooth induction, possibly without crying or agitation (e.g., patients with cardiac disease)

Before examining the most frequently used drugs for premedication, it should be noted that its risks are respiratory depression, loss of airway reflexes, paradoxical response to the drug, and obviously potential allergic reactions. These risks are generally influenced not only by age but also by underlying medical conditions (furthermore in this chapter, we refer to elective surgery, but there are special circumstances such as full stomach, head or abdominal trauma, etc., that require different considerations). Although risks are mainly connected to a relative overdose (or coadministration of another drug) and can therefore be minimized using a high degree of attention, the conditions that may require close monitoring after premedication are:

- Upper airway obstruction and/or obstructive sleep apnea syndrome
- Neurological disorders
- Dysphagia or gastroesophageal reflux
- Infants
- Heart disease (especially cyanotic heart defects)

The goal of premedication in children should be individualized: a mild sedation, while not able to eliminate anxiety completely, can be effective in a child who is not very agitated and could therefore make the induction mild and pleasant. Conversely, a heavier sedation may be necessary in the case of a very agitated child.

The factors to be considered when choosing the drug(s) are therefore age, weight, medication history of the patient (allergies), comorbidities, expectations of the child and family, level of psychological maturity, anxiety, and cooperativeness.

Table 3.1 Drugs and doses commonly administered for premedication

Drug	Route	Dose (mg/kg)
Midazolam	Oral	0.3–0.7 (up to 20 mg)
	Nasal	0.2
	Rectal	0.5–1
	Intramuscular	0.1–0.15
Ketamine	Oral	3–8
	Nasal	3–6
	Rectal	5–10
	Intramuscular	2–5
Clonidine	Oral	0.002–0.004
	Nasal	0.002–0.004
	Rectal	0.002–0.005
Dexmedetomidine	Oral	0.001–0.004
	Nasal	0.001–0.004

Another important point to consider is the route of administration of the drug. Although parenteral administration (especially intravenous) can be faster, can be more effective, and have a greater predictability in terms of clinical response, the majority of pediatric anesthesiologists refrain from this route of administration unless there is a venous access in place. In fact, most of the children reported needle puncture as their worst experience in hospital.

For this reason, enteral or transmucosal premedication is better accepted by the child, parents, and hospital staff. A noteworthy exception to this general rule (according to the experience of the authors) is for children born with spina bifida who generally do not have sensitivity in the buttock region. The same children on the other hand are often hostile to inhalation induction, often already have experience during previous surgeries. The doses of the two main drugs (midazolam and ketamine) used intramuscularly as premedication in Italy are disclosed in Table 3.1.

In spite of the relative abundance of literature about the different drugs/routes of administration, we can state that the ideal drug (or the ideal combination of drugs) for premedication in children has unfortunately yet to be invented. In this brief review, we will focus on oral, nasal, and rectal routes by examining midazolam, α-2 agonists, and ketamine.

3.2.1 Oral Route

Although the oral route of administration does not always produce predictable and consistent effects because of fluctuations in the bioavailability and a substantial first-pass effect, it still remains the most accepted and widespread way of administration [19].

Although in the past it was feared that oral premedication might increase gastric residual volume and therefore increase the risk of reflux with subsequent inhalation, this was later denied, as long as a large amount of fluid is not ingested [20].

3.2.1.1 Midazolam

Midazolam administered orally still remains the method of choice in 90% of cases in the USA according to a recent survey [21]. The usual dose of 0.5 mg/kg up to a maximum of 20 mg causes a constant anxiolysis in the presence of a large safety margin, whereas the increase above 0.5 mg/kg does not result in an increase of its sedative or anxiolytic properties [22]. The sedative and anxiolytic effect starts after 10' and is present after 20' in the vast majority of children [23]. The peak effect is observed at 30', but after 45' the effect on separation anxiety starts to disappear [24], even with a possible sedative/light anxiolytic effect up to 2 h.

The effect on awakening times seems to be minimal, while there have been conflicting data on discharge time over years. A recent review [25] has shown that premedication with midazolam 0.5 mg/kg 30' before surgery reduces separation anxiety at induction but does not increase recovery times, while opposite results were found in a previous study [26].

It is essential for the anesthesiologist to be careful about the timing of midazolam administration to prevent the child from arriving in the operating room not properly sedated (due to either a late or an early administration). In this last case, however, a re-administration of midazolam at a reduced dose (e.g., 0.25 mg/kg) can be attempted.

The main problem of oral midazolam is its bitter taste. In 1998, the FDA approved a syrup with a more pleasant taste and a lower pH than the intravenous formulation, thus increasing its bioavailability. A coadministration with a more pleasant tasting syrup may be useful.

In another study, oral midazolam did not result in an increased frequency of delirium and agitation after awakening [26]. On the other hand, the effects on behavioral outcomes such as nightmares, nocturnal enuresis, etc., are contradictory. Doses greater than 0.5 mg/kg are associated with side effects such as alterations in balance, posture, vision, and dysphoric reactions in the postoperative period [26]. Of note, these reaction can easily be controlled and antagonized by the administration of flumazenil 10 µg/kg up to 1 mg iv.

Midazolam (0.5 mg/kg) has been compared to clonidine (4 µg/kg) for premedication in children undergoing tonsillectomy and has been found to be better in terms of preoperative anxiety and postoperative analgesia, with no difference in awakening and discharge times [27]. When compared to oral ketamine 5 mg/kg, midazolam has displayed similar effects but with a better recovery and discharge profile [28]. Similarly, a better sedation and anxiolysis has been observed with midazolam (0.5 mg/kg) compared to the combination diazepam-droperidol (0.25 mg/kg each) [29]. After sevoflurane anesthesia, midazolam was found to be as effective as clonidine and melatonin in reducing postoperative agitation [30].

3.2.1.2 Ketamine

Despite its marked first-pass effect, the usual dose of 6 mg/kg makes the children quiet and calm at the time of separation from their parents within 30' and provides good conditions at the time of induction [31]. Oral ketamine does not generally produce effects like tachycardia, respiratory depression, agitation during awakening, or nightmares [23], even though episodes of hallucinations and laryngo-spasm have been reported [32].

3.2.1.3 α_2-Agonists

In recent years, there has been a sort of "rediscovery" of α_2-agonists although cloni-dine has been used for years for premedication in children. It has anxiolytic, seda-tive, and analgesic properties, tastes better than midazolam, and displays a high rate of satisfaction among both the medical care team and parents.

Clonidine results in sedation, amnesia, perioperative hemodynamic stability, and intraoperative (in terms of reduction of anesthetics) and postoperative analgesia, when orally administered at the dose of 1–4 µg/kg. In addition, premedication with clonidine 4 µg/kg before adenotonsillectomy was as effective as the administration of fentanyl 3 µg/kg perioperatively as far as postoperative analgesia (VAS and mor-phine consumption) was concerned [33]. The effectiveness of premedication with clonidine in reducing postoperative pain has been confirmed by a Cochrane meta-analysis in 2014 [34].

Due to its pharmacodynamic effect, clonidine produces a state of sedation more similar to fatigue and physiological sleep when compared to midazolam. This is also demonstrated by the ability of patients to be easily awakened to perform a vari-ety of cognitive tests [35, 36].

One of the disadvantages of premedication with clonidine is its markedly delayed onset, up to 90'. Still, many pediatric anesthesiologists accept this delay as it is largely offset by its beneficial perioperative clinical effect. In particular, what is valued and desirable in pediatric anesthesia is its reduction of sympathetic outflow without the simultaneous reduction of compensatory homeostatic reflexes. In fact, although bradycardia and hypotension are potentially dangerous side effects, they do not actually occur if the total dose of clonidine is below 10 µg/kg.

The more recently introduced dexmedetomidine is an α_2-agonist with an α_2/α_1 specificity eight times greater than clonidine (1600:1 vs. 200:1). This greater selectiv-ity, together with its limited cardiorespiratory effects, could theoretically offer some advantages even though data are still limited. Preliminary and retrospective data indi-cate that dexmedetomidine can be used for both premedication and procedural seda-tion at a dose of 1–4 µg/kg [37]. An important paper comparing premedication with oral midazolam(0.5 mg/kg), oral clonidine (4 µg/kg), and transmucosal dexmedeto-midine (1 µg/kg) showed no difference in terms of anxiety and postoperative sedation but greater intraoperative hemodynamic stability and reduced postoperative pain in the clonidine and dexmedetomidine group compared to midazolam [38].

3.2.2 Nasal Route

The drugs most frequently administered through the nasal route are midazolam, ketamine, and more recently dexmedetomidine.

Nasal absorption is usually faster than the oral route. It is generally true that any side effects (such as respiratory depression) could occur more rapidly, and therefore, this route of administration should only be used when there is personnel with equipment readily available to intervene.

Traditionally premedication through the nasal route included both drops and sprays. Considering the widespread diffusion of devices such as atomizers, nowadays sprays seem more widespread than drops. For this reason, a proper and precise dose must be administered to generate a rapid and predictable onset. The only real disadvantage of nasal sprays is the possible uncomfortable feeling for patients which can sometimes be associated with anxiety and fear, even though the discomfort linked to nasal adminis-tration of midazolam can be reduced by pre-administration of a lidocaine puff.

3.2.2.1 Midazolam

At the dose of 0.2–0.3 mg/kg, nasal midazolam has proven effective in the reduction of separation anxiety and during induction, while not increasing recovery and dis-charge times even after short surgeries. In a direct comparison between 0.2 mg/kg and 0.3 mg/kg, the higher dose resulted in a higher efficacy without an increase in side effects [39].

Nasal midazolam (0.5 mg/kg) has been compared to a combination of ketamine-midazolam and has proven as effective as the combination in reducing separation anxiety in all patients even if its effect took twice as much time (5 min vs. 2.5 min) as the combination of drugs [40].

In a comparison between midazolam 0.2 mg/kg and dexmedetomidine 1 μg/kg, both administered nasally, both drugs were similar with respect to separation anxi-ety, but midazolam was superior for the achievement of satisfactory conditions dur-ing induction of anesthesia [41].

Nasal midazolam 0.2 mg/kg has been recently compared to two different doses of intranasal ketamine (0.5 and 3 mg/kg, respectively) and was superior to ketamine in reducing preoperative anxiety in pediatric patients [42].

3.2.2.2 Ketamine

Nasal ketamine has been used as premedication in pediatric patients. In doses up to 6 mg/kg, it has been proven effective in reducing separation anxiety and during mask induction, without increasing recovery times.

The addition of nasal ketamine 2 mg/kg after oral administration of midazolam (both used for premedication) is superior to intranasal alfentanil 10 μg/kg for reduction of pre-operative anxiety and quality of recovery (agitation) after sevoflurane anesthesia [43].

Ketamine (10 mg/kg) has been compared to nasal midazolam (0.2 mg/kg) and their combination (7.5 mg/kg and 0.1 mg/kg, respectively). Even though sedation was adequate in the midazolam group, reduction of separation anxiety and, above all, compliance during the insertion of venous cannula were superior in the two ketamine groups, with no significant differences between the combination and ket-amine alone [44].

3.2.2.3 α₂-Agonists

Nasal clonidine 4 μg/kg has been proven to be as effective as the same dose adminis-tered orally, even with a paradoxically lower onset [45]. It has been proven effective not only as premedication but also to treat agitation/hallucination episodes following oral midazolam administration, as well as to treat hypertension preoperatively [46].

A prospective, randomized trial compared clonidine 4 μg/kg vs. midazolam 0.3 mg/kg and showed that even though midazolam produced a faster onset of sedation, both drugs displayed a similar onset of anxiolysis with reduced side effects in the clonidine group [47].

Dexmedetomidine displays the same properties as clonidine with greater selectivity on presynaptic receptors. At the same dose, it is actually more effective when administered nasally rather than orally in terms of sedation, anxiety reduction, and tolerability of the mask during induction [48]. Dexmedetomidine has been shown to have analgesic properties since 2 μg/kg administered before induction can reduce the EC50 of sevoflurane (LMA positioning) by 21 % [31].

When compared at low doses (1 μg/kg) with oral midazolam (0.2 mg/kg) as a premedication before general anesthesia, it confers (despite its slower onset) a significantly greater degree of sedation at the time of separation from parents, greater compliance with the application of the mask, and a reduced incidence of shivering and excitement in the postoperative period. Notably, while about one third of children in the midazolam group showed signs of nasal irritation, this side effect was not present in any child in the dexmedetomidine group [49].

3.2.3 Rectal Route

3.2.3.1 Midazolam
The effective dose of rectally administered midazolam ranges from 0.3–0.5 mg/kg [50, 51]. The effective dose shown to make mask induction acceptable by a child is 0.35 mg/kg, even though 1 mg/kg did not seem to increase PACU discharge times [51]. The dose usually administered in our center is 0.5 mg/kg up to 20 mg.

3.2.3.2 Ketamine
The ketamine dose used in most of the literature ranges from 5 to 10 mg/kg. A study by Tanaka et al. compared different doses of rectal ketamine within this range to midazolam 1 mg/kg. They showed that only ketamine 10 mg/kg and midazolam 1 mg/kg resulted in a significantly greater proportion of children with reduced separation anxiety and mild induction. On the other hand, ketamine 10 mg/kg resulted in a longer recovery when compared to lower doses [52]. Low doses of the $(_{S+})$ enantiomer did not show any benefit compared to the combination ketamine-midazolam or rectal midazolam 0.75 mh/kg [53].

3.2.3.3 α$_2$-Agonists
The most frequently tested drug is clonidine. When administered rectally, it has a half-life similar to that in adult patients. The rectal route is associated with an almost total (95%) bioavailability and a time-to-peak plasma concentration of 50 minutes, and even though only 20 minutes after the rectal administration of clonidine 2.5 μg/ kg, a plasma concentration in the range known as effective in adults is reached [54].

Clonidine 5 μg/kg resulted in a significant reduction of postoperative pain after adenotonsillectomy when compared to midazolam 0.3 mg/kg, together with a moderately increased sedation during the first 24 h after surgery. This finding was in agreement with the finding of a parental preference for a sedated child [35].

3.3   Preoperative Fasting

The awareness about fasting before surgery has increased over time even in pediatric anesthesia. While solids leave the stomach following zero-order kinetics (slower emptying), liquids follow a first-order kinetics (faster emptying).

After combining different studies on gastric emptying in children, it has been shown that clear liquids can be ingested up to 2 h before surgery without any problem. Children should be encouraged to drink clear fluids (including water, pulp-free juice, and tea or coffee without milk) up to 2 h before elective surgery. Rather than ensuring a minimal fasting interval has been achieved, it is important to encourage patients to keep drinking up until 2 h before surgery in order to reduce their discomfort and improve their well-being [55, 56].

It remains common practice to avoid solid food for at least 6 h before elective surgery. There is no clear benefit to reduce the fasting time for solids below 6 h. Cow's milk and formula are generally treated as solids (proteins coagulate once in the stomach), while breast milk is considered for the most part similar to a liquid and therefore requires a time of fasting somewhat intermediate between that for solids and liquids. It is recommended to finish breast feeding 4 h before anesthesia and to stop infant formula 4–6 h prior to anesthesia depending on the age. Both cow's milk and powdered milk are considered as solid food [55, 56].

There is no consensus on the effects of the trauma on the stomach empty times. The volume of gastric contents may depend on the nature of the trauma, but gastric content may not be related to the length of fasting. Gastric volume is better linked to the interval between the last meal and the trauma. Thus, the injured child should be considered as a patient with a full stomach [57].

However, in malnourished or debilitated patients and patients with important comorbidities, as well as in emergency situations, fasting times must be individualized and optimized according to the individual case. An increasing number of minor surgical procedures are done under sedation in the emergency department or in other suites outside the operating theater. The available literature does not provide sufficient evidence to conclude that pre-procedure fasting results in a decreased incidence of adverse outcomes in children undergoing either moderate or deep sedation [58].

For more extensive discussion regarding the preoperative fasting, we recommend the guidelines of the American Society of Anesthesiologists and of the European Society of Anaesthesiology [55, 56].

Acknowledgments   The authors would like to thank Carolyn David for her support and English review of the chapter.

References

1. Section on Anesthesiology and Pain Medicine (2014) The pediatrician's role in the evaluation and preparation of pediatric patients undergoing anesthesia. Pediatrics 134:634–641. doi:10.1542/peds.2014-1840
2. Kain ZN, Mayes LC, Cicchetti DV et al (2007) Measurement tool for preoperative anxiety in young children: the yale preoperative anxiety scale. Child Neuropsychol 1:203–210. doi:10.1080/09297049508400225
3. Kain ZN, Caramico LA, Mayes LC et al (1998) Preoperative preparation programs in children: a comparative examination. Anesth Analg 87:1249–1255
4. Fell D, Derbyshire DR, Maile CJ et al (1985) Measurement of plasma catecholamine concentrations. An assessment of anxiety. Br J Anaesth 57:770–774
5. Kain ZN, Caldwell-Andrews AA, Maranets I, et al (2004) Preoperative anxiety and emergence delirium and postoperative maladaptive behaviors. Anesth Analg 99:1648–54– table of contents. doi:10.1213/01.ANE.0000136471.36680.97
6. Kain ZN, Wang SM, Mayes LC et al (1999) Distress during the induction of anesthesia and postoperative behavioral outcomes. Anesth Analg 88:1042–1047
7. Armstrong TS, Aitken HL (2000) The developing role of play preparation in paediatric anaesthesia. Paediatr Anaesth 10:1–4
8. Melamed B, Siegel L, Franks C, Evans F (1980) Psychological preparation for hospitalization. In: Franks C, Evans F (eds) Behavioral medicine: practical applications in health care. Springer, New York, pp 307–355
9. Kain ZN, Caldwell-Andrews AA, Mayes LC et al (2007) Family-centered preparation for surgery improves perioperative outcomes in children: a randomized controlled trial. Anesthesiology 106:65–74
10. Fortier MA, Kain ZN (2015) Treating perioperative anxiety and pain in children: a tailored and innovative approach. Pediatric Anesthesia 25:27–35. doi:10.1111/pan.12546
11. Kain ZN, Caldwell-Andrews AA, Krivutza DM et al (2004) Interactive music therapy as a treatment for preoperative anxiety in children: a randomized controlled trial. Anesth Analg 98:1260–1266, – table of contents
12. Seiden SC, McMullan S, Sequera-Ramos L et al (2014) Tablet-based Interactive Distraction (TBID) vs oral midazolam to minimize perioperative anxiety in pediatric patients: a noninferiority randomized trial. Pediatric Anesthesia 24:1217–1223. doi:10.1111/pan.12475
13. Gauderer MW, Lorig JL, Eastwood DW (1989) Is there a place for parents in the operating room? J Pediatr Surg 24:705–706, – discussion 707
14. Kain ZN, Caramico LA, Mayes LC, Genevro JL, Bornstein MH, Hofstadter MB. Preoperative preparation programs in children: a comparative examination. Anesth Analg 1998;87(6):1249–1255
15. Kain ZN, Mayes LC, Wang SM et al (2000) Parental presence and a sedative premedicant for children undergoing surgery: a hierarchical study. Anesthesiology 92:939–946
16. Lerman J (2000) Anxiolysis – by the parent or for the parent? Anesthesiology 92:925–927
17. Serafini G, Ingelmo PM, Astuto M et al (2014) Preoperative evaluation in infants and children: recommendations of the Italian Society of Pediatric and Neonatal Anesthesia and Intensive Care (SARNePI). Minerva Anestesiol 80:461–469
18. Sigurdsson GH, Lindahl S, Nordén N (1983) Influence of premedication on the sympathetic and endocrine responses and cardiac arrhythmias during halothane anaesthesia in children undergoing adenoidectomy. Br J Anaesth 55:961–968
19. Brzustowicz RM, Nelson DA, Betts EK et al (1984) Efficacy of oral premedication for pediatric outpatient surgery. Anesthesiology 60:475–477
20. Rajkumar (2007) A comparative study of volume and pH of gastric fluid after ingestion of water and sugar-containing clear fluid in children. Indian J Anaesthesia 51:117
21. Kain ZN, Caldwell-Andrews AA, Krivutza DM et al (2004) Trends in the practice of parental presence during induction of anesthesia and the use of preoperative sedative premedication in the United States, 1995–2002: results of a follow-up national survey. Anesth Analg 98:1252–1259, – table of contents

22. Coté CJ, Cohen IT, Suresh S et al (2002) A comparison of three doses of a commercially prepared oral midazolam syrup in children. Anesth Analg 94:37–43, – table of contents
23. Levine MF, Spahr-Schopfer IA, Hartley E et al (1993) Oral midazolam premedication in children: the minimum time interval for separation from parents. Can J Anaesth 40:726–729. doi:10.1007/BF03009769
24. Weldon BC, Watcha MF, White PF (1992) Oral midazolam in children: effect of time and adjunctive therapy. Anesth Analg 75:51–55
25. Cox RG, Nemish U, Ewen A, Crowe M-J (2006) Evidence-based clinical update: does premedication with oral midazolam lead to improved behavioural outcomes in children? Can J Anesth/J Can Anesth 53:1213–1219. doi:10.1007/BF03021583
26. Viitanen H, Annila P, Viitanen M, Yli-Hankala A (1999) Midazolam premedication delays recovery from propofol-induced sevoflurane anesthesia in children 1–3 yr. Can J Anaesth 46:766–771
27. Fazi L, Jantzen EC, Rose JB et al (2001) A comparison of oral clonidine and oral midazolam as preanesthetic medications in the pediatric tonsillectomy patient. Anesth Analg 92:56–61
28. Alderson PJ, Lerman J (1994) Oral premedication for paediatric ambulatory anaesthesia: a comparison of midazolam and ketamine. Can J Anaesth 41:221–226. doi:10.1007/BF03009834
29. Patel D, Meakin G (1997) Oral midazolam compared with diazepam-droperidol and trimeprazine as premedicants in children. Paediatr Anaesth 7:287–293
30. Özcengiz D, Gunes Y, Ozmete O (2011) Oral melatonin, dexmedetomidine, and midazolam for prevention of postoperative agitation in children. J Anesth 25:184–188. doi:10.1007/s00540-011-1099-2
31. Savla JR, Ghai B, Bansal D, Wig J (2014) Effect of intranasal dexmedetomidine or oral midazolam premedication on sevoflurane EC50 for successful laryngeal mask airway placement in children: a randomized, double-blind, placebo-controlled trial. Pediatric Anesthesia 24:433–439. doi:10.1111/pan.12358
32. Gingrich BK (1994) Difficulties encountered in a comparative study of orally administered midazolam and ketamine. Anesthesiology 80:1414–1415
33. Reimer EJ, Dunn GS, Montgomery CJ et al (1998) The effectiveness of clonidine as an analgesic in paediatric adenotonsillectomy. Can J Anaesth 45:1162–1167. doi:10.1007/BF03012457
34. Lambert P, Cyna AM, Knight N, Middleton P (2014) Clonidine premedication for postoperative analgesia in children. Cochrane Database Syst Rev (1):CD009633. doi:10.1002/14651858.CD009633.pub2
35. Bergendahl HTG, Lönnqvist PA, Eksborg S et al (2004) Clonidine vs. midazolam as premedication in children undergoing adeno-tonsillectomy: a prospective, randomized, controlled clinical trial. Acta Anaesthesiol Scand 48:1292–1300. doi:10.1111/j.1399-6576.2004.00525.x
36. Hall JE, Uhrich TD, Ebert TJ (2001) Sedative, analgesic and cognitive effects of clonidine infusions in humans. Br J Anaesth 86:5–11
37. Zub D, Berkenbosch JW, Tobias JD (2005) Preliminary experience with oral dexmedetomidine for procedural and anesthetic premedication. Paediatr Anaesth 15:932–938. doi:10.1111/j.1460-9592.2005.01623.x
38. Schmidt AP, Valinetti EA, Bandeira D et al (2007) Effects of preanesthetic administration of midazolam, clonidine, or dexmedetomidine on postoperative pain and anxiety in children. Paediatr Anaesth 17:667–674. doi:10.1111/j.1460-9592.2006.02185.x
39. Baldwa NM, Padvi AV, Dave NM, Garasia MB (2012) Atomised intranasal midazolam spray as premedication in pediatric patients: comparison between two doses of 0.2 and 0.3 mg/kg. J Anesth 26:346–350. doi:10.1007/s00540-012-1341-6
40. Weber F, Wulf H, el Saeidi G (2003) Premedication with nasal s-ketamine and midazolam provides good conditions for induction of anesthesia in preschool children. Can J Anaesth 50:470–475. doi:10.1007/BF03021058
41. Akin A, Bayram A, Esmaoglu A et al (2012) Dexmedetomidine vs midazolam for premedication of pediatric patients undergoing anesthesia. Pediatric Anesthesia 22:871–876. doi:10.1111/j.1460-9592.2012.03802.x

42. Hosseini Jahromi SA, Hosseini Valami SM, Adeli N, Yazdi Z (2012) Comparison of the effects of intranasal midazolam versus different doses of intranasal ketamine on reducing preoperative pediatric anxiety: a prospective randomized clinical trial. J Anesth 26:878–882. doi:10.1007/s00540-012-1422-6

43. Bilgen S, Köner Ö, Karacay S et al (2014) Effect of ketamine versus alfentanil following midazolam in preventing emergence agitation in children after sevoflurane anaesthesia: a prospective randomized clinical trial. J Int Med Res 42:1262–1271. doi:10.1177/0300060514543039

44. Gharde P, Chauhan S, Kiran U (2006) Evaluation of efficacy of intranasal midazolam, ketamine and their mixture as premedication and its relation with bispectral index in children with tetralogy of fallot undergoing intracardiac repair. Ann Card Anaesth 9:25–30

45. Almenrader N, Passariello M, Coccetti B et al (2007) Steal-induction after clonidine premedication: a comparison of the oral and nasal route. Paediatr Anaesth 17:230–234. doi:10.1111/j.1460-9592.2006.02080.x

46. Stella MJ, Bailey AG (2008) Intranasal clonidine as a premedicant: three cases with unique indications. Paediatr Anaesth 18:71–73. doi:10.1111/j.1460-9592.2007.02349.x

47. Mitra S, Kazal S, Anand LK (2014) Intranasal clonidine vs. midazolam as premedication in children: a randomized controlled trial. Indian Pediatr 51:113–118

48. Cimen ZS, Hanci A, Sivrikaya GU et al (2013) Comparison of buccal and nasal dexmedetomidine premedication for pediatric patients. Pediatric Anesthesia 23:134–138. doi:10.1111/pan.12025

49. Sheta SA, Al-Sarheed MA, Abdelhalim AA (2014) Intranasal dexmedetomidine vs midazolam for premedication in children undergoing complete dental rehabilitation: a double-blinded randomized controlled trial. Pediatric Anesthesia 24:181–189. doi:10.1111/pan.12287

50. Spear RM, Yaster M, Berkowitz ID et al (1991) Preinduction of anesthesia in children with rectally administered midazolam. Anesthesiology 74:670–674

51. Saint-Maurice C, Estève C, Holzer J et al (1984) Premedication using intrarectal midazolam. Study of effective dosage in pediatric anesthesia. Ann Fr Anesth Reanim 3:181–184

52. Tanaka M, Sato M, Saito A, Nishikawa T (2000) Reevaluation of rectal ketamine premedication in children: comparison with rectal midazolam. Anesthesiology 93:1217–1224

53. Marhofer P, Freitag H, Höchtl A et al (2001) S(+)-ketamine for rectal premedication in children. Anesth Analg 92:62–65

54. Lönnqvist PA, Bergendahl HT, Eksborg S (1994) Pharmacokinetics of clonidine after rectal administration in children. Anesthesiology 81:1097–1101

55. Smith I, Kranke P, Murat I et al (2011) Perioperative fasting in adults and children: guidelines from the European Society of Anaesthesiology. Eur J Anaesthesiol 28:556–569

56. NA (2011) Practice guidelines for preoperative fasting and the use of pharmacologic agents to reduce the risk of pulmonary aspiration: application to healthy patients undergoing elective procedures. Anesthesiology 114:495–511. doi:10.1097/ALN.0b013e3181fcbfd9

57. Bricker SR, McLuckie A, Nightingale DA (1989) Gastric aspirates after trauma in children. Anaesthesia 44:721–724

58. Green SM, Roback MG, Miner JR et al (2007) Fasting and emergency department procedural sedation and analgesia: a consensus-based clinical practice advisory. Ann Emerg Med 49:454–461

Preoperative Consideration in Common Pathological and Nonpathological Conditions

4

Marinella Astuto, Gianpaolo Serafini, Simonetta Baroncini,
Fabio Borrometi, Luciano Bortone, Cristina Ceschin,
Andrea Gentili, Elisabetta Lampugnani, Giovanni Mangia,
Luisa Meneghini, C. Minardi, Giovanni Montobbio,
Francesca Pinzoni, Barbara Rosina, Carlotta Rossi,
Marina Sammartino, Emre Sahillioğlu, Rita Sonzogni,
Valter Sonzogni, Simonetta Tesoro, Costanza Tognon,
Tiziana Tondinelli, Nicola Zadra, and Pablo M. Ingelmo

4.1   Upper Respiratory Infections: URI

Adverse respiratory events are of the most frequent causes of perioperative morbidity and mortality in children undergoing general anesthesia [1, 2]. Children with recent upper respiratory tract infections (upper respiratory infections – URI), undergoing general anesthesia, have an increased risk of complications such as lung and

M. Astuto (✉)
Anesthesia, Intensive Care, University of Catania, Policlinico Hospital, Catania, Italy

Dipartimento di Anestesia e Rianimazione, Ospedale Universitario Policlinico, Catania, Italy
e-mail: astmar@tiscali.it

G. Serafini
Anestesia e Rianimazione 1, Fondazione IRCCS Policlinico S. Matteo, Università di Pavia,
Pavia, Italy

S. Baroncini • A. Gentili
Dipartimento di Anestesia e Rianimazione Pediatrica, Ospedale S. Orsola-Malpighi,
Università di Bologna, Bologna, Italy

F. Borrometi
Servizio di Cure Palliative e Terapia del Dolore, Ospedale Santobono Pausilipon, Napoli, Italy

L. Bortone
First Service of Anesthesia and Intensive Care, Parma Hospital, Parma, Italy

Dipartimento di Anestesia e Rianimazione, Azienda Ospedaliera di Parma, Parma, Italy

© Springer International Publishing Switzerland 2016
M. Astuto, P.M. Ingelmo (eds.), *Perioperative Medicine in Pediatric Anesthesia*,
Anesthesia, Intensive Care and Pain in Neonates and Children,
DOI 10.1007/978-3-319-21960-8_4

airway laryngospasm, bronchospasm, hypoxia, atelectasis, and post-extubation airway obstruction [3–6].

Respiratory symptoms, eczema or a family history of asthma, rhinitis, and exposure to passive smoking were associated with an increased risk of adverse respiratory events [6].

The risks of respiratory complications, especially laryngospasm, are age related, with a relative risk reduction of 11 % for each year of increasing age [7]. The risk of bronchospasm is ten times higher in patients with nocturnal dry cough and a history of eczema, a disease frequently associated with atopy, wheezing, and asthma [8]. Symptoms of respiratory infection such as cough, purulent nasal secretions, and fever within two weeks prior to surgery are associated with an increased frequency of respiratory adverse events [6].

Propofol anesthesia was associated with a lower incidence of perioperative respiratory complications, particularly that of laryngospasm, when compared with sevoflurane maintenance [6].

Instrumentation of the airways (endotracheal tube or LMA) is an independent risk factor for the occurrence of adverse respiratory events, especially laryngospasm. LMA was associated with a higher risk of laryngospasm when compared with the face mask, but with a lower risk when compared with the endotracheal tube. [6, 9–11].

C. Ceschin • C. Rossi
Servizio di Anestesia e Rianimazione, Dolo Hospital, Mirano, Italy

E. Lampugnani • G. Montobbio
Dipartimento di Anestesia e Rianimazione, IRCCS Ospedale dei Bambini G. Gaslini, Genova, Italy

G. Mangia • T. Tondinelli
Dipartimento di Anestesia, Ospedale S. Camillo, Rome, Italy

L. Meneghini • C. Minardi • C. Tognon • N. Zadra
Dipartimento di Anestesia e Rianimazione, Università di Padova, Padova, Italy

F. Pinzoni • B. Rosina
Dipartimento di Anestesia Pediatrica, Ospedali Civili, Brescia, Italy

M. Sammartino
Dipartimento di Anestesia e Rianimazione, Ospedale Universitario A. Gemelli, Università Cattolica del Sacro Cuore, Rome, Italy

E. Sahillioğlu
Department of Anesthesiology and Reanimation, Acibadem University, Istanbul, Turkey

R. Sonzogni • V. Sonzogni
Primo Servizio di Anestesia e Rianimazione, Ospedali Riuniti di Bergamo, Bergamo, Italy

S. Tesoro
Sezione di Anestesia, Analgesia e Rianimazione, Dipartimento di Medicina Clinica e Sperimentale, Università di Perugia, Perugia, Italy

Department of Anesthesia, Analgesia and Intensive Care, University of Perugia, Perugia, Italy

P.M. Ingelmo
Deparment of Anesthesia, Montreal Children's Hospital, MUHC, McGill University, Montreal, QC, Canada

The preoperative administration of salbutamol (2.5 mg in children weighing < 20 kg, 5 mg in those > 20 kg) in children with recent URI reduced the incidence of respiratory adverse events, such as laryngospasm, bronchospasm, and desaturation (<95 %) and severe cough by at least 35 % [12]. This data confirmed previous observations in children with asthma [13, 14].

In conclusion, children at high risk for perioperative respiratory adverse events should be systematically identify during the preoperative assessment. The following factors were associated with an increased risk of perioperative respiratory adverse events:

- History of recent respiratory tract infection
- Onset of wheezing during physical activity
- More than three episodes of wheezing in the last 12 months
- Nocturnal dry cough
- History of eczema
- Asthma or family history of asthma
- Rhinitis
- Exposure to secondhand smoke

Children with the risk factors listed above, but with moderate symptoms (clear runny nose, dry cough), may benefit from an anesthetic approach that includes:

- Preoperative premedication with salbutamol
- Induction and maintenance with propofol anesthesia

Surgical procedures of children with purulent rhinitis, productive cough, lower respiratory tract involvement, and general symptoms (fever > 38.5 ° C, headache, malaise, poor feeding, irritability) should be postponed for 2–3 weeks [3, 6, 15–17].

4.2 Asthma and Bronchial Hyperresponsiveness

The inflammation of the airways is a distinctive feature of asthma. The inflamed airway become hyperreactive to irritating stimuli. In patients with asthma, many procedures routinely used in anesthesia, such as laryngoscopy and tracheal intubation, may induce bronchospasm.

An episode of intraoperative bronchospasm is a serious adverse event and can make ventilation difficult or impossible. It also produces hypercapnia, acidosis, hypoxia, and, rarely, cardiovascular collapse and death. The airways are more prone to bronchospasm within 6 weeks after an attack of asthma. A thorough preoperative optimization of medical treatment may prevent or limit asthma complications. Thus, a recent exacerbation of asthma that has required hospitalization or emergency therapy within 6 weeks of surgery precludes elective surgery [18, 19].

Asthma is characterized by episodes of variable and intermittent airway obstruction, and children present tachypnea, wheezing, and coughing and use accessory

Table 4.1 Stepwise management in children aged 5–12 years

Level	Step	Steroids	Add therapy
1	Mild intermittent asthma	No	Inhaled short-acting β2-agonist as required
2	Regular preventer therapy	Up to 400 mcg/die BDP	LABA
3	Initial add-on therapy	Up to 400 mcg/die BDP	LTRA
4	Persistent poor control	Up to 800 mcg/die BDP	LABA/LTRA/aminofillina
5	Continuous or frequent use of oral steroids	Other doses of BPD (≥800 mcg/die) and per os steroids	Use daily steroid tablet in lowest dose providing adequate control

Patients should start treatment at the step most appropriate to the initial severity of their asthma. Check concordance and reconsider diagnosis if response to treatment is unexpectedly poor. *BPD* beclomethasone dipropionate, *LABA* long-acting β2-agonist, *LTRA* leukotriene-receptor antagonist

respiratory muscles. Older children may complain of shortness of breath, wheezing, or discomfort. [20].

The diagnosis of asthma could be done in a patient with four or more episodes of wheezing per year, associated to a parent with asthma, atopic dermatitis, or sensitization to inhalant allergens, and two of the following: food sensitization, wheezing outside of infectious episodes, or eosinophilia [21].

Most radiological studies have a reasonable positive predictive value, but poor negative predictive value [22]. A chest radiograph is rarely useful in mild asthma, but may be useful in more severe cases to exclude acute infection, hyperinflation, or pneumothorax in an acute exacerbation [18]. Similarly, a computed tomography (CT scan) can show bronchomalacia or a dilation of bronchial wall in children with chronic asthma [23, 24].

Pulmonary function tests as flow expiratory volume (FEV_1) are able to determine the degree of reversibility of respiratory resistance and to measure the extent of improvement after treatment in collaborative children usually beyond 7 years of age [18]. Diurnal variation in FEV_1 may indicate poor disease control. In general, pulmonary function tests are still of limited use in the preoperative evaluation children with asthma [25].

The differential diagnosis are fixed obstructions, suppurative lung diseases (cystic fibrosis, ciliary dyskinesia), post viral bronchitis, and bronchial or tracheomalacia. In these circumstances asthma may be misdiagnosed [26, 27].

It is essential to establish the severity and measures for control asthma because both aspects are closely linked. Asthma of mild severity, but poorly controlled, may seem harsh in terms of frequent and persistent symptoms. In contrast, severe asthma may seem well controlled but requires high doses of inhaled corticosteroids to maintain control. Poorly controlled asthma is defined by various aspects such as the frequency of symptoms, the use of symptomatic drugs, frequent emergency admissions, and the use of oral corticosteroids (Table 4.1) [20, 22].

A difficult asthma is a poorly controlled asthma despite high doses of inhaled steroids (≥800 µg/day of beclomethasone dipropionate (BDP) or belonging to levels 4 and 5). Although some asthmatic children may be unresponsive to steroids, the most common reasons for a "difficult asthma" are the low compliance to treatment, inadequate technical capacity with the inhaler, or an incorrect diagnosis of asthma [28].

A small group of children with severe asthma may be at risk of life. Those children may have a poorly controlled asthma or a "fragile" asthma with asthma attacks of sudden onsets, which simulate an asphyxiating or anaphylactic reaction. A history of serious recent exacerbations especially if they required admission to the ICU is indicative that a child is particularly vulnerable to a sudden attack, which may be precipitated by nonsteroidal analgesics or anesthetic vapors [29].

Children who take medication only during exacerbation should start taking the same drugs (inhaled β2-agonists or oral medications) and doses used during exacerbation, on a regular basis 3–5 days before surgery [30]. The benefits on airway reactivity are evident after 6–8 h with a maximum effect between 12 and 36 hours.

Children receiving asthma medication on regular basis should continue with usual administered treatment. The administration of β2-agonists (e.g., salbutamol) before the induction of anesthesia may prevent the increase of airway resistance associated with halogenated anesthesia [13] and URIs [12].

Children under steroid medication and those who have been taking steroids in the previous two months should receive corticosteroids as during exacerbation (e.g., prednisone $1 \text{ mg} \cdot \text{kg}^{-1} \cdot \text{day}^{-1}$) [30]. There is no need for perioperative supplemental doses of steroids as inhaled steroids alone do not cause adrenal suppression [31].

Finally, a child with "difficult" asthma who regularly takes bronchodilators and/or corticosteroids may require an intensification of the frequency of bronchodilators, an increase in the dosage of corticosteroids, or occasionally all these measures [28].

4.3 Bronchopulmonary Dysplasia (BPD)

Bronchopulmonary dysplasia (BPD) is the most common cause of chronic lung disease in infants.

It mostly affects premature infants weighting about 1000 g at birth that still need oxygen therapy for more than 28 days and after the 36 gestational week [32, 33].

Northway first described BPD in 1967 in a group of infants with respiratory failure after prolonged mechanical ventilation and administration of high concentrations of oxygen [33]. The lung of these infants presented emphysema, atelectasis, fibrosis, epithelial metaplasia, and marked hypertrophy of smooth muscles in the airways and pulmonary vessels.

The uses of less aggressive ventilation modes and postnatal surfactant therapy have significantly reduced the severity of respiratory distress syndrome and, consequently, the severity of BPD. Actually BDP is characterized mainly by pulmonary inflammation a decrease of the process of septation of the alveoli and an alteration in vascular development [34–36], with a framework characterized by diffused X-ray opacity [37].

The triad airway obstruction, bronchial hyperreactivity, and lung hyperinflation determine inhomogeneous distribution of ventilation, reduced compliance, increased work of breathing, and gas exchange impairment [38]. The clinical manifestations of BPD are tachypnea, wheezing, coughing, frequent febrile episodes, episodes of desaturation, and bradycardia [38, 39].

Patients with BPD have high respiratory resistance, decreased lung volumes, lower functional residual capacity, airway obstruction, and lung hyperinflation. During the first year of life, infants with BPD are at increased risk of laryngospasm, bronchospasm, and desaturation due to bronchial hyperreactivity. Moreover bronchial secretions may lead to occlusion of the endotracheal tube. Finally, in the presence of hypothermia, pain, acidosis, or hypoxia, infants with BPD may develop pulmonary hypertension resulting in pulmonary hypoperfusion, hypoxemia, and cardiac failure [40].

These respiratory alterations are mostly evident during the first 3 years of life. After 5–8 years infants with a medium form of severe BPD can be asymptomatic, while the airway's hyperresponsiveness may persist.

Nutritional support and therapy with bronchodilators, antibiotics, diuretics, and corticosteroids should be optimized before surgery [40]. Preoperative echocardiography is recommended, in order to assess cardiac contractility and the presence of an associated right ventricular dysfunction [37, 40]. If a BPD patient is taking diuretics, the concentration of electrolytes should be evaluated before surgery [40].

Patients with BPD may require monitoring and ventilation up to 24–48 hours after surgery. The risks of general anesthesia with intubation in infants with BPD may possibly be reduced or prevented by the use of regional anesthesia techniques and/or with the use of a laryngeal mask airway (LMA) [19, 41].

4.4   Allergies

In most industrialized countries, the immediate hypersensitive reactions to anesthetics and drugs used in the perioperative period are being reported with increasing frequency. Muscle relaxants and latex are the two main causes responsible for these intraoperative allergic events [42, 43]. In most cases, the reactions are of immunologic origin (IgE-mediated reactions, anaphylactic reactions) or due to the direct stimulation of histamine release (anaphylactoid reactions) [44, 45].

The clinical history may reveal a history of atopy and allergy to medications, to latex, or to tropical fruits.

Atopy is a hereditary predisposition in which the patient synthesizes IgE antibodies to various allergens: pollen, dust, animal hair, and foods. Clinically it presents with asthma, allergic rhinitis, conjunctivitis, fever, and eczema [46]. Gualdagen H et al. suggested an association between anaphylactic shock during anesthesia and atopy. The basophils of atopic patients easily release histamine [47]. Atopy may be a risk factor when drugs that induce histamine release (atracurium, mivacurium, etc.) are injected rapidly.

Table 4.2 Groups of patients at risk for developing latex allergy

Group	Incidence %
Spina bifida [87, 88]	18–72
Urogenital tract malformations [89]	17–71
Repeated gastrointestinal tract surgery [90, 91]	17–20
Extensive or repeated neurosurgical procedures [92]	36
More than five surgical procedures at neonatal stage or before the age of one [93]	55
Atopic subject [49]	9–36
Tetraplegic patients	a
History of anaphylactic reaction of unknown etiology [94]	a
Allergy to fruits and vegetables, especially the tropical variant [95]	35–55

[a]Numerous case reports with no objective definition of a percentage than the general population

An unexplained episode characterized by cardiovascular collapse, broncho-spasm, and edema, during a previous anesthesia, could be interpreted as an allergic reaction. Allergy to local anesthetics is quite exceptional. In a series of 208 patients who had a suspected reaction to local anesthetics, IgE-mediated mechanism was demonstrated in only four cases. In other patients, the causes were vasovagal phenomena, possible reactions to additives, panic episodes, or intervascular injection of adrenaline [48]. There is a high incidence of cross-reactions between neuromuscular-blocking agents. It is recommended to avoid administering neuromuscular-blocking agents to patients with previous allergic reactions to this class of drugs before an allergy test has been performed.

Preoperative identification of patients at risk is the first element of prevention against latex allergy. In the operating room, the main objective is to ensure the patient at risk avoids coming in contact with latex, for, e.g., the gloves. The prevention of this contact and/or the repeated exposure to latex is the cornerstone in preventing patients from developing anaphylaxis during surgery[49–53].

The incidence of latex allergy in the pediatric population varies from 0.8 to 6.7 % (Table 4.2). Common features of groups at risk of presenting an allergic reaction are atopy, early contact with latex (within the first year of life), and the frequent and prolonged exposure to latex [54, 55]. An allergy skin tests with specific IgE + before surgery could be justified in [56]:

- Patients with a documented allergy to an anesthetic drugs or latex
- Patients with a history of unexplained reactions during general anesthesia (i.e., severe hypotension, bronchospasm, edema)
- Patients who claim to have an allergy toward local anesthetics
- Patients who belong to a group at high risk for latex allergy (Table 4.2)

The skin prick test (SPT) remains the gold standard for IgE-mediated reactions evaluation. To prevent a false-negative result due to the depletion of mast cells, STP should be performed 6 weeks after an acute allergic event. The sensitivity to latex is

70–100 % and specificity of 74–100 %. Muscle relaxant allergy sensitivity is greater than 95 %, and specificity is still a matter of debate [52, 57]:

The radioallergosorbent test (RAST) is an in vitro-specific IgE test and is currently restricted to the diagnosis of anaphylaxis to muscle relaxants, thiopental, or latex. The RAST sensitivity to latex varies between 53 and 97 % with specificity of 33–87 %. The RAST specificity may not exclude a false-negative case of latex sensitization. Nevertheless, because of the absence of the risk of anaphylaxis and the simplicity of execution, the RAST is one of the most widely used test. Some studies report that serum levels of IgE are well correlated with the number of surgeries. The patient is considered sensitized if the IgE antibody concentrations of $>0:35$ kU / L [54, 58].

Some studies support the prophylaxis with diphenhydramine, cimetidine, and methylprednisolone [18, 54]. Pharmacological prophylaxis may only mitigate early immune response or may not prevent anaphylaxis at all [58, 59]. However, there is no evidence to support the use of pharmacological premedication [60].

The term latex-safe defines a path that must be applied to patient with latex allergy during the perioperative period. Latex-safe strategies designed to prevent patients at risk to be in contact with latex must be a priority of health-care facilities [49, 54, 61]. The term latex-free defines an instrument or tool in which the manufacturer certifies the absolute absence of latex [60].

If the patient presented a severe allergic reaction of unknown origin, characterized by unexplained hypotension or circulatory collapse, bronchospasm, and edema during a previous general anesthesia, it is recommended to adopt a latex-safe environment with a regional anesthesia technique or general anesthesia without neuromuscular-blocking drugs [46, 62].

4.5   Heart Murmurs

Heart murmurs are a common finding in childhood, and about 50–72 % of these murmurs are normal or innocents [63, 64]. Every child with a heart murmur requires a thorough clinical examination with assessment of peripheral pulses, blood pressure, and SaO2, ECG, and in selected cases an echocardiography [65–67].

The anamnesis should look for history of prematurity, the presence of congenital malformations, respiratory symptoms including repeated infections, cyanosis, chest pain, syncope, or family history of sudden death. Table 4.3 includes some useful questions to determine the clinical effect of a murmur [68].

The physical examination includes auscultation of the heart, both when supine or sitting, as the intensity of an innocent murmur increases in the supine position for increased end-diastolic volume and stroke volume. The intensity of the most of the pathological murmurs doesn't vary during changes on the patient position. The only exception is the murmur of the hypertrophic cardiomyopathy (HCM), which increases in intensity from supine to sitting position [69]. Table 4.4 shows the characteristics of innocent murmurs and pathological ones [64, 65, 70].

Both arms' brachial pulses in infants or radial pulses in children should be examined and compared with femoral pulses. Small femoral pulses, especially if discrepant with respect to the quality of brachial or radial or associated with radio-femoral

Table 4.3 Evaluation of the clinical effects a murmur [68]

Children
Does he/she run? Like peers?
Is he/she calmer or slower than peers?
Cyanosis
Does he/she turn blue? During feeding/when crying?
Does he/she lose consciousness?
Does he/she stop playing and squat?
Infant
Is feeding prolonged?
Does he/she sweat during normal care?
Does he/she have swollen eyes in the morning?

Table 4.4 Characteristics of innocent murmurs and pathological ones [64, 65, 70]

Murmur	Characteristics
Innocent	Systolic or a continuous Increases and decreases Mild or moderately mild (2/6 or less) Increase in intensity from sitting to supine position
Pathological	Diastolic, pansystolic, or late systolic Generally intense (3/6 or more) Associated with tremors Associated with signs or symptoms of heart disease Does not vary significantly going from sitting to supine position (except CMI murmur)

delay, are suggestive of aortic coarctation or aortic arch obstruction and require further investigation [66].

The value of ECG and chest radiography in the diagnosis of congenital heart disease is limited. Both tests have a very low sensitivity and specificity. Chest X-rays also expose the child to ionizing radiation and its routine application can be defined as inappropriate in an asymptomatic child [71–73].

ECG has a low sensitivity in identifying congenital heart lesions in children with asymptomatic heart murmur.

Echocardiography remains the gold standard for diagnosis of congenital heart disease and its role in the diagnosis of asymptomatic murmurs has changed radically in the last 10 years. In the presence of a murmur, it is recommended to perform an echocardiogram if [65–67]:

- The child is less than 1 year old.
- The murmur has the characteristics of a pathological murmur.
- Signs and symptoms of heart disease are presented.
- There is evidence on the ECG of right or left hypertrophy.

Nonurgent surgery in infants under 1 year of age, with pathological murmur, and/or signs and symptoms of congenital heart disease, and/or ECG with evidence of right or left hypertrophy, should be delayed until an echocardiogram with a cardiology consultation identifies or excludes a pathological condition [64, 68].

4.6 Vaccination

Vaccination represents the most efficient and reliable prevention of primary infectious diseases [74].

Anesthesia and surgery may interfere with the immune response [75–77]. However, the immune-modulatory effect of general anesthesia and surgery may not modify the efficacy of recently given vaccine [31, 78–81].

Adverse effects to vaccines can occur on the day of administration during the following 90 days [82]. The most common complications of vaccination (fever, malaise, crying, pain) can be wrongly interpreted as particularly infectious complications after surgery. Then there are two questions that need to be answered [81]:

1. Should vaccination be postponed in children scheduled for surgery?
2. Should anesthesia be postponed in recently vaccinated children?

There are no clear answers to these questions [83]. The Italian Schedule of Vaccination from Ministry of Health did not provide recommendations regarding anesthesia or surgery [74]. The handbook on vaccinations of Great Britain states that "anesthesia and surgery are not contraindications to routine immunization but in some of these situations, additional precautions may be required" like in case of asplenia or splenic dysfunction [84]. The Australian handbook on vaccinations specifies "that surgery should be postponed for a week after an inactivated vaccine and three weeks after a live attenuated vaccine". A vaccination should be postponed for a week after an operation under general anesthesia [85]. The Ministry of Health of New Zealand stated that "there is no evidence that anesthetic reduces the immune response to a vaccine or increases the risk of adverse events following immunization (AEFI)."

Immunization with inactive vaccines should be avoided for 3 days prior to an anesthetic (12 days for a live vaccine such as MMR) in case an AEFI occurs and results in the postponement of the anesthetic [86].

It seems reasonable to accept that there is a risk, albeit vague and theoretical, associated with anesthesia in recently vaccinated children. This small risk can be reduced to zero by ensuring that surgery, anesthesia, and vaccinations do not coincide. The following has been recommended [83]:

- Postpone an elective procedure that requires anesthesia rather than vaccination, especially in neonates and infants.
- Postpone vaccinations, one week after general anesthesia.
- Postpone anesthesia to a week after vaccination with inactivated vaccine (diphtheria, tetanus, pertussis (DTPa)), inactive polio vaccine (IPV), *Haemophilus influenzae* type b (Hib) vaccine, and vaccine against meningitis C.
- Postpone anesthesia to three weeks after vaccination with live attenuated vaccine: measles, mumps, rubella (MMR), polio, and BCG (against TB).

References

1. Bhananker SM et al (2007) Anesthesia-related cardiac arrest in children: update from the Pediatric Perioperative Cardiac Arrest Registry. Anesth Analg 105(2):344–350
2. Mamie C et al (2004) Incidence and risk factors of perioperative respiratory adverse events in children undergoing elective surgery. Paediatr Anaesth 14(3):218–224
3. Tait AR et al (2001) Risk factors for perioperative adverse respiratory events in children with upper respiratory tract infections. Anesthesiology 95(2):299–306
4. Murat I, Constant I, Maud'huy H (2004) Perioperative anaesthetic morbidity in children: a database of 24,165 anaesthetics over a 30-month period. Paediatr Anaesth 14(2):158–166
5. Olsson GL, Hallen B (1984) Laryngospasm during anaesthesia. A computer-aided incidence study in 136,929 patients. Acta Anaesthesiol Scand 28(5):567–575
6. von Ungern-Sternberg BS et al (2010) Risk assessment for respiratory complications in paediatric anaesthesia: a prospective cohort study. Lancet 376(9743):773–783
7. von Ungern-Sternberg BS et al (2007) Laryngeal mask airway is associated with an increased incidence of adverse respiratory events in children with recent upper respiratory tract infections. Anesthesiology 107(5):714–719
8. Arshad SH et al (2005) Early life risk factors for current wheeze, asthma, and bronchial hyperresponsiveness at 10 years of age. Chest 127(2):502–508
9. Tait AR et al (1998) Use of the laryngeal mask airway in children with upper respiratory tract infections: a comparison with endotracheal intubation. Anesth Analg 86(4):706–711
10. Harnett M et al (2000) Airway complications in infants: comparison of laryngeal mask airway and the facemask-oral airway. Can J Anaesth 47(4):315–318
11. Rachel Homer J et al (2007) Risk factors for adverse events in children with colds emerging from anesthesia: a logistic regression. Paediatr Anaesth 17(2):154–161
12. von Ungern-Sternberg BS et al (2009) Salbutamol premedication in children with a recent respiratory tract infection. Paediatr Anaesth 19(11):1064–1069
13. Scalfaro P et al (2001) Salbutamol prevents the increase of respiratory resistance caused by tracheal intubation during sevoflurane anesthesia in asthmatic children. Anesth Analg 93(4):898–902
14. Zachary CY, Evans R 3rd (1996) Perioperative management for childhood asthma. Ann Allergy Asthma Immunol 77(6):468–472
15. Tait AR, Reynolds PI, Gutstein HB (1995) Factors that influence an anesthesiologist's decision to cancel elective surgery for the child with an upper respiratory tract infection. J Clin Anesth 7(6):491–499
16. Tait AR, Malviya S (2005) Anesthesia for the child with an upper respiratory tract infection: still a dilemma? Anesth Analg 100(1):59–65
17. Parnis SJ, Barker DS, Van Der Walt JH (2001) Clinical predictors of anaesthetic complications in children with respiratory tract infections. Paediatr Anaesth 11(1):29–40
18. Black AE (1999) Medical assessment of the paediatric patient. Br J Anaesth 83(1):3–15
19. Maxwell LG (2004) Age-associated issues in preoperative evaluation, testing, and planning: pediatrics. Anesthesiol Clin North America 22(1):27–43
20. British Thoracic Society and Scottish Intercollegiate Guidelines Network (2012) http://www.sign.ac.uk/pdf/sign101.pdf [cited 2012 16/02/2012]
21. Liccardi G et al (2012) Bronchial asthma. Curr Opin Anaesthesiol 25(1):30–37
22. Services, U.S.D.o.H.a.H., Expert Panel Report: Guidelines for the Diagnosis and Management of Asthma - Update on Selected Topics 2002. National Asthma Education and Prevention Program, 2002. http://www.nhlbi.nih.gov/guidelines/archives/epr-2_upd/asthmafullrpt_archive.pdf [cited 2012 18/04/2012]
23. James A, King G (2004) The computed tomographic scan: a new tool to monitor asthma treatment? Am J Med 116(11):775–777

24. Takemura M et al (2004) Bronchial dilatation in asthma: relation to clinical and sputum indices. Chest 125(4):1352–1358
25. Doherty GM et al (2005) Anesthesia and the child with asthma. Paediatr Anaesth 15(6): 446–454
26. de Jongste JC, Shields MD (2003) Cough. 2: chronic cough in children. Thorax 58(11):998–1003
27. Thomson F, Masters IB, Chang AB (2002) Persistent cough in children and the overuse of medications. J Paediatr Child Health 38(6):578–581
28. Balfour-Lynn I (1999) Difficult asthma: beyond the guidelines. Arch Dis Child 80(2):201–206
29. Plaza V et al (2002) Frequency and clinical characteristics of rapid-onset fatal and near-fatal asthma. Eur Respir J 19(5):846–852
30. Pien LC, Grammer LC, Patterson R (1988) Minimal complications in a surgical population with severe asthma receiving prophylactic corticosteroids. J Allergy Clin Immunol 82(4): 696–700
31. Mattila-Vuori A et al (2000) Local and systemic immune response to surgery under balanced anaesthesia in children. Paediatr Anaesth 10(4):381–388
32. Northway WH Jr, Rosan RC, Porter DY (1967) Pulmonary disease following respirator therapy of hyaline-membrane disease. Bronchopulmonary dysplasia. N Engl J Med 276(7):357–368
33. Northway WH Jr (1992) An introduction to bronchopulmonary dysplasia. Clin Perinatol 19(3):489–495
34. Bancalari E, Claure N, Sosenko IR (2003) Bronchopulmonary dysplasia: changes in pathogenesis, epidemiology and definition. Semin Neonatol 8(1):63–71
35. Bancalari E, Claure N (2006) Definitions and diagnostic criteria for bronchopulmonary dysplasia. Semin Perinatol 30(4):164–170
36. Jobe AJ (1999) The new BPD: an arrest of lung development. Pediatr Res 46(6):641–643
37. Coalson JJ, Winter V, deLemos RA (1995) Decreased alveolarization in baboon survivors with bronchopulmonary dysplasia. Am J Respir Crit Care Med 152(2):640–646
38. Vassallo SA, Goudsouzian NG (1990) In: Rogers MC (ed) Current practice in anesthesiology. Current therapy series. University of Michigan, B.C. Decker. pp 222–225
39. Bhutani VK, Abbasi S (1992) Long-term pulmonary consequences in survivors with bronchopulmonary dysplasia. Clin Perinatol 19(3):649–671
40. Jobe AH, Bancalari E (2001) Bronchopulmonary dysplasia. Am J Respir Crit Care Med 163(7):1723–1729
41. Ferrari LR, Goudsouzian NG (1995) The use of the laryngeal mask airway in children with bronchopulmonary dysplasia. Anesth Analg 81(2):310–313
42. Murat I (1993) Anaphylactic reactions during paediatric anaesthesia; results of the survey of the French Society of Paediatric Anaesthetists (ADARPEF) 1991–1992. Pediatr Anesth 3(6):339–343
43. Karila C et al (2005) Anaphylaxis during anesthesia: results of a 12-year survey at a French pediatric center. Allergy 60(6):828–834
44. Johansson SG et al (2004) Revised nomenclature for allergy for global use: Report of the Nomenclature Review Committee of the World Allergy Organization, October 2003. J Allergy Clin Immunol 113(5):832–836
45. Moneret-Vautrin DA et al (1993) Prospective study of risk factors in natural rubber latex hypersensitivity. J Allergy Clin Immunol 92(5):668–677
46. Bouaziz H, Laxenaire MC (1998) Anaesthesia for the allergic patient. Curr Opin Anaesthesiol 11(3):339–344
47. Guldager H, Sondergaard I (1987) Histamine release from basophil leukocytes in asthma patients after in vitro provocation with various neuromuscular blocking drugs and intravenous anaesthetic agents. Acta Anaesthesiol Scand 31(8):728–729
48. Fisher MM, Bowey CJ (1997) Alleged allergy to local anaesthetics. Anaesth Intensive Care 25(6):611–614
49. Murat I (2000) Latex allergy: where are we? Paediatr Anaesth 10(6):577–579

50. Gentili A et al (2001) Latex allergy in pediatric age: an interdisciplinary perioperative management and case reports. Minerva Anestesiol 67(1–2):29–40
51. Konrad C et al (1997) The prevalence of latex sensitivity among anesthesiology staff. Anesth Analg 84(3):629–633
52. Mazon A et al (1997) Factors that influence the presence of symptoms caused by latex allergy in children with spina bifida. J Allergy Clin Immunol 99(5):600–604
53. Brehler R et al (1997) "Latex-fruit syndrome": frequency of cross-reacting IgE antibodies. Allergy 52(4):404–410
54. De Queiroz M et al (2009) Latex allergy in children: modalities and prevention. Paediatr Anaesth 19(4):313–319
55. Degenhardt P et al (2001) Latex allergy in pediatric surgery is dependent on repeated operations in the first year of life. J Pediatr Surg 36(10):1535–1539
56. Mertes PM et al (2005) Reducing the risk of anaphylaxis during anaesthesia: guidelines for clinical practice. J Investig Allergol Clin Immunol 15(2):91–101
57. Hamburger RN (1996) Diagnosis of latex allergy. Ann Allergy Asthma Immunol 76(3):296
58. Hepner DL, Castells MC (2003) Latex allergy: an update. Anesth Analg 96(4):1219–1229
59. Setlock MA, Cotter TP, Rosner D (1993) Latex allergy: failure of prophylaxis to prevent severe reaction. Anesth Analg 76(3):650–652
60. Holzman RS (1997) Clinical management of latex-allergic children. Anesth Analg 85(3):529–533
61. Taylor JS, Erkek E (2004) Latex allergy: diagnosis and management. Dermatol Ther 17(4):289–301
62. Kroigaard M et al (2007) Scandinavian Clinical Practice Guidelines on the diagnosis, management and follow-up of anaphylaxis during anaesthesia. Acta Anaesthesiol Scand 51(6):655–670
63. Hurrell DG, Bachman JW, Feldt RH (1989) How to evaluate murmurs in children. Postgrad Med 86(2):239–241, 243
64. McEwan AI, Birch M, Bingham R (1995) The preoperative management of the child with a heart murmur. Paediatr Anaesth 5(3):151–156
65. Coleman EN, Doig WB (1970) Diagnostic problems with innocent murmurs in children. Lancet 2(7666):228–232
66. Johnson R, Holzer R (2005) Evaluation of asymptomatic heart murmurs. Curr Paediatr 15(7):532–538
67. Von Ungern-Sternberg BS, Habre W (2007) Pediatric anesthesia – potential risks and their assessment: part I. Paediatr Anaesth 17(3):206–215
68. Diedericks J (2008) Should I do this case? The paediatric murmur. Contin Med Educ 26(3):141–144
69. McConnell ME, Adkins SB 3rd, Hannon DW (1999) Heart murmurs in pediatric patients: when do you refer? Am Fam Physician 60(2):558–565
70. Rosenthal A (1984) How to distinguish between innocent and pathologic heart murmurs in children. Pediatr Clin North Am 31(6):1229–1239
71. Swenson JM et al (1997) Are chest radiographs and electrocardiograms still valuable in evaluating new pediatric patients with heart murmurs or chest pain? Pediatrics 99(1):1–3
72. Danford DA et al (2000) Effects of electrocardiography and chest radiography on the accuracy of preliminary diagnosis of common congenital cardiac defects. Pediatr Cardiol 21(4):334–340
73. Birkebaek NH et al (1999) Chest roentgenogram in the evaluation of heart defects in asymptomatic infants and children with a cardiac murmur: reproducibility and accuracy. Pediatrics 103(2), E15
74. Salute Md, Piano Nazionale Prevenzione Vaccinale (PNPV) 20012-2014. http://www.salute.gov.it/imgs/C_17_pubblicazioni_1721_allegato.pdf [cited 2012 12/04/2012]
75. Lecky JH (1975) Anesthesia and the immune system. Surg Clin North Am 55(4):795–799
76. Hunter JD (1999) Effects of anaesthesia on the human immune system. Hosp Med 60(9):658–663
77. Hogan BV et al (2011) Surgery induced immunosuppression. Surgeon 9(1):38–43

78. Correa-Sales C, Tosta CE, Rizzo LV (1997) The effects of anesthesia with thiopental on T lymphocyte responses to antigen and mitogens in vivo and in vitro. Int J Immunopharmacol 19(2):117–128
79. Hauser GJ et al (1991) Immune dysfunction in children after corrective surgery for congenital heart disease. Crit Care Med 19(7):874–881
80. Puri P, Brazil J, Reen DJ (1984) Immunosuppressive effects of anesthesia and surgery in the newborn: I short-term effects. J Pediatr Surg 19(6):823–828
81. Siebert JN et al (2007) Influence of anesthesia on immune responses and its effect on vaccination in children: review of evidence. Paediatr Anaesth 17(5):410–420
82. Williams SE et al (2011) Overview of the Clinical Consult Case Review of adverse events following immunization: Clinical Immunization Safety Assessment (CISA) network 2004–2009. Vaccine 29(40):6920–6927
83. Short JA, van der Walt JH, Zoanetti DC (2006) Immunization and anesthesia – an international survey. Paediatr Anaesth 16(5):514–522
84. Fortier MA et al (2010) Perioperative anxiety in children. Paediatr Anaesth 20(4):318–322
85. (ATAGI), A.T.A.G.o.I., The Australian Immunisation Handbook (2013) http://www.health.gov.au/internet/immunise/publishing.nsf/Content/Handbook-specialrisk237 [cited 2012 18/04/2012]
86. Khattab AM et al (2010) Sevoflurane-emergence agitation: effect of supplementary low-dose oral ketamine premedication in preschool children undergoing dental surgery. Eur J Anaesthesiol 27(4):353–358
87. Bernardini R et al (1999) Risk factors for latex allergy in patients with spina bifida and latex sensitization. Clin Exp Allergy 29(5):681–686
88. Cremer R et al (1998) Latex allergy in spina bifida patients--prevention by primary prophylaxis. Allergy 53(7):709–711
89. Ricci G et al (1999) Latex allergy in subjects who had undergone multiple surgical procedures for bladder exstrophy: relationship with clinical intervention and atopic diseases. BJU Int 84(9):1058–1062
90. Gentili A et al (2003) Latex allergy in children with oesophageal atresia. Paediatr Anaesth 13(8):668–675
91. Cremer R et al (2007) Natural rubber latex sensitisation and allergy in patients with spina bifida, urogenital disorders and oesophageal atresia compared with a normal paediatric population. Eur J Pediatr Surg 17(3):194–198
92. Nieto A et al (1996) Allergy to latex in spina bifida: a multivariate study of associated factors in 100 consecutive patients. J Allergy Clin Immunol 98(3):501–507
93. Porri F et al (1997) Association between latex sensitization and repeated latex exposure in children. Anesthesiology 86(3):599–602
94. Lieberman P (2002) Anaphylactic reactions during surgical and medical procedures. J Allergy Clin Immunol 110(2 Suppl):S64–S69
95. Makinen-Kiljunen S (1994) Banana allergy in patients with immediate-type hypersensitivity to natural rubber latex: characterization of cross-reacting antibodies and allergens. J Allergy Clin Immunol 93(6):990–996

Part II

Perioperative Care During Surgery

Perioperative Care in Day Hospital Surgery

5

Simonetta Tesoro and Laura Marchesini

5.1 Introduction

The pediatric patient is best suited for intervention in outpatient surgery since he/she rarely suffers from severe systemic disease and the procedures most commonly performed are minor surgery. During the last ten years, many procedures, previously performed as inpatient, were shifted to outpatient bringing many benefits for both patients and national health systems. The minimum separation of the child from the family, the decreased risk of in-hospital infections, and the necessary active participation of parents caring for their children are the main benefits of the day-surgery (DS) patient. Reduction in costs for institutions and the greater availability of beds and staff for more severe cases represent the advantages for health systems.

A surgical procedure and anesthesia should be understood as processes at risk requiring high-quality performances providing maximum safety and reduced hospitalization. Advances in the field of anesthesia and surgery and the increasing need to reduce health-care costs have encouraged DS also in patients previously excluded. The evolution of techniques, such as minimally invasive surgery and the introduction of new drugs together with high levels of professional competence and organizational skills, allows to create a care pathway that leads to high-quality performance associated with the highest levels of safety.

The effectiveness and efficiency of the care pathway depend on two factors: clinical practice and the organizational model. Best clinical practice is the ability to administer the most appropriate care derived from the best scientific evidence available throughout

S. Tesoro, MD (✉)
Sezione di Anestesia, Analgesia e Rianimazione, Dipartimento di Medicina Clinica e Sperimentale, Università di Perugia, Perugia, Italy

Department of Anesthesia, Analgesia and Intensive Care, University of Perugia, Perugia, Italy
e-mail: simonettatesoro@gmail.com

L. Marchesini, MD
Department of Anesthesia, Analgesia and Intensive Care, University of Perugia, Perugia, Italy

© Springer International Publishing Switzerland 2016   55
M. Astuto, P.M. Ingelmo (eds.), *Perioperative Medicine in Pediatric Anesthesia*,
Anesthesia, Intensive Care and Pain in Neonates and Children,
DOI 10.1007/978-3-319-21960-8_5

the care pathway. In other words, the clinical appropriateness is the ability to choose the "right procedure," the "right patient," and the "right time." Choosing the "right environment" is part of organizational appropriateness that may be national, regional, or institutional, in which the "right professionals" bring their skills with the proper evaluation and synthesis of evidence and allow application in the specific organizational model [1]. This will lead to high quality, high performance, and a high turnover rate.

This chapter reviews the fundamental concepts concerning the most appropriate care for safe and effective outpatient anesthesia.

5.2   Epidemiology

The number of pediatric outpatient procedures has increased by almost 50 % during the period 1996–2006 [2]. In 2012, 64 % of pediatric surgical activity was performed on an outpatient basis in France [3].

The data show a large day-surgery activity worldwide; however, there are few scientific societies that have specific Guidelines or Recommendations for the management of pediatric DS from a clinical and organizational point of view. The Association des Anesthésistes Réanimateurs Pédiatriques d'Expression Française (ADARPEF) published the French Guidelines in 2010 [4].

A systematic review of the literature showed that the rate of perioperative complications related to anesthesia for the various types of pediatric DS was overall very low [5]. Specifically, there appeared to be no deaths related to DS anesthesia. As for the occurrence of adverse cardiorespiratory intra- and postoperative (within 24 hours) events, a 19–24 % incidence was recorded for various procedures. Adverse events included laryngospasm, bronchospasm, desaturation <90 %, bradycardia, arrhythmia, hypotension, or hypertension requiring therapeutic intervention. As for bleeding, another major adverse event, the incidence within the first 24 hours was low even for adenotonsillectomies (0.6 % tonsillectomy, <1 % adenoidectomy). Bleeding in adenotonsillectomies was recorded at one week with an incidence of 5/826 patients, of these 4 to 5 were recorded as major bleeding [6]. The incidence of other perioperative complications may vary according to the type of surgery. For example, in strabismus surgery, there is an incidence of 34–79 % of postoperative nausea and vomiting (PONV), where the incidence of 16–36 % in the pool of procedures [7].

Another complication is the perioperative/postoperative agitation that may occur in 11–25 % of cases [8].

Complications in pediatric DS are very low with a tendency toward zero for very serious complications. However, if not managed properly, may cause the loss of benefit of the care process.

In this chapter, the paragraph *Special Considerations* will focus on patients undergoing adenotonsillectomy with a higher incidence of postoperative complications.

5.3   Organizational Aspects

The organizational aspect plays an important role in the success of the care pathway and the different models adopted by the numerous national health systems. An organizational model is the set of rules used to carry out the activities, protocols, or procedures. To date, there is no scientific evidence proving the superiority of an organizational model over another. Any facility that provides services in DS should use an organizational model created according to local legislation and the available resources. In any case, the care pathway must be accredited by the standards of accreditation of health facilities in order to minimize clinical risks.

There are three organizational models:

1. Free-standing DS unit with acceptance, wards, operating rooms, and independent administrative offices, geographically linked or not to a referral hospital
2. DS unit located inside a hospital organizational structure in a continuous cycle either public or private
3. Beds dedicated to DS incorporated in the inpatient unit

In the last two organizational models, use of the operating room can be scheduled together with other units or there may be operating rooms exclusively for DS.

As previously stated, there is no great organizational model; however, the division of inpatients and outpatients leads to better care due to the different needs of the patients undergoing DS, including rapid turnover. When children must be cared for in an adult unit, they should be nursed in customized and specifically designed pediatric day-care units; a separate area must be organized for them and their parents/caregivers.

Another important organizational aspect is the perioperative environment in which the patient and the family are welcomed. It should be comfortable, practical, and designed for children, with a multidisciplinary staff able to handle the children and families from both a clinical and psychological point of view [9].

The word "outpatient" does not mean minor procedure but rather a complex process that requires detailed organization and optimal clinical management of the whole perioperative period. The anesthesiologist, responsible for the pivotal moments, must have adequate experience and training in the care of infants and children.

The key role in all major care processes, particularly in DS, is the multidisciplinary team of professionals who collaborate according to protocols and standardized procedures, the reference physicians being the surgeon and the anesthesiologist.

5.4   Selection Criteria

Appropriate patient selection is the cornerstone of DS. Factors contributing to the selection are related to the patient, the procedure, and the social context.

5.4.1 Patient

5.4.1.1 ASA Physical Status
Children with no known systemic diseases and classified as American Society of Anesthesiologists Physical Status I and II are eligible for DS.

However, children classified as ASA III, with good control of the disease, can be eligible for DS, at the discretion of the unit that is in charge. It is advisable to present them as the first case in order to have more time for monitoring prior to discharge.

There is little scientific evidence on this topic, so recommendations are considered from a methodological point of view, grade IV recommendations, or experts' opinion.

Specifically, patients with seizure disorders under control can be regarded as outpatients. In the case of anticonvulsant therapy, the therapeutic range should be controlled as well as the functionality of organs that could be implicated in the metabolism of chronic therapy drugs or anesthesia, including liver and kidney function in case of valproic acid administration.

Blood glucose in patients with diabetes mellitus should be closely monitored during hospitalization, and regular food and fluid intake should be reestablished prior to discharge.

In some circumstances, such as the presence of stable chronic diseases, early discharge is recommended to avoid complications related to hospitalization. This is the case in patients with immunosuppressive diseases in which hospitalization could trigger hospital-acquired infection or patients psychologically disturbed, mentally retarded, in which the distance from home could generate major trauma.

Obesity, OSA (obstructive sleep apnea syndrome), and sleep disorders, with or without associated adenotonsillar hypertrophy, are more and more frequently found in the pediatric population, and very often these children undergo adenotonsillectomy. For special assessment and management of these patients, see the paragraph *Special Considerations.*

5.4.1.2 Age

Age itself is not an absolute contraindication to DS. However, because of the increased risk of respiratory complications in infants, children born at term (over 38 weeks) less than one month old are excluded [10]. It remains at the discretion of the structure whether to admit patients in DS under 1 month of age who will undergo surface interventions such as frenulectomia lingual or finger supernumerary, usually without complications. The former preterm children should not be included in the DS program unless they are in excellent condition and have passed the 60 weeks postconceptual age (PCA) [11] for increased risk of postoperative apnea and bradycardia [12]. More recent studies [13, 14] have shown that apnea occurs in 25 % of infants but that this is inversely related to PCA: in patients with PCA > 60 weeks, the incidence is <5 %, and 44–46 weeks PCA are sufficient to prevent postoperative apnea and bradycardia. The incidence of apnea and bradycardia is low after 52 weeks PCA. Literature data show that after 60 weeks, PCA former preterm children may be admitted to DS provided that they will not be subject to situations that could increase the risk of apnea (i.e., anemia) and that there will be postoperative monitoring depending on postconceptual age. Specifically, with PCA <46 weeks, continuous monitoring is required for at least 12 hours, excluding the possibility to be admitted to DS. Between 46 and 60 weeks PCA, six hours of monitoring could be enough.[13]

Because of the instability of these children and the need for possible intensive postoperative monitoring, these patients should be treated in high specialty level III hospitals.

5.4.1.3 Malignant Hyperthermia

Treatment in DS may not be completely ruled out for patients with suspected or known susceptibility to malignant hyperthermia, if trigger-free anesthesia is performed and postoperative monitoring of at least 6–8 hours is guaranteed [15]. However, it may be safer to monitor for at least 12 hours in view of late-onset reaction due to the use of new-generation halogenated anesthetics (sevoflurane and desflurane) and the possibility that stress alone could trigger this adverse reaction.

5.4.1.4 Sudden Infant Death Syndrome

It is contraindicated to admit siblings of children who have died from SIDS as outpatients unless they have passed 60 weeks PCA, although there is no evidence of a correlation between anesthesia and SIDS [16].

5.4.1.5 Sickle Cell Disease

Patients with thalassemia may be admitted in DS.

5.4.1.6 Incidental Heart Murmurs

Patients with severe heart disease are excluded from DS. There is a large pediatric population in which occasionally a heart murmur is found. An innocent murmur typically soft, early systolic with no abnormal symptoms or signs is eligible for DS. The murmur varies in intensity with position. Regardless of DS, a murmur in a child <1 year of age, loud or continuous murmurs, all diastolic, pansystolic, late systolic, and other signs as failure to thrive, recurrent chest infections, syncope, cyanosis or hypertension require more in-depth investigation.

5.4.1.7 Upper Respiratory Infection (URI)

Upper respiratory tract infection (URI) is common in the pediatric patient and poses a dilemma whether to proceed with surgery, particularly in the DS regime. URI is associated with an increased incidence of respiratory complications in anesthesia: cough, desaturation, bronchospasm, and laryngospasm. Although these can be readily managed and without sequelae [17–19], preoperative evaluation on the day of surgery must focus on the general health of the patient and assess whether the patient is feverish, tired, overwhelmed, with disordered breathing and tachycardia. The preoperative saturation control could be discriminatory to evaluate whether the infection is confined to the upper respiratory tract or if it involves the lower respiratory tract. Other risk factors for respiratory complications in patients with URI are use of the endotracheal tube, prematurity, asthma, exposure to secondhand smoke, copious secretions, nasal congestion, and airway surgery [20].

Surgery should be postponed for two weeks when a child is symptomatic with or without association of additional risk factors [21].

When symptoms are mild or moderate:

- Age < one year: postpone
- Age > 1 year: consider other risk factors and evaluate the risk/benefit of the procedure [22]

5.4.1.8 Asthma

Asthma is the most common chronic disease in children but may not be considered a contraindication to DS. If the disease is adequately controlled with therapy and there are no other risk factors such as respiratory tract infections, the patient can be treated by slightly increasing the basic therapy. The administration of beta-agonists is recommended in the immediate preoperative period. At discharge, there should be no breath sounds and eupnea. In case of poor control of the disease or in the presence of severe asthma (requiring daily therapy), DS is not recommended for the patient.

5.4.2 Procedure

Each structure can define the list of procedures to be performed in DS, according to local legislation. In general, all surface interventions and all diagnostic tests requiring analgosedation or anesthesia are recommended for DS. In the past, criteria regarding the general characteristics of the procedures were defined [23]:

- No intracranial, intrathoracic, or major intraabdominal surgery
- Minimal risk of bleeding
- Ability to adequately control pain at home
- Simple nursing care that can be provided by parents
- No major limitation on the child's activity

The duration of the procedure (two hours considering the cutoff) is not a contraindication to discharge, provided that 4 hours of postoperative observation are guaranteed. Discharge is not excluded even for orthopedic operations requiring cast; however, it is recommended to avoid motor block. With the increase in minimally invasive techniques in pediatrics, an increasing number of children undergo laparoscopic surgery. In literature, there are many papers proving the feasibility of laparoscopic procedures in DS; however, the lack of large randomized controlled clinical trials does not allow to draw strong recommendations on the feasibility of interventions classified as DS. The most frequent appears to be the correction of inguinal hernia in the newborn or infant, often ex-premature. The indication is to diagnose and treat metachronous contralateral hernia in a single session without surgical exploration. These patients require endotracheal intubation.

The final decision remains at the discretion of the multidisciplinary team, based on the patient's general conditions, the anesthetic technique adopted, the surgical time, and the satisfaction of discharge criteria after 4–6 hours of observation. Performing laparoscopy as the first case of the session is recommended.

5.4.3   Social Factor

Parents have an active role in care management. They should be responsible and be able to communicate and get to the hospital by themselves. The possibility of reaching a hospital within 1 hour (50 km) is recommended. Weather and other obstacles that could cause delay in reaching the hospital should also be taken into account.

5.5   Patient Preparation and Premedication

The surgeon is the first professional who meets the patient, posing indication for surgery and defining the eligibility for DS, based on the type of procedure.

The preoperative evaluation, carried out under the direct responsibility of the anesthesiologist, consists of clinical evaluation of the patient before anesthesia is performed. The evaluation of an outpatient is the same as that of an inpatient (to this regard, see Chap. 2).

The benefits, with regard to DS, resulting from a preoperative anesthetic assessment include the safety of perioperative care with improved outcome and reduction of complications. Indeed, it is through an adequate preoperative evaluation that the patient can be clinically and socioculturally framed, and, if necessary, preoperative investigations can be prescribed.

In DS, a preoperative evaluation allows the anesthesiologist to declare eligible this path to care. It also provides information on the anesthetic technique of postoperative pain management and home care, the timetable for the day, and how to behave with regard to fasting and therapies. It allows to have informed written consent.

As for the organization and manner of the preoperative visit, it is up to each individual to find the best feasible organizational model: preprepared questionnaires for the anamnesis filled out by the parents or primary care physician, or for ASA I and II patients, evaluation could be performed the morning of surgery (one-stop anesthesia). There is no scientific evidence on the "timing" of the evaluation, although it is recommended in proximity of the operation, especially in patients younger than 2 years of age, when the physiological evolution is fast. A very important developmental phase, both from the medical history and clinical point of view, is the difference between non-walking and walking.

The use of a well-written and understandable (cultural mediators) brochure on the conduct of the entire process is recommended to avoid misunderstandings or cancelations that could alter an organization built on detail. Cancelation or non-presentation of the patient has a high cost for the institution [24], so many actually call the day before to check on the health of the child (patient medically fit) and remind the parents about arrival time, place of admission, and preoperative fasting.

Proper detailed and written information for parents has the power to reduce parental anxiety. It has been shown that children with anxious parents are more likely to display signs of perioperative anxiety themselves [25]. It is important that the child is aware of what he/she will experience and provide a correct explanation of all stages of the day, in particular, the oral premedication, induction, and awakening and the possibility of minimum postoperative pain. Tools such as videotapes, brochures with animated characters, or even a guided tour of the unit could be helpful.

5.5.1 Fasting

The most common complications in DS are PONV and agitation on awakening. Keeping a child fasting from midnight means inducing and then awakening an irritated child because of thirst and hunger and in addition with a gastric residual volume greater than 0.4 ml/kg with a pH less than 2.5. This increases the risk of aspiration, PONV, and agitation on awakening. Clear liquids should be administered 2–3 hours before induction so that the gastric residual volume will reduce and the pH will increase [26, 27].

Please refer to the Guidelines [28] and Chap. 3.

5.5.2 Premedication

The three main goals of premedication are the reduction of preoperative anxiety, easy separation from parents, and easy induction either intravenously or by mask. There are several techniques of premedication, pharmacological and not, but none can take the place of the other. In addition, "one cannot fit like a glove for all." It depends on previous experience, age and character of the child, ability of the parents to control their anxiety, and the experience of the team.

For example, in children undergoing repeated procedures requiring anesthesia, very often the presence of a parent at the moment of induction is of great help and usually the child asks not to be sedated but to have a parent with him/her. That in this case can become a valuable ally for the team and can help smooth the experience for the child, for the staff, and for themselves. In other cases, the parental presence at induction could create more problems to the parents who see their child having "strange reactions". If the induction is to be done in the presence of the parents, it must be planned with adequate counseling.

The presence of a parent at induction will be of help in reducing the child's anxiety. Children under 6 months generally do not require premedication, but some practical precautions could help maintain the child's comfort such as maintaining the child dressed and wrapped in his/her blanket, or using a pacifier.

If you opt for intravenous induction, the use of anesthetic ointments (EMLA) for venipuncture is recommended; however, using EMLA to eliminate pain during venipuncture does not eliminate the fear of needles.

In our experience, patients should be adequately premedicated because this will facilitate the work of the staff, who will have a calm and collaborative patient able to separate from his/her parents and enter the operating room.

5.5.3   Pharmacological Premedication

The ideal premedication is one that does not interfere with the recovery and the discharge.

Oral administration is the most widely used, but for more reluctant children, intramuscular administration can be used.

Midazolam is the benzodiazepine of choice for premedication, exploiting its main anxiolytic and, most of all, anterograde amnesia effects. It can be administered through different routes and dosage depending on the route chosen. The most widely used is the oral route at a dose of 0.5 mg/kg (max 15 mg). Because of its bitter taste, it should be given with sugar or fruit juice without pulp. The oral onset is 10–30 min. In children less collaborative, the intranasal route can be used at the same dose as the oral route.

Ketamine is usually used in cases of poor collaboration during oral therapy assumption and is administered parenterally. It can be taken orally at a dose of 6 mg/kg or intramuscularly 2–4 mg/kg to achieve a sedative effect in 10–15 minutes.

5.6   Anesthesia

The purpose of DS is rapid recovery in order to quickly reach the criteria of discharge and minimize side effects of anesthesia.

In light of this need, the anesthetic conduct should aim to discharge patients as quickly as possible. The main complications that may interfere with discharge include PONV, behavioral disorders, and respiratory and cardiovascular complications. The choice anesthetic technique depends on several factors, including the type of surgery and the patient's conditions. When treating a pediatric population, local or regional anesthesia is rarely performed in the absence of sedation. Therefore, it is important to find the anesthetic technique with the lowest impact on recovery times and with minimal side effects so as not to delay discharge. A recent systematic review [29] did not provide strong evidence on reduction of side effects, such as PONV and behavioral disturbances, using induction and maintenance of intravenous anesthesia with propofol compared to inhaled anesthesia.

5.6.1   Drugs

When choosing an inhaled induction, which is of great help with noncollaborative children or with difficult intravenous access, the drug most widely used today is sevoflurane that ensures fast and smooth induction with minimum side effects. Another halogenated agent that can be used is halothane, but this is disappearing from operating theaters because it is linked to hepatitis and sensitizes the myocardium to catecholamines.

As for intravenous medications, propofol or thiopental is to be preferred because recovery from other agents, such as benzodiazepines and ketamine, is too long.

The use of muscle relaxants is not precluded in DS, as long as they are antagonized based on the monitoring of the neuromuscular junction. Currently, sugammadex, that can antagonize neuromuscular block when using nondepolarizing aminosteroid muscle relaxants. Its use is registered in the pediatric field [30] and can be a viable alternative to neostigmine, to eliminate the possibility of side effects such as PONV and increased secretions.

There is limited space today for the pediatric use of succinylcholine, which can be used in emergency situations, but is not recommended routinely in pediatrics because of its numerous side effects (triggers malignant hyperthermia, life-threatening hyperkalemic cardiac arrest, masseter muscle rigidity).

Opioids are not ideal for pediatric day cases as they may produce ventilatory depression, excessive sedation and PONV. Intraoperative opioids with shorter duration of action, such as fentanyl and remifentanil, are recommended. The most important side effects are rigidity of the chest, for which slow administration is recommended, and overdose, for which an adequate titration is recommended.

5.6.2 Locoregional Anesthesia

The use of local anesthetics in pediatric anesthesia is recommended at the minimum effective dose. The success of regional anesthesia means administering the right dose of the right drug in the right place, particularly in DS where the primary benefit of locoregional anesthesia is postoperative pain relief without unwanted motor block [31]. Its applicability depends on the type of surgery, the experience of the team, and the means/tools available.

In children, administration of locoregional anesthesia without sedation is very rare. A major benefit of combined general and regional anesthetic technique is that general anesthesia or sedation can be maintained at a lower level and perioperative opioid requirements can be reduced. In addition, use of local anesthetics at an analgesic and non-anesthetic dose is recommended.

Ultrasound-guided blocks allow a minimum dose of local anesthetic while reducing the risk of systemic toxicity and accidental intravascular administration of the drug.

Some current regional anesthetic techniques that may be successfully used in this context are:

5.6.3 Spinal Block

The duration of spinal anesthesia is much shorter in small children than in adults and may not be sufficient for bilateral procedures. It is not recommended in DS because of poor postoperative analgesic coverage compared to alternative techniques.

5.6.4 Caudal Block

This block represents the most commonly used regional technique in children and can be used successfully for all subumbilical procedures. To achieve adequate postoperative pain relief without unwanted postoperative motor block, the correct concentration of long-lasting local anesthetics needs to be used. Ivani et al. [32] have shown that administration of 1 ml/kg of levobupivacaine 0.25 % and ropivacaine 0.2 % produces adequate postoperative analgesia. The limitation of the technique is the duration of effective analgesia when used in surgery involving the lower thoracic dermatomes (inguinal hernia and hydrocele repair) because of its known regression to craniocaudal fashion. The risk for urinary retention is approximately 2 % and is similar to that after general anesthesia without caudal block [33].

5.6.5 Ilioinguinal/Iliohypogastric Nerve Block

The use of this block has been popular in association with inguinal hernia and hydrocele repair. Weintraud et al. demonstrated that with traditional landmark-based technique, the local anesthetic is deposited at a suboptimal anatomical location [34]. Thus, this block should be performed under ultrasound guidance to achieve an acceptable success rate as well as to avoid unintentional puncture of the nearby peritoneum and bowel. Using ultrasound guidance, the volume of local anesthetic needed for a successful block is slightly less than 0.1 ml/kg. Its limit is adequate analgesia for orchidopexy. Even if perfect ultrasound-guided ilioinguinal/iliohypogastric nerve block has been performed, it will not influence the testicular pain that is responsible for the deep, nauseating pain that represents the major problem after orchidopexy. For testicular pain, it is necessary to anesthetize the lower thoracic segments.

5.6.6 Paravertebral Block

It represents a useful alternative to ilioinguinal/iliohypogastric nerve block for inguinal hernia and is more effective for orchidopexy when performed at a low thoracic level. At this level, the low risk of unintentional pleural puncture is almost completely abolished. It is most frequently used as a unilateral technique.

5.6.7 Lower and Upper Extremity Nerve Blocks

The aim is to avoid the motor block. A longer duration is often desirable, so the use of continuous peripheral catheter technique is becoming increasingly popular, and recent publications describe the use in outpatients. However, these techniques are best applied in slightly older children [35] and in the absence of motor block.

5.6.8 Penile Block

Indicated for circumcision, this block can be used also for postoperative analgesia following minor hypospadias repair.

5.6.9 Opioids as Adjuvants in Locoregional Anesthesia

Use of morphine to increase the duration of locoregional anesthesia in outpatients is discouraged.

The most effective drug to prolong the analgesic effect of the caudal block is ketamine (S-ketamine 1 mg/kg), but the use of clonidine (1 mcg/kg) has not been excluded.

For peripheral blocks, only clonidine has been found to be effective in prolonging the block.

5.6.10 Fluid Therapy

For short-term procedures (<1 h), it may not be necessary to administer intraoperative fluids as long as the child drinks clear liquids up to two hours before induction. In DS, it is desirable to restore spontaneous oral hydration as soon as possible, but some authors have shown that children forced to drink tend to vomit more frequently than those that resume oral hydration spontaneously [36]. Intraoperative hydration could have a rationale for interventions at high risk of PONV, such as strabismus and adenotonsillectomy in which pain could limit swallowing or in infants and babies when even the minimum interval of fasting necessary for administration of anesthesia appears to be long (3 hours). In any case, administration of polyelectrolyte solutions is recommended, leaving glucose solutions for very young children more prone to hypoglycemia.

5.6.11 Airway

The choice of airway management should be assessed on a case-by-case basis depending on the procedure, the patient's age, and the experience of the anesthesiologist. Sedation is required for many outpatient interventions, so it may be sufficient to maintain spontaneous or assisted breathing by face mask. The laryngeal mask airway (LMA) helps maintain airway patency unless endotracheal intubation is obtained. In the past, intubation was not recommended in DS patients because of the risk of post-extubation croup. Today, with the use of muscle relaxants and a safe antagonist and next-generation devices, the risk is very low. It usually occurs within 1 hour from extubation; therefore, a closer postoperative monitoring is recommended.

5.6.12 Temperature

Even for short interventions, monitoring and precautions should be taken to keep the body temperature stable in pediatric patients by heating the operating room, using mattresses or blankets, and administrating heated fluids.

5.7 Analgesia

Pain control is a cornerstone in pediatric surgery whether dealing with inpatients or outpatients. The challenge is to provide a pain-free emergence and recovery by starting analgesics in the intraoperative period, especially when using a rapid recovery anesthesia as in DS.

Patients should be discharge after adequate analgesia has been achieved. Furthermore, medications to control pain at home should be prescribed. All techniques and medications available can be used, as long as these do not increase the side effects and allow postoperative analgesia. The multimodal approach is probably the gold standard of therapy because it exploits the power of the drugs. Each drug with a different mechanism of action can be used at a lower dose.

The most commonly used analgesic drug is paracetamol (acetaminophen). The recommended dose is 10–15 mg/kg every 6 hours, reaching a maximum daily dose of no more than 100 mg/kg [37]. It can be considered the base drug that can be associated with other therapies for the multimodal approach. Oral administration is the most effective route because of its predictable systemic absorption. When possible, oral use should be encouraged. Another recommendation is the dosing interval, which must be respected even at night, especially in DS patients requiring stable pain coverage.

The NSAIDs are not contraindicated in pediatrics. Acetylsalicylic acid is no longer used because of its association with the Reye syndrome. The main side effect of NSAIDs is platelet antiaggregation. Oral use is encouraged. The most frequently used are ibuprofen 5–10 mg/kg and ketorolac 0.3–0.5 mg/kg which can be used parenterally. Ketoprofene can be used parenterally in 1–2 mg/kg dose [38].

5.7.1 Locoregional Anesthesia

Locoregional anesthesia appears to meet the requirements of good management of postoperative analgesia in DS. Correctly used regional anesthetic techniques are feasible and often associated with superior postoperative analgesia when compared to other options [39].

It is the analgesic of choice since it blocks pain transmission, and produce adequate analgesia up to 6–8 hours. A major benefit of a combined general and regional anesthetic technique is the reduction in perioperative opioid requirements and, consequently, reduced postoperative emesis. Kokinsky [40] shows that the administration of fentanyl 1 mcg/kg to children undergoing outpatient surgery under general anesthesia combined with a caudal block did not improve analgesia but caused a very significant increase in PONV compared to saline placebo (36 vs. 0 %).

Using continuous peripheral catheter appears very promising in order to extend analgesia after the return home.

5.8   Postoperative Nausea and Vomiting

Postoperative nausea and vomiting (PONV) are the most common complications in anesthesia. The medical complications of PONV include pulmonary aspiration, dehydration, electrolyte imbalance, fatigue, and wound disruption. Postoperative vomiting (POV) is an expensive complication in DS because it delays discharge, it causes discomfort in the patient and causes anxiety in both the children and parents, and increases medical care.

Eberhart [41] identified 4 independent predictors of POV: duration of surgery >30 minutes; age > 3 years; history of POV in the patient, parent, or sibling; strabismus surgery; and ear-nose-throat surgery. Based on the presence of 0,1, 2, 3, 4 factors, the risk of POV was 9 %, 10 %, 30 %, 55 %, and 70 %, respectively. The incidence of POV when prophylaxis was not used was 3.4 %, 11.6 %, 28.2 %, and 42.3 %, respectively, in the presence of 0, 1, 2, or 3 factors.

The management approach is multifactorial and involves proper preoperative preparation, risk stratification, and rational selection of antiemetic prophylaxis.

The main factor in preoperative preparation for reducing PONV is to avoid preoperative dehydration and encourage the patient to take clear liquids up to two hours before induction. PONV can be reduced by avoiding nitrous oxide and volatile anesthetics and by reducing postoperative opioids. However, a recent Cochrane study[29] showed that there is no PONV reduction when comparing intravenous anesthesia to inhalation anesthesia in outpatients.

The rational selection of antiemetic prophylaxis is derived from a proper risk stratification in the pediatric population.

The most recent guidelines [42] identify, according to risk stratification, the most effective single antiemetic therapy and combination therapy regimens for PONV prophylaxis for most pediatric patients at high risk for POV.

Children who are at moderate or high risk of POV should receive a combination therapy with at least 2 prophylactic drugs from different classes.[42]

- Ondansetron 0.05 mg/kh + dexamethasone 0.015 mg/kg
- Ondansetron 0.1 mg/kg + droperidol 0.015 mg/kg
- Tropisetron 0.1 mg/kg + dexamethasone 0.5 mg/kg

New data on pharmacokinetics of ondansetron in children <2 years of age are now available. Dolasetron is not recommended for cardiac arrhythmia risk. Caution should be used when administering 5-HT3 antagonist in children with prolonged QT syndrome.

The incidence of post-discharge nausea and vomiting (PDNV) in children is 20 % after tonsillectomy.

In a recent review by Hohne [43], for outpatients who had short anesthesia with surgery lasting less than 30 min, with rare use of perioperative opioids, a single prophylaxis is recommended; for strabismus or ear-nose-throat surgery or high-risk patients, a double prophylaxis is to be preferred.

5.9   Discharge

Reduction of hospitalization times (pre- and postoperative) is the most effective tool to reduce the cost of the care process. However, time of observation reductions should not affect the safety of patients, therefore the phase of postoperative observation should be ensured by the standards of accreditation which include taking care of the patient from admission to discharge (chapter access to care and continuity of care -ACC 1- Joint Commission [44]). Currently, especially in the fast track of surgery at short cycle, the focus has increasingly shifted to the process of taking charge of the patient even at home.

Discharge is the culmination of DS care and, as all other phases, consists of two components: clinical management and organizational management.

Modalities for discharge vary depending on the type of organizational model adopted. There are facilities where patients are transferred from the recovery room to a hospital ward (short-stay area) where they are discharged. Others are discharged directly from the recovery room.

In any case, clinical criteria for discharge must be respected. Scoring systems make the discharge process easier and more efficient. The Aldrete scoring system and postanesthetic discharge scoring system (PADSS) [45] have received widespread consensus in assessing postanesthetic recovery (Table 5.1).

The first is essentially based on the assessment of vital signs (respiratory and cardiovascular) and is used for recovery from anesthesia for the assessment of restoration of consciousness, protective reflexes, and motility. It is indicated for recovery phase I, that is, for the discharge of the patient from the recovery room to the ward for observation. The second system evaluates the vital parameters in a single item and associates the evaluation of other functions that can ensure the restoration of activities which will allow the return home, such as the ability to stand stably, the presence of nausea and vomiting, adequate pain control, and bleeding of the surgical wound. The PADSS is used for discharge home phase II recovery. Patients achieving a total score of 9 or 10 are considered fit for transfer or discharge to the next phase of recovery.

Recently, the Société Française d'Anesthésie et de Réanimation (SFAR) published a prospective observational study in which PADSS is applied in the pediatric

Table 5.1 Aldrete scoring system

Respiration	
Able to take deep breath and cough = 2	
Dyspnea/shallow breathing = 1	
Apnea = 0	
O2 saturation	
Maintains >92 % on room air = 2	
Needs O2 inhalation to maintain O2 saturation > 90 % = 1	
O2 saturation >90 % even with supplemental oxygen = 0	
Consciousness	
Fully awake = 2	
Arousable on calling = 1	
Not responding = 0	
Circulation	
BP ± 20 mmHg pre-op = 2	
BP ± 20–50 mmHg pre-op = 1	
BP ± 50 mmHg pre-op = 0	
Activity	
Able to move 4 extremities = 2	
Able to move 2 extremities = 1	
Able to move 0 extremities = 0	

population, defining Ped-PADSS pediatric discharge score in ambulatory surgery [46] (Table 5.2).

An analysis of the literature does not provide data on the minimum time of postoperative observation. Previously, a postoperative observation period of at least 4 hours was required; today, as reported by SFAR, 95 % of patients have the Ped-PADSS ≥9 after two hours of observation. A more recent study [47] including 1060 children and using Ped-PADSS, 97.2 % of children could be discharged one hour after returning from the operating room, and 99.8 % of children were dischargeable two hours after. Therefore, it is advisable, but not required, that patients remain in the hospital for at least four hours postoperatively, but the time may vary depending on the organizational model, as long as the scoring system is used and patients are fully satisfied at discharge.

Discharge must be decided by the surgeon or the anesthesiologist but, according to the Joint Commission Accreditation, can be carried out by educated and empowered personnel according to the procedure in use in the institution.

The child should be entrusted to a responsible adult who can take the patient back to the hospital for any need. Means of transportation and/or the possibility of a telephone to call for help should be available.

Postoperative management indications must be written, may be differentiated by type of procedure, should be handed to the parents or the adult responsible, and explained in a comprehensible manner with the aid of a mediator, if needed.

Table 5.2 Postanesthetic discharge scoring system (PADSS)	Vital signs
	BP and pulse within 20 % pre-op = 2
	BP and pulse within 20–40 % pre-op = 1
	BP and pulse within >40 % pre-op = 0
	Activity
	Steady gait, no dizziness, or meets pre-op level = 2
	Requires assistance = 1
	Unable to ambulate = 0
	Nausea and vomiting
	Minimal/treated with p.o. medication = 2
	Moderate/treated with parenteral medication = 1
	Severe/continues despite treatment = 0
	Pain
	Controlled with oral analgesics and acceptable to patient:
	Yes = 2
	No = 1
	Surgical bleeding
	Minimal/no dressing changes = 2
	Moderate/up to two dressing changes required = 1
	Severe/more than three dressing changes required = 0

Prescriptions for pain therapy, including the rescue dose, must be clear and precise. Could the family report difficulty in finding the first home administration, the structure should provide it.

A telephone follow-up could be made the day after surgery to determine the frequency of complications, including minor ones not requiring hospitalization, and to report on the child's condition and resumption of daily activity (information on meals, sleep disorders, recovery motor activity). Monitoring pain control at home is also part of patient care according to the standards of the Joint Commission of Accreditation.

5.10   Special Consideration for Tonsillectomy

Tonsillectomy is the most performed pediatric surgery in the world. As previously stated, it is one of the interventions with increased incidence of minor postoperative complications, as well as major complications. Common complications are:

- Respiratory
- PONV
- Hemorrhage

Because of the higher incidence of complications, the indication for surgery in DS varies according to criteria related to the patient, but also to the organization and to the legislation of the institutions. The criteria attached to the patient for which the tonsillectomy with or without adenoidectomy can be performed in DS are:

- Age > 3.
- ASA I and II.
- Lack of comorbidities that may increase the risk of respiratory complications (OSAS, severe obesity, craniofacial deformities, neuromuscular disorders with pharyngeal hypotonia, signs of heart failure or pulmonary hypertension, metabolic diseases, recent upper or lower respiratory tract infections). The presence of just one of these conditions is enough to exclude the patient from DS.
- Normal coagulation tests.

Any facility deciding to perform ATC surgery must adhere to a specific protocol and must have the ability to shift the patient to inpatient and provide intensive care for 24 hours. For children under three years of age or with comorbidities (see above), surgery is recommended in hospitals with ICU. If surgery is performed in DS, some special precautions must be considered:

- Consensus among the surgeon, anesthesiologist, and parents on postoperative course.
- At least 6 hours of postoperative surveillance is recommended to check absence of pharyngeal bleeding, assess and treat postoperative pain, prevent and treat any PONV, and ensure resumption of feeding. Any adverse event observed during surveillance may lead to conventional admission.
- Prophylaxis for PONV: these patients are at high risk of PONV, so a combination therapy with at least two prophylactic drugs from different classes is recommended.
- Plan adequate postoperative analgesia for at least a few days after surgery: the importance of systematic scheduled administration of paracetamol and a rescue dose for at least a few days. NSAID prescription following tonsillectomy is not widespread recomended due to a suspected elevation of hemorrhage risk, even if Cardwell in a systematic review [48] concluded that NSAID do not increase bleeding after tonsillectomy/adenoidectomy procedures.
- Specific and detailed instructions about food (cold, smooth, and nonspiced) and drinks (cold and nonacid).

References

1. Qaseem A, Forland F, Macbeth F, Ollenschlager G, Phillips S, van der Wees P (2012) Guidelines International Network: toward international standards for clinical practice guidelines. Ann Intern Med 156:525–531
2. Rabbitts JA et al (2010) Epidemiology of ambulatory anesthesia for children in United States: 2006 and 1996. Anesth Analg 111:1011–1015
3. Ètats des lieux 2012 sur l'activitè de chirurgie ambulatoire (2013) Agence technique de l'information sur l'hospitalisation, http://www.atih.sante.fr/sites/default/files/public/content/1504/gdr_ca_analyse_atih2012.pdf

4. www.ADARPEF.org. One day surgery in children less than 18 years old: French Guidelines 2010
5. Majholm B et al (2012) Is day surgery safe? A Danish multicentre study of morbidity after 57,709 day surgery procedures. Acta Anaesthesiol Scand 56:323–331
6. Segerdahl M et al (2008) Children in day surgery: clinical practice and routines. The results from a nation-wide survey. Acta Anaesthesiol Scand 52:821–828
7. Villeret I et al (2002) Incidence of postoperative nausea and vomiting in paediatric ambulatory surgery. Paediatr Anaesth 12(8):712–717
8. Ortiz AC et al (2014) Intravenous versus inhalational anaesthesia for paediatric outpatient surgery Cochrane Database Sys Rev (2):CD009015. doi:10.1002/14651858.CD009015.pub2
9. American Academy of Pediatrics (1999) Section on anesthesiology: guidelines for the pediatric perioperative anesthesia environment. Pediatrics 103:512
10. Smith I (2014) Anaesthesia services for day surgery 2014 in Guidelines for the provision of anaesthetic services. chapter 6. www.rcoa.ac.uk/gpas2014
11. Wilkinson KA, Brennan L, Rollin A-M (2015) Paediatric anaesthesia services in guidelines for the prevision of anaesthetic services. www.rcoa.ac.uk
12. Short J, Bew S (2011) Paediatric day surgery. In: Smith I, McWhinnie D, Jackson I (eds) Oxford specialist handbook of day surgery. Oxford University Press, pp 161–197
13. Walther –Lansen S, Rasmussen L (2006) The former preterm infant and risk of post-operative apnoea: recommendations form management. Acta Anaesthesiol Scand 50:888–893
14. Cote CJ, Zaslavky A, Dowes JJ (1995) Postoperative apnoea in former preterm infants after inguinal herniorrhaphy. A combined analysis. Anesthesiology 82:809–822
15. Yentis SM et al (1992) Should all children with suspected or confirmed malignant hyperthermia susceptibility be admitted after surgery? A 10-year review. Anesth Analg 75:345
16. Rubens D, Sarnat HB (2013) Sudden Infant Deaths Syndrome: un update ad new perspectives of etiology. Handb Clin Neurol. doi:10.1016/B978-0-444-52910-7.00008-8
17. Issues in paediatric day surgery (2007) BADS, London (www.daysurgeryuk.net/en/shop/handbooks/issues-in-paediatric-day-surgery)
18. Rolf N, Cotè CJ (1992) Frequency and severity of desaturation events during general anesthesia in children with and without upper respiratory infections. J Clin Anesth 4:200–203
19. Parnis SJ, Barker DS, Van Der Walt JH (2001) Clinical predictors of anaesthetic complications in children with respiratory tract infections. Paediatr Anaesth 11:29–40
20. Tait AR, Malviya S (2005) Anesthesia for the child with an upper respiratory tract infection: still a dilemma? Anesth Analg 100:59–65
21. von Ungern-Sternberg BS et al (2010) Risk assessment for respiratory complications in paediatric anaesthesia: a prospective cohort study. Lancet 376(9743):773–783
22. World Federation of Society of Anesthesiologists (2010) ATOTW 203 Paediatric anaesthesia for day surgery
23. Lawrie R (1964) Operating on children as day-cases. Lancet 2:1289
24. Haana V et al (2009) Case cancellation on the day of surgery: an investigation in an Australian paediatric hospital. ANZ J Surg 79:636–640
25. Hmed MI, Farrell MA, Parrish K, Karla A (2011) Preoperative anxiety in children risk factors and non-pharmacological management. Middle East J Anaesthesiol 21(2):153–164
26. Brady MC et al (2009) Preoperative fasting for preventing perioperative complications in children. Cochrane Libr (4)
27. Schmidt AR (2015) Gastric pH and residual volume after 1 and 2 h fasting time for clear fluids in children. Br J Anaesth 114(3):477–482. doi:10.1093/bja/aeu 399
28. Smith I et al (2011) Perioperative fasting in adults and children: guidelines from the European Society of Anaesthesiology. Eur J Anaesthesiol 28(8):556–569
29. Ortiz AC et al (2014) Intravenous versus inhalational anaesthesia for paediatric outpatient surgery (review). Cochrane Libr (2) 2014;2:CD009015. doi: 10.1002/14651858.CD009015.pub2
30. Meretoja OA (2010) Neuromuscular block and treatment strategies for its reversal in children. Paediatr Anaesth 20(7):591–604. doi:10.1111/j.1460-9592.2010.03335.x

31. Bosenberg A (2012) Benefits of regional anesthesia in children. Paediatr Anaesth 22:10–18
32. Ivani G et al (2002) Comparison of racemic bupivacaine, ropivacaine, and levo-bupivacaine for pediatric caudal anesthesia: effects on postoperative analgesia and motor block. Reg Anesth Pain Med 27:157–161
33. Pappas AL et al (1997) Caudal anesthesia and urinary retention in ambulatory surgery. Anesth Analg 85:706
34. Weintraud M et al (2009) Ultrasound versus landmark-based technique for ilioinguinal-iliohypogastric nerve blockade in children: the implications on plasma levels of ropivacaine. Anesth Analg 108:1488–1492
35. Ludot H et al (2008) Continuous peripheral nerve block for postoperative pain control at home: a prospective feasibility study in children. Reg Anesth Pain Med 33:52–56
36. Schreiner MS et al (1992) Should children drink before discharge from day surgery? Anesthesiology 76:528
37. Anderson BJ, Pons G, Autret-Leca E, Allegaert K, Boccard E (2005) Pediatric intravenous paracetamol (propacetamol) pharmacokinetics: a population analysis. Paediatr Anaesth 15(4):282–292
38. Baley K, Michalov K, Kossick MA, McDowell M (2014) Intravenous acetaminophen and intravenous ketorolac for management of pediatric surgical pain: a literature review. AANA J 82(1):53–64
39. Ecoffey C et al (2010) Association des Anesthésistes Réanimateurs Pédiatriques d'Expression Française (ADARPEF). Epidemiology and morbidity of regional anesthesia in children: a follow-up one-year prospective survey of the French-Language Society of Paediatric Anaesthesiologists. Paediatr Anaesth 20:1061–1069
40. Kokinsky E, Nilsson K, Larsson LE (2003) Increased incidence of postoperative nausea and vomiting without additional analgesic effects when a low dose of intravenous fentanyl is combined with a caudal block. Paediatr Anaesth 13:334–338
41. Eberhart LH et al (2004) The development and validation of a risk score to predict the probability of postoperative vomiting in pediatric patients. Anesth Analg 99:1630–1637
42. Gan TJ et al (2014) Consensus guidelines for the management of postoperative nausea and vomiting. Anesth Analg 118(1):85–113
43. Hohne C (2014) Postoperative nausea and vomiting in pediatric anesthesia. Curr Opin Anesthesiol 27:303–308
44. www.jointcommissioninternation.org
45. Ead H (2006) From Aldrete to PADSS: reviewing discharge criteria after ambulatory surgery. J Peri Anesth Nurs 21(4):259–267
46. Biedermann S et al (2014) Paediatric discharge score in ambulatory surgery. Ann Fr Anesth Réanim 33:330–334
47. Moncel JB et al (2015) Evaluation of the pediatric post anesthesia discharge scoring system in an ambulatory surgery unit. Paediatr Anaesth. doi:10.1111/pan.12612. Epub ahead of print
48. Cardwell et al (2013) Nonsteroidal anti-inflammatory drugs and perioperative bleeding in paediatric tonsillectomy. Cochrane Database Syst Rev 7:CD003591

Perioperative Care in Remote Locations

6

Maria Sammartino, Fabio Sbaraglia,
and Francesco Antonio Idone

A significant number of children receive some kind of nonoperating room anesthesia (NORA) for painful or uncomfortable procedures [1]. Several advantages are reported for NORA even if risks and adverse events are described by some authors [1, 2]. Determination of safety standards in this particular pediatric field must be considered a priority in clinical research to ensure high quality of care.

The current status of pediatric NORA is even undefined because of the wide overlapping in literature with sedation, the variety of locations (with different levels of intensity of care), the different techniques utilized, and the performers involved. In the matter of this last point, there is a strong debate about who should be performing sedation in children [3, 4], which reflects the existence of an evolving situation that does not concern the objective of this chapter.

Independendtly of the degree, the provider must be able to choose a comfortable sedation plan, and to manage adverse events related to drugs and techniques utilized [5]. The Joint Commission for Accreditation of Healthcare Organization has stated that every provider has to be able, when needed, to rescue the patient for that level of sedation and for one deeper level [6]. Our intent is to examine current practice, highlighting potential gray areas in the three steps of anesthesia: pre-procedural assessment, anesthesiological management, and discharge.

M. Sammartino (✉)
Department of Anesthesia and Intensive Care, Catholic University of Sacred Heart,
Training Hospital "A. Gemelli", Rome, Italy

Dipartimento di Anestesia e Rianimazione, Ospedale Universitario A. Gemelli, Università
Cattolica del Sacro Cuore, Rome, Italy
e-mail: marinasammartino@libero.it

F. Sbaraglia • F.A. Idone
Department of Anesthesia and Intensive Care, Catholic University of Sacred Heart,
Training Hospital "A. Gemelli", Rome, Italy

© Springer International Publishing Switzerland 2016
M. Astuto, P.M. Ingelmo (eds.), *Perioperative Medicine in Pediatric Anesthesia*,
Anesthesia, Intensive Care and Pain in Neonates and Children,
DOI 10.1007/978-3-319-21960-8_6

6.1 Pre-procedural Assessment

NORA is required for several diagnostic and therapeutic procedures. The feasibility in these cases is dependent on a multidimensional evaluation by the anesthesiologist, who will consider the clinical status of the child, the invasivity (pain, duration, risks, etc.) of the procedure, and the location facilities.

Even if there are not absolute contraindications to procedural sedation outside the operating room, the quality of care of the operating room should be transferred also to a remote location.

Location of NORA should be overviewed by the anesthesiologist before the procedure. The setup should guarantee the presence of a certain number of items that could be remembered with the acronym SOAPME (Table 6.1). An adequate number of sockets are important to connect monitors, suction, infusion pumps, etc. Also a reliable contact trough phone, pager, or mobile is mandatory. Whether one of these standards is missing, performing NORA is not safe, even if dealing with a mild sedation.

Children who have to undergo the procedures should be evaluated concerning their physical and behavioral status (just as for anesthesia in the operating room), and the correlated suitability for sedation should be investigated. The history should include comorbidities and previous hospitalization, sedation or general anesthesia, current therapies, relevant familiar history, and possible allergies. Particular attention should be dedicated to the risk of obstructive sleep apnea, for obese or snoring children [7]. Physical examination should include auscultation of the heart and lungs and evaluation of the neck and airways. Evidence specific for children regarding identification and management of difficult airways is limited [8]. Nevertheless, a systematic approach for children can be developed from experience with adults in the operating room using the acronym LEMON (Table 6.2).

Table 6.1 SOAPME mnemonic acronym

S	Suction	Suction device with child-sized suction catheters
O	Oxygen	Availability of adequate oxygen delivery
A	Airway	Age-appropriate airway equipment
P	Pharmacy	Sedation and emergency drugs
M	Monitors	Standard monitors for vital parameters (SaO_2, EKG, NiBP, $EtCO_2$)
E	Equipment	Special equipment in child size

Table 6.2 LEMON mnemonic acronym

L	Look at him	Look for external indicators for difficult airways
E	Evaluation	Evaluate mouth opening, thyromental distance, mandibular space
M	Mallampati	Mallampati score
O	Obstruction	Signs of airway obstruction or OSAS
N	Neck	Neck mobility

Table 6.3 Fasting rules by ASA [71]

2 h	Clear liquids
4 h	Breast milk
6 h	Infant formula and light meal
8 h	Fatty food or meat

Certain patient factors have been associated with failed sedations, like the presence of upper respiratory infection (URI) that mainly causes cancellation and rescheduling of the procedure. URIs are responsible of higher incidence of complications, but serious events are rare in literature [9]. Whether infectious secretions are present, the operation should be postponed at least for 2 weeks.

During pre-anesthesiological assessment, provider must present the sedation/anesthesia plan to parents and child (depending on the age) describing the benefits (minimizing pain, anxiety, and physiological trauma) and the possible risks often agent specific but commonly including potential for airway compromise, hypoxia, and vomiting. An informed consent has to be signed by both parents.

The patient fasting status is a key consideration when assessing the risk index. The American Society of Anesthesiologists (ASA) suggestions for fasting in children undergoing sedation for elective procedures are universal and are showed in Table 6.3. However, the degree of fasting for urgent/emergent procedures is controversial, and disparate recommendations have been proposed by the ASA and the American College of Emergency Physicians [10, 11].

Evidence regarding the optimum duration of fasting required to reduce risk of aspiration during sedation is limited [12]. No relationship has been proved between the duration of fasting prior to procedural sedation and the amount of content found in the stomach [13–17]. Furthermore, there are some evidences that the more is the fasting, the more is the residual gastric volume [18].

Approach to fasting time needs some flexibility when facing with pathologies that modify children metabolism or digestive tract mobility. In some cases, as in concomitance of dumping syndrome [19], the provider should consider that the risk of hypoglycemia is more important than the risk of aspiration. On the other hand, a slow emptying, as in the case of achalasia or ileus, requires a longer fasting [20].

As reported by recent recommendations of the Italian Society of Pediatric and Neonatal Anesthesia, the systematic use of complementary tests in children, should be replaced by a selective prescription, based on the preoperative evaluation [21].

6.2   Anesthesiological Management

Differently from inside the operating room, anesthesiological management cannot be based only on patient status and on the procedure, but it should be decided also on the actual environment.

Flexibility is a key factor in the good outcome of NORA. Most of the procedures are scheduled in remote locations, which often do not guarantee a wide space of action and cannot allow the use of some drugs or equipment. Anesthesiologists have to tailor an anesthesia service to the particular requirements imposed by the actual context. For example, procedures performed directly in neonatal intensive care unit often do not allow the use of halogenated vapors for the absence of adequate anesthesia machines, vaporizers, and scavenger systems so that only intravenous drugs can be utilized; MRI and many radiologic exams do not allow to remain close to the patient, reducing the direct control on his ventilation and other vital signs; dentistry and endoscopy oblige the anesthesiologist to share airways with the co-workers (more challenging when outside the operating room); some electrophysiological retinal exams require a dark room without possibility to look at the child, etc. In these challenges, a right choice of drugs and an efficient and reliable monitoring is essential for a safe outcome.

Although respiratory adverse events are the most common [2, 22], a basic hemodynamic monitoring (EKG, NiBP) is recommended in every patient, independent from procedure, location, and clinical status. If deep sedation is performed, or if a patient has significant underlying illness, vital signs should be measured at least every 5 min.

Experience and evidence suggest that respiratory complications are the most reported and are likely to occur within 5–10 min after administration of intravenous medications and immediately after the procedure when the painful stimuli are removed.

Provided that continuous visual observation of the face, mouth, and chest wall movements is not reliable, adequate respiratory monitoring is recommended throughout the procedure [23, 24]. The use of SaO_2 is mandatory but does not give a value in real time. $EtCO_2$ monitoring, on the contrary, better by Microstream Sensor particularly in neonates, is strongly recommended [25]. Microstream monitors have a sampling chamber of 15 mcl and work well even with low flow of 50 ml.

$EtCO_2$ monitoring is increasingly available in many settings for non-intubated patients and may be helpful to assess ventilation during sedation and analgesia. Increases in $EtCO_2$ may be detected in children undergoing respiratory depression before hypoxemia is noted, particularly in those who are receiving supplemental oxygen. Different approaches to preoxygenation and to the use of continuous supplemental oxygen during procedural sedation are reported in literature [26]. A FiO_2 higher than 0.21 can allow to maximize O_2 lung storage [27] and a longer maintenance of a good level of PaO_2 during occurrence of apnea. However, continuous supplemental oxygen can delay desaturation and apnea detection unless capnographic monitoring is available [28]. Furthermore, there is no evidence that preoxygenation or increasing FiO_2 is associated with improved safety in NORA [29].

An additional monitoring is represented by the cerebral activity monitoring. The most utilized technology is the bispectral index (BIS). It is able to quantify the level of consciousness ranging from 0 (no brain activity) to 100 (alert), obtained by continuous EEG monitoring through probes placed on the forehead. It has shown good sensitivity in children older than 6 months, and it can be useful to guide adequate drug administration and to avoid overdosage [30] that could delay awakening. It should be considered that BIS index is not sensitive to drugs that have site effect out of the cerebral cortex, as ketamine, dexmedetomidine, remifentanil, and N_2O [31].

Other brain activity monitoring devices, as entropy [32] and cerebral state index [33], are under validation for pediatric age, but results are even controversial.

Table 6.4 Definitions to describe the depth of sedation

Minimal sedation	The patient responds normally to verbal commands. Cognitive function and coordination may be impaired, but ventilatory and cardiovascular function is unaffected
Moderate sedation/ analgesia	The patient has depression of consciousness but can respond purposefully to verbal commands either alone or accompanied by light touch. Maintains airways and adequate ventilation without intervention. Cardiovascular function is maintained
Deep sedation	The patient cannot be easily aroused but responds purposefully to noxious stimulation. May require assistance to maintain airway and adequate ventilation. Cardiovascular function is usually maintained
General anesthesia	The patient cannot be aroused. May require airway assistance and ventilation. Cardiovascular function may be impaired

Table 6.5 Principal routes of administration

Inhalation	Halogenated, N_2O
Intravenous	All opiates, propofol, midazolam, ketamine, flumazenil, naloxone
Intramuscular	Ketamine, benzodiazepine
Rectal	Ketamine, benzodiazepine
Intranasal	Midazolam, flumazenil, dexmedetomidine, fentanyl, ketamine
Buccal	Midazolam, ketamine, sufentanil, dexmedetomidine
Transmucosal	Fentanyl

Various drugs and techniques can be chosen: clinicians who administer sedation must understand the pharmacology of the drugs used. Because sedation is a continuum in which responses to medications vary greatly upon developmental, behavioral, and clinical status, type of procedure, need to cover painful maneuvers or only immobility, clinicians must identify the appropriate level of sedation/analgesia for the single child (Table 6.4). Careful titration of the chosen medication is often necessary to safely achieve the desired depth of sedation. A wide range of short-acting sedative-hypnotic and analgesic medications are available [24, 34, 35], and many of these agents have multiple routes of administration (Table 6.5). Procedures that are not painful and require only immobility can usually be performed with sedation alone. Children undergoing painful procedures require also analgesia. It has to be underlined that every performer must be able to deal with possible complications, and competence in emergency airway management is mandatory [5, 24, 36].

6.3 Inhalation Techniques

Historically, children have been anesthetized in operating rooms by halogenated vapors. The increasing demand of procedures in NORA has transferred this technique even outside of the operating room. The recent attention to the environmental pollution and to the occupational safety has restricted the use of inhalation anesthesia inside the locations equipped by specific scavenger systems.

The most used vapor in this field is sevoflurane that guarantees a safe profile for maintenance of spontaneous breathing and stabile hemodynamic. It is also advantageous for its rapid onset and the possibility to find a venous access in not cooperating children. It can be used trough facial mask or even by nasal probes, very useful in procedures performed on the eyes or on the face where the mask could result cumbersome.

Other halogenated (as desflurane or isoflurane) are not indicated for this use, due to their irritating effect on the tracheobronchial system, when used in spontaneous ventilation.

Nitrous oxide (N_2O) is an old gas which recently has been proposed again, in a new formulation. It is commercialized as a mixture with O_2 50 % in portable tanks. It is delivered through a demand valve mask or continuous flow system [37]. Because the demand valve mask requires cooperation and may be difficult to be activated by smaller children, N_2O is used primarily in patients older than 4 years of age. To prevent excessive exposure, dedicated facial masks connected with a scavenger system can be utilized. A continuous delivery system (a mask strapped over the nose and/or mouth) has been used in younger children with variable success. This system indeed is more frequently associated with emesis [38, 39]. N_2O provides good analgesia, sedation, amnesia, and anxiolysis [40, 41], and it is a widely used analgesic for acute, short-term pain relief in a diverse range of clinical situations. Contraindications to nitrous oxide include nausea and vomiting and trapped gas within body cavities (e.g., bowel obstruction, pneumothorax, middle ear infection). Deeper sedation than anticipated can occur with prolonged inhalation and when N_2O is combined with opioids or benzodiazepines [42]. It is reported that fasting is not mandatory using 50 % N_2O/O_2 mixture [43]. In the absence of a clear evidence, every physician should identify the best choice according to his experience or skill.

6.4 Intravenous Techniques

Children are usually afraid of needles, and often in NORA, there is no possibility to use inhalation induction, so the cooperation of the child for finding a venous access is important. Application of anesthetic transdermic cream 45 min earlier can be very useful, in association with administration of midazolam 0.4–0.5 mg/kg (for a maximum of 15 mg) by mouth or better through the more rapid nasal route, thanks to the high mucosal vascularization [44].

Over the last decade, intravenous techniques are developed even in pediatrics with successful outcome. The marketing of new short-acting drugs and the safer profile of pharmacodynamics allows to calibrate anesthesia in real time with respect to the procedure.

The development of pediatric pharmacokinetic models for target-controlled infusion (TCI), Paedfusor and Kataria, has been a further boost to better utilize propofol in children.

TCI technique is particularly advantageous in NORA, allowing to perform sedation in spontaneous breathing assuring a constant propofol plasma concentration [45]. When compared with manual controlled infusion or intermittent bolus, TCI provides reduced apnoeic events and shorter awakening time [46].

For these reasons, propofol currently is the commonest intravenous agent (alone or in combination) administered in NORA. Safety profile is very comfortable even in smaller children [47], despite propofol infusion syndrome has been described after longer or high-dose infusion [48]. However, high doses administered by mistake for short procedures have not shown fatal outcome, despite a transient alteration in the metabolic pattern [49].

Remifentanil shows a pharmacokinetic profile even more advantageous in general anesthesia due to the efficacy of plasmatic esterases, which seems already mature even in premature babies [50]. Among opiates, remifentanil is the most indicated for a rapid recovery and discharge, even if the apnoeic effect requires a strict capnographic monitoring when spontaneous breathing is performed.

Outside the operating room, other opioids have proven useful. Alfentanil has been utilized by bolus in association with propofol or midazolam in short painful procedures as bone marrow aspiration or lumbar puncture [51]. Opioids with longer half-life are less recommended, as unique sedation agent, due to the increased interindividual variability and difficult titration. Recently sufentanil has been experimented successfully in a preliminary study by nasal route in dentistry [52], but this technique still needs major validation.

Ketamine, which came back to our attention in the last years, provides sedation, analgesia, and immobilization while usually preserving upper airway muscle tone and spontaneous breathing [53–55]. Its use in small doses in association with hypnotic agents is common, particularly for the possibility of administration by several routes.

Dexmedetomidine can be considered the future of sedation also in NORA. It causes minimal respiratory depression and, in healthy children, has been found generally safe and effective for nonpainful procedures [56], and in some sedation service, it is already the preferred agent for diagnostic imaging [57, 58].

Further molecules are going to be investigated. Among these, remimazolam, an ultra short-acting benzodiazepine, is actually in phase II and represents something new on the horizon [59, 60].

Ketofol, a combination of propofol and racemic ketamine mixed in the same syringe, for sedation and analgesia in short procedures is still under investigation. The best ratio between the two drugs is not yet well established: a ratio of 1:3 for bolus and 1:4 for infusion seems to be a reliable combination [61].

Reversing agent availability is mandatory during NORA, but their use should be limited to rare and specific situations. Flumazenil, antagonist of benzodiazepines, could be useful even in the absence of venous access [62]. Naloxone should be used with extreme prudence as suggested by American Academy of Pediatric Committee on Drugs guidelines on the use in children [63].

6.5 Complementary Techniques

Complementary and alternative medicines are described for sedation in children. Sweetening agents like sucrose has been utilized to reduce stress response in neonates [64], as well as the simply sensorial stimulation from skin-to-skin contact with the mother [65].

Hypnotherapy, acupuncture, and Chinese traditional medicine are proposed as alternative treatment, but evidence is very poor. Certainly the creation of a reassuring environment and a good interaction with patient and parents assures an easy approach to NORA.

6.6   Discharge

After the procedure, children need a stay in recovery room during which monitoring must be carried out. As reported above, minor adverse events are common in the first minutes after the end of the procedure when stimuli associated with the procedure are removed [24], but serious adverse events rarely occur after 25 min from the final drugs administration [66].

Sedation scales modified for children are used to assure a safe discharge: the University of Michigan Sedation Scale (UMSS) [67], the Dartmouth Operative Conditions Scale [68], and the Modified Maintenance of Wakefulness Test-MMWT [69] are the unique scales validated in children.

NORA requires specific criteria for the discharge of the patients, which should be approved by local protocols. As general suggestion, we have to achieve different requirements in case of inpatient or outpatient procedures.

Inpatients may not need a long stay in recovery room (some procedures are carried out even at bedside), and clinical and multiparametric monitoring could continue at minor intensity in the ward. On the other hand, outpatients need to assess discharge readiness before leaving the hospital. It is undeniable that a sedation scale is a useful and simple measure to optimize recovery time.

However, additional elements in this decision should be considered. Several children undergoing NORA are affected by neurological or respiratory diseases, and recovery from anesthesia cannot be ensured by traditional scores; the surgical procedure can need a longer stay; outdoor logistics (home environment, distance from medical center, etc.) are also to be considered. Discharge should be based on standardized criteria, but this general rule should be applied with flexibility. In any case, it is mandatory that discharge process appears in the chart and that parents get clear instructions in post-procedural care.

Depending on the procedure, cooperation between anesthesiologist and surgeon/physician should be desirable at discharge. NORA is a field in rapid growth due to increasing sensibility to pediatric pain and an increasing offer of diagnostic and, particularly, therapeutic procedures that can enhance the standard of care: often these need to be performed outside the operating room necessarily for logistic reasons or preferably for economic motivations.

The increased availability of short-acting drugs along with accurate noninvasive monitoring and improved sedation training (including simulation programs) has enabled effective and safe management of sedation also outside the operating room [70].

References

1. Metzner J, Domino KB (2010) Risks of anesthesia or sedation outside the operating room: the role of the anesthesia care provider. Curr Opin Anaesthesiol 23(4):523–531
2. Cravero JP, Beach ML, Blike GT, Gallagher SM, Hertzog JH, Pediatric Sedation Research C (2009) The incidence and nature of adverse events during pediatric sedation/anesthesia with propofol for procedures outside the operating room: a report from the Pediatric Sedation Research Consortium. Anesth Analg 108(3):795–804
3. Baxter AL, Bernard PA, Berkenbosch JW et al (2008) Society for pediatric sedation reply to Dr Cote's editorial. Paediatr Anaesth 18(6):559–560; author reply 560–561
4. Cote CJ (2008) Round and round we go: sedation – what is it, who does it, and have we made things safer for children? Paediatr Anaesth 18(1):3–8
5. Sury M, Bullock I, Rabar S, Demott K, Guideline Development G (2010) Sedation for diagnostic and therapeutic procedures in children and young people: summary of NICE guidance. BMJ 341:c6819
6. Organizations JCoAoHC (2000) Comprehensive accreditation manual for hospitals. JACHO, Oakland
7. Brown KA (2011) Outcome, risk, and error and the child with obstructive sleep apnea. Paediatr Anaesth 21(7):771–780
8. Gruppo di Studio SVAD, Frova G, Guarino A et al (2006) Recommendations for airway control and difficult airway management in paediatric patients. Minerva Anestesiol 72(9):723–748
9. Tait AR, Malviya S, Voepel-Lewis T, Munro HM, Seiwert M, Pandit UA (2001) Risk factors for perioperative adverse respiratory events in children with upper respiratory tract infections. Anesthesiology 95(2):299–306
10. American Society of Anesthesiologists Task Force on S, Analgesia by N-A (2002) Practice guidelines for sedation and analgesia by non-anesthesiologists. Anesthesiology 96(4):1004–1017
11. Green SM, Roback MG, Miner JR, Burton JH, Krauss B (2007) Fasting and emergency department procedural sedation and analgesia: a consensus-based clinical practice advisory. Ann Emerg Med 49(4):454–461
12. Agrawal D, Manzi SF, Gupta R, Krauss B (2003) Preprocedural fasting state and adverse events in children undergoing procedural sedation and analgesia in a pediatric emergency department. Ann Emerg Med 42(5):636–646
13. Brady M, Kinn S, Stuart P (2003) Preoperative fasting for adults to prevent perioperative complications. Cochrane Database Syst Rev (4):CD004423
14. Miner JR, Burton JH (2007) Clinical practice advisory: emergency department procedural sedation with propofol. Ann Emerg Med 50(2):182–187, 187 e181
15. Sandhar BK, Goresky GV, Maltby JR, Shaffer EA (1989) Effect of oral liquids and ranitidine on gastric fluid volume and pH in children undergoing outpatient surgery. Anesthesiology 71(3):327–330
16. Soreide E, Eriksson LI, Hirlekar G et al (2005) Pre-operative fasting guidelines: an update. Acta Anaesthesiol Scand 49(8):1041–1047
17. Brady M, Kinn S, Ness V, O'Rourke K, Randhawa N, Stuart P (2009) Preoperative fasting for preventing perioperative complications in children. Cochrane Database Syst Rev (4):CD005285
18. Schmitz A, Kallenberger CJ, Neuhaus D, Schroeter E, Deanovic D, Prufer F, Studhalter M, Vollmer L, Weiss M (2011) Fasting times and gastric contents volume in children undergoing deep propofol sedation: an assessment using magnetic resonance imaging. Paediatr Anaesth 21(6):685–690
19. Calabria AC, Gallagher PR, Simmons R, Blinman T, De Leon DD (2011) Postoperative surveillance and detection of postprandial hypoglycemia after fundoplasty in children. J Pediatr 159(4):597–601, e591

20. Kelly CJ, Walker RW (2015) Perioperative pulmonary aspiration is infrequent and low risk in pediatric anesthetic practice. Paediatr Anaesth 25(1):36–43
21. Serafini G, Ingelmo PM, Astuto M et al (2014) Preoperative evaluation in infants and children: recommendations of the Italian Society of Pediatric and Neonatal Anesthesia and Intensive Care (SARNePI). Minerva Anestesiol 80(4):461–469
22. Mallory MD, Baxter AL, Yanosky DJ, Cravero JP, Pediatric Sedation Research C (2011) Emergency physician-administered propofol sedation: a report on 25,433 sedations from the pediatric sedation research consortium. Ann Emerg Med 57(5):462–468, e461
23. American Academy of P, American Academy of Pediatric D, Cote CJ, Wilson S, Work Group on S (2008) Guidelines for monitoring and management of pediatric patients during and after sedation for diagnostic and therapeutic procedures: an update. Paediatr Anaesth 18(1):9–10
24. Krauss B, Green SM (2006) Procedural sedation and analgesia in children. Lancet 367(9512):766–780
25. Sammartino M, Volpe B, Sbaraglia F, Garra R, D'Addessi A (2010) Capnography and the bispectral index-their role in pediatric sedation: a brief review. Int J Pediatr 2010:828347
26. Shavit I, Leder M, Cohen DM (2010) Sedation provider practice variation: a survey analysis of pediatric emergency subspecialists and fellows. Pediatr Emerg Care 26(10):742–747
27. Campbell IT, Beatty PC (1994) Monitoring preoxygenation. Br J Anaesth 72(1):3–4
28. Fu ES, Downs JB, Schweiger JW, Miguel RV, Smith RA (2004) Supplemental oxygen impairs detection of hypoventilation by pulse oximetry. Chest 126(5):1552–1558
29. Green SM, Krauss B (2008) Supplemental oxygen during propofol sedation: yes or no? Ann Emerg Med 52(1):9–10
30. Powers KS, Nazarian EB, Tapyrik SA et al (2005) Bispectral index as a guide for titration of propofol during procedural sedation among children. Pediatrics 115(6):1666–1674
31. Johansen JW (2006) Update on bispectral index monitoring. Best Pract Res Clin Anaesthesiol 20(1):81–99
32. Davidson AJ, Kim MJ, Sangolt GK (2004) Entropy and bispectral index during anaesthesia in children. Anaesth Intensive Care 32(4):485–493
33. Disma N, Tuo P, Astuto M, Davidson AJ (2009) Depth of sedation using Cerebral State Index in infants undergoing spinal anesthesia. Paediatr Anaesth 19(2):133–137
34. Kennedy RM, Luhmann JD (2001) Pharmacological management of pain and anxiety during emergency procedures in children. Paediatr Drugs 3(5):337–354
35. Sahyoun C, Krauss B (2012) Clinical implications of pharmacokinetics and pharmacodynamics of procedural sedation agents in children. Curr Opin Pediatr 24(2):225–232
36. Cravero JP, Blike GT (2004) Review of pediatric sedation. Anesth Analg 99(5):1355–1364
37. Mace SE, Brown LA, Francis L et al (2008) Clinical policy: critical issues in the sedation of pediatric patients in the emergency department. Ann Emerg Med 51(4):378–399, 399 e371–357
38. Luhmann JD, Kennedy RM, Porter FL, Miller JP, Jaffe DM (2001) A randomized clinical trial of continuous-flow nitrous oxide and midazolam for sedation of young children during laceration repair. Ann Emerg Med 37(1):20–27
39. Krauss B (2001) Managing acute pain and anxiety in children undergoing procedures in the emergency department. Emerg Med 13(3):293–304
40. Gamis AS, Knapp JF, Glenski JA (1989) Nitrous oxide analgesia in a pediatric emergency department. Ann Emerg Med 18(2):177–181
41. Kanagasundaram SA, Lane LJ, Cavalletto BP, Keneally JP, Cooper MG (2001) Efficacy and safety of nitrous oxide in alleviating pain and anxiety during painful procedures. Arch Dis Child 84(6):492–495
42. Babl FE, Oakley E, Seaman C, Barnett P, Sharwood LN (2008) High-concentration nitrous oxide for procedural sedation in children: adverse events and depth of sedation. Pediatrics 121(3):e528–e532
43. Morton N, Scottish Intercollegiate Guidelines N (2004) Sedation in children. SAAD Dig 21(2):20–26

44. Wolfe TR, Braude DA (2010) Intranasal medication delivery for children: a brief review and update. Pediatrics 126(3):532–537
45. Constant I, Rigouzzo A (2010) Which model for propofol TCI in children. Paediatr Anaesth 20(3):233–239
46. Lerman J (2010) TIVA, TCI, and pediatrics: where are we and where are we going? Paediatr Anaesth 20(3):273–278
47. Sepulveda P, Cortinez LI, Saez C et al (2011) Performance evaluation of paediatric propofol pharmacokinetic models in healthy young children. Br J Anaesth 107(4):593–600
48. Hatch DJ (1999) Propofol-infusion syndrome in children. Lancet 353(9159):1117–1118
49. Sammartino M, Garra R, Sbaraglia F, Papacci P (2010) Propofol overdose in a preterm baby: may propofol infusion syndrome arise in two hours? Paediatr Anaesth 20(10):973–974
50. Welzing L, Ebenfeld S, Dlugay V, Wiesen MH, Roth B, Mueller C (2011) Remifentanil degradation in umbilical cord blood of preterm infants. Anesthesiology 114(3):570–577
51. Chiaretti A, Ruggiero A, Barone G et al (2010) Propofol/alfentanil and propofol/ketamine procedural sedation in children with acute lymphoblastic leukaemia: safety, efficacy and their correlation with pain neuromediator expression. Eur J Cancer Care 19(2):212–220
52. Hitt JM, Corcoran T, Michienzi K, Creighton P, Heard C (2014) An evaluation of intranasal sufentanil and dexmedetomidine for pediatric dental sedation. Pharmaceutics 6(1):175–184
53. Bassett KE, Anderson JL, Pribble CG, Guenther E (2003) Propofol for procedural sedation in children in the emergency department. Ann Emerg Med 42(6):773–782
54. Green SM, Rothrock SG, Harris T, Hopkins GA, Garrett W, Sherwin T (1998) Intravenous ketamine for pediatric sedation in the emergency department: safety profile with 156 cases. Acad Emerg Med 5(10):971–976
55. Green SM, Rothrock SG, Lynch EL et al (1998) Intramuscular ketamine for pediatric sedation in the emergency department: safety profile in 1,022 cases. Ann Emerg Med 31(6):688–697
56. Kost S, Roy A (2010) Procedural sedation and analgesia in the pediatric emergency department: a review of sedative pharmacology. Clin Pediatr Emerg Med 11(4):233–243
57. Mason KP, Robinson F, Fontaine P, Prescilla R (2013) Dexmedetomidine offers an option for safe and effective sedation for nuclear medicine imaging in children. Radiology 267(3):911–917
58. Mason KP, Prescilla R, Fontaine PJ, Zurakowski D (2011) Pediatric CT sedation: comparison of dexmedetomidine and pentobarbital. AJR Am J Roentgenol 196(2):W194–W198
59. Gin T (2013) Hypnotic and sedative drugs–anything new on the horizon? Curr Opin Anaesthesiol 26(4):409–413
60. Borkett KM, Riff DS, Schwartz HI et al (2015) A phase IIa, randomized, double-blind study of remimazolam (CNS 7056) versus midazolam for sedation in upper gastrointestinal endoscopy. Anesth Analg 120(4):771–780
61. Coulter FL, Hannam JA, Anderson BJ (2014) Ketofol dosing simulations for procedural sedation. Pediatr Emerg Care 30(9):621–630
62. Heard C, Creighton P, Lerman J (2009) Intranasal flumazenil and naloxone to reverse oversedation in a child undergoing dental restorations. Paediatr Anaesth 19(8):795–797; discussion 798–799
63. American Academy of Pediatrics Committee on Drugs (1990) Naloxone dosage and route of administration for infants and children: addendum to emergency drug doses for infants and children. Pediatrics 86(3):484–485
64. O'Sullivan A, O'Connor M, Brosnahan D, McCreery K, Dempsey EM (2010) Sweeten, soother and swaddle for retinopathy of prematurity screening: a randomised placebo controlled trial. Arch Dis Child 95(6):F419–F422
65. Lago P, Garetti E, Merazzi D et al (2009) Guidelines for procedural pain in the newborn. Acta Paediatr 98(6):932–939
66. Newman DH, Azer MM, Pitetti RD, Singh S (2003) When is a patient safe for discharge after procedural sedation? The timing of adverse effect events in 1367 pediatric procedural sedations. Ann Emerg Med 42(5):627–635

67. Malviya S, Voepel-Lewis T, Tait AR, Merkel S, Tremper K, Naughton N (2002) Depth of sedation in children undergoing computed tomography: validity and reliability of the University of Michigan Sedation Scale (UMSS). Br J Anaesth 88(2):241–245
68. Cravero JP, Blike GT, Surgenor SD, Jensen J (2005) Development and validation of the Dartmouth Operative Conditions Scale. Anesth Analg 100(6):1614–1621
69. Malviya S, Voepel-Lewis T, Ludomirsky A, Marshall J, Tait AR (2004) Can we improve the assessment of discharge readiness? A comparative study of observational and objective measures of depth of sedation in children. Anesthesiology 100(2):218–224
70. Howard RF (2003) Current status of pain management in children. JAMA 290(18): 2464–2469
71. American Society of Anesthesiologists Committee (2011) Practice guidelines for preoperative fasting and the use of pharmacologic agents to reduce the risk of pulmonary aspiration: application to healthy patients undergoing elective procedures: an updated report by the American Society of Anesthesiologists Committee on Standards and Practice Parameters. Anesthesiology 114(3):495–511

Perioperative Care in Paediatric Orthopaedic Surgery

7

A.U. Behr

7.1 Clinical Practice

7.1.1 Preoperative Evaluation in Orthopaedic Surgery

The orthopaedic paediatric patient includes all stages of development, from birth to adolescence, and ranges from a normal healthy child to a child with multiple congenital malformations, neuromuscular diseases or metabolic disorders. Children with cerebral palsy, dysmorphic syndromes, myelomeningocele, trisomy 21, autism or other congenital or acquired development diseases offer several clinical challenges to the anaesthetist. The aims of preanaesthetic assessment are to identify the most appropriate anaesthetic techniques for each case, to ensure the safety of perioperative care and an optimal use of resources and to improve the outcome and patient satisfaction, while considering the individual and person-related risk factors and circumstances. Many children in the orthopaedic setting are operated in day surgery and the adequate preparation of the patients and their parents plays an important role. The healthy child does not usually need any preoperative investigation or laboratory tests, but the situation changes significantly when congenital abnormalities or familiar disorders are present. Children with developmental disorders (Fig. 7.1) frequently experience complications such as seizures, dysphagia or reactive airway diseases, and they need an interdisciplinary assessment for optimal surgical outcome.

A.U. Behr
Istituto di Anestesia e Rianimazione, Azienda Ospedaliera Università, Padova, Italy
e-mail: astridursula.behr@gmail.com

© Springer International Publishing Switzerland 2016
M. Astuto, P.M. Ingelmo (eds.), *Perioperative Medicine in Pediatric Anesthesia*,
Anesthesia, Intensive Care and Pain in Neonates and Children,
DOI 10.1007/978-3-319-21960-8_7

Fig. 7.1 An 8-year-old
(12 kg) female affected by
osteogenesis imperfecta

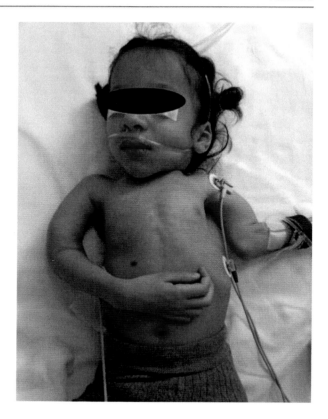

7.1.2   Ambulatory Orthopaedic Surgery in Children

Ambulatory surgery is a somewhat lighter burden for health services, resulting in considerable cost reduction and resource saving. Paediatric orthopaedic surgery seems to be rarely done in an outpatient setting, mainly because of the postoperative pain, which all parents fear. The anaesthetic management is challenging because young children lack the ability to communicate pain, and analgesic need is often difficult to determine. Therefore, provision of adequate postoperative analgesia and parents' education are important elements of the care plan. Inclusion criteria for ambulatory surgery proposed by Khoury et al. [1] are summarised in Table 7.1. Parents must be adequately informed on how to deal with cast, including possible complications. They should be given written instruction and a staff contact number should be available as well. Of the utmost importance is to provide the family detailed information about postoperative pain management and consequences of regional anaesthesia. For example, if the child undergoes a nerve block, parents should be aware of what is an acceptable time for resumption of active motion. The most frequent orthopaedic ambulatory procedures are cast change, arthroscopy, closed fracture reduction and manipulation, hardware removal, percutaneous tenotomies and arthrograms.

Table 7.1 Inclusion criteria for orthopaedic paediatric ambulatory surgery

Social and geographic factors
Surgery schedule compatible with day-care unit opening hours
Parents able to follow pain management and follow-up instructions
Availability of a phone at home
Ability to return to hospital in less than 30 min
Surgical criteria
Surgery lasting <90 min
Minimal estimated blood loss or fluid shifts (<10 % of total BV)
Few operative complications anticipated
Patient conditions
Child of >4 months of age if preterm or born at term if ageing <4 months
ASA physical status classification I or II
Absence of apnoea syndrome

Adapted from Khoury et al. [1]

7.1.3 Preoperative Fasting and Premedication

Every child has to be treated individually and it is therefore difficult to establish fixed rules regarding the perioperative anaesthetic management. For preoperative fasting, the orthopaedic setting shares the same rules of any other surgical specialty, but in this arena, trauma patients are frequent and the stomach of traumatised children is assumed never to be empty. Nonetheless, it may be necessary to treat the child as fast as possible, mandating for focused attention to advanced airway management. Preoperative anxiety may be reduced by premedication similarly to other surgical settings, but non-pharmacological strategies are available as well. Indeed, there is evidence that the viewing of animated cartoons by paediatric surgical patients is an inexpensive, easy to administer, comprehensive intervention that can be very effective in alleviating preoperative anxiety and "needle phobia" in this special surgical population [2]. Furthermore, it may be useful to apply EMLA tapes not only at the venous puncture site but also at the insertion site of the plexus or nerve block.

7.1.4 Procedural Sedation

Anaesthetic services are commonly required for sedation during diagnostic procedures, non-invasive treatment of fractures and other short but painful procedures. Reposition or manipulation of a fractured limb without sufficient analgesia is inhuman, and, to some extent, it is comparable to severe personal injury. Closed reduction and cast immobilisation in the emergency department are usually eased by deep sedation to reduce procedure-related stress.

Deep sedation for both emergent and elective orthopaedic procedures is associated with several, rare but potentially serious adverse events like apnoea or hypotension, which require continuous monitoring and several dedicated staff members [3]. Furthermore, in these cases, preoperative fasting is mandatory, and postprocedural observation in adequate recovery area may be prolonged with relatively long time to discharge. Performing an analgesic or anaesthetic nerve block (Fig. 7.2) of the interested area based on anatomical considerations results in lighter sedation, reduced risks and shorter postoperative observation time. Indeed, the patients can be discharged 2 h after uncomplicated procedures, even with persistent sensory block. With regard to postoperative pain management, regional anaesthesia combined with postoperative non-opioid analgesics, like paracetamol, NSAIDs, or weak opioid, such as codeine or tramadol, are regularly used after ambulatory surgery.

Procedural sedation is also required for non-intrusive approaches for correction of early-onset scoliosis. This treatment in infants and toddlers is based on sequential, repeated body cast positioning, which may initiate as early as at 4 months of age. After the child is positioned on the frame, distraction and derotation of the spine will be performed in general anaesthesia or deep sedation. Plaster application, particularly around the hip, should allow bowel and bladder function, avoid skin breakdown and permit access to epidural or perineural catheters. These infants and toddlers with scoliosis, as well as other children with chronic diseases, present repeatedly for surgical or diagnostic procedures and should be treated with particular sensibility and compassion. Indeed, even a single negative experience can indelibly ruin patient and family attitude toward anaesthesia.

Fig. 7.2 US-guided infraclavicular nerve block for non-invasive treatment of upper limb fracture

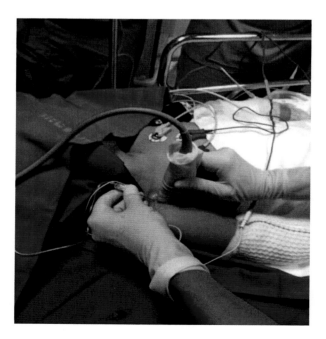

7.1.5   Intraoperative Positioning

Anaesthetists, surgeons and nurses are all responsible for the safe positioning of surgical patients to prevent position-related complications. Paddings, pillows and special jelly frames are required for achieving the best posture on the surgical bed and to protect the patient against damage from inadvertent pressure ischemia. Nerve injuries and skin pressure injuries result from poor positioning, with direct pressure causing ischemia to that area. Spine surgery involving vertebral fusion and instrumentation often requires special operating tables and the patient in a prone position. Special attention must be paid in these cases, because cardiovascular and respiratory functions may be compromised in this position. Body weight should be distributed unburdening the abdomen in order to minimise venous congestion, and direct pressure on the eyeballs must be carefully avoided. The arms should not be abducted or extended greater than 90° from the natural position, and the weight of the arms should be evenly distributed across the forearm to avoid ulnar nerve compression at the elbow. Positioning may be even more challenging in children with important deformities and particular caution is warranted. The use of intraoperative radiologic imaging is common, radioprotective barriers should be used, and radiation exposure must be monitored by the anaesthetist, as well.

7.1.6   Intraoperative Warming

The detrimental effects of hypothermia include increased rates of wound infection, increased blood loss and increased length of stay in recovery room and hospital. Hypothermia exacerbates blood loss by decreasing platelet function, interfering with coagulation factors' activity and slowing vasoconstriction. Therefore, the monitoring of patient's core temperature is advisable, and several precautions help maintaining normothermia in the perioperative period. They include active patient warming using forced-air devices, the preservation of a comfortable temperature in the operating room at least until the patient is positioned and covered and an adequate warming of intravenous fluids and blood products before infusion [4]. Furthermore, some diseases, such as osteogenesis imperfecta or arthrogryposis multiplex congenita, may be associated with altered baseline temperature regulation. In these patients, core temperature monitoring is mandatory and special attention must be addressed to its perioperative maintenance (Fig. 7.3).

7.1.7   Tourniquet

Tourniquets are commonly used in surgery to establish and maintain a bloodless surgical field, allowing the surgeon to work with greater technical precision and safety. Nonetheless, the widespread use of tourniquets in orthopaedic surgery in adults and children is not without risks, and the surgical literature includes numerous reports of injuries and hazards associated with tourniquet overpressurization,

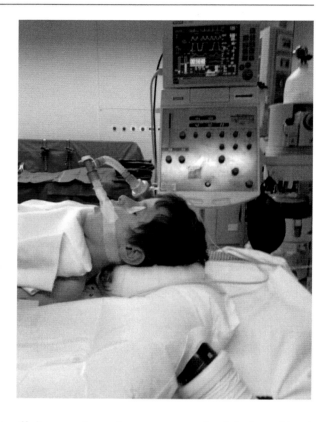

like pain at the tourniquet cuff site; muscle weakness; compression injuries to blood vessels, nerves, muscles or skin and extremity paralysis. Underpressurization, vice versa, may result in blood leakage in the surgical field and venous congestion of the limb. Overall, the risk of tourniquet-related injuries can be reduced minimising tourniquet inflation time, using automatic tourniquet instruments and cuffs that allow accurate pressure delivery, control and monitoring and maintaining tourniquet cuff pressure near the minimum level required to stop arterial blood flow in the operated limb. Indeed, significantly lower tourniquet cuff pressures based on limb occlusion pressure (LOP) and the use of wide contour cuffs can be used effectively and safely in the paediatric population without compromising the quality of a bloodless surgical field [5]. LOP is the minimal cuff pressure required to occlude arterial blood flow into a patient's limb with a specific tourniquet cuff at a specific moment. LOP may be determined manually by slowly increasing tourniquet cuff pressure until distal arterial pulsations cease at the Doppler stethoscope or with a recently developed automated plethysmographic system. Previous studies in children showed that tourniquet cuff pressures based on LOP measurements before cuff inflation significantly decreased mean tourniquet cuff pressures and were sufficient to maintain a satisfactory surgical field [6]. Before tourniquet application, a flat rubber bandage named Esmarch's bandage will be wrapped repeatedly around the limb to

Table 7.2 Recommendations for pneumatic tourniquet use in paediatric limb surgery

1. Use the widest cuff suitable for the selected limb location, and use a contoured cuff able to match the taper of the thigh
2. Select a limb protection sleeve specifically designed for the selected cuff. If such sleeve is not available, apply two layers of elastic bandage sized such that its basal compression is minor than venous pressure ($\approx$20 mmHg) and less than a snugly applied cuff
3. Accurately apply the tourniquet cuff over the sleeve, avoiding fluid collection between the cuff or the sleeve and the patient's skin
4. Using the applied cuff, measure the LOP and set tourniquet pressure, respectively, 50, 75 or 100 mmHg above LOP for LOP < 130 mmHg, 131 < LOP < 190 mmHg or >190 mmHg. To measure the occlusion pressure, use a plethysmographic tourniquet system or a Doppler stethoscope. For manual measurement, locate an arterial pulse distal to the tourniquet, slowly inflate the cuff until arterial pulse stops for several heartbeats, then deflate and confirm that the pulse resumes. Measurement must be done once systemic blood pressure is stable at the level expected during surgery. Note that the limb should remain horizontal and motionless
5. Exsanguinate the limb by elevation or elastic bandage
6. Inflate the tourniquet cuff and monitor the tourniquet during use
7. If arterial blood flow over the tourniquet cuff is observed, increase cuff pressure in 25 mmHg increments until flow stops
8. Minimise tourniquet inflation time
9. Remove the cuff and the sleeve of the tourniquet immediately after the deflation

Adapted from Reilly et al. [5]

make it bloodless, and a soft dressing will be applied to the limb at the tourniquet site to avoid wrinkles and blisters (Table 7.2). Adequate exsanguination can also be achieved by elevation of the limb at 90° or 45° for the upper or the lower extremities, respectively. Also the anaesthetic conduct may influence the effects of tourniquet application. In fact, both the continuous propofol infusion and regional anaesthesia techniques attenuate lipid peroxidation and decrease tourniquet-related injuries in paediatric limb surgery [7]. Also intraoperative temperature regulation may be affected by tourniquet application owing to a combination of decreased heat loss from the ischemic limb and a reduced heat transfer from the central to the ischemic peripheral compartment.

7.1.8   Blood Management

Paediatric patients undergoing major orthopaedic surgery are at risk of significant intraoperative blood loss. The judicious use of blood transfusion is imperative both because of limited blood bank supply and because transfusions can lead to various complications. Awareness of infectious hazards of transfusion prompted a more thoughtful approach to blood product administration, greater tolerance of asymptomatic anaemia, more attention to medical, preoperative treatment of anaemia and greater attention to surgical haemostasis. Whenever possible, a cost-effective approach is based on the identification and treatment of preoperative anaemia, and, in most circumstances, it can be accomplished with nothing more than oral iron therapy. Fortunately, the amount of blood transfused for many surgical procedures has decreased in recent years. A close observation (or surveillance) of the operative field helps to estimate blood loss, while the monitoring of vital signs, haematocrit, urine output and central venous pressure is valuable to assess the adequacy of volume replacement and are useful tools in blood-sparing strategies [8, 9].

7.1.8.1 Preoperative Donation of Autologous Blood

As the hazard gap between allogeneic and autologous transfusions narrows (the risk of bacterial infection and mistransfusion are almost the same for the two alternatives), a balanced appraisal of the beneficial and detrimental effects of both is appropriate. Importantly, autologous blood donation (ABD) should not be attempted in children with significant ischaemic cardiac disease or in paediatric patients with an active infection, because bacteria can contaminate the collected unit and overgrow during storage. ABD should be discouraged before procedures for which RBC transfusion is unlikely and in children with needle phobia and limited collaboration capacity. Erythropoietin proved to be useful in a wide variety of patients, including preterm infants, children on chemotherapy, children with renal failure and children undergoing elective major reconstructive surgery, spine surgery, liver transplantation, cardiac surgery and Jehovah's witnesses. Erythropoietin stimulates erythropoiesis by the bone marrow. Recommended is recombinant erythropoietin, 600 U/kg sc, once or twice weekly, 3–4 weeks before surgery with supplementation of iron, vitamin B12, vitamin E and folic acid oral supplementation. Coordination with the haematology unit, blood bank and the primary patient care team is required to take full advantage of this therapy, especially if ABD is programmed. Common practice is to donate one unit per week, but the last unit should be donated at least 5–7 days prior to surgery to allow plasma proteins to normalise, to restore intravascular volume and to allow adequate erythropoiesis so that the patient will not be anaemic on the day of surgery. Banked units of autologous blood may be stored for 35–42 days in the liquid state. Because of the risk of incorrect patient identification and possible bacterial contamination, also autologous blood has to be transfused only if strictly indicated.

7.1.8.2 Intraoperative Blood Recovery and Reinfusion

Acute normovolaemic haemodilution involves withdrawal of a calculated volume of the patient's blood after the induction of anaesthesia with simultaneous volume replacement with crystalloid or colloid infusion. The patient's own fresh blood is carefully stored in a refrigerator and reinfused in the final phase of surgery. The two major advantages of intraoperative haemodilution are the following: blood lost during surgery has a low haematocrit and fresh, whole autologous blood is available for transfusion.

Intraoperative red cell salvage (CS), i.e. the process of collecting shed blood during surgery and reinfusing it to the patients, is often used as an effective blood conservation strategy, and CS has been linked with reduced ABT. The blood recovered from the surgical field will be washed, centrifugated and reinfused. In this way, infectious and immunologic risks of allogeneic transfusion and the risk of mistransfusion will be avoided. Intraoperative blood recovery compared with allogeneic blood transfusion proved cost saving and cost-effective also in paediatric orthopaedic surgery [10]. Nonetheless, this CS is not widely used in paediatric patients, probably because of the capital investment for the devices, the significant costs of disposable parts and the need for a trained operator. CS may be particularly useful to minimise allogeneic blood transfusion in scoliosis surgery, and it may also be used in conjunction with preoperative autologous blood donation, further reducing the need for allogeneic RBC transfusions. The development of paediatric-sized equipment should make this technique more widely used and more cost-effective even in small children. Major contraindications to CS are infection or contamination of the surgical field, sickle cell disease and surgery for malignancies.

7.1.8.3 Antifibrinolytics

The fibrinolytic system is the most important antithrombotic mechanism that maintains vascular patency. Major surgery and trauma cause extensive tissue injury and release large amounts of tissue activators (tissue plasminogen activator, kallikrein and urokinase) leading to a shift from physiological fibrinolysis to hyperfibrinolysis, which decreases clot stability and increases tendency to bleeding, leading to coagulopathy, fibrinogen and clot factor consumption. Antifibrinolytic drugs reduce fibrin degradation through inhibition of plasmin generation, therefore decreasing surgical bleeding and the need for transfusion in adults and children [11]. Tranexamic acid (TXA) is worldwide the most used synthetic antifibrinolytic agent. TXA has a higher and more sustained antifibrinolytic activity in tissue (i.e. ten times stronger) compared to ε-aminocaproic acid, and it is more effective at reducing postoperative and total blood loss in spine surgery. The half-life of TXA is about 80–90 min in patients with normal renal function, and for this reason, a maintenance infusion or repeated administration is generally required to achieve an optimal haemostatic effect. Dosage schemes are not based on pharmacokinetic studies, and there is a large variability in initial loading dose, varying between 2 and 100 mg/kg and a continuous infusion of 3–10 mg/kg/h. Our dosage scheme for paediatric population is 50 mg/kg of intravenous TXA as loading dose (2 g max), followed by an infusion of 5 mg/kg/h.

7.1.8.4 Transfusion Trigger

The "absolute" threshold for red blood cell transfusion is a controversial topic, especially in the paediatric population. Most of the actual recommendations are based on expert opinion or derived from adult studies, and, as observed in adults, the trend in paediatric patients has been toward a lower absolute transfusion trigger. As important as the preoperative preparation of the patient to optimise the Hb level is the awareness that there is no universal trigger for the administration of allogeneic blood products, and clinical decision must be based on the single patient. In the absence of co-morbidities which compromise organ oxygenation or limit the compensatory mechanisms for anaemia, Hb levels as low as 7 g/dL are generally well tolerated and transfusion is recommended if the Hb is lower than 6 g/dL [12].

7.1.9   Postoperative Care

The absence of a family member, the strange environment, hunger, changes in body temperature, the presence of peripheral venous access or a cast are factors that may all contribute to increase the discomfort of the paediatric patient awakening from anaesthesia. A recovery room that permits awaking in the presence of parents and adequate pain control is essential in orthopaedic paediatric surgery. Caring for an alert, calm and cooperative child reduces the workload for nurses in the recovery room because children who are pain-free are less inclined to be uncooperative, and it is less likely that they interfere with the operation site (Fig. 7.4), removing dressings, drainage tubes or urinary catheters [13].

7.1.9.1 Pain Treatment

Acute perioperative pain in infants and children is still undertreated, although intraoperative and postoperative analgesia significantly improved in the last decades. Intense pain without adequate analgesia will not only cause unacceptable pain at the time of intervention, it will also produce long-lasting pain memory and behavioural disorders [14]. Orthopaedic surgery is one of the most painful and it is frequently described to be more painful than expected. To counteract pain in the immediate postoperative period in infants and children, an adequate multimodal pain therapy concept must be implemented, and local or regional anaesthesia (Fig. 7.5) should be performed whenever possible [15]. Acetaminophen (paracetamol) and NSAIDs are the most common analgesics prescribed for moderate pain in orthopaedics and they should be regularly administered after any painful intervention. Regular, round-the-clock administration of these drugs decreases the need of opioid rescue, and their intravenous administration assures the analgesic effect before the child is able to do oral intake. Opioids should be given immediately and sufficiently whenever necessary, and they may be administered by the intravenous, oral, transmucosal and transdermal route. Long-term pain associated with limb-lengthening techniques, like the Ilizarov frame, or paediatric oncologic orthopaedic surgery, may require oral intake

Fig. 7.4 Ilizarov frame in a 9-year-old female affected by Cornelia de Lange syndrome

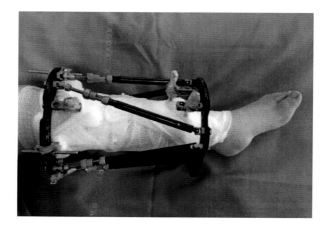

Fig. 7.5 Continuous sciatic nerve block for pain treatment in septic arthritis of the ankle

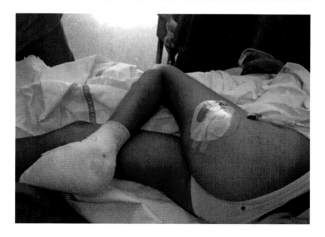

of opioids after hospital discharge. Opioids may also be added to neuraxial anaesthesia through the epidural or spinal route for postoperative pain treatment. Benzodiazepines provide sedative, anxiolytic and amnesic effect; they have no analgesic properties but are synergic with pain medication when muscle spasm is a component of pain.

Regional anaesthesia in children is an evolving technique with many advantages in perioperative management compared with systemic analgesia. Indeed, the profound analgesia delivered by regional anaesthesia provides ideal psychological conditions for the recovering children and their family, reducing emergence agitation and anxiety often present in the orthopaedic setting. Unfortunately, even for established regional techniques, such as the caudal block, the evidence for procedure-specific indications is not currently well defined [16, 17]. Nowadays, we are able to use regional anaesthesia techniques in more than 80 % of orthopaedic procedures in children. There is significant evidence on a transition from neuraxial to peripheral nerve blocks in clinical practice. The main concern regarding single-shot nerve blocks, even with adjuvant, is the limited duration of analgesia, which is usually sufficient for a large number of orthopaedic procedures, but insufficient in many cases of major surgery. Continuous peripheral nerve blocks (CPNBs) are one of the most recent developments in paediatric regional anaesthesia, and it is a valuable alternative to parenteral opioids or continuous neuraxial blockade for several types of surgery [18, 19].

CPNBs proved superior to traditional opioid-based analgesia in terms of improved analgesia with reduced sedation, nausea, pruritus and length of hospital stay [20]. The multimodal pre-emptive analgesia involves the use of low concentration, motor-sparing blocks in conjunction with other analgesics such as opioids, NSAIDs and acetaminophen. This technique aims to facilitate early ambulation by providing excellent analgesia without accompanying motor weakness. Dadure demonstrated that CPNBs are feasible in the paediatric setting and that in skilled hands they promote prolonged analgesia in the majority of patients without major adverse events. The most common minor adverse events are catheter-related mechanical problems dominated by leakage of local anaesthetic around the catheter and catheter dislodgment [21]. Other minor adverse events are less common in CPNBs compared to continuous epidural infusion.

CPNBs are indicated after major orthopaedic surgery in children, for complex regional pain syndromes, for phantom limb pain prevention and for managing vasospasm. Ropivacaine is the local anaesthetic most commonly administered in CPNBs, and the doses for continuous infusion range from 0.2 to 0.4 mg/kg/h at a concentration of 0.2 %. Specific indications for continuous analgesic treatment include hip, femoral, tibial and humeral osteotomies; traction of femoral shaft fracture; congenital foot or hand malformation; limb elongation; osteosynthesis and exostosis; toe, hand or foot amputation; club foot repair; hallux valgus repair; chronic oncologic pain but also painful physical therapy after knee and ankle arthrolysis or knee ligamentoplasty. Otherwise, painful rehabilitation and physiotherapy are other main indications to catheter positioning, because only if pain is under control, good rehabilitation will be performed [22]. A significant advantage of CPNBs over single injection nerve blocks is the ability to provide prolonged analgesia with relatively low doses of local anaesthetics. Patient-controlled regional anaesthesia is feasible also in paediatric patients, and it was demonstrated that patient-controlled regional anaesthesia with boluses of ropivacaine 0.2 % provides adequate postoperative analgesia with smaller doses of ropivacaine or levobupivacaine and lower total plasma concentrations of local anaesthetics than continuous infusion [23]. Low doses of local anaesthetics remain an important precaution for potential complications such as local anaesthetic systemic toxicity (LAST) and permit the use of these devices even at home after hospital discharge.

7.1.9.2 Compartment Syndrome

Compartment syndrome is a condition in which increased pressure within a closed compartment compromises tissue function and perfusion within that space. It occurs most commonly in an osteofascial compartment of the leg or the forearm, but it may occur in the upper arm, thigh, foot, buttock, hand and abdomen as well. The most common cause of compartment syndrome is a trauma, usually when a fracture occurred [24]. Acute compartment syndrome requires prompt diagnosis and management. Plaster cast immobilisation can cause compartment syndrome and pressure sores. In case of persisting pain, the cast should be removed and the area carefully examined. Delays in treatment can result in significant disability including neurological deficit, muscle necrosis, amputation and death. Severe pain and paraesthesia are often reported as cardinal symptoms, but many authors consider these symptoms unreliable, as they are subjective and variable. These symptoms are particularly difficult to assess at extreme ages or in patients with neurologic compromise, and there is unconvincing evidence that PCA, opioids or RA might delay the diagnosis of compartment syndrome. Main clinical signs are tense, swollen compartments, sensory loss and pulselessness of distal segments. Objective monitoring may be the measurement of compartment pressure by needle or catheter, the monitoring of tissue oxygenation by near-infrared spectroscopy (NIRS) or the dosage of serum creatine phosphokinase (CK) as an indicator of muscle necrosis [25]. High clinical suspicion, ongoing assessment of patients and compartment pressure measurements are essential for early diagnosis. The outcome is related to the time from diagnosis to fasciotomy, which allows tissue decompression and must be performed within 8 h. Delay in diagnosis may be a concern of surgeons when plexus blockade is performed in cases of fractures. It is important to highlight that compartment syndrome is one of the most painful experiences, and it cannot be masked by opioids or other drugs or diluted concentrations of local anaesthetics used for postoperative infusion. Nonetheless, it is nowadays inacceptable that the diagnosis of compartment syndrome is made thank to children's pain, especially when sufficient diagnostic tools are available [26]. Importantly, surgeries at risk for developing compartment syndrome must be excluded from ambulatory paediatric protocols.

7.1.9.3 Fat Embolism
Fat embolism (FES) has been rarely described in paediatric population, only case reports and small series are published, but it could be a fatal event [27]. The classic presentation includes neurologic abnormalities such as confusion, drowsiness, lethargy, convulsions, coma and hypoxia resulting from impaired respiratory function. These manifestations usually arise 12–24 h after the injury. A petechial rash on mucous membranes and skin, mainly of the thorax and neck region, often appears later, but it could be absent in about 50 % of the cases. Minor symptoms of FES are fever as high as 38.5 °C, decreased haematocrit, retinal changes and tachycardia. Patients may show severe hypoxia progressing to acute respiratory distress syndrome (ARDS) with pulmonary hypertension. Diagnosis is primarily clinical, but biological tests (serum lipase presence or elevation in urine or sputum, thrombocytopenia or blood coagulation disorders), echocardiography and imaging studies of brain and chest are useful diagnostic tools. Respiratory failure often dominates the clinical picture of FES and it represents the main cause of death for these patients. Treatment is based on supportive pulmonary therapy and on other resuscitative measures. Severe cases require mechanical ventilation and analgesia, fluids and cardiovascular supportive therapy. Caution in mobilisation and an early fixation of the fracture site are suggested to reduce the risk of FES. Despite its low incidence in children, FES has to be suspected in all patients that show hypoxia and altered consciousness after traumatic long-bone fracture or surgery.

7.1.9.4 Thromboprophylaxis
Venous thromboembolism (VTE) in children is a rare complication mainly because of limited direct evidence in paediatric population. Besides, about 50 % of currently available drugs are used unlicensed or off-label in these patients, reflecting the paucity of specific trials in children. Most recommendations are extrapolated from adults, and there is evidence that such approach may, in many circumstances, be inappropriate [28]. Rates of VTE associated with elective paediatric orthopaedic procedures seem to have a total incidence of 0.05 %, ranging from 0.02 to 0.33 %

in the paediatric trauma population [29]. Spine or spinal cord injuries, pelvic fracture and lower extremity fractures have an increased risk for VTE. Although rare, VTE is associated with 2.2 % mortality rate, while thrombosis recurs in about 8 % of the cases, and postphlebitic or postthrombotic syndrome occurs in 12–50 % of the patients. Besides, hospital costs are increased and length of stay in hospital is frequently prolonged. Interestingly, the development of a VTE is more frequently related to patients' co-morbidities, such as metabolic condition or syndrome, obesity, complications of implanted devices, older age and admission as an inpatient, more than to the kind of surgical procedure [30]. In addition to patients' age, clinicians need to consider factors such as physical development, stage of puberty and emotional and intellectual development. In absence of clear guidelines for VTE prophylaxis in paediatrics patient, low dose of unfractionated heparin or low-molecular-weight heparin combined with intermittent pneumatic compression may be a good choice in selected high-risk patients.

7.2 Peripheral Paediatric Orthopaedic Surgery

Peripheral paediatric orthopaedic surgery is defined as any surgery on muscles, tendons, bones or joints of children's limbs from the ileum or scapular to toes or fingers. Ambulatory surgery may be possible in appropriately selected patients undergoing a limited number of procedures, but frequently the anaesthetist have to take into account major orthopaedic surgery with intense postoperative pain. Children with skeletal abnormalities repeatedly present for orthopaedic procedures and often had previous experience of operating rooms (Fig. 7.6). Prophylactic, systematic and multimodal approach for pain control including regional anaesthesia assures high quality of postoperative analgesia. Regional anaesthesia is very useful in case of peripheral surgery in children, and it is generally performed in combination with general anaesthesia or deep sedation. This combination permits to reduce anaesthetic requirements. Most of

Fig. 7.6 Preprocedural scan for sacral plexus block in stump regulation after leg amputation in a 13-year-old female with Charge syndrome

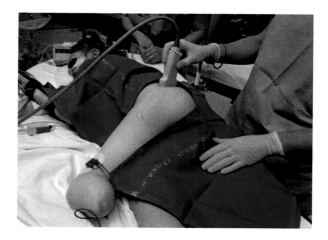

the anaesthetic agents produce a dose-related decrease in cardiorespiratory mechanics and central ventilatory control, particularly in neonates, infants and young children. The reduction of MAC offers several advantages including avoidance of airway instrumentation, and respiratory assistance is not usually required. Therefore, regional anaesthesia reduce the need for muscle relaxants, opioids and hypnotics; it allows smoother and more comfortable emergence, reduced wake-up times, more rapid discharge from recovery and earlier return of appetite. Importantly, RA will decrease the risks associated with deeper planes of general anaesthesia. Regional anaesthesia provides profound analgesia for orthopaedic surgery with minimal physiological perturbations and side effects. Spinal, epidural and peripheral nerve blocks are effective in obtunding the neuroendocrine stress response to surgical trauma, avoiding autonomic, hormonal, metabolic, immunologic, inflammatory and neurobehavioral consequences. Stress hormones (epinephrine, norepinephrine, adrenocorticotropic hormones, cortisol, prolactin) and blood glucose levels are lower following regional anaesthesia than after general anaesthesia, independently from opiate analgesia, and this occurs also when the central or regional block is placed at the end of surgery. Regional anaesthesia is an effective alternative to systemic analgesics, particularly when systemic opiates are contraindicated, such as in children at risk of opiate-induced respiratory depression (acute) or in patients that have become tolerant to their analgesic effects (chronic pain). General anaesthesia supplemented with pre-emptive regional anaesthesia produces better operating conditions and reduced risks of surgical blood loss in children, and this may contribute to shorter operating time. Wound infiltration with local anaesthetic has additional beneficial effects on the inflammatory response and stimulates the activity of natural killer cells. Single-shot blocks are limited by the duration of the local anaesthetic agent used. However, with the recent development and application of continuous peripheral nerve catheters, prolonged analgesia is possible. The decision to intubate the trachea or to use a supraglottic device like a laryngeal mask should be based on the usual criteria, such as a full stomach, intraoperative positioning, need to maintain adequate ventilation and the expected duration of the surgical procedure. If indicated, the trachea should be intubated before the block is performed. The difficult airway is not uncommon in children and the laryngeal mask may be an invaluable alternative. Various types of supraglottic devices (Fig. 7.7) are widely used for securing and maintaining a patent airway in orthopaedic surgery as an alternative to tracheal intubation in patients requiring general anaesthesia or very deep sedation. The main advantages of these devices include less or no need for muscle relaxation and the need for lower doses of anaesthetic drugs. Furthermore, these airway devices are less invasive and are applicable also in spontaneously breathing anaesthetised patients. The supraglottic devices can be inserted also if the space is limited and in children with head and neck vascular malformations. Pierre-Robin, Treacher-Collins, Goldenhar, cri-du-chat syndromes, and mucopolysaccharidoses are examples of conditions that have been successfully managed with these devices in different paediatric surgical settings. This approach avoids excessive airway instrumentation, minimises the risk of trauma and further airway obstruction due to bleeding or oedema, circumvents the "can't intubate, can't ventilate" scenario and can also act as a conduit to facilitate flexible fibreoptic bronchoscopy for

Fig. 7.7 Insertion of i-gel mask for airway management

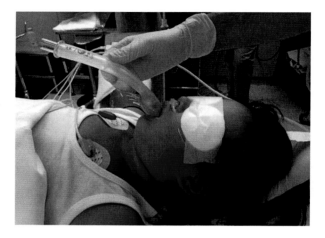

diagnostic or interventional purposes and to aid tracheal intubation [31]. The i-gel airway, an innovative supraglottic non-inflatable device made of a medical-grade thermoplastic elastomer (soft, gel-like and transparent), assures a high success rate of correct positioning at the first attempt, a short median insertion time, good oropharyngeal sealing pressure, ease of gastric tube placement and rare postoperative complications, like blood staining and sore throat. It seems to be safe, efficient and cost-effective [30, 32], and it may be extremely popular in children undergoing minor therapeutic and diagnostic procedures or short orthopaedic surgery not requiring controlled ventilation with muscle relaxants, like surgery of the upper and lower limbs.

7.2.1 Upper Limb

All kinds of upper extremity surgery can be managed with brachial plexus blockade, but these cases are still frequently managed in general anaesthesia in most of the institutions because of interdisciplinary and other organisational reasons. Forearm fractures and supracondylar humeral fractures are frequent findings in the paediatric emergency department, and they may require close reduction or open surgery. Closed reduction and cast immobilisation are usually facilitated by deep sedation of the paediatric patients. A variety of techniques have been used to induce analgesia in children with closed fractures requiring manipulation, including haematoma block, Bier block (intravenous regional anaesthesia) or peripheral nerve blocks [33]. Each technique has related advantages and disadvantages and the choice must be tailored on each child. Nonetheless, regional nerve block during manipulation has several benefits such as the significantly reduced need for sedation and systemic opiate analgesia, with less nausea and emesis. Motor blockade provides good muscle relaxation and makes the manipulation easier and faster. PNBs have a good safety profile, particularly with the use of ultrasound guidance, and provide better pain control in the postoperative period. Importantly, if the surgeon has to change strategy and convert to open reduction, the anaesthesia is just done and the surgeon can switch to open osteosynthesis. The duration of analgesia depends on the type of administered local anaesthetic, and it may last as long as 6 to 8 hours with long-acting agents like ropivacaine and levobupivacaine.

Elective surgery of the upper limb in paediatric orthopaedics includes correction of hand disorders like polydactyly, syndactyly and upper limb function and restoration for life care in arthrogryposis like humeral elongation, shoulder arthroscopy in the adolescent, humeral osteotomy, resection and treatment of tumours of the cephalic end of the humerus or upper extremity amputation.

All upper extremity blocks may be performed also in children, and in the recent Pediatric Regional Anesthesia Network (PRAN), it was found that most upper extremity blocks (82 %) were placed using US guidance [19]. Interscalenic block in paediatric orthopaedic surgery is less frequently adopted in clinical practice compared to the adult patients, because it is indicated only in case of shoulder luxation, shoulder arthroscopy in the adolescent, fracture of the proximal humerus and treatment of rare oncological pathologies. The surgical procedures below the mid-humeral level can be managed with axillary, infraclavicular or supraclavicular approaches. Infraclavicular and supraclavicular approaches are particularly recommended in patients with injured or fractured arm in order to avoid painful arm abduction. The supraclavicular approach is preferred because of the easily identified sonoanatomy, the ability to perform the block with a single injection and the low incidence of significant complications, but it is imperative to perform it with US guidance to avoid complications, such as pneumothorax and intravascular injection.

7.2.2 Lower Limb

Foot, ankle and long-bone osteotomies for correction of congenital or acquired lower limb abnormalities in children (Fig. 7.8) are common orthopaedic procedures. Regional anaesthesia in paediatric patients really improved in recent years, thanks to technical development, the availability of new equipment and increased information on the safety and pharmacology of local anaesthetics in children and infants. Caudal blocks, lumbar epidural and spinal anaesthesia are the neuraxial techniques applied as single or continuous injection in infants and children for surgery of the lower limb and the pelvis. Central neuraxial block in young children is characterised by remarkable hemodynamic stability, and clinical hypotension is seldom observed in children younger than 8 years of age [34]. Unlike in adults, in children, the adoption of ultrasound for central nerve blocks is increasing in clinical practice. Without considering the better resolution for more superficial structures that is generally observed in children, the very limited ossification of bony structures allows good visual resolution of central neuraxial anatomy, perception of the inserted needle and the spread of injected solutions [35]. Few, small studies proved that there may be benefits from ultrasound guidance, but there is still insufficient evidence. Ultrasound imaging during and/or before performing neuraxial block may reliably

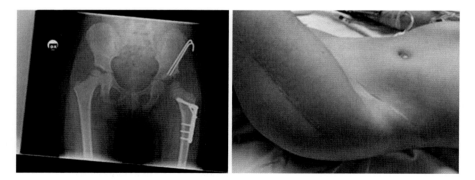

Fig. 7.8 Hardware removal after pelvic osteotomy acc. Salter and femoral varus derotation osteotomy in a 4-year-old female (16 kg)

predict the expected depth for loss of resistance, and it may enable dynamic view during the procedure. For unilateral lower limb surgery in adults, alternatives to epidural analgesia are CPNBs, and they probably represent the gold standard for postoperative analgesia after major unilateral surgery. CPNBs are associated with a reduced incidence of side effects when compared with epidural analgesia, and anaesthesia is restricted to the involved area [36]. In adults, the use of CPNBs is increasing in parallel with the evidence for their efficacy. In some meta-analyses, postoperative analgesia provided with perineural analgesia was superior to opioids at all time periods and for all catheter locations [37]. Unfortunately, there is extreme paucity of medical literature regarding feasibility, safety and efficacy of continuous nerve blockade in the paediatric population. Benefits for children include, even if performed in general anaesthesia, site-specific analgesia, reduced side effects, early discharge from hospital and significant reduction in healthcare resource utilisations [38]. The use of ultrasound guidance is recommended for increasing the success and safety of both single and continuous peripheral nerve blocks.

The lumbar plexus or psoas compartment block (PSCB) is useful for hip, thigh, femur and knee surgery (Fig. 7.9). This plexus of nerves travels between the dorsal and the intermediate portion of the psoas muscle and comprises the ventral rami of the first four lumbar roots, frequently including a branch of T12. These spinal nerves divide into ventral and dorsal branches as the plexus runs distally. Relevant nerves derived from this plexus include femoral, lateral femoral cutaneous and obturator nerves. The use of PSCB in experienced hands combined with general anaesthesia is considered a safe technique for open hip reduction and osteotomies for hip dysplasia in small children, and it is considered superior to single-shot caudal block for postoperative analgesia [39]. Compared to epidural anaesthesia, PSCB is associated with significantly less adverse events and lower total ropivacaine doses and plasma concentration [40]. A valid and more simple alternative for postoperative pain treatment in pelvic osteotomy may be a catheter surgically placed in the fascia iliaca compartment with subsequent continuous fascia iliaca block infusing larger volumes of local anaesthetics at lower concentrations [41].

Fig. 7.9 US-guided
continuous PSCB for hip
surgery

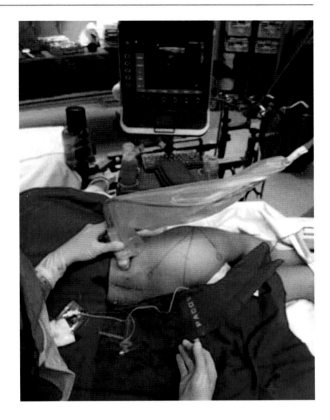

More distal types of peripheral surgeries below the knee level, such as leg fracture and foot surgery, like club foot surgery, mostly require saphenous or femoral
(FN) and sciatic nerve (SN) blocks. For anterior knee procedures like knee arthroscopy, an FN block may be sufficient (Fig. 7.10). However, consideration should be
given to adding an obturator nerve (ON) block for coverage of the medial aspect of
the knee, while lateral femoral cutaneous nerve (LFCN) blockade is advisable
when the lateral aspect of the knee is involved. Similarly, the SN should be blocked
when surgery involves the posterior aspect of the knee, such as in the case of anterior cruciate ligament repair when hamstring allograft is performed. FN block has
been used to provide analgesia for femur fractures in paediatric patients. However,
surgical repair of femur fractures usually requires an incision within the distribution
of the LFCN. Ultrasound-guided LFCN and FN block have been reported in paediatric patients for postoperative analgesia following surgical repair of femur
fractures.
  Many complications in infants and non-verbal children are difficult to diagnose
for impossibility to describe their symptoms accurately. Nevertheless, the incidence
of serious complications detected in the PRAN study was extremely small, and no
sequelae lasting >3 months were reported. Problems such as catheter dislodgement,

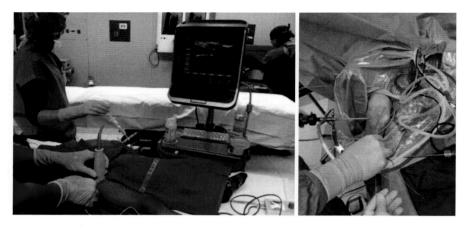

Fig. 7.10 US-guided femoral nerve block for knee arthroscopy

kinking and malfunction were especially common, accounting for one-third of all postoperative adverse events, suggesting that devising better methods of placement and fixation should be a high priority. This study confirmed the reduced performance of neuraxial anaesthesia in favour of peripheral nerve blocks for lower limb surgery in recent years. Peripheral regional anaesthesia proved effective in paediatric patients, and it was burdened with less complications and adverse events. Most of these procedures were performed with ultrasound guidance augmenting procedural safety.

7.3 Scoliosis Surgery

Currently, scoliosis is defined as lateral deviation of the normal vertical line of the spine greater than 10° when measured on a radiograph. Because the lateral curve of the spine is associated with rotation of the vertebrae, a three-dimensional deformity occurs. Procedures involving the spinal column and surgery for scoliosis repair became common in the paediatric age group during the last decades and provide a multitude of challenges to the anaesthetist. Spinal deformities requiring orthopaedic surgical intervention may be the result of congenital, acquired or traumatic conditions. Children often present concomitant diseases that affect the cardiovascular and respiratory function. Operating time may be protracted, significant blood loss is possible and strategies for blood sparing and blood product management are warranted. Surgical procedures on the paediatric spine may involve one or several vertebral levels with an incision at any level of the vertebral column (cervical, thoracic, lumbar, sacral). Further variations include an anterior approach, a posterior approach or, in the case of thoracic and lumbar spine procedures, a combined anteroposterior procedure (Fig. 7.11).

The magnitude of the scoliotic curve is commonly measured using the Cobb method. Measurement is made from an anteroposterior radiography, identifying all the vertebrae involved within the curve. The apical vertebra is the one with the

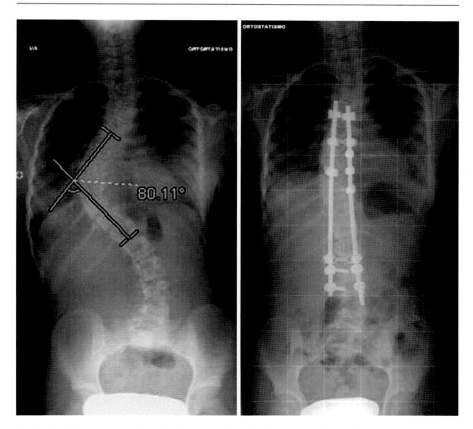

Fig. 7.11 Measurement of scoliosis curve using the Cobb method in a 10-year-old female with idiopathic scoliosis before and after spinal surgery (Images courtesy of D.A. Fabris Monterumici, Spine Surgery Unit, University General Hospital, Padua, Italy)

greatest body rotation and displacement from the ideal alignment. The top and bottom vertebrae of the curved or scoliotic segment are then identified. These vertebrae have the most evident tilt but the least degree of rotation and displacement. They are located above and below the apical vertebra, respectively. A line is drawn along the edge of these two vertebrae and extended out. On the top vertebra, the line is drawn along the upper edge and slopes downward according to the angle of the vertebra. On the bottom vertebra, the line is drawn along the lower edge in an upward direction. Perpendicular lines are then drawn from both lines so that they cross at the level of the apical vertebra. The Cobb angle is the angle formed by these two intersecting lines, and if it exceeds 40°, surgery will be frequently indicated. Vertebral rotation and rib cage deformity usually accompany any lateral curve [42]. There are various classifications of scoliosis, but from an anaesthetic perspective, the etiologic classification is more useful. Two main etiological groups of paediatric scoliosis exist: neuromuscular scoliosis (NMS) secondary to a wide range of underlying pathologies such as cerebral palsy, Duchenne muscular dystrophy, spinal muscular dystrophy, Friedrich ataxia, Marfan syndrome or osteogenesis imperfecta, and idiopathic scoliosis (IS), a genetically modulated growth abnormality, which tends to be more common in girls. While the latter is a diagnosis of exclusion, the former has defined criteria and subgrouping, of which cerebral palsy is the most common form. Children with scoliosis of early onset (<5 years) or with independent cardiac or pulmonary diseases appear to have increased risk of respiratory failure. Vertebral rotation and rib cage deformity result in distortion in the thorax and can cause restrictive lung defect, with restriction of lung volume and function for impaired movement and reduced compliance. In the long term, this may lead to hypoxemia, hypercarbia, recurrent lung infections and pulmonary hypertension. Spinal instrumentation for the treatment of scoliosis is performed when conservative treatment measures have failed to arrest the progression of the spinal curvature (Fig. 7.12). Patients with NMS are often younger and sicker at the time of surgery. In addition, the skeletal deformity is usually more severe and extended than in patients with idiopathic disease. Children with NMS add mechanical distortion to deteriorating muscle function, and the natural history of the specific neuromuscular disease must be considered. In these children, respiratory complications are five times more common than in patients with IS. Furthermore, pneumonia, pulmonary oedema and upper airway obstruction are more common when scoliosis is associated with

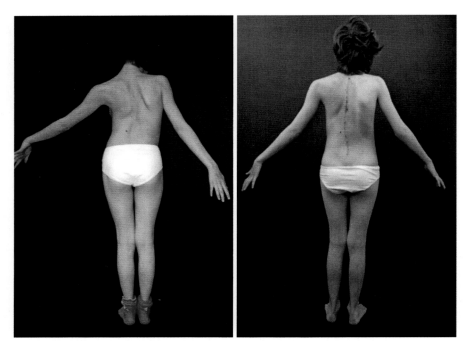

Fig. 7.12 The same patient with IS before and after spine surgery (Images of D.A. Fabris Monterumici, Spine Surgery Unit, University General Hospital, Padua, Italy)

mental retardation and developmental delay. Among these patients, those with cerebral palsy have the highest complication rate [43, 44].

Surgery for scoliosis correction is a major undertaking associated with significant blood loss and cardiac and pulmonary complications related to the effects of the patient's distorted anatomy. Important preoperative variables are pulmonary function, Cobb angle and number of fused vertebra, which may predict the outcome of the immediate postoperative period. In some medical centres, patients are admitted to the intensive care unit following scoliosis surgery because of the prolonged anaesthesia, the need for efficient pain control and the known immediate postoperative complications, which are most commonly pulmonary (atelectasis, pneumothorax), gastrointestinal (paralytic ileus) and infective, although the most feared and unpredictable are the neurological complications. A relationship between intraoperative blood loss and postoperative complications was established; ICU admission for patients with one or more of the above-mentioned complications is probably justified, but it may be unnecessary in many patients. Co-morbidity, the time of day and staffing level on the orthopaedic ward should also be taken into account. Especially in elective paediatric spine deformity surgery, many efforts should focus on minimising allogeneic blood transfusion. The estimated blood loss (EBL) is 60–150 ml per vertebral segmented fused in children with IS. In children with cerebral palsy, this estimation is significantly higher, ranging from 100 to 190 ml per level while it may reach 200–280 ml per vertebral level in children with DMD. Factors implicated in the increased blood loss include neuromuscular aetiology, degree of spine curvature, number of fused spinal segments, weight and height of the patient, surgical complexity including reoperation and more complex anteroposterior approach or lumbosacral fusion, coexisting pulmonary disease, intraoperative arterial blood pressure control and dilution coagulopathy [45, 46].

A large-bore intravenous access with a fluid warmer and an arterial line for invasive blood pressure and arterial blood gases monitoring must be routinely applied. A central line should be placed if massive blood loss is expected (e.g. >1 blood volume) or if vascular access is limited. The long preparation time and exposure of an undraped child on the spinal frame may predispose to hypothermia and require additional effort for maintaining normothermia for optimal clotting and hemodynamic stability. It will be useful to position a warming blanket underneath the frame so that warming from below occurs. Some spinal table or frame may negatively impact cardiac function, and correct positioning without abdominal compression is important to minimise venous congestion and intraoperative bleeding (Fig. 7.13). Direct control of bleeding via mechanical occlusion and topical haemostatic agents may be blood sparing as well. Routine complete blood count, electrolytes and clotting studies must be performed during surgery. Consumption of clotting factors as well as dilution of clotting factors enhances the blood loss. Normal saline, autologous blood recovery and transfusion of blood and fresh frozen plasma must be given according to estimated blood loss, intraoperative blood test results and hemodynamic status. Patients treated with TXA lost significantly less blood and received significantly fewer blood transfusions than the control group without significant differences in intra- and postoperative complications. Controlled hypotension with

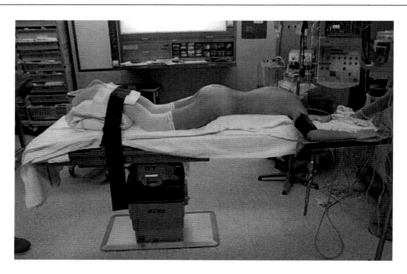

Fig. 7.13 Intraoperative prone position for posterior approach in spine surgery

a targeted mean arterial pressure of 50–60 mmHg is recommended. The use of remifentanil enabled better achievement of permissive hypotension during surgery, shorter operation times and early postoperative spontaneous ventilation with reduced need for ICU hospitalisation and no increase in significant complications. In a retrospective analysis (25 years) of paediatric patients undergoing elective scoliosis surgery at the Mayo Clinic [47], a significant change in blood management strategies was observed with lower transfusion trigger, a significant increase in allogeneic RBC transfusion and a significant increase in preoperative autologous donation and intraoperative autotransfusion. Although the patients had worse baseline co-morbidities and lower perioperative Hb level, they did not observe any increase in morbidity or mortality.

Early detection of spinal cord injury during surgery requires intraoperative spinal cord monitoring with neurophysiologic monitoring of the motor evoked potentials (MEPs) end somatosensorial evoked potentials (SSEPs). Utility of wake-up test, consisting in decreasing the depth of anaesthesia almost to awaking and asking the child to respond to verbal commands, is limited by the fact that it may be conducted a significant time after neurologic insult and delay the correction of the spinal instrumentation; it is less specific and it may be performed only in neurologically normal children. Somatosensory and motor evoked potentials are useful to record, but they request specific anaesthetic regimen with monitoring of anaesthetic depth by bispectral analysis (BIS) [48]. Although inhalational anaesthetics and most intravenous anaesthetics markedly depress SSEPs and MEPs, ketamine and etomidate seem to enhance the amplitude of both, possibly by attenuating inhibition. During MEP monitoring, neuromuscular blockade must be limited, and in many centres, neuromuscular blocking drugs are not given after intubation, initial incision and muscle dissection, especially if children suffered preoperative neuromuscular dysfunction.

Extubation criteria are the commonly accepted: awake, calm and cooperative patient, hemodynamic stability, negative inspiratory force >20 cm H2O, respiratory rate <30 min, $PaCo2 < 50$ mmHg and $PaO2 > 70$ mmHg with $FiO2 < 0.4$. No active bleeding from the operative site or from the drains. Relatively young and healthy children with IS operated on propofol and remifentanil and fused posteriorly can be successfully managed in a regular ward in the postoperative period. Postoperative visual loss in spine surgery is extremely rare, but it remains a dreaded complication despite significant efforts to identify risk factors and a pathophysiological mechanism. The vast majority of cases are related to ischemic optic neuropathy [49].

Spinal fusion surgery for correction of scoliosis is considered one of the most invasive procedures performed in paediatrics. Because of the significant length of the surgical incision and the degree of bony and soft tissue dissection, there may be significant postoperative pain, and if it is not treated adequately, it may contribute to chronic postsurgical pain. In many cases, the experience of pain is relatively transient and declines predictably over time with recovery from surgery, while in other cases, pain persists for several months engendering problems in everyday functioning. Currently, there is an increasing trend toward the use of pre-emptive multimodal analgesia as well as a significant interest in the application of regional anaesthetic techniques as a means of controlling pain following spine surgery in children using intrathecal or epidural single-shot or catheter technique [50]. Effective analgesia is generally best provided using a pre-emptive multimodality approach, which includes analgesic agents (paracetamol, NSAIDs, ketamine and opioids), anxiolytic agents and medications to control muscle spasms. Muscle spasms may be particularly problematic in patients with underlying cerebral palsy. Options for the provision of analgesia include also the use of patient-controlled analgesia (PCA). Although young patients or those with developmental disabilities may not be able to activate the device, nurse-controlled or parent-controlled analgesia may be provided. Using the device in this manner, the bedside parent or nurse has ready access to a supply of opioid to provide an immediate rescue dose. Importantly, prior to instituting PCA, an appropriate level of analgesia must be achieved by careful opioid titration. This is generally done in the operating room on completion of the surgical procedure. A choice may be fixed doses of intravenous paracetamol every 6 h, administration of NSAIDs at fixed intervals and PCA with morphine.

References

1. Khoury C et al (2009) Combined regional and general anesthesia for ambulatory peripheral orthopedic surgery in children. J Pediatr Orthop B 18:37–45
2. Jeongwoo L et al (2012) Cartoon distraction alleviates anxiety in children during induction of anesthesia. Anesth Analg 115:1168–1173
3. Stone MB et al (2008) Ultrasound-guided supraclavicular brachial plexus nerve block vs procedural sedation for the treatment of upper extremity emergencies. Am J Emerg Med 26:706–710
4. Warttig S et al (2014) Interventions for treating inadvertent postoperative hypothermia. Cochrane Database Syst Rev 20(11):CD009892

5. Reilly CW et al (2009) Minimizing tourniquet pressure in pediatric anterior cruciate ligament reconstructive surgery. J Pediatr Orthop 29:275–280
6. Lieberman JR et al (1997) Tourniquet pressures on pediatric patients: a clinical study. Orthopedics 20:1143–1147
7. Budić I et al (2010) The effects of different anesthesia techniques on free radical production after tourniquet-induced ischemia-reperfusion injury at children's age. Vojnosanit Pregl 67(8):659–664
8. Hyatt Sherman C, MacIvoe DC (2012) Blood utilization: fostering an effective hospital transfusion culture. J Clin Anesth 24:155–163
9. Goobie SM, Haas T (2014) Bleeding management for pediatric craniotomies and craniofacial surgery. Paediatr Anaesth 24:678–689
10. Samnaliev M et al (2013) Economic evaluation of cell salvage in pediatric surgery. Paediatr Anaesth 23:1027–1034
11. Faraoni D, Goobvie SM (2014) The efficacy of antifibrinolytic drugs in children undergoing non cardiac surgery: a systematic review of the literature. Anesth Analg 118(3):628–636
12. Secher EL et al (2013) Transfusion in critically ill children: an ongoing dilemma. Acta Anaesthesiol Scand 57:684–691
13. Bosenberg A (2012) Benefits of regional anesthesia in children. Paediatr Anaesth 22:10–18
14. Lonnquist PA, Morton NS (2005) Postoperative analgesia in infants and children. Br J Anaesth 95:59–68
15. Schultz-Machata AM et al (2014) What's new in pediatric acute pain therapy? Curr Opin Anaesthesiol 27:316–322
16. Suresh S et al (2014) Regional anaesthesia to improve pain outcomes in paediatric surgical patients: a qualitative systematic review of randomized controlled trials. Br J Anaesth 113(3):375–390
17. Marhofer P et al (2012) Everyday regional anesthesia in children. Paediatr Anaesth 22:995–1001
18. Ivani G, Mossetti V (2010) Continuous central and perineural infusions for postoperative pain control in children. Curr Opin Anaesthesiol 23:637–642
19. Dadure C, Capdevila X (2012) Peripheral catheter techniques. Paediatr Anaesth 22:93–101
20. Swenson JD (2010) Use of catheters in the postoperative patient. Orthopedics 33(9):20–22
21. Polaner DM et al (2012) Pediatric regional anesthesia network (PRAN): a multi-institutional study of the use and incidence of complications of pediatric regional anesthesia. Anesth Analg 115(6):1353–1364
22. Ludot H et al (2008) Continuous peripheral nerve block for postoperative pain control at home: a prospective feasibility study in children. Reg Anesth Pain Med 33:52–56
23. Duflo F et al (2006) Efficacy and plasma levels of ropivacaine for children: controlled regional anesthesia following lower limb surgery. Br J Anaesth 97:250–254
24. Mar GJ et al (2009) Acute compartment syndrome of the lower limb and the effect of postoperative analgesia and diagnosis. Br J Anaesth 102(1):3–11
25. Tobias JD (2007) Near-infrared spectroscopy identifies compartment syndrome in an infant. J Pediatr Orthop 27:311–313
26. Marhofer P et al (2012) Ultrasound-guided upper extremity blocks – tips and tricks to improve the clinical practice. Paediatr Anaesth 22:65–71
27. Stroud MH et al (2006) Fatal pulmonary fat embolism following spinal fusion surgery. Pediatr Crit Care Med 7:263–266
28. Monagle P et al (2012) Antithrombotic therapy in neonates and children: antithrombotic therapy and prevention of thrombosis, 9th ed: American College of Chest Physicians Evidence-Based Clinical Practice Guidelines. Chest 141(2 Suppl):737–801
29. Thompson AJ et al (2013) Venous thromboembolism prophylaxis in the pediatric trauma population. J Pediatr Surg 48:1413–1421
30. Georgopoulus G et al (2015) Incidence of deep vein thrombosis and pulmonary embolism in the elective pediatric orthopaedic patient. J Pediatr Orthop (Epub ahead of print)

31. Patel B, Bingham R (2009) Laryngeal mask airway and other supraglottic airway devices in paediatric practice. Contin Educ Anaesth Crit Care Pain 9(1):6–9
32. Smith P, Bailey CR (2015) A performance comparison of the paediatric i-gelTM with other supraglottic airway devices. Anesthesia 70:84–92
33. Kriwanek KL et al (2006) Axillary block for analgesia during manipulation of forearm fractures in the pediatric emergency department. J Pediatr Orthop 26(6):737–740
34. Murat I et al (1987) Continuous epidural anesthesia in children. Clinical haemodynamic implications. Br J Anaesth 59:1441–1450
35. Tsui B, Suresh S (2010) Ultrasound imaging for regional anesthesia in infants, children and adolescents: a review of current literature and its application in the praxis of neuraxial blocks. Anesthesiology 112:719–728
36. Fowler SJ et al (2008) Epidural analgesia compared with peripheral nerve blockade after major knee surgery: a systematic review and meta-analysis of randomized trials. Br J Anaesth 100:154–164
37. Richman JM et al (2006) Does continuous peripheral block provide superior pain control to opioids? A meta-analysis. Anesth Analg 102:248–257
38. Illfeld BM et al (2004) Continuous regional analgesia following ambulatory pediatric orthopedic surgery. Am J Orthop 33:405–408
39. Omar AM et al (2011) Psoas compartment block for acute postoperative pain management after hip surgery in pediatrics. A comparative study with caudal analgesia. Reg Anesth Pain Med 36:121–124
40. Dadure C et al (2010) Continuous epidural block versus continuous psoas compartment block for postoperative analgesia after major hip or femoral surgery in children: a prospective comparative randomized study. Ann Fr Anesth Reanim 29:610–615
41. Lako SJ et al (2009) Incisional continuous fascia iliaca block provides more effective pain relief and fewer side effects than opioids after pelvic osteotomy in children. Anesth Analg 109:1799–1803
42. Cunin V (2015) Early-onset scoliosis – current treatment. Orthop Traumatol Surg Res 101:109–118
43. Abu-Kishk I et al (2013) Pediatric scoliosis surgery – is postoperative intensive care unit admission really necessary? Paediatr Anaesth 23:271–277
44. Sullivan DJ et al (2014) Complications in pediatric scoliosis surgery. Paediatr Anaesth 24:406–411
45. Carreon LY et al (2007) Non neurological complications following surgery for adolescent idiopathic scoliosis surgery. J Bone Joint Surg Am 89:2427–2432
46. Vitale MG et al (2002) Quantifying risk of transfusion in children undergoing spine surgery. Spine J 2:166–172
47. Long TR, Stans AA, Shaughnessy WJ et al (2012) Changes in red blood cell transfusion practice during the past quarter century: a retrospective analysis of pediatric patients undergoing elective scoliosis surgery using the Mayo database. Spine J 12:455–462
48. Martin DP et al (2014) A preliminary study of volatile agents or total intravenous anesthesia for neurophysiological monitoring during posterior spinal fusion in adolescents with idiopathic scoliosis. Spine 39:E1318–E1324
49. Nickels TJ et al (2014) Perioperative visual loss after spine surgery. World J Orthop 5(2):100–106
50. Borgeat A, Blumenthal S (2008) Postoperative pain management following scoliosis surgery. Curr Opin Anaesthesiol 21:313–316

Perioperative Care of the Pediatric Neurosurgical Patient

8

Massimo Lamperti

The improvement in diagnosis, treatment, and outcome in infants and children treated for neurosurgical procedures has increased in the last years due to the new technologies available for neuromonitoring, standardized protocols for anesthesia maintenance, improved postoperative acute care, and highly specialized anesthesiologist taking care of these patients. The anesthesiologist taking care for neurosurgical patients has to keep in mind that neurological diseases are often long-term diseases and their management has to include since the beginning patients' families, psychologists, and an integrated social care system as these diseases can be associated with mild to severe disabilities.

The developing brain of a child has specific aspects to be considered such as age-dependent differences in anatomy, metabolism, cerebrovascular physiology, and locations of neurologic lesions. The perioperative management of children undergoing neurosurgical procedures is based on the acknowledgments of the differences on the pediatric neurophysiology, the neurosurgical procedures, and treatment of related complications.

8.1 Neurophysiology of the Pediatric Brain

8.1.1 Cerebral Blood Flow

Cerebral blood flow (CBF) varies with age. CBF of newborns and premature infants is lower than adults (40–42 ml 100 g^{-1} min^{-1}), while in term infants and older children, values become higher than in adults. From 6 months to 3 years, the CBF is thought to be 90 ml 100 g^{-1} min^{-1} and from 3 to 12 years at 100 ml 100 g^{-1} min^{-1} [1, 2].

M. Lamperti, MD
Anesthesiology Institute, Cleveland Clinic Abu Dhabi (CCAD), Swing Wing L7-207,
P O Box# 112412, Al Maryah Island, Abu Dhabi, United Arab Emirates (UAE)
e-mail: LamperM@ClevelandClinicAbuDhabi.ae

© Springer International Publishing Switzerland 2016
M. Astuto, P.M. Ingelmo (eds.), *Perioperative Medicine in Pediatric Anesthesia*,
Anesthesia, Intensive Care and Pain in Neonates and Children,
DOI 10.1007/978-3-319-21960-8_8

8.1.2   Brain Energy Metabolism

The brain requires large amounts of energy to maintain its cellular integrity and support neurotransmission. The pediatric brain has a higher glucose consumption (6.8 mg of glucose per 100 g^{-1} min^{-1}) compared to an adult brain (5.5 mg per 100 g 100 g^{-1} min^{-1}). The brain has no reserve of glucose to face this large requirement. Glucose is stored as glycogen and enters the glial cells (mostly astrocytes) using a facilitated ATP Na+ −K+ transport system. This membrane transport system is limited by its kinetic constant, and the amount of glucose transported into the astrocytes actually decreases when the plasma glucose level increases. This could provide some protection to the brain tissue against excessive intracellular hyperglycemia in the normal brain. However, the glucose transport system could be altered in case of brain injury leading to hyperglycemia and secondary brain tissue damage. As a consequence a tight glycemic control is mandatory to prevent and treat the injured brain [3, 4].

8.1.3   Cerebral Oxygen Metabolism

With the only exception of the glomic cells in the carotid body, the brain is the organ with the highest rate of oxygen consumption. It is 3.5 ml $O2 \times min^{-1} \times 100$ g^{-1} in adult and 5.5 ml $O2 \times min^{-1} \times 100$ g^{-1} in children. When this is compared with the overall oxygen consumption rate of the body (0.3 ml $O2 \times min^{-1} \times 100$ g^{-1}), it is more evident why the brain is very sensitive to hypoxia. Most of the oxygen consumption in the brain is used to maintain cellular integrity and electrogenesis and sustain cellular transport mechanism such as reuptake of neurotransmitters. When the supply of oxygen decreases, electrogenesis is impaired and quickly ceases. Cerebral autoregulation and cerebrovascular reactivity are impaired and the neuronal integrity is jeopardized. In the presence of hypoxia, ion pump impairment prevents normal membrane repolarization and leaves the neuron in a constant refractory state. Neuronal integrity is initially maintained, and if oxygen supply is restored, neuronal function resumes rapidly (zona pellucida). With ongoing lack of oxygen, however, neuronal viability and integrity deteriorate with increasing duration of hypoxia (zona penumbra). In this brain tissue area, neuronal damage will become irreversible if hypoxia persists at normothermia.

8.1.4   Arterial Carbon Dioxide/Oxygen Tension (Pa$_{CO2}$/Pa$_{O2}$)

Arterial Pa_{CO2} has a major vasodilatory effect on cerebral blood vessels, leading to an increase in CBF, which is linear between a Pa_{CO2} of 3.5 and 8 kPa. At birth, the cerebrovascular response to changes in Pa_{CO2} is incompletely developed. For this reason, moderate hypocapnia has mild effects on the newborn brain compared to adults and CBF has only moderate changes until severe hypocapnia occurs. Brain ischemia due to hypocapnia is thought to be caused by the effect of pH and CO_2 on cerebral vascular tone. The association between hypocapnia and clinical adverse outcome in various studies in adults and children has resulted in the advice to apply therapeutic hypocapnia only after careful consideration of the risks and the potential benefits. Special attention should be given to avoid accidental hypocapnia [5].

Capnography is standard in anesthesia monitoring and to prevent hypo- and hypercapnia. It is of crucial importance to be aware of the limitations of the end-tidal measurement of carbon dioxide ($ETCO_2$) in the neonate and small infants. Although the $ETCO_2$ value is in general lower than the corresponding Pa_{CO2} value, in some patients, the $ETCO_2$ overestimates Pa_{CO2}. The frequent evaluation of the capillary or arterial blood CO_2 trend is mandatory for the prevention of clinical hypocapnia in long procedures, major surgery, and compromised neonates.

The cerebral vasculature of adults is less sensitive to changes in Pa_{O2} and CBF does not increase until Pa_{O2} decreases below 50 mmHg, when it increases exponentially. In neonates, CBF is more sensitive to hypoxia and increases even in response to smaller decreases in Pa_{O2} [6].

8.1.5 Blood Pressure and Cerebral Autoregulation

The lower limits of cerebral autoregulation in neonates are not precisely known, and there is likely a wide range of variability in infants. Several studies have shown that the lower limit of cerebral autoregulation for some infants is indeed fairly close to the definition of hypotension using the infant's age in gestational weeks although there is also evidence that some premature infants are able to demonstrate cerebral autoregulation at a MAP level considerably lower than their gestational age in weeks [7, 8]. Vavilala et al [9] found that in infants older than 6 months of age undergoing a sevoflurane anesthesia, the lower limit of cerebral autoregulation for mean arterial pressure (MAP) was found to be 59 mmHg, which was 11 mmHg lower than baseline blood pressures. The lower limit of cerebral autoregulation of older children was also found to be 60 mmHg, but was 22 mmHg lower than baseline blood pressures. A study of children younger than 2 years undergoing sevoflurane anesthesia found that in infants <6 months of age, the lower limit of autoregulation occurred at 38 mmHg or a 20 % decrease from baseline awake MAP [10]. In contrast the same authors found that, in infants older than 6 months, the lower limit of autoregulation did not occur until blood pressure had decreased 40 %. These studies demonstrate that infants have less cerebral autoregulatory reserve and may be at the risk of inadequate cerebral perfusion following a decrease in blood pressure after anesthetic induction.

Inadequate perfusion from hypotension can lead to partial asphyxia. Most general anesthetics are associated with some degree of hypotension, which can be ameliorated by surgical stimulation. Prolonged inductions or surgical preparation times may lead to prolonged periods of hypotension in neonates. Ideally, general anesthesia should decrease cerebral metabolic rate and thus decrease the need for intraoperative neuronal substrate. However, it is not known whether common volatile and intravenous general anesthetics, which are gamma-aminobutyric acid (GABA) receptor agonists, lead to a lowered cerebral metabolic rate in young infants.

The difficulties of anesthetizing young infants can be compounded by inaccurate blood pressure monitoring. It is essential to assure a proper noninvasive blood pressure monitoring during induction and maintenance or before an invasive arterial monitoring is placed.

8.1.6   Intracranial Pressure

The Monro-Kellie doctrine states that the skull is a closed box containing the brain, blood, and cerebrospinal fluid (CSF). An increase in volume of one of these components, with an increase in intracranial pressure (ICP), will result in a compensatory reduction in the other components to counteract the change. In the infant, before cranial suture fusion, decompression can occur through an increase in skull size. The posterior fontanelle closes at about 6 months of age, and the anterior fontanelle at around 12–18 months. The final cranial suture closure may be as late as 10 years old. Increases in intracranial volume can only be accommodated if the change is gradual. Acute increases, such as after traumatic brain injury, will still result in raised ICP as in adults.

The infant may not demonstrate signs typically associated with intracranial hypertension, because the cranium can substantially expand in response to an expanding intracranial brain mass or process causing hydrocephalus, before coming to clinical attention. Early in the course, infants and young children often do not exhibit the traditional signs of intracranial hypertension such as bradycardia, elevated systemic blood pressure, dilation of the pupils, and papilledema. If present, these signal severe progression with poor outcomes. Neonates and infants may present with increased head circumference, bulging fontanelles, widened cranial sutures, "sundowning" of the eyes, irritability, drowsiness, poor feeding, or lower motor deficits.

8.1.7   Brain and Inflammation

The brain was thought not to be involved in the inflammatory processes. New studies suggest that in traumatic brain injury [11] subarachnoid hemorrhage [12], a severe cerebral inflammatory reaction, is activated. Systemic inflammatory reactions affect the brain while cerebral inflammatory processes lead to significant systemic effects. Cerebral ischemia and reperfusion injury are the main causes of brain damage because of the inflammatory reactions they start.

Currently, there is no clinical evidence to suggest that direct inflammatory modulation reduces the incidence of mortality or morbidity in patients affected with a cerebral insult [13]. The secondary effects of an inflammatory reaction such as hypoxia, hypotension, hyperthermia, and hyperglycemia are known to induce secondary brain injury and should be prevented.

8.1.8 Pediatric Electrophysiology

Children develop different pathological conditions from adults that are often age specific. The electroencephalogram (EEG) recording is different in children than adults because the brain, meninges, skull, scalp, head size, and the child's behavior and ability to cooperate all change over time.

Therefore, pediatric EEGs must be recorded and interpreted with special attention given to the child's age and developmental level. An EEGer must be aware of normal age-specific characteristics. For example, the normal pediatric EEG activity has more variation than the adult EEG. Focalities are not always abnormal but lack of change between states is abnormal in infants. As EEG varies greatly by age, its interpretation needs to be conceptually age specific [14–17].

8.1.9 Anesthesia and Neurotoxicity

Data supporting anesthetic neurotoxicity have been presented more than 10 years ago [18, 19]. Researchers found that exposure of developing rodents to ethanol, a known N-methyl-D-aspartate (NMDA) receptor antagonist and gamma-aminobutyric acid (GABA) receptor agonist, during a critical period of development resulted in widespread neuroapoptosis of the central nervous system [20]. Most anesthetic agents were studied for their potential negative effects via these receptors. Further studies tried to confirm the potential role of general anesthetics in neurodegeneration [21] and long-term deficits in developing monkeys [22–24]. The histologic changes induced by anesthetics exposure not only damage neurons but even oligodendrocytes [22].

Although there are evidences, it should be almost impossible to extrapolate those results to humans as any randomized controlled trial would deserve ethical consequences if the same methods should applied in neonates and children. All studies reported in the literature on general anesthetics' neurotoxicity in children are retrospective. Most studies supporting the association between neurocognitive outcome and exposure to anesthetics showed hazard ratios less than 2 [25–28]. At the current time, retrospective human data remain hypotheses generating, rather than conclusion generating.

8.2 Perioperative Management

8.2.1 Preoperative Assessment

The preoperative assessment of the pediatric neurosurgical patient includes understanding of the underlying neurological pathology and a thorough assessment of any coexisting diseases, medications, intravascular volume status, and anesthetic history.

Children with brain tumors can have a variety of signs and symptoms that may affect the conduct of anesthesia such as drowsiness, lethargy, seizures, cranial nerve palsies, focal muscle weakness, hypothalamic-pituitary axis hormonal deficiencies, nausea, and vomiting.

Intracranial hypertension should be kept great consideration, as it can become a life threatening during induction and early phases of the anesthesia. Intense crying or screaming or fighting can cause significant elevations in ICP. Premedication with oral midazolam has shown significant benefits with no respiratory depression or change in Pa_{CO2}. Opioids may produce respiratory depression and should be used with caution in patients with elevated ICP. Ketamine should be avoided in patients with elevated ICP as it increases both cerebral blood flow (CBF) and cerebral metabolic rate.

The intravascular blood volume could be contracted because of poor intake or recurrent vomiting. Children may have abnormal airways because of associated craniofacial abnormalities. Pediatric patients have a higher risk for perioperative respiratory and cardiovascular morbidity and mortality than adults [29].

8.2.2 Induction

Infants and children without intravenous access will undergo inhalational induction. As volatile anesthetics can increase in CBF, it is important to support or control the ventilation to prevent the Pa_{CO2} increase and offset the rise in CBF. Non-depolarizing neuromuscular blocking agent could also be administered to facilitate endotracheal intubation and prevents the increase of ICP.

Patients with lethargy or nausea and vomiting are at risk for aspiration of gastric contents and will benefit from a modified rapid sequence induction technique.

8.2.3 Monitoring

Intracranial surgery may be associated with sudden cardiovascular changes and the potential for rapid blood loss. Routine monitoring includes capnography, pulse oximetry, electrocardiography, temperature, and invasive arterial pressure. Urethral catheterization and the measurement of urine output are necessary for prolonged procedures and especially those associated with diabetes insipidus or the requirement for mannitol. A central venous catheter (CVC) provides large-bore access and allows for central administration of vasoactive drugs and potentially treatment of venous air embolism (VAE). Readings can be unreliable in small children in the prone position but trends may be useful.

Precordial Doppler ultrasonography could be useful for VAE detection.

Neurophysiological monitoring may be utilized with the aim to improve outcome and reduce morbidity by early detection of neurological injury at a point when damage can be limited or reversed. In brief, the modalities for monitoring include EEG, somatosensory evoked potentials (SSEPs), motor evoked potentials (MEPs), and transcranial Doppler (TCD).

8.2.4   Positioning

Proper position of the patient for pediatric neurosurgical procedures is imperative to ensure both patient safety and comfort. Most patients undergoing neurosurgery are in a supine position. The flexion of the neck may result in downward migration of the endotracheal tube or occlusion of jugular venous drainage, causing cerebral venous hypertension and increased intracranial volume and pressure. The prone position raises the risk of eye injury from direct ocular pressure and hypoperfusion. The park-bench position is utilized for lateral or midline incisions and when quick access to the patient is needed. Appropriate padding and stabilization is required to prevent stretch, ischemia, and pressure injury to the axilla as well as other parts of the body. The sitting position requires careful attention to padding pressure points as well as securing the patient on the bed to ensure patient safety and surgical stability.

8.2.5   Maintenance of General Anesthesia

Maintenance of anesthesia commonly is accomplished with a balanced anesthetic technique of opioids, volatile anesthetic, and neuromuscular blockade. Volatile anesthetics may significantly blunt cerebral autoregulation in a dose-dependent manner by producing cerebral vasodilatation and exacerbate intracranial hypertension. Inhalational anesthetics also alter the evoked potentials that are used in neurological monitoring. These agents are typically avoided or used at low concentration of 0.5 MAC or less.

Infusions of short-acting opioids such as sufentanil or remifentanil can provide adequate intraoperative analgesia and rapid emergence, permitting postoperative neurological assessment. A remifentanil infusion commenced at the induction of anesthesia can readily be titrated to response and avoids the hypotension and bradycardia associated with boluses of remifentanil in children. Remifentanil usually obviates the need for repeated doses of neuromuscular blocking agents.

Total intravenous anesthesia (TIVA) with propofol may be used in older children, but its widespread use in younger children has been limited due to the original weight restrictions on target controlled infusion devices.

Dexmedetomidine can be used as an adjunct. It does not significantly affect most intraoperative neurophysiologic monitoring and reduces opioid requirements.

Neuromuscular blockade is typically used unless the case requires intraoperative assessment of motor nerve function, as in spinal cord or epilepsy surgery.

8.2.6   Fluid Management

Glucose-containing and hypotonic solutions should not be used in pediatric patients. Hyperglycemia worsens reperfusion injury, and hypotonic infusions increase cerebral edema. However, the dangers of hypoglycemia particularly in the neonate or ex-premature infant should be considered and blood glucose monitored closely. The commonly used isotonic crystalloids are Ringer's lactate and 0.9 % sodium chloride. Excessive quantities of normal saline can result in hypernatremia and hyperchloremic metabolic acidosis. For these reasons, electrolytes and blood glucose should be monitored especially during long procedures.

Blood loss can be difficult to assess during craniotomies due to constant oozing onto the surgical drapes and irrigation. There is a potential for sudden and drastic losses, so cross-matched blood should always be available. Transfusion of 10 ml/kg of packed red blood cells increases hemoglobin concentration by 2 g/dl. Pediatric patients are susceptible to dilutional thrombocytopenia in the setting of massive blood loss and multiple red blood cell transfusions. Administration of 5–10 ml/kg of platelets increases the platelet count by 50,000–100,000/mm^3. The routine use of the antifibrinolytic agent, tranexamic acid, in surgical procedures with excessive blood loss, such as posterior spine fusions and craniofacial reconstructive procedures, has been shown to decrease blood loss in pediatric patients [30].

8.2.7 Body Temperature

Mild hypothermia (34–35 °C) decreases in CMRO2 and may help to attenuate raised ICP. However, it is essential to appreciate the complications of hypothermia (e.g., disordered coagulation), the importance of normothermia for adequate emergence from anesthesia, and the time required to rewarm even a mildly hypothermic child, especially an infant. Fluid warmers, warm air devices, and heated mattresses are required.

8.2.8 Venous Air Embolism (VAE)

VAE is a major risk in patients in sitting position or in those with the head of bed significantly elevated. Continuous precordial Doppler ultrasound allows early detection of a VAE and normovolemia minimizes this risk. In case of VAE producing significant reduction of the ETCO2 and hemodynamic instability, the operating table must be placed in the Trendelenburg position to prevent further embolism of intravascular air. Significant rotation of the head can also impair venous return through a compression of the jugular veins. However these measures can reduce cerebral perfusion, increased intracranial pressure, and venous bleeding. Special risks exist in neonates and young infants as right-to-left cardiac mixing lesions can result in paradoxical emboli.

8.2.9 Postoperative Care

Postoperative care is determined by the complexity of the surgical procedure and the physiologic alterations that may occur during the operative course. Generally extracranial procedures usually need routine postoperative care.

Intracranial procedures and other major neurosurgical cases may require postoperative care in the pediatric intensive care unit (PICU).

In the past, many clinicians avoided morphine analgesia due to the side effects of vomiting, sedation, and its potential effect on pupil size. However, strong opioids provide effective analgesia without increase in complications. Acetaminophen is usually started intraoperatively and continued regularly after operation.

8.3   Main Postoperative Complications

8.3.1   Hyponatremia

Hyponatremia is the most common electrolyte disturbance in patients undergoing neurosurgery. Severe hyponatremia may result in brain swelling and the symptoms reflect its effects on the central nervous system. Initial symptoms may include headache, nausea, and vomiting; as hyponatremia worsens, mental confusion, seizures, stupor, and coma may develop.

Hyponatremia of neurosurgical patients is often associated with a syndrome of inappropriate antidiuretic hormone secretion (SIADH) or with the salt-wasting brain syndrome (SWS). The differential diagnosis between these two clinical conditions is essential, since treatment strategies are completely different.

Patients with SIADH need fluid restriction of approximately 70 mL/100 kcal and may need furosemide and/or increased sodium supply due to an excess ADH secretion. Volume replacement with an isotonic solution and increased sodium supply are mandatory in the salt-wasting syndrome to prevent severe dehydration.

8.3.2   Diabetes Insipidus

The removal of brain lesions in the suprasella could affect the pituitary function and impaired the ADH secretion. The reduced secretion of ADH causes hypernatremia due to intravascular volume depletion, polyuria, and dehydration. This complication usually occurs within the first postoperative hours, when the urine output is higher than 3 ml/kg/h. Patients with diabetes insipidus typically present hypernatremia ($Na > 150$ mEq/L), urinary sodium levels below 20 mEq/L, and dehydration. Treatment is based on the administration of intranasal or intravenous desmopressin.

8.3.3   Hyperglycemia

This complication can be not uncommon in neurosurgical patients [31] and must be treated although it is not related to a worse outcome.

8.3.4   Brain Edema

Surgical manipulation of the brain and nervous tissues may cause perilesional edema in several grades, impacting the postoperative clinical symptomatology. There is lack of evidence warranting a benefit of systemic corticosteroid to reduce brain edema. Corticosteroid adverse effects, such as hyperglycemia, infection, and slow wound healing, are well known.

8.4   Perioperative Prophylaxis

Perioperative antibiotic prophylaxis by intravenous administration reduces the risk of surgical wound infection, although there is no consensus on short or extended time protocol [32]. Postoperative seizure prophylaxis is still debated. The current consensus is to continue the antiepileptic drugs if the patient had seizures before the neurosurgical intervention. There is no evidence on the prophylactic use of antiepileptic drugs in patients with brain tumors, and the use of these drugs is highly related to an increased risk of adverse events [33].

8.5   Main Neurosurgical Conditions in Pediatric Patients

8.5.1   Hydrocephalus and Shunt Procedures

The need for CSF drainage can be caused by an acute or chronic mismatch in cerebral fluid content circulation and related increase in ICP. CSF can be diverted commonly from cerebral ventricles to the peritoneal cavity or the right atrium. In some cases, if the CSF circulation is altered by an endoventricular problem, an endoscopic third ventriculostomy could be sufficient.

The main problem related to shunt procedures is heat conservation related to a large skin exposure especially in neonates. Fluid and body warmers and a strict core body temperature monitoring are mandatory in these patients.

8.5.2   Brain Tumors

Brain tumors are the most common solid tumor of childhood. Two-thirds of them arise infratentorially. The anesthetic implications of posterior fossa pathology include an increased likelihood of raised ICP due to CSF outflow obstruction and a higher occurrence of postoperative airway problems due to perioperative compromise of brainstem respiratory centers and lower cranial nerve function. The hemodynamic response to laryngoscopy and fixation of the head in pins may lead to a detrimental increase in ICP that should be attenuated by a potent opioid such as remifentanil.

A reinforced tracheal tube is recommended to aid positioning airway from the surgical field and avoid kinking associated with positioning and surgery duration. A throat pack aids in stabilizing the tube position.

Most patients require postoperative monitoring in a high dependency units or PICU to detect early changes in consciousness and neurological impairment.

8.5.3 Epilepsy Surgery

Medically intractable seizures have now several possible surgical options such as insertion of vagal stimulator, craniotomy for resection of epileptic foci, or hemispherectomy. Perioperative anesthetic considerations have to deal with developmental delay, perioperative seizures, and coexisting diseases. Intraoperative neurophysiologic monitoring useful for surgical removal of the epileptic foci can be impaired by volatile anesthetics. Nitrous oxide can precipitate pneumocephalus after a recent craniotomy (up to 3 weeks later) and should be avoided until after the dura is opened.

Awake craniotomy offers the advantage of allowing EEG mapping intraoperatively, minimizing unnecessary tissue resection, but this is usually possible only when children are mature and psychologically prepared to participate in this particular procedure. In the "sleep-awake-asleep" technique, the patient undergoes general anesthesia for the surgical exposure. The patient is then awakened for functional testing, and general anesthesia is recommended when patient's collaboration is not anymore necessary. Most cooperative patients will tolerate sedation with propofol or dexmedetomidine. Propofol does not interfere with EEG, if it is discontinued 20 min before monitoring in children undergoing an awake craniotomy [34]. Supplemental opioids are administered to provide analgesia.

Cerebral hemispherectomy techniques for medically intractable seizures have changed in the last decade, with a trend from anatomic (total) toward minimally invasive functional resections [35]. Significant intraoperative blood loss and hemodynamic instability of both techniques have an impact on the anesthetic management of these patients [36].

8.5.4 Craniosynostosis Repair

Craniosynostosis is the premature fusion of one or more cranial sutures. Single-suture craniosynostosis usually occurs in otherwise healthy children. Multiple suture disease often occurs also as part of a craniofacial syndrome such as Apert's, Crouzon's, or Pfeiffer's.

Techniques for cranial remodeling are varied and involve removal of the skull vault by the neurosurgical team followed by refashioning by plastic or maxillofacial surgeons.

Manipulation of the skull vault alters the skull shape to promote uniform growth in sagittal and coronal planes. The management of more complex multiple suture craniosynostosis with craniofacial anomalies has to be referred to tertiary centers.

Anesthetic management of craniofacial surgery has to consider the following aspects:

1. Blood loss: surgery for correction of these malformations has to be scheduled in a period of physiological anemia between 2 and 6 months. Bleeding comes from scalp wounds and bones, making it difficult to quantify accurately as it is hidden in surgical sponges. Blood products are invariably required perioperatively according surgical technique used. Tranexamic acid has been recently shown to attenuate massive blood loss and has been administered in surgical procedures associated with massive blood loss [37].
2. VAE: the patient is at risk during retraction of the scalp over the orbital ridge as the scalp veins are at an upper level than the right atrium. The current monitoring for VAE in neonates and children is precordial Doppler.
3. Oculocardiac reflex: profound bradycardia may result from orbital manipulation. It usually responds to removal of the stimulus and administration of antimuscarinic agents.
4. Airway: surgery below the orbital ridge is associated with excessive facial edema and may involve the use of a rigid extraction device frame. This may present the anesthesiologist with problems at the initial and subsequent surgeries.
5. Positioning: this will vary for individual procedures; particular care is needed around the eyes and to guard against excessive neck extension/flexion.

8.5.5 Congenital Spinal Lesions

Failure of the neural tube to close during the first trimester results in a disease spectrum ranging from spina bifida occulta to anencephaly.

The most common conditions presenting for neurosurgical correction are lumbosacral meningoceles. If posterior herniation includes neural structure (myelomeningocele), the distal neurological function is often severely impaired.

These defects require correction within the first few days of life to minimize bacterial contamination and sepsis. Main aspects in surgery for neural tube defects repair are:

1. Surgery in the first days after birth.
2. Bleeding: if a skin grafting is required, there may be a need for blood replacement.
3. Positioning: care must be taken to minimize pressure on the cystic structure, leading to further damage or rupture. Induction of anesthesia may be carried out in the lateral decubitus or more commonly supine, with a ring-shaped sponge to

support and relieve pressure from the herniation. Surgery is conducted in the prone position, and particular care is required to avoid abdominal compression and venous congestion of the operating site.

4. Latex allergy prevention: children with myelodysplasia have an increased risk of latex allergy and a latex-free environment is mandatory.

8.5.6 Vascular Malformations

The primary goal of anesthetic management during cerebrovascular surgery is to optimize cerebral perfusion while minimizing the risk of bleeding. Large arteriovenous malformations (AVMs) may be associated with high output congestive heart failure requiring vasopressors during general anesthesia. Hypertensive crisis after embolization or surgical resection of the AVMs should be rapidly treated with vasodilators as sodium nitroprusside.

These lesions are often managed by combined neurointerventional and neurosurgical approach, which start with endovascular occlusion of the lesion followed by surgical resection and ending with a postoperative angiography.

Management of patients with Moyamoya syndrome is targeted to optimize cerebral perfusion with aggressive preoperative hydration and maintaining normotension or mild hypertension during surgery and the postoperative period.

Intraoperative normocapnia is essential because both hypercapnia and hypocapnia can lead to steal phenomenon from the ischemic region. Intraoperative EEG monitoring may be utilized during surgery to detect cerebral ischemia. Optimization of cerebral perfusion should be extended into the postoperative period by maintaining euvolemia and maintaining sedation and analgesia in the PICU to prevent hyperventilation induced by pain and crying.

8.5.7 Neuro-Endoscopy and Anesthesia

Children undergoing third ventriculostomy surgery will be positioned in a Mayfield headrest. Warmed Ringer's lactate fluid is used to irrigate the operating site; measuring the volume of fluid infused and drained is imperative to avoid rapid increases in ICP. Hypertension, arrhythmias, and neurogenic pulmonary edema have been reported in conjunction with acute intracranial hypertension.

Conclusions

A comprehensive anatomical and physiological acknowledgment of pediatric brain function is essential to allow the anesthesiologist to maintain a balance in brain metabolism during anesthesia for neurosurgical procedures.

A specific training and a dedicated team of anesthesiologist, neurosurgeons, and nurses for those patients are crucial not only for perioperative management but also to create a special environment for children and their families.

References

1. Chiron C, Raynaud C, Maziere B et al (1992) Changes in regional cerebral blood flow during brain maturation in children and adolescents. J Nucl Med 33:696–703
2. Mackersie A (1999) Paediatric neuroanaesthesia. Balliere's Clin Anaesthesiol 13:593–604
3. Feinendegen LE, Herzog H, Thompson KH (2001) Cerebral glucose transport implies individualized glial cell function. J Cereb Blood Flow Metab 21:1160–1170
4. Weir CJ, Murray GD, Dyker AG et al (1997) Is hyperglycaemia an independent predictor of poor outcome after acute stroke? Results of a long-term follow up study. BMJ 314:1303–1306
5. Curley G, Kavanagh BP, Laffey JG (2011) Hypocapnia and the injured brain: evidence for harm. Crit Care Med 39:229–230
6. Krane EJ, Phillip BM, Yeh KK, Domino KB (1986) Anaesthesia for paediatric neurosurgery. In: Smith RM, Mototyama EK, Davis PJ (eds) Smith's anaesthesia for infants and children, vol 2006, 7th edn. Mosby, Philadelphia, pp 651–684
7. Munro MJ, Walker AM, Barfield CP (2004) Hypotensive extremely low birth weight infants have reduced cerebral blood flow. Pediatrics 114:1591–1596
8. Tyszczuk L, Meek J, Elwell C et al (1998) Cerebral blood flow is independent of mean arterial blood pressure in preterm infants undergoing intensive care. Pediatrics 102:337–341
9. Vavilala MS, Lee LA, Lam AM (2003) The lower limit of cerebral autoregulation in children during sevoflurane anesthesia. J Neurosurg Anesthesiol 15:307–312
10. Torvik A (1984) The pathogenesis of watershed infarcts in the brain. Stroke 15:221–223
11. Whalen MJ, Carlos TM, Kochanek PM et al (2000) Interleukin-8 is increased in cerebrospinal fluid of children with severe head injury. Crit Care Med 28:929–934
12. Chyatte D, Bruno G, Desai S et al (1999) Inflammation and intracranial aneurysms. Neurosurgery 45:1137–1146; discussion 1146–1147
13. Bracco D, Ravussin P (2000) Neuroinflammation and infection. Curr Opin Anaesthesiol 13:523–528
14. Blume WT (1982) Atlas of pediatric encephalography. Raven, New York
15. Holmes GL (1989) Diagnosis and management of seizures in children. W.B. Saunders Company, Philadelphia
16. Petersen I, Eeg-Olofsson O (1971) The development of the electroencephalogram in normal children from the age of 1 through 15 years. Neuropadiatrie 2:247–304
17. Novotny EJ (1998) The role of clinical neurophysiology in the management of epilepsy. J Clin Neurophysiol 15(2):98–108
18. Stratmann G (2011) Review article: neurotoxicity of anesthetic drugs in the developing brain. Anesth Analg 113:1170–1179
19. Pruett D, Waterman EH, Caughey AB (2013) Fetal alcohol exposure: consequences, diagnosis, and treatment. Obstet Gynecol Surv 68:62–69
20. Ikonomidou C, Bittigau P, Ishimaru MJ et al (2000) Ethanol-induced apoptotic neurodegeneration and fetal alcohol syndrome. Science 287:1056–1060
21. Jevtovic-Todorovic V, Hartman RE, Izumi Y et al (2003) Early exposure to common anesthetic agents causes widespread neurodegeneration in the developing rat brain and persistent learning deficits. J Neurosci 23:876–882
22. Brambrink AM, Back SA, Riddle A (2012) Isoflurane-induced apoptosis of oligodendrocytes in the neonatal primate brain. Ann Neurol 72:525–535
23. Brambrink AM, Evers AS, Avidan MS (2012) Ketamine-induced neuroapoptosis in the fetal and neonatal rhesus macaque brain. Anesthesiology 116:372–384
24. Brambrink AM, Evers AS, Avidan MS (2010) Isoflurane-induced neuroapoptosis in the neonatal rhesus macaque brain. Anesthesiology 112:834–841
25. Flick RP, Katusic SK, Colligan RC (2011) Cognitive and behavioral outcomes after early exposure to anesthesia and surgery. Pediatrics 128:e1053–e1061

26. Hansen TG, Pedersen JK, Henneberg SW (2011) Academic performance in adolescence after inguinal hernia repair in infancy: a nationwide cohort study. Anesthesiology 114:1076–1085
27. Ing C, DiMaggio C, Whitehouse A (2012) Long-term differences in language and cognitive function after childhood exposure to anesthesia. Pediatrics 130:e476–e485
28. Walker K, Halliday R, Holland AJ (2010) Early developmental outcome of infants with infantile hypertrophic pyloric stenosis. J Pediatr Surg 45:2369–2372
29. Cohen MM, Cameron CB, Duncan PG (1990) Pediatric anesthesia morbidity and mortality in the perioperative period. Anesth Analg 70:160–167
30. Faraoni D, Goobie SM (2014) The efficacy of antifibrinolytic drugs in children undergoing noncardiac surgery: a systematic review of the literature. Anesth Analg 118:628–636
31. Mekitarian Filho E, Carvalho WB, Cavalheiro S, Horigoshi NK, Freddi NA (2011) Hyperglycemia and postoperative outcomes in pediatric neurosurgery. Clinics 66:1637–1640
32. Barker F II (2007) Efficacy of prophylactic antibiotics against meningitis after craniotomy: a meta-analysis. Neurosurgery 60:887–894
33. Tremon-Lukats IW, Ratilal BO, Armstrong T, Gilbert MR (2008) Antiepileptic drugs for preventing seizures in people with brain tumors. Cochrane Database Syst Rev (2):CD004424
34. Soriano SG, Eldredge EA, Wang FK et al (2000) The effect of propofol on intraoperative electrocorticography and cortical stimulation during awake craniotomies in children. Paediatr Anaesth 10:29–34
35. Beier AD, Rutka JT (2013) Hemispherectomy: historical review and recent technical advances. Neurosurg Focus 34:E11
36. Flack S, Ojemann J, Haberkern C (2008) Cerebral hemispherectomy in infants and young children. Paediatr Anaesth 18:967–973
37. Sethna NF, Zurakowski D, Brustowicz RM et al (2005) Tranexamic acid reduces intraoperative blood loss in pediatric patients undergoing scoliosis surgery. Anesthesiology 102:727–732

Pain After Surgical Correction of Congenital Chest Wall Deformities

9

Robert Baird and Pablo M. Ingelmo

9.1 Pectus Excavatum

9.1.1 Background

This most common chest wall deformity involves posterior encroachment of the sternum and lower costal cartilages. While the precise incidence remains subjective, as many as 1–2 % of individuals may be affected, with boys typically presenting more frequently. In most instances, patients are asymptomatic and chiefly concerned with their cosmetic appearance; rarely, cardiopulmonary function may be compromised by the constraints of the chest wall. Some patients will have associated musculoskeletal conditions – Marfan and Loeys-Dietz syndrome are classic examples that should be ruled out when clinical suspicions arise [1].

The preoperative assessment of patients with PE involves a complete history and physical exam, paying particular attention for stigmata of an inheritable musculoskeletal condition. Patients should also be screened for metal allergies whenever an implant is expected. In addition, a CT scan for objective measurement of the defect and pulmonary function tests and echocardiography are standard evaluations in

R. Baird, MDCM, MSc, FRCSC, FACS (✉)
Department of Pediatric Surgery, MUHC, Montreal Children's Hospital, McGill University, Montreal, QC, Canada
e-mail: robert.baird@mcgill.ca

P.M. Ingelmo
Department of Anesthesia, Montreal Children's Hospital, MUHC, McGill University, Montreal, QC, Canada
e-mail: pablo.ingelmo@mcgill.ca

© Springer International Publishing Switzerland 2016
M. Astuto, P.M. Ingelmo (eds.), *Perioperative Medicine in Pediatric Anesthesia*,
Anesthesia, Intensive Care and Pain in Neonates and Children,
DOI 10.1007/978-3-319-21960-8_9

Fig. 9.1 CT scan of a
patient with severe PE
(Haller Index of 7) as
well as significant
sternal tilt

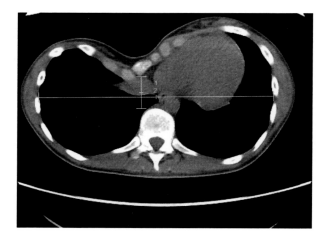

most high-volume centers (Fig. 9.1). Finally, a preoperative visit with the anesthesiology team is crucial to review perioperative pain-control strategies.

9.1.2 Surgical Technique

The standard approach to repair of PE is the thoracoscopic-assisted Nuss procedure.
Championed by Dr. Nuss and the team from Virginia, this procedure involves the
transthoracic insertion of a metal bar with affixation to the lateral chest wall [2, 3].
Briefly, after surgical marking and prophylactic antibiotic administration, oblique
skin incisions are made in the anterior axillary line at the point of deepest sternal
depression (typically T5–6). A second small incision is then made in the right chest,
and a port is inserted into the thoracic space followed by gentle insufflation and
insertion of a thoracoscope. A tunneler is then use to dissect from lateral to medial,
entering the chest just medial to the ridge above the point of maximal depression.
Once intrathoracic, the tunneler is then gradually advanced under direct vision
above the pericardium until the opposite chest is reached. Once brought through,
heavy suture material is affixed to both the tunneler and the chosen bar – after it has
been bent to shape. The tunneler is then slowly withdrawn, bringing the suture and
Nuss bar with it. Once the Nuss bar is in position, it is then flipped, immediately
correcting the deformity. Care is then taken to ensure the bar is adequately secured
to the lateral chest – a stabilizer is typically used on one side. Pneumothorax is then
ceased, air is allowed to egress from the chest, and wounds are closed in layers.

An alternative technique for repair of PE involves an open approach to remove
abnormal costal cartilages, performance of a wedge osteotomy to elevate the sternum, and insertion of a retrosternal strut to maintain the reconfigured sternum in
place. This modified Ravitch repair continues to have applications in patients with
stiff chest walls or those that have had prior attempts at a chest wall reconstruction.
It remains the procedure of choice for some surgeons [4].

9.1.3 Analgesic Considerations

Comparative studies have suggested that the Nuss procedure is associated with increased postoperative pain compared with the modified Ravitch procedure [5–7]. Nonetheless, no differences have been noted in patient satisfaction or overall outcomes between the two groups [8]. In both cases, the length of hospitalization is typically dictated by the ability to adequately achieve effective analgesia. A recent large multi-institutional observational study has demonstrated that pain typically crescendos at 8/10 (median) during hospitalization and improves to 3/10 before discharge with a variety of different analgesic techniques [9]. Importantly, this cohort of patients demonstrates improved body image and perceived ability for physical activity after surgery [10].

Three main options exist for early postoperative pain relief: thoracic epidural (TE), patient-controlled analgesia (PCA), and a continuous paravertebral nerve block (PVNB). Elective repair of pectus excavatum is an ideal indication for placement of a TE catheter – a recent global survey of 108 pediatric institutions revealed that 91 % of respondents used thoracic epidurals as the primary mode of analgesia [11]. While these allow for sparing systemic narcotics, concerns remain about rare but devastating complications like paraplegia [12]. Older prospective trials comparing epidural catheters with intravenous PCA have demonstrated equivalency in pain relief and length of stay [13, 14]. This has resulted in several centers publishing their preference for PCA, especially given the significant number of patients with failed epidurals [15, 16]. A recent randomized trial of 110 patients receiving either epidural or PCA revealed a 22 % failure rate for epidural and an increase in resource utilization for epidural patients with only modest differences in very early pain scores compared to PCA patients [17]. A subsequent meta-analysis of available literature confirmed a small improvement in pain scores through to 48 h after surgery, without significant differences in secondary outcomes [18].

Thus, it is currently unclear whether epidural or PCA is the optimal analgesic strategy given the apparent small benefit but small increased risk associated with epidural. An attractive alternative is a continuous paravertebral nerve block – potentially marrying the improved analgesia of an epidural without the increased risk [19]. Two recent retrospective comparisons of PVNB to standard epidural have suggested equivalent efficacy without the need for urinary catheterization [20, 21]. Clearly, further prospective evaluations of PVNB for pectus excavatum repair are required prior to widespread adoption.

Chronic pain after Nuss procedure remains a rare but devastating consequence after an elective operation. Twenty-two percent of anesthesiologists responding to a survey on the subject disclose referring at least one patient per year for chronic pain treatment [11]. The true rate of chronic pain after Nuss procedure is difficult to ascertain as is it not commonly reported in surgical reports. Every effort must be taken to adequately treat early postoperative pain with multimodal therapy in order to avoid the transition to long-term pain. Should this occur, dedicated treatment in a pain clinic should be considered mandatory.

9.2 Pectus Carinatum

9.2.1 Background

This deformity is generally believed to be less common than pectus excavatum, with centers reporting PC to be half as common as PE [22]. The deformity is manifest as overgrowth of the cartilaginous costo-sternal junctions. The deformity can be symmetric or asymmetric and occasionally involves protrusion of the manubrium as well. It is associated with other musculoskeletal conditions only very rarely and an extensive workup is typically unnecessary. Unlike PE, the treatment of choice for PC has rapidly become compression bracing. While reports of corsets and other binders have been in existence for many years, the modern era of bracing began with the description of dynamic compression bracing from Dr. Martinez-Ferro in Argentina [23]. This device gradually reduces the anteroposterior chest dimension while allowing room for lateral expansion. It (or variations of it) has been widely adopted and has made the operative repair of PC much less frequent [24]. Nonetheless, a subset of patients either desire immediate or delayed correction while others fail compression bracing and subsequently undergo surgery.

9.2.2 Surgical Techniques

Pectus carinatum is traditionally treated by the Ravitch procedure [25]. This involves excision of multiple offending costal cartilages followed by one or several osteotomies to achieve an appropriate chest contour. Typically, a large dissection is required and a closed-suction drain is left in the operative field and only removed once the output decreases. More recently, a "reverse Nuss" has been described. Also known as the Abramson based on its originator, a Nuss bar is passed in front of the deformation and secured under tension to the lateral thoracic wall in order to retract the protrusion [26]. This technique has shown promise; however further studies are required before it can be considered generalizable.

9.2.3 Analgesic Considerations

The Ravitch procedure is generally considered to be less painful than the Nuss procedure [5–7]. As a consequence, less effort has been placed in investigating analgesic strategies in the perioperative period. Although the reporting is incomplete, Fonkalsrud et al. report a series of Ravitch procedures without epidural placement and minimal analgesics required at the time of discharge to hospital [27]. For patients undergoing the "reverse Nuss," the most appropriate analogous operation is the Nuss and not the Ravitch. As such, the debate about thoracic epidural versus PCA versus the emerging option of PVNB is highly relevant. Further investigations will be required to evaluate this patient subset in further detail.

Conclusions

The correction of a chest wall deformity is very often a pivotal moment in the life of an adolescent. It is a decision designed to enhance a patient's quality of life and self-esteem; the pain associated with this choice should never be underestimated or minimized. Multiple options remain available to the conscientious clinician and ongoing research efforts will continue to clarify optimal analgesic options that best balance patient comfort with procedural risk. Ultimately, the choice of pain-control strategy should be based on patient and parental desires and past experiences, as well as individual and institutional practice patterns.

References

1. Kelly RE (2008) Pectus excavatum: historical background, clinical picture, preoperative evaluation and criteria for operation. Semin Pediatr Surg 17(3):p181–p193
2. Nuss D et al (1998) A 10-year review of a minimally invasive technique for the correction of pectus excavatum. J Pediatr Surg 33(4):545–552
3. Kelly RE et al (2010) Twenty-one years of experience with minimally invasive repair of pectus excavatum by the Nuss procedure in 1215 patients. Ann Surg 252(6):1072–1081
4. Fonkalsrud EW, Dunn JC, Atkinson JB (2000) Repair of pectus excavatum deformities: 30 years of experience with 375 patients. Ann Surg 231(3):443
5. Fonkalsrud EW et al (2002) Comparison of minimally invasive and modified Ravitch pectus excavatum repair. J Pediatr Surg 37(3):413–417
6. Molik KA et al (2001) Pectus excavatum repair: experience with standard and minimal invasive techniques. J Pediatr Surg 36(2):324–328
7. Papic JC et al (2014) Postoperative opioid analgesic use after Nuss versus Ravitch pectus excavatum repair. J Pediatr Surg 49(6):919–923
8. Nasr A, Fecteau A, Wales PW (2010) Comparison of the Nuss and the Ravitch procedure for pectus excavatum repair: a meta-analysis. J Pediatr Surg 45(5):880–886
9. Kelly RE et al (2007) Prospective multicenter study of surgical correction of pectus excavatum: design, perioperative complications, pain, and baseline pulmonary function facilitated by internet-based data collection. J Am Coll Surg 205(2):205–216
10. Kelly RE et al (2008) Surgical repair of pectus excavatum markedly improves body image and perceived ability for physical activity: multicenter study. Pediatrics 122(6):1218–1222
11. Muhly WT, Maxwell LG, Cravero JP (2014) Pain management following the Nuss procedure: a survey of practice and review. Acta Anaesthesiol Scand 58(9):1134–1139
12. Skouen JS, Wainapel SF, Willock MM (1985) Paraplegia following epidural anesthesia. Acta Neurol Scand 72(4):437–443
13. Walaszczyk M et al (2011) Epidural and opioid analgesia following the Nuss procedure. Med Sci Monit 17(11):PH81–PH86
14. Butkovic D et al (2007) Postoperative analgesia with intravenous fentanyl PCA vs epidural block after thoracoscopic pectus excavatum repair in children. Br J Anaesth 98(5):677–681
15. Peter S, Shawn D et al (2008) Is epidural anesthesia truly the best pain management strategy after minimally invasive pectus excavatum repair? J Pediatr Surg 43(1):79–82
16. Bogert JN et al (2013) Patient-controlled analgesia-based pain control strategy for minimally-invasive pectus excavatum repair. Surg Pract 17(3):101–104
17. St Peter SD et al (2012) Epidural vs patient-controlled analgesia for postoperative pain after pectus excavatum repair: a prospective, randomized trial. J Pediatr Surg 47(1):148–153
18. Stroud AM et al (2014) Epidural analgesia versus intravenous patient-controlled analgesia following minimally invasive pectus excavatum repair: a systematic review and meta-analysis. J Pediatr Surg 49(5):798–806

19. Qi J, Du B, Gurnaney H, Lu P, Zuo Y. (2014) A prospective randomized observer-blinded study to assess postoperative analgesia provided by an ultrasound-guided bilateral thoracic paravertebral block for children undergoing the Nuss procedure. Reg Anesth Pain Med. 39(3):208–13
20. Pontarelli EM et al (2013) On-Q® pain pump versus epidural for postoperative analgesia in children. Pediatr Surg Int 29(12):1267–1271
21. Hall Burton DM, Boretsky KR (2014) A comparison of paravertebral nerve block catheters and thoracic epidural catheters for postoperative analgesia following the Nuss procedure for pectus excavatum repair. Paediatr Anaesth 24(5):516–520
22. Westphal FL, Lima LC, Lima Neto JC et al (2009) Prevalence of pectus carinatum and pectus excavatum in students in the city of Manaus, Brazil. J Bras Pneumol 35(3):221–226
23. Martinez-Ferro M, Fraire C, Bernard S (2008) Dynamic compression system for the correction of pectus carinatum. Semin Pediatr Surg 17(3):194–200
24. Emil S et al (2012) Pectus carinatum treatment in Canada: current practices. J Pediatr Surg 47(5):862–866
25. Ravitch MM (1949) The operative treatment of pectus excavatum. Ann Surg 129(4):429
26. Abramson H, D'Agostino J, Wuscovi S (2009) A 5-year experience with a minimally invasive technique for pectus carinatum repair. J Pediatr Surg 44(1):118–124
27. Fonkalsrud EW, Anselmo DM (2004) Less extensive techniques for repair of pectus carinatum: the undertreated chest deformity. J Am Coll Surg 198(6):898–905

General Approach to Abdominal and Pelvic Procedures

10

Jean-Francois Courval

Abdominal and pelvic procedures are characterized by a wide range of pathological processes which have their unique preoperative considerations, intraoperative management issues, postoperative pain control techniques, as well as special monitoring requirements (intraoperative or postoperative). Also typical of these procedures is the wide age and weight variation which ranges from extreme prematurity with very low birth weight in neonates to the near adult population who may be morbidly obese. Adding to this, changing physiology, disease-specific considerations, possible associated syndromes, and the challenging clinical practice of pediatric anesthesiologists involved in such procedures becomes evident. In this context, keeping a flexible and varied approach, adapted to the clinical settings of abdominal and pelvic procedures, is more important than a rigid specific recipe. This chapter will explore some of the common preoperative, intraoperative and postoperative considerations for the pediatric population in need of an abdominal or pelvic procedure.

10.1 Common Preoperative Considerations

An awareness of possible congenital anomalies or syndromes associated with abdominal and pelvic procedures is essential in a pediatric practice. Common congenital anomalies such as a Meckel's diverticulum (an embryological remnant of the omphalomesenteric duct) may not significantly alter anesthetic management; however, it may completely alter the surgical procedure. A common abdominal procedure such as an appendectomy for acute appendicitis may be transformed into a Meckel's diverticulum resection [1]. On occasion, the likeliness of associated syndrome or congenital anomalies will be raised by the age of presentation or clinical

J.-F. Courval
Anesthesia Department, Montreal Children's Hospital, Montreal, QC, Canada
e-mail: jf.courval@gmail.com

© Springer International Publishing Switzerland 2016
M. Astuto, P.M. Ingelmo (eds.), *Perioperative Medicine in Pediatric Anesthesia*,
Anesthesia, Intensive Care and Pain in Neonates and Children,
DOI 10.1007/978-3-319-21960-8_10

history. Intussusceptions are usually idiopathic; however, if recurrent or occurring in a child older than 3 years old, the incidence of associated cystic fibrosis, Burkitt lymphoma, or Peutz-Jeghers syndrome is increased [1]. At the other extreme, the abdominal pathologies will have significant associated anomalies which will have an impact on the anesthetic plan. Omphaloceles have been associated with chromosomal anomalies, bladder/cloacal exstrophy, neurological and cardiac defects, Beckwith-Wiedemann syndrome, and Down syndrome. These have significant anesthetic implications and they must be taken into consideration [2–4].

Trisomy 21 (i.e., Down syndrome) and Beckwith-Wiedemann syndrome are a reoccurring theme when it comes to abdominal and pelvic procedures. The range of abdominal and pelvic pathologies that have been associated with either or both is extensive and includes omphalocele, umbilical hernias, Hirschsprung disease, Wilms' tumor, as well as others [3–6]. Specific airway considerations and possible associated congenital cardiac malformations with their physiological impact will add to the complexity of the anesthetic management in such patients. VACTERL (Vertebral, Anal, Cardiovascular, TransEsophageal, Renal, and Limb) anomalies are another possible association that the pediatric anesthesiologist should be aware of. A VACTERL association is more common with higher and more complex anorectal malformations; however, in a review by Rollins et al., a complete workup was felt to be warranted even with more benign lesion such as rectoperineal fistula [7].

Also important to consider is an understanding of the disease process as well as its possible complications or evolution. This may prompt the pediatric anesthesiologist to make additional preparation or plan for additional monitoring. Knowing that complex gastroschisis (commonly associated with bowel atresia) has an increased risk of morbidity and mortality [2], or that abdominal pathologies such as necrotizing enterocolitis, appendicitis, anorectal malformations, and intussusception have the potential to cause bowel necrosis and bowel perforation [1, 8], are good examples. Anticipating possible complications such as peritonitis and septic shock is very important and improves the chances of survival of the pediatric patient which could succumb to associated cardiovascular collapse, renal dysfunction, anemia, thrombocytopenia, and coagulopathy. Knowledge of the potential complications secondary to chemotherapy or radiotherapy when dealing with the pediatric oncologic abdominal or pelvic masses is also important. Myocardial damage resulting in cardiac dysrhythmias or acute cardiomyopathy, myelosuppression, hepatic failure, pulmonary fibrosis, or neuronal damages are some of the considerations inerrant to the anesthetic management of this population [6]. The mass or hormonal effects of neoplasm should also be considered. For example, Wilms' tumors have been associated with systemic complications such as hypertension and acquired von Willebrand's disease; in addition, vascular extension of this tumor may complicate the surgical procedure as well as anesthetic management due to possible pulmonary embolism and inferior vena cava or tricuspid valve obstruction from the mass itself [6].

Finally, electrolytes imbalance and volume status are common perioperative concerns with abdominal and pelvic procedures. Loss of gastrointestinal fluid due to excessive vomiting or diarrhea with abdominal pathologies such as appendicitis, intussusception, or pyloric stenosis may lead to abnormal electrolyte values. Certain tumor such as Wilms' tumor may produce excessive amount of renin which can result in polydipsia and aldosterone-induced wasting of potassium [6]. This may also occur with pheochromocytoma and the secretion of excessive amount of catecholamines. Catecholamine secretions have also been associated with hyperglycemia which may require insulin therapy [9]. The electrolytes anomalies may also be related to genito-urinary anomalies and renal dysfunction which is common in patient with anorectal malformations, gastroschisis, or Beckwith-Wiedemann syndrome [4, 10–12] Hypovolemia may result from various mechanisms: gastrointestinal bleeding third spacing, and large evaporative loss [3] are common in this patient population. Although early and aggressive fluid resuscitation (from 50 ml/kg up to 200 ml/kg) has been reported to improve outcome in sepsis [13], this may prove insufficient in pathol-ogies such as a toxic megacolon syndrome and enteric bacteremia, where the combi-nation of fluid as well as vasopressor support may be lifesaving measures [14].

10.2   Intraoperative Management

Overall outcome and complication rate of abdominal and pelvic pathologies have greatly improved over the past 50 years. Gastroschisis, isolated omphalocele, and Wilms' tumor are examples of pathologies that were associated with significant mortality rate which now have a survival rate of 90 % or more [10, 14]. The reasons leading to these remarkable improvements are probably multifactorial and multidis-ciplinary; total parenteral nutrition, neonatal and surgical care, oncology protocols, better diagnostic tools, identification of associated pathologies, and improved peri-operative monitoring are some of the factors that may have contributed to these results. The practice of anesthesia has also evolved significantly over the past years, and patients have benefited from increased safety protocols and improved monitor-ing in the operating room.

A better understanding of the risk associated with a full stomach and the serious-ness of aspiration pneumonitis has led to the adoption of strict rules regarding inges-tion of fluid or solids during the perioperative period. Unfortunately, these rules should not be viewed as an assurance of an empty stomach since poor children compliance or delayed gastric emptying secondary to intestinal obstruction in pyloric stenosis or intussusception may interfere with normal gastric emptying. Direct assessment of gastric content with ultrasound has been looked at and may have future applications; however, it remains unproven at this time [16, 17]. Therefore, anesthesiologists still have to resort to the use of the rapid sequence induction (RSI) technique to minimize the risk of aspiration during the induction period. Gastric decompression with a nasogastric tube insertion prior to induction has been advocated to prevent or minimize the risk of aspiration [4, 18]. However, the classic RSI may represent a significant challenge in a pediatric population par-ticularly when patients may be hypovolemic without IV access and may not want to cooperate for preoxygenation or an awake intubation [14, 16].

As was previously mentioned, Beckwith-Wiedemann and Down syndromes are frequent consideration with abdominal and pelvic procedures. Airway assessment prior to induction is important in order to evaluate the potential risk of a difficult intubation. Macroglossia is common with Beckwith-Wiedemann syndrome and may complicate airway management [4]. Down syndrome has a number of features which may also lead to difficulty in securing the airway: short neck, macroglossia, mandibular hypoplasia, cervical spine instability, subglottic stenosis, and poor cooperation due to possible mental retardation. In addition, Down syndrome patients may have associated congenital cardiac anomalies and are at risk for bradycardia with inhalational induction with sevoflurane [19, 20]. Combining all of those clinical features (acute abdomen, full stomach, difficult airway, cervical spine instability, congenital heart anomalies, bradycardia on induction, difficult or absent IV access) and managing these patients becomes a challenge even for the most experience pediatric anesthesiologist.

Certain pathologies such as pyloric stenosis, gastroschisis, necrotizing enterocolitis, or Hirschsprung disease are more prevalent during the neonatal period in patient who may be born prematurely. Appropriate ventilation becomes very important in these patients in order to avoid hypoxemia, oxygen toxicity or barotrauma. Tidal volume should not exceed 8 ml/kg, and the inspiratory oxygen concentration should be adjusted to maintain an oxygen saturation of 88–92 % [13]. Pulmonary hypoplasia should also be considered and may lead to prolonged mechanical ventilation and tracheostomy in this population [2, 21]. As an increased number of abdominal and pelvic procedures are being done laparoscopically, the reduced pulmonary compliance, increased airway pressure, and increased CO_2 load must also be considered during the operation [22]. In addition, given the relative short distance between the end of the endotracheal tube and the carina in small pediatric patients, the increased intra-abdominal pressure from gas insufflation during laparoscopy, can lead to the cephalad displacement of the carina [14] resulting in possible endobronchial intubation orsevere bronchospasm. Adequacy of ventilation should also be reassessed postoperatively since the procedure itself may have impacts on the ventilatory parameters. For example, after primary closure of a gastroschisis, the resultant increase in intra-abdominal pressure could negatively affect postoperative ventilation.

The need for invasive monitoring will vary greatly depending on the abdominal and pelvic procedure. While certain procedures will be performed with standard monitoring, others may mandate the full spectrum of what is available in modern anesthesia (i.e. arterial line, central venous catheter, pulmonary artery wedge catheter, transesophageal echocardiography, etc.). The potential for rapid changes in hemodynamic stability, need for frequent blood sampling and diagnostic accuracy, are important factors when deciding which monitors should be added to standard monitoring. The pediatric anesthesiologists involved in such procedures must be prepared for potential massive blood loss and sudden hypotension with a Wilms' tumor invading the inferior vena cava [6] as well as severe hypertensive crisis from massive catecholamine release associated with secreting neuroblastoma or pheochromocytoma [23, 24]. The maintenance of an adequate mean arterial pressure is further complicated by the fact that this value will vary depending on the age of the patient [25]. Invasive monitoring will facilitate perioperative management of complex intra-abdominal pathologies; however, will this result to improved outcome remains controversial. With pheochromocytoma going from a perioperative mortality of 50 to 3 % [9], associating this impressive result solely on improved monitoring would be an oversimplification since there have been significant concomitant improvements in surgical techniques as well as preoperative medical management. Unfortunately, the entire arsenal of adult invasive monitoring may not be possible in the pediatric population. It is often necessary to modulate monitoring according to possible size limitation, technical difficulties, and/or lack of experience with a specific monitoring device and consider the potential benefit of such tools [9].

Intraoperative fluid management will vary according to the weight of the patient, the disease process, the duration of the surgery, as well as the surgical approach. Losses from third spacing can be minimal for a laparoscopic hernia repair, may reach 20–30 mL/kg for intussusception [13] or be in excess of 50 mL/kg for necrotizing enterocolitis [26]. Adequate evaluation and management of intraoperative fluid can be a challenge; however, it is important since it may lead to improved outcome [27]. Unfortunately, the opposite is also true, particularly for patient with pheochromocytoma. The chronic hypertension in these patients may lead to an uncertain intravascular volume status and acute myocardial dysfunction. Aggressive fluid resuscitation in this clinical setting would be unwise and could lead to congestive heart failure or pulmonary edema [9]. It is also important to consider which fluid will be used to replace losses. By far, crystalloids are the most common fluid used in abdominal and pelvic procedures. However, colloid, packed red blood cells, fresh frozen plasma, cryoprecipitate, and others may be indicated depending on the clinical setting. The importance of early replacement with massive blood loss is of critical importance. The pediatric anesthesiologist providing care to this population must keep in mind that massive blood loss may not be a large volume, particularly in the context of a very low birth weight premature neonate with necrotizing enterocolitis.

Positioning for gastrointestinal and genitourinary procedures is usually in the supine or lithotomy position. On occasion, the prone position is encountered for procedures such as a posterior sagittal anorectoplasty, a procedure introduced by Peña in 1982 for the correction of anorectal malformation [8]. Particular attention to pressure points and temperature control during positioning is crucial since this patient population may have very sensitive skin where minimal pressure may result in damages and the procedure may be prolonged. When the bowel is exposed as in gastroschisis or omphalocele, measures to reduce evaporative fluid and heat loss are essential. Covering the bowel with a sterile plastic wrapping is helpful in that setting, and it also prevents desiccation of the viscera [3, 13]. However, with the introduction of a laparoscopic approach to increasingly complex abdominal and pelvic procedures, third spacing and evaporative loss have been significantly reduced. An unfortunate consequence of this approach has been the increased duration of procedures and the potential risk of significant perioperative hypothermia. However, the overall popularity of the laparoscopic approach has increased to the point that the McBurney incision for appendicitis is now a rare event in major pediatric centers

[1]. With increased experience, the increased surgical duration of laparoscopic procedure has been steadily reduced, and the gains on length of hospital stay, when compared to laparotomy, far outweigh the possible increase in surgical time [28]. This tendency toward less invasive correction of various pathologies has been growing and now mandates that the pediatric anesthesiologist learns to work in environments outside of the traditional operating room. For example, the correction of intussusception is now frequently performed in the radiology suite, either pneumatically or with enema. In addition to facilitating the procedure, general anesthesia has also improved the overall success rate for this approach [6, 29].

10.3   Postoperative Management

When it comes to postoperative care, the postanesthesia care unit (PACU) is where most patients will recover from their surgery. For most abdominal or genitourinary procedures, the PACU will be the intermediate step before being discharged home. The PACU stay is usually limited and discharge home commonly occurs within 3 or 4 h. For some patients, an overnight stay will be required to determine whether the patient can be discharged home or needs to be admitted for further monitoring. Down syndrome being commonly associated with many abdominal and genitourinary pathologies, obstructive sleep apnea becomes a significant concern in this patient population.

There has been a constant push to perform more complex procedure in a day surgery setting. A combination of improved surgical technique, anesthesia monitoring, and risk stratification has been instrumental in this evolution [30]. The impact of laparoscopic surgery, interventional radiology, and cardiology has certainly been impressive over the past two decades in the pediatric as well as the adult population. The delivery of improved medical care at a lower cost is certainly an incentive for this approach. Procedures may have become more expensive; however, the shortened length of hospital stay offsets this additional cost and contributes to improve the overall efficiency of care. For example, an appendectomy for acute appendicitis will now be discharged within 24 h and will only be admitted if prolong antibiotic therapy is necessary [1]. The complexity of patients observed in the PACU has also seen a significant increase. This is particularly true in environments where access to the intensive care unit (ICU) may be limited or at times when the number of admission to the ICU is unusually large. As discussed above and given the numerous potential complications, the need for postoperative admission to the pediatric or neonatal intensive care unit remains. The importance of postoperative risk evaluation and an assessment of possible prolong monitoring must be done early.

Postoperative pain control management for abdominal and pelvic procedures has improved significantly in the past two decades. High-dose narcotics have been associated with postoperative nausea and vomiting which may result in delayed discharge home. Finding the most effective peripheral nerve block to obtain the best pain relief has been the subject of a number of research projects. The benefits of peripheral nerve blocks may even be extended after discharge home with the placement of a catheter connected to an elastomeric pump [31]. In major pediatric centers, inguinal hernia repair and orchidopexy are now associated with minimal pain, whereas patients undergoing tonsillectomy are still reported to have significant pain up to 7 days postoperatively [32, 33].

Conclusion

When providing anesthesia care to patient undergoing an abdominal or pelvic procedure, it is important to look for possible associated syndromes and to understand the disease process. Particular attention to volume status, electrolytes balance, and blood loss can be challenging and may mandate additional monitoring intraoperatively or postoperatively. Communication with the surgical team prior to incision will help you anticipate and prepare for potential intraoperative complications. Finally, in this era, it should be possible to provide excellent pain relief to the vast majority of these patients and avoid having to resort to high-dose narcotics.

References

1. Pepper VK, Stanfill AB, Pearl RH (2012) Diagnosis and management of pediatric appendicitis, intussusception, and meckel diverticulum. Surg Clin North Am 92:505–526
2. Islam S (2012) Advances in surgery for abdominal wall defects. Clin Perinatol 39:375–386
3. Kelly K, Ponsky T (2013) Pediatric abdominal wall defects. Sug Clin North Am 93:1255–1267
4. Ledbetter D (2012) Congenital abdominal wall defects and reconstruction in pediatric surgery. Surg Clin North Am 92:713–727
5. Langer J (2013) Hirschsprung disease. Curr Opin Pediatr 25:368–378
6. Whyte S, Ansermino J (2006) Anesthetic considerations in the management of Wilms' tumor. Pediatr Anesth 16:504–513
7. Rollins M, Russel K, Schall K et al (2014) Complete VACTERL evaluation is needed in newborns with rectoperineal fistula. J Pediatr Surg 49:95–98
8. Sharma S, Gupta D (2012) Delayed presentation of anorectal malformation for definitive surgery. Pediatr Surg Int 28:831–834
9. Hack H (2000) The perioperative management of children with phaeochromocytoma. Paediatr Anaesth 10:463–476
10. Giuliani S, Midrio P, De Filippo R et al (2013) Anorectal malformation and associated endstage renal disease: management from newborn to adult life. J Pediatr Surg 48:635–641
11. Islam S (2008) Clinical care outcomes in abdominal wall defects. Curr Opin Pediatr 20:305–310
12. Mastroiacovo P, Lisi A, Castilla E et al (2007) Gastroschisis and associated defects: an international study. Am J Med Genet A 143:660–671
13. McDougall R (2013) Pediatric emergencies. Anaesthesia 68(Suppl 1):61–71
14. Lerman J, Kondo Y, Suzuki Y et al (2013) General abdominal and urologic surgery. In: Coté CJ, Lerman J, Anderson BJ (eds) A practice of anesthesia for infants and children. Elsevier Saunders, Philadelphia, pp 569–589
15. Davidoff A (2012) Wilms tumor. Adv Pediatr 59:247–267
16. Davidson A (2013) Anesthetic management of common pediatric emergencies. Curr Opin Anesthediol 26(3):304–309
17. Schmitz A, Thomas S, Melanie F et al (2012) Ultrasonographic gastric antral area and gastric contents volume in children: a pro-con debate. Paediatr Anaesth 22:144–149

18. Cook-Sather SD, Tulloch HV, Cnaan A et al (1998) A comparison of awake versus paralyzed tracheal intubation for infants with pyloric stenosis. Anesth Analg 86:945–951
19. Shapiro N, Huang R, Sangwan S et al (2000) Tracheal stenosis and congenital heart disease in patients with Down syndrome: diagnostic approach and surgical options. Int J Pediatr Otorhinolaryngol 54:137–142
20. Kraemer F, Stricker P, Gurnaney H et al (2010) Bradycardia during induction of anesthesia with sevoflurane in children with Down syndrome. Anesth Analg 111:1259–1263
21. Edwards E, Broome S, Green S et al (2007) Long-term respiratory support in children with giant omphalocele. Anaesth Intensive Care 35:94–98
22. Whalley D, Berrigan M (2000) Anesthesia for radical prostatectomy, cystectomy, nephrectomy, pheochromocytoma, and laparoscopic procedures. Anesth Clin North America 18:899–917
23. Seefelder C, Sparks J, Chirnomas D et al (2005) Perioperative management of a child with severe hypertension from a catecholamine secreting neuroblastoma. Pediatr Anaesth 15:606–610
24. Kalra Y, Agarwal H, Smith A (2013) Perioperative management of pheochromocytoma and catecholamine-induced dilated cardiomyopathy in a pediatric patient. Pediatr Cardiol 34:2013–2016
25. Lee J, Rajadurai V, Tan K (1999) Blood pressure standards for very low birthweight infants during the first day of life. Arch Dis Child Fetal Neonatal Ed 81:168–170
26. Murat I, Dubois M (2008) Perioperative fluid therapy in pediatrics. Pediatr Anesth 18:363–370
27. Carcillo J, Davis A, Zaritsky A (1991) Role of early fluid resuscitation in pediatric septic shock. J Am Med Ass 266:1242–1245
28. Apelt N, Featherstone N, Giuliani S (2013) Laparoscopic treatment of intussusception in children: a systematic review. J Pediatr Surg 48:1789–1793
29. Purenne E, Franchi-Abella S, Branchereau S et al (2012) General anesthesia for intussusception reduction by enema. Paediatr Anaesth 22:1211–1215
30. Qadir N, Smith I (2007) Day surgery: how far can we go and are there still any limits? Curr Opin Anaesthesiol 20:503–505
31. Fredrickson M, Praine C, Hamill J (2010) Improved analgesia with the ilioinguinal block compared to the transversus abdominis plane block after pediatric inguinal surgery: a prospective randomized trial. Paediatr Anaesth 20:1022–1027
32. Stewart D, Ragg P, Sheppard S et al (2012) The severity and duration of postoperative pain and analgesia requirements in children after tonsillectomy, orchidopexy, or inguinal hernia repair. Paediatr Anaesth 22:136–143
33. Kost-Byerly S, Jackson E, Yaster M et al (2008) Perioperative anesthetic and analgesic management of newborn bladder exstrophy repair. J Pediatr Urol 4:280–285

Perioperative Care of Children with a Difficult Airway

11

Alan Barnett and Thomas Engelhardt

11.1 Introduction

Airway problems are a leading cause of perioperative morbidity and mortality in healthy children without any signs or symptoms of airway anomalies but also frequently encountered in children with an impaired airway [1, 2].

Mortality due to perioperative hypoxia is a consequence of prolonged airway obstruction. Transient perioperative hypoxia may result in apparent short-term postoperative morbidity. However, long-term consequences of transient hypoxemia are only poorly understood.

Neonates and young children are at a particular high risk as are children undergoing emergency procedures [3, 4]. Children in general have a decreased oxygen reserve and increased oxygen consumption when compared with adults. Their apnoea tolerance is, therefore, very low (measured in seconds) [5, 6]. Even a transient airway obstruction develops rapidly into significant hypoxemia and profound bradycardia compromising the well-being of the child.

This chapter describes essential anatomical and physiological information and their direct clinical consequences. A pragmatic approach is suggested for the management of different paediatric airway problems including a list of minimum airway equipment available.

A. Barnett
Department of Surgery, Radiology, Anaesthesia and Intensive Care,
The University of the West Indies, Mona, Kingston 7, Jamaica, West Indies

T. Engelhardt (✉)
Department of Anaesthesiology, Royal Aberdeen Children's Hospital,
Foresterhill, Aberdeen AB25 2ZN, UK
e-mail: tomkat01@yahoo.com

© Springer International Publishing Switzerland 2016
M. Astuto, P.M. Ingelmo (eds.), *Perioperative Medicine in Pediatric Anesthesia*,
Anesthesia, Intensive Care and Pain in Neonates and Children,
DOI 10.1007/978-3-319-21960-8_11

11.2 The Paediatric Airway

11.2.1 Anatomical Considerations

As the child develops from birth and progresses to adulthood, there are significant changes, which occur in the airway and lungs. The head is large relative to the body in infants and young children, and facial structures are small when compared to the neurocranium. The oral cavity is small at birth and increases in size in the first year of life following a substantial growth of the mandible and teeth. The neonatal tongue is flat with limited lateral mobility.

The larynx is loosely embedded in the surrounding structures when compared with adults and more anterior. External manipulation allows positioning during direct laryngoscopy. The epiglottis is long, narrow and frequently U-shaped, obscuring the glottic view on direct laryngoscopy. The glottis is higher in relation to the spine in neonates (C2/C3) and descends to its usual position at C5 after 2 years. The vocal cords are shorter in the neonate and comprise about half of the anterior glottis [7].

The neonatal larynx is thought to be conically shaped and approximately cylindrical in an older child. In addition, the larynx is thought to be widest at the supraglottic and narrowest at the subglottic level. However, this view has been challenged in MRI studies indicating that the narrowest part is in fact at the glottis. Most importantly, the cricoid ring is functionally the narrowest (unyielding) part of the neonatal airway. The cricoid ring is not circular but has an ellipsoid shape and a mucosal layer highly susceptible to trauma. Pressure or trauma at the cricoid ring results in oedema, increase in airway resistance and airway obstruction [8].

Tracheal length is related to the patient's age and height. Alteration of the head position changes the tracheal tube position and requires reassessment by clinical or other means.

11.2.2 Physiological Considerations

Young children have a very low functional residual capacity and increased closing capacity. In addition, children have a higher oxygen demand as well as increased carbon dioxide production. The direct consequence is a very low apnoea tolerance leading to significant hypoxemia and respiratory acidosis. Even optimal pre-oxygenation does not generate a sufficiently long 'safety period'. The younger the child, the less time there is [5, 6].

The laryngeal reflexes are the most powerful protective reflexes in humans and are designed to prevent pulmonary aspiration. They are functional reflexes. The recurrent laryngeal nerve and the external and internal branches of the superior laryngeal nerve (vagus) innervate the larynx. The former supplies the afferent innervation of the subglottic part of the larynx and all muscles with the exception of the cricothyroid muscle which is innervated by the external branch of the superior laryngeal nerve. The internal branch of the superior laryngeal nerve provides sensory innervation to the epiglottis and larynx above the vocal cords. Stimulation results in coughing, laryngospasm and bradycardia.

The larynx is very sensitive to mechanical or chemical stimulation induced by liquids or solids. It is relatively insensitive to inhaled irritants such as volatile anaesthetic agents [9]. Laryngospasm is defined as complete closure of the larynx. A mechanical stimulus (secretions/blood/foreign body) is the primary cause and frequently observed in children with upper respiratory tract infections. A 'true' or 'complete' laryngospasm is in contrast to glottic spasm or 'partial' laryngospasm, a strong approximation of the vocal cords only. A partial laryngospasm leaves a small lumen at the posterior commissure, potentially allowing minimal oxygenation with high inflation pressures.

A complete laryngospasm results in silent chest movements but no movement of the reservoir bag. Face mask ventilation is not possible. In partial laryngospasm, there is chest movement, but there is a stridulous noise with a mismatch between the patient's respiratory effort and the small amount of movement of the reservoir bag [10].

Laryngospasm must also be differentiated from postextubation stridor, commonly due to trauma of the paediatric airway and mucosal injury with subsequent oedema.

11.2.3 Clinical Consequences of Airway Obstruction

Airway obstruction may occur at any time in the perioperative period in any child and may be described as either anatomical or functional (Table 11.1).

Anatomical airway obstructions are caused by poor technique such as incorrect use of the face mask, suboptimal positioning of the patient's head, mandible and upper thorax and failure to recognise airway obstruction caused by large adenoids and tonsils.

Table 11.1 Airway obstructions during anaesthesia are generally divided into anatomical (mechanical) and functional airway obstructions

Anatomical airway obstructions	Functional airway obstructions
Causes	*Causes*
Inadequate head position	Inadequate anaesthesia
Poor face mask technique	Laryngospasm
Large adenoids/tonsils/obesity	Muscle rigidity
Secretions	Bronchospasm
Treatment	*Treatment*
Repositioning/reopening/Guedel	Deepen anaesthesia
Two-hand/two-person technique	Muscle relaxation
Suction	Epinephrine

This distinction necessitates different treatments: anaesthetic technique for anatomical airway obstructions and pharmacological interventions for functional airway obstructions

Simple mouth opening and the application of the 'triple airway manoeuvre' (head-tilt, chin-lift, jaw-thrust) or alternatively the use of an appropriately sized oropharyngeal airway will usually overcome these problems. Mechanical obstruction due to secretions, blood, regurgitation or foreign bodies necessitates suction removal under direct vision. Gastric distension secondary to forceful bag-mask ventilation requires decompression by orogastric suctioning. Unexpected subglottic or other tracheal mechanical obstructions (inhaled foreign bodies) can be overcome by bypassing with a smaller tracheal tube. Prolonged and/or failed tracheal intubation attempts in small neonates and small infants result in peripheral lung collapse. Careful lung recruitment manoeuvres are required in order to restore optimal oxygenation and ventilation. If no mechanical obstruction is detected during direct laryngoscopy and the trachea cannot be intubated, a supraglottic airway device must be inserted as an alternative in order to overcome any potentially overlooked anatomical supraglottic airway problems [7].

Functional upper airway obstructions are frequent in children and may be caused by insufficient depth of anaesthesia, laryngospasm or opioid-induced glottic closure. Functional lower airway obstructions are caused by bronchospasm or opioid-induced muscle rigidity of the thoracic wall. Treatment options of functional airway obstructions are primarily pharmacological. Additional hypnotics may be used in the child without co-morbidities which is not already deeply hypoxic and bradycardic. The administration of muscle relaxation overcomes most functional airway obstructions with the exception of bronchospasm for which epinephrine may be used in the impending peri-arrest situation [11].

11.3 Classification of the Paediatric Airway

The paediatric airway may be classified under three headings: normal, impaired normal and an expected difficult airway (Table 11.2). This pragmatic classification in conjunction with the presented urgency of the situation determines the anaesthetic approach.

11.3.1 Normal (Unexpected Difficult)

Children in this category are encountered on a daily basis. These children are usually healthy and have no previous symptoms or signs indicative of a difficult airway. Problems encountered are either due to an anatomical (mechanical) or functional airway obstruction (Table 11.1).

11.3.2 Impaired Normal (Suspected Difficult)

Swelling, trauma and infections can turn the normal airway of otherwise healthy children rapidly into an impaired normal airway. The severity of symptoms and

Table 11.2 Simple and pragmatic classification of the paediatric airway

Normal paediatric airway: 'unexpected'	Time: critical
	Place: anywhere
	Who: anyone
	Comment: established paediatric airway algorithm essential
Impaired normal paediatric airway: 'suspected'	Time: urgent
	Place: anywhere, consider transfer to specialist centre
	Who: expertise required, consider ENT
Known abnormal paediatric airway: 'expected'	Time: normally elective, planning essential
	Place: paediatric specialist centres only
	Who: specialist expertise required, ENT support essential

After Marin and Engelhardt [12]
The vast majority of children have a normal airway. The known difficult paediatric airway is the domain of the experienced paediatric anaesthetist

speed of deterioration dictate the urgency and need of the anaesthetic intervention. The underlying disorder – infectious (epiglottitis), allergic or mechanical (inhaled foreign body, bleeding tonsil) – requires swift recognition and treatment. Most children, however, tolerate a certain delay in order to allow resuscitation, organisation and preparation of appropriate staff, location and equipment.

11.3.3 Expected Difficult Airway

This refers to children who have a known or obvious difficult/abnormal airway.

Examples include but are not limited to head, neck and airway anomalies. They may be congenital (associated with syndromes) or acquired (burns, scars), associated with tumours and other masses and more rare causes such as subglottic and tracheal disorders or anterior mediastinal mass syndrome.

Unless there is an immediate threat to life or limb, these patients must be transferred to a specialised hospital with appropriate experience, personnel and equipment available to guarantee optimal safety.

11.3.4 Approach to the Paediatric Airway

The clear distinction between 'normal', 'impaired normal' and 'known abnormal' allows the non-specialist paediatric anaesthetist to determine the optimal approach to the child requiring airway interventions (Fig. 11.1). Whereas the 'normal' paediatric airway may be managed in most centres with appropriate staffing and resources, the establishment of simple, locally adapted, easy memorisable and rehearsed algorithms is essential for safe paediatric airway management (see below). The acutely

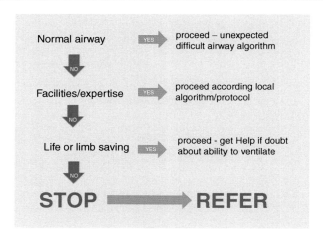

Fig. 11.1 Flow chart for approaching paediatric airway management (After Marin and Engelhardt [12])

impaired normal paediatric airway requires experience and skill. If these are available, the paediatric airway can be managed locally. The gravity of the underlying disease process (infectious, allergic swelling, trauma or burn) and speed of deterioration will guide the anaesthetic intervention. Resuscitation, organisation and preparation of appropriate staff, location and equipment should be arranged if the condition of the child allows. All other patients should be transferred to a dedicated paediatric unit unless intervention is critical. Surgical (ENT) support is required if the anaesthetist is not experienced enough or has doubts about the ability to oxygenate and ventilate.

11.4 Management of the Paediatric Airway

11.4.1 Managing the Unexpected Difficult Airway

Routine paediatric airway management is usually easy in experienced hands. However, as outlined above, children have an increased oxygen consumption and a lower oxygen reserve when compared with adults. Therefore, preparation, regular training and education are essential to prevent and recognise early unexpected difficulties in the otherwise 'normal' paediatric airway. Time critical concepts are required based on simple, forward only, easy memorisable, locally adapted and rehearsed algorithms. Such a simple proposal for the paediatric patient was published recently and is reproduced in an adapted form (Fig. 11.2).

Maintenance of the ability to oxygenate and ventilate is the key to successful airway management. Good daily clinical practice is required to achieve this. Anatomical/mechanical airway obstructions need to be recognised and treated first as described. No pharmacological intervention will solve this problem. If the

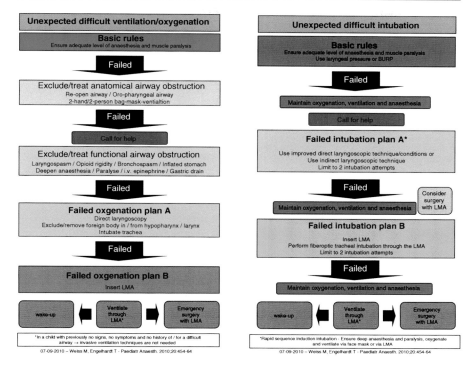

Fig. 11.2 Simplified 'open-box' proposal for the management of the unexpected difficult paediatric airway (Adapted from Weiss and Engelhardt [13]). A clear separation between oxygenation/ventilation problems and difficult intubation is essential. Oxygenation/ventilation (and anaesthesia) must be guaranteed

situation does not improve early, call for help immediately. Recognition and treatment of functional airway obstruction using either an additional dose of hypnotic, muscle relaxant or epinephrine is essential. Limited and as of yet unpublished evidence suggests that all otherwise normal children can be oxygenated and ventilated if anatomical and functional airway problems are recognised and treated [11]. An unexpected foreign body (food/chewing gum – a mechanical obstruction) occluding the glottis must be removed or bypassed following muscle relaxation. A supraglottic airway device may be helpful in overcoming unexpected/unknown anatomical airway obstructions. Unexpected difficult tracheal intubation may occur, and similarly a simple, stepwise, forward only and locally adapted algorithm must be in place. It is essential to realise that repeated traumatic airway instrumentation will convert a difficult paediatric airway into an impossible situation.

A 'rescue' option is frequently incorporated into the management of the 'cannot oxygenate-cannot ventilate' algorithms. Principally, the choice is between a surgical airway, needle cricoidotomy and rigid bronchoscopy. There is currently only insufficient evidence to firmly endorse any of these options in children. Emphasis must be on prevention of this situation in the otherwise normal child through the early recognition and treatment of anatomical and functional airway obstructions through dedicated teaching and training.

11.5 Managing the Suspected Difficult (Previously Normal) Airway

In contrast to the unexpected difficult airway, the suspected (previously normal) paediatric airway presents unique challenges to the anaesthetist. Previous training and experience as well as existing facilities dictate the approach. Frequently, there is sufficient time to allow optimisation of the patient, planning as well as organisation of additional help.

Optimisation of the patient includes specific treatment directed at the underlying cause and may include antimicrobial cover in case of bacterial infections, administration of corticosteroids in children with croup-like symptoms and inhalational trauma as well as appropriate resuscitation if required.

Prior to any intervention a short, rapid evaluation, directed at the characteristics of the onset of the illness and the course of development of respiratory signs, must be performed in order to exclude trauma and foreign body aspiration. Clinical signs of acute airway obstruction should be assessed and include stridor, cyanosis, dyspnoea, suprasternal recession, use of auxiliary respiratory muscles, presence of apnoeic episodes as well as the posture of the patient. Frequent observations and assessments are recommended [14].

A concise plan (method of induction and spontaneous ventilation versus controlled ventilation) needs to be formulated prior to starting induction of anaesthesia, with all instruments and drugs available and ready to use. The most experienced anaesthetist should perform airway procedures in the child with the compromised airway. In life-threatening situations and situations in which there are doubts about the ability to ventilate, the presence of an experienced (ENT) surgeon ready to intervene immediately is mandatory. Anatomical and functional airway obstructions can occur at any time and must be treated as previously outlined.

11.6 Managing the Expected Difficult Airway

The management of the expected difficult airway is the domain of the experienced paediatric anaesthetist and requires a specialised setup. Management of these children is challenging. Preparation for a child with an expected difficult airway includes a quiet environment, anaesthetists proficient in advanced airway management techniques including fibre-optic intubation as well as trained anaesthetic nurses/assistants and suitable paediatric equipment.

Similarly to the previous descriptions, expected difficulties for mask ventilation and tracheal intubation may need to be catered for separately.

Inhalational induction or incremental doses of intravenous hypnotics (propofol) can be used to establish a depth of anaesthesia.

Depending on the anaesthetist's preference and experience, this is followed by one of the two options for further airway manipulations:

1. (Assisted) spontaneous ventilation using inhalational or total intravenous anaesthesia
2. Positive pressure ventilation with muscle paralysis (if bag-mask ventilation is possible)

An experienced ENT surgeon must be on standby ready to intervene if difficulty with mask ventilation occurs as rigid bronchoscopy or establishing a surgical airway may be urgently required.

Direct laryngoscopy should be attempted, and access to the larynx (Cormack and Lehane grading) must be documented for future anaesthetic interventions.

Fibre-optic tracheal intubation remains the gold standard despite the advent of alternatives such as videolaryngoscopes or other techniques [15]. It is, therefore, essential to maintain skills and expertise in fibre-optic intubation in children. A tracheostomy is the final option and must be considered during complicated and failed intubation attempts before swelling and bleeding make mask ventilation impossible. It may be necessary to secure the airway with a prophylactic tracheostomy if a repeated subsequent tracheal intubation is unlikely to succeed [16]. Awake direct laryngoscopy may only be considered in extreme circumstances (grotesque hygroma, lymphagioma or tumours of the head and neck). The EXIT procedure during birth represents a special option to oxygenate the newborn until conventional or invasive airway has been established [17]. A reversible extubation strategy using an airway exchange catheter should be planned in patients with a difficult airway [18].

11.7 Paediatric Airway Equipment

Safe paediatric airway management of the paediatric airway necessitates availability of suitable equipment. Safe anaesthesia does not have to be expensive. In every operating theatre and wherever a child is anaesthetised, there is an essential minimum equipment requirement (Table 11.3). Maker and manufacturer are of little relevance, but the equipment must be suitable for children and acceptable to the anaesthetist in charge.

There is an ever expanding range of desirable paediatric airway equipment on the market, and individual departments need to decide their best options based on their needs and affordability. These include (but are not limited to) endoscopy masks, second-generation supraglottic airway devices and videolaryngoscopes. It is essential that this equipment is regularly maintained and that regular training of all staff occurs.

In addition, a difficult/emergency airway trolley should be available in every suite where children are managed. This must be adapted to locally accepted difficult airway algorithms. A one-stop 'airway trolley' may be the best option for some

Table 11.3 Essential minimum airway equipment requirements for paediatric anaesthesia

Equipment	Comment
Face masks	All age-appropriate sizes must be available
Self-inflating bag	Connection possible to face mask
Oropharyngeal airway	All age-appropriate sizes must be available
Nasopharyngeal airway	All age-appropriate sizes must be available. A tracheal tube may be cut and used
Supraglottic airway device	All age-appropriate sizes must be available (1, 1½, 2, 2½, 3, 4 and 5)
	First-generation devices are adequate
Tracheal tube	All age-appropriate sizes must be available. If Microcuff tracheal tubes are used, cuff pressure must be monitored
Direct laryngoscope	Selection of straight and curved blades
Alternative laryngoscope	Select one alternative option to visualise the larynx
Other equipment	Intubating stylet, introducer, gastric drains, tapes and syringes (throat pack)

Table 11.4 Difficult/emergency airway trolley setup, arrange according to locally adapted airway algorithm

Drawer 1 label: failed oxygenation/ventilation
LMA: sizes 1, 1.5, 2, 2.5, 3, 4 and 5 (in duplicate)
Alternative masks and supraglottic airway devices
Magill forceps
Drawer 2 label: failed intubation plan A
Selection of 'alternative' laryngoscopy blades (s.a. McCoy, Wisconsin, Miller)
Gum elastic bougies (sizes 5 and 10 F)
Malleable stylet (sizes 2 and 5 F)
Choice of visualisation or intubating aid (depending on local preference)
Drawer 3 label: failed intubation plan B
Airway exchange catheters of assorted sizes
7 F, ID 2.5 mm; 8 F, ID 3.0 mm; 11 F, ID 4.0 mm; 14 F, ID 5.5 mm; and 19 F, ID 7.0 mm
Endoscopy masks
(Drawer 4 label: rescue)
Cricoidotomy needle kit (Melker) label: age > 8 years
Surgical cricoidotomy kit label: age < 8 years
Different-sized cannulae for cannula cricoidotomy and connection tubing
Scalpel (x 2)
Tracheal hook
Artery forceps
Surgical gloves

departments, with equipment separated according to age/weight. Other departments who have a dedicated 'difficult airway' trolley for elective procedures may choose an additional simplified 'airway rescue' trolley equipped according to departmental rescue algorithms. Simplicity is the key to success and overstocking must be avoided at all costs (Table 11.4).

All paediatric difficult/emergency airway equipment must be regularly checked and operators must be familiar with its content. Availability and signage must be guaranteed.

11.8 Summary

Paediatric airway management can be challenging. However, if clear concepts and local protocols for the management of the unexpected, suspected and expected difficult airway are established and expertise and training are maintained, significant airway-related morbidity and mortality can be avoided.

References

1. Bhananker SM, Ramamoorthy C, Geiduschek JM, Posner KL, Domino KB, Haberkern CM, Campos JS, Morray JP (2007) Anesthesia-related cardiac arrest in children: update from the Pediatric Perioperative Cardiac Arrest Registry. Anesth Analg 105:344–350
2. Woodall NM, Cook TM (2011) National census of airway management techniques used for anaesthesia in the UK: first phase of the Fourth National Audit Project at the Royal College of Anaesthetists. Br J Anaesth 106:266–271
3. de Graaff JC, Bijker JB, Kappen TH, van Wolfswinkel L, Zuithoff NP, Kalkman CJ (2013) Incidence of intraoperative hypoxemia in children in relation to age. Anesth Analg 117(1):169–175
4. Gencorelli FJ, Fields RG and Litman RS. Complications during rapid sequence induction of general anesthesia in children: a benchmark study. Paediatr Anaesth 2010;20:421–424. Anesth Analg. 2013;117: 169–75
5. Sands SA, Edwards BA, Kelly VJ, Davidson MR, Wilkinson MH, Berger PJ (2009) A model analysis of arterial oxygen desaturation during apnea in preterm infants. PLoS Comput Biol 5, e1000588
6. Hardman JG, Wills JS (2006) The development of hypoxaemia during apnoea in children: a computational modelling investigation. Br J Anaesth 97:564–570
7. Schmidt AR, Weiss M, Engelhardt T (2014) The paediatric airway: basic principles and current developments. Eur J Anaesthesiol 31:293–299
8. Litman RS, Weissend EE, Shibata D, Westesson PL (2003) Developmental changes of laryngeal dimensions in unparalyzed, sedated children. Anesthesiology 98:41–45
9. Nishino T, Isono S, Tanaka A, Ishikawa T (2004) Laryngeal inputs in defensive airway reflexes in humans. Pulm Pharmacol Ther 17:377–381
10. Hampson-Evans D, Morgan P, Farrar M (2008) Pediatric laryngospasm. Paediatr Anaesth 18:303–307
11. Weiss M, Engelhardt T (2012) Cannot ventilate--paralyze! Paediatr Anaesth 22:1147–1149
12. Marin PCE, Engelhardt T (2014) Algoritmo para el manejo de la vía aérea difícil en pediatría. Rev Colomb Anestesiol 42:325–335
13. Weiss M, Engelhardt T (2010) Proposal for the management of the unexpected difficult pediatric airway. Paediatr Anaesth 20:454–464

14. Engelhardt T, Machotta A, Weiss M (2013) Management strategies for the difficult paediatric airway. Trends Anaesth Crit Care 3:183–187
15. Wallace C, Engelhardt T (2015) Videolaryngoscopes in paediatric anaesthesia. Curr Treat Options Pediatr. doi:10.1007/s40746-014-0007-z
16. Wrightson F, Soma M, Smith JH (2009) Anesthetic experience of 100 pediatric tracheostomies. Paediatr Anaesth 19:659–666
17. Olutoye OO, Olutoye OA (2012) EXIT procedure for fetal neck masses. Curr Opin Pediatr 24:386–393
18. Loudermilk EP, Hartmannsgruber M, Stoltzfus DP, Langevin PB (1997) A prospective study of the safety of tracheal extubation using a pediatric airway exchange catheter for patients with a known difficult airway. Chest 111:1660–1665

Perioperative Care of Children with Neuromuscular Disease

12

Fabrizio Racca and Chiara Robba

12.1 Introduction

Children with neuromuscular disorders (NMDs) (Table 12.1) are at high risk of intraoperative and postoperative complications. Indeed, this peculiar group of patients may have altered vital functions (e.g., weakness of the respiratory muscles, scoliosis, cardiac involvement), which increase the risk of surgical procedures requiring general anesthesia (GA) or sedation. Moreover, in children with some types of NMDs, succinylcholine and halogenated agents can trigger life-threatening reactions, such as malignant hyperthermia (MH), rhabdomyolysis, or hyperkalemic cardiac arrest secondary to denervation. On the other hand, survival rate of these children has progressively improved, increasing the need for surgical procedures related or unrelated to NMDs.

An intensive, proactive, multidisciplinary approach should be instituted before, during, and after any surgical procedure requiring GA or sedation. Thus, surgery in this children population should be performed in a fully equipped hospital with extensive experience in NMD management.

This chapter will review the pathophysiology of life-threatening complications of anesthesia in NMDs and the assessment and management of these children before, during, and after anesthesia.

F. Racca, MD (✉)
Anesthesiology and Intensive Care Unit, S.C. Anestesia e Rianimazione Pediatrica Azienda Ospedaliera SS Antonio Biagio e Cesare Arrigo Hospital, Via Venezia 16,
Alessandria 15100, Italy
e-mail: fracca7766@gmail.com

C. Robba
Anesthesiology and Intensive Care Unit, SS Antonio Biagio e Cesare Arrigo Hospital,
Alessandria, Italy

© Springer International Publishing Switzerland 2016
M. Astuto, P.M. Ingelmo (eds.), *Perioperative Medicine in Pediatric Anesthesia*,
Anesthesia, Intensive Care and Pain in Neonates and Children,
DOI 10.1007/978-3-319-21960-8_12

Table 12.1 Neuromuscular disorders of childhood

1. Motoneuron diseases		Spinal muscular atrophy (SMA), SMA with respiratory distress (SMARD) Spinobulbar muscular atrophy (Kennedy disease) Poliomyelitis
2. Peripheral neuropathies		Guillain–Barrè Syndrome (GBS) Chronic inflammatory demyelinating polyneuropathy (CIDP) Hereditary sensory and motor neuropathies (i.e., Charcot–Marie–Tooth disease) Hereditary sensory and autonomic neuropathies (HSAN) Critical illness polyneuropathy
3. Neuromuscular junction diseases		Myasthenia gravis (MG) Congenital autoimmune myasthenia gravis Congenital myasthenias Botulism
4. Muscle diseases	*Progressive muscular dystrophies*	Dystrophinopathies: Duchenne (DMD) and Becker (BMD) type Limb-girdle muscular dystrophies (LGMD) Facioscapulohumeral muscular dystrophy (FSHD) Oculopharyngeal muscular dystrophy (OPMD) Myotonic dystrophy (DM): DM type 1 (DM1), DM type 2 (DM2 or PROMM disease)
	Congenital muscular dystrophies	Ullrich CMD, Bethlem myopathy Emery–Dreifuss dystrophy Merosin-deficient CMD Alpha-dystroglycanopathies (e.g., Fukuyama CMD)
	Congenital myopathies	Central core disease/malignant hyperthermia Nemaline/rod myopathies Centronuclear/myotubular myopathy Fiber-type disproportion myopathy Myofibrillar myopathies
	Metabolic myopathies	Mitochondrial encephalomyopathies Glycogen storage disorders (i.e., GSD type II or Pompe disease, McArdle disease) Lipid storage myopathies

12.2 Life-Threatening Complications of Anesthesia in NMDS

12.2.1 Respiratory Failure

Respiratory involvement can vary significantly between different NMDs and within each type of disorder. Reduction of inspiratory muscle strength results initially in restrictive pulmonary impairment with a progressive decrease of forced vital capacity (FVC). Subsequently, ineffective alveolar ventilation may occur, leading to nocturnal hypercapnia and eventually to diurnal hypercapnia. In addition, weakness of expiratory muscles leads to inadequate clearance of airway secretions. Hypoventilation, coupled with an impaired cough, predisposes to atelectasis and respiratory failure. Furthermore, patients with NMDs often experience mild to moderate bulbar dysfunction, affecting their ability to swallow. Children with type 1 spinal muscular atrophy (SMA), myasthenia gravis (MG), and with other rapidly progressive NMDs may develop a more severe bulbar dysfunction with an increased likelihood of aspiration. Finally, respiratory status can be further impaired by sleep apneas, nutritional problems, gastroesophageal reflux, or progressive scoliosis. In patients with compromised respiratory function, anesthetic agents may further decrease respiratory muscle strength, exacerbating hypoventilation, airway secretion retention, aspiration, and obstructive and central apneas. These conditions may lead to nosocomial infections, prolonged intubation, tracheotomy, and eventually death.

12.2.2 Cardiovascular Failure

Several NMDs are associated with cardiac dysfunctions (cardiomyopathies and/or abnormality of the conduction system) as shown in Table 12.2. However, clinical manifestations of heart failure are often unrecognized until very late stage, owing to musculoskeletal limitations. All children with relevant cardiac dysfunctions have a limited ability to increase cardiac output in response to stress. Consequently, they are at high risk for perioperative cardiac side effects due to negative inotropic effect of volatile and i.v. anesthetic agents, positive pressure ventilation, hypoxemia, and acute anemia. Volatile anesthetics may also induce arrhythmia resulting from sensitization of the heart to catecholamines and from inhibitory effects on voltage-gated K^+ channels. Finally, children with NMDs with respiratory involvement leading to nocturnal hypoxemia may be affected by right ventricular changes because of pulmonary hypertension.

Table 12.2 Cardiac dysfunction in children with neuromuscular disorders

Disorder	Cardiac dysfunction
Guillain–Barrè syndrome, SMA type 1, a subgroup of hereditary neuropathies	Dysautonomia may enhance cardiovascular instability (i.e., bradycardia, blood pressure shifts)
Dystrophinopathies	Dilated cardiomyopathy (*very common; broad spectrum of severity including severe cardiac failure*); arrhythmias and conduction defects (*<10 % of patients*)
Limb-girdle muscular dystrophies (LGMD)	Arrhythmias and conduction defects (*common*); dilated cardiomyopathy (*rare in LGMD type 2A, 2D*)
Myotonic dystrophies	Arrhythmias and conduction defects (*common*); dilated cardiomyopathy (*rare*)
Congenital myopathies	Arrhythmias and conduction defects; dilated cardiomyopathy
Mitochondrial encephalomyopathies	Arrhythmias and conduction defects; dilated cardiomyopathy
Glycogen storage diseases type II	Cardiomyopathy (hypertrophic cardiomyopathy in the infantile form)
Lipid storage myopathies	Cardiomyopathy

12.2.3 Malignant Hyperthermia (MH)

It is a rare inherited drug-induced disorder of the skeletal muscle characterized by an increased muscle metabolism with excessive heat, carbon dioxide and lactate production, high oxygen consumption, contractures of the muscles, and myofiber breakdown. It is usually triggered when an MH-susceptible individual is exposed to a halogenated agent or succinylcholine and in rare cases to strenuous exercise and/ or heat exposure.

12.2.3.1 Patients at Risk
- Diagnosis of ryanodine receptor 1 (RYR1) mutations or central core disease (CDC)
- Relatives of MH or CCD patients
- Few muscle diseases:
  - Central core disease
  - Core-rod myopathy
  - King–Denborough syndrome

12.2.3.2 Prevention
- Choice of anesthesia: "trigger-free" anesthetic and "clean" anesthesia machine for halogenated agents. The anesthesia machine must be prepared by using a disposable circuit, a fresh CO_2 absorbent, disconnecting the vaporizers and flushing with O_2 at a rate of 10 L min for at least 20 min before use. However, these recommendations are derived from older-style anesthetic machines, and modern anesthetic workstations may need longer cleaning times to wash out residual inhalational anesthetics in order to establish an acceptable concentration below 5 ppm.
- Availability of sufficient quantities of dantrolene in order to treat MH: dantrolene (vials, 20 mg each).
- Adequate intra- and postoperative monitoring: carefully monitoring for signs of rhabdomyolysis (i.e., serial plasma CK and myoglobin and urine myoglobin), capnometry, and measurement of body temperature.

12.2.3.3 Management of Acute Crisis
- Discontinue inhalational agents and use non-triggering agents for the remainder of the procedure.
- Hyperventilate with 100 % oxygen and intubate with endotracheal tube.
- Give dantrolene: loading bolus of 2.5 mg/kg i.v., with subsequent bolus doses of 1 mg/kg i.v. until the signs of acute MH have abated; 1 mg/kg every 6 h should be continued for 48 h after the last observed sign of acute MH to prevent recrudescence.
- Give sodium bicarbonate for acidosis.
- Cool the patient (cold saline for infusion, ice to body surface); lavage body cavities (e.g., stomach, bladder, rectum). Maintain temperature <39 °C.

- Treat hyperkalemia:
  - To antagonize the myocardial effects of hyperkalemia, give immediately calcium chloride i.v. (repeat the dose after 5 min if ECG changes persist).
  - To shift potassium back into muscle cells hyperventilate, give sodium bicarbonate and insulin with 10 % dextrose (monitor finger stick glucose closely).
- Treat dysrhythmias: usually responds to treatment of acidosis and hyperkalemia; use standard ACLS protocols; calcium channel blockers are contraindicated in the presence of dantrolene.

12.2.4 Rhabdomyolysis

It is an uncommon but potentially fatal disorder triggered by succinylcholine or halogenated agents in susceptible patients, characterized by muscle necrosis with release of intracellular muscle constituents (i.e., myoglobin, potassium, and creatine kinase) into the circulation. It can be acute, resulting in hyperkalemic cardiac arrest, or subacute, presenting as dark urine, acute kidney failure, or cardiac arrest in the postanesthetic care unit.

12.2.4.1 Patients at Risk
- Succinylcholine may cause rhabdomyolysis in almost all neuromuscular diseases but especially if muscles are denervated, progressively dystrophic, or metabolically altered.
- Halogenated agents may cause rhabdomyolysis in patients with myopathies (especially dystrophinopathies and metabolic myopathies).

12.2.4.2 Prevention
- "Trigger-free" anesthetic and "clean" anesthesia machine for halogenated agents (see malignant hyperthermia)
- Adequate intra- and postoperative monitoring: carefully monitoring for signs of rhabdomyolysis up to 12 h postoperatively (i.e., serial plasma CK and myoglobin and urine myoglobin)

12.2.4.3 Management of Acute Crisis
- Treat hyperkalemia (see malignant hyperthermia).
- Prevent heme pigment-induced acute kidney injury:
  - Early and aggressive fluid resuscitation with isotonic saline to maintain the urine output greater than 1 mL/kg/h.
  - Loop diuretics may be given to patients who develop volume overload as a result of aggressive volume administration.
  - Alkalinization of urine: administration of an alkaline solution to maintain the urine pH above 6.5, providing the patient is not severely hypocalcemic and has an arterial pH less than 7.5 and a serum bicarbonate less than 30 meq/L.
- Treat acute kidney injury: dialysis may be necessary for control of hyperkalemia and correction of acidosis or for the treatment of volume overload.

12.2.5 Hyperkalemic Cardiac Arrest Secondary to Denervation

It is a cardiac arrest due to hyperkalemia triggered by succinylcholine in the presence of striated muscle denervation hypersensitivity (upregulation of nicotinic acetylcholine receptors).

12.2.5.1 Pathologies at Risk
- Motoneuron diseases
- Peripheral neuropathies

12.2.5.2 Prevention
Avoid succinylcholine in children with motoneuron diseases or peripheral neuropathies.

12.2.5.3 Management of Acute Crisis
- Use standard ACLS protocols.
- Shift potassium back into muscle cells, give sodium bicarbonate and insulin with 10 % dextrose, and hyperventilate.
- Continue cardiopulmonary resuscitation until serum potassium levels are lowered to a near normal level.

12.3 Preoperative Assessment and Management

12.3.1 Neurological Assessment

Detailed diagnosis is essential to assess the risk during surgery and anesthesia. Thus, preoperative assessment must include a neurological examination to confirm the diagnosis, when feasible, and to identify the level of progression of the disease in each patient. However, diagnostic process may be complex and some patients may lack a definite diagnosis, particularly those manifesting only with isolated elevated creatine kinase levels with or without minor signs. These children are particularly at risk of life-threatening complications related to anesthesia and should be treated as subjects at highest risk level.

12.3.2 Pulmonary Assessment

In all children with NMDs, preoperative pulmonary evaluation is strongly recommended to assess the risk of respiratory complications and the need for specific perioperative and postoperative management.

Assessment of respiratory function should include an accurate medical history and physical examination, a chest x-ray, an evaluation of sleep-disordered breathing, and the measurements of respiratory function and cough effectiveness. Evaluation of respiratory function and cough effectiveness includes measurement of FVC, peak cough flow (PCF), and diurnal pulse oximetry (SpO_2). SpO_2 less than

95 % in room air has been established as a clinically significant threshold of abnormality, requiring carbon dioxide (PCO_2) level measurement. Preschool or older patients with developmental delay may not be able to perform evaluation tests of respiratory function and cough effectiveness. In these cases, the measurement of the crying vital capacity (i.e., FVC obtained from a tightly fitted mask over the nose and mouth with in-line spirometer) can approximate FVC.

It is crucial to optimize the patient's respiratory status before surgery. When respiratory function measurements and sleep studies are abnormal, noninvasive ventilation (NIV) and manual or mechanically assisted cough techniques may be indicated. Therefore, planning and coordination with the hospital respiratory therapists is crucial. In particular, mechanical insufflator–exsufflator (MI-E) can increase coughing, promote deep lung inflation, and treat or prevent atelectasis. Consequently, patients with limited respiratory reserve should be trained in these techniques before surgery and assisted with these devices during sedation, regional anesthesia, and in the postoperative period. This strategy is also recommended for patients already using assisted cough techniques and long-term NIV.

Recently, preoperative training in the use of NIV has been recommended for patients with Duchenne muscular dystrophy (DMD) with preoperative FVC <50 % of predicted value and especially for patients at high risk of respiratory failure, defined by an FVC <30 % of predicted value. Moreover, for children over 12 years of age, if PCF is less than 270 L/min, training in assisted cough techniques is advocated before surgery. This strategy has the potential to be applied to adults and children with respiratory involvement resulting from diagnosis other than DMD.

12.3.3 Cardiac Assessment

Children with NMDs should undergo a careful assessment of cardiac function as well as optimization of therapy before anesthesia or sedation. In all children with NMDs, an electrocardiogram and echocardiogram should be performed before anesthesia or sedation, if not done in the previous 12 months. Moreover, signs or symptoms of arrhythmias should be promptly investigated with a Holter test. In addition, patients with a high degree of AV blocks may need a cardiac pacemaker before GA.

In all patients with severe cardiac dysfunctions, invasive arterial pressure should be monitored during GA and in the postoperative period.

In children with NMDs without primary myocardial dysfunction (e.g., SMA), preoperative cardiologic evaluation is suggested only if pulmonary hypertension is suspected.

12.3.4 Other Issues

Nutritional status should be optimized before surgery. In case of poor nutritional balance, wound healing can be delayed and the patient could be too weak to adequately clear secretions or maintain ventilation.

Patients with NMDs have an increased sensitivity to *premedication drugs*, which could induce apnea and hypoventilation.

For patients *chronically treated with steroids* (i.e., DMD, MG), consideration has to be paid to their administration during surgery. In fact, this therapy can suppress the hypothalamic–pituitary–adrenal axis, and during a phase of stress, such as surgery, the adrenal glands may not respond appropriately.

The preoperative evaluation should also include the assessment for a *difficult intubation* due to jaw ankylosis, atrophy of the masseter muscle and/or other masticatory muscles, macroglossia, or limited mobility of the cervical spine. If any of these conditions is present, intubation should be performed taking into account children guidelines for difficult airway management.

Moreover, in those patients, obtaining an appropriate *intravenous line* could be difficult. Ultrasound may assist peripheral cannulation. Besides, ultrasound-guided venous access is considered the gold standard for any patient for whom central vascular access is necessary. In this case, a peripherally inserted central venous catheter utilizing a cephalic or basilic venous approach under ultrasonic guidance may provide a safe alternative to the standard approach.

In addition, children with NMDs with NMDs are predisposed to *hypothermia* because of reduced heat production in atrophic or dystrophic muscle. Negative effects of hypothermia are preventable by heating the skin with heated blankets or blown hot air.

Postoperative admission to a pediatric intensive care unit (PICU) should be considered in any patient at risk for respiratory complications, with weak cough, severe bulbar dysfunction, severe cardiac dysfunction, or morphine infusions. In fact, PICU setting allows intensive cardiovascular and respiratory monitoring and use of adjuvant therapy, including NIV and cough-assisted and suctioning devices.

Finally, a very important preoperative issue is to establish whether the benefit of surgery outweighs the anesthetic risk and *discuss risks and benefits* of surgical procedures with the patients and/or their family.

12.3.5 Preoperative Considerations in Specific NMDs

12.3.5.1 Myasthenia Gravis
Pharmacologic therapy should be optimized. If the patient is poorly controlled, a preoperative course of plasmapheresis or i.v. immunoglobulins could be beneficial. However, there is little evidence that supports this strategy in order to reduce anesthetic complication. Oral anticholinesterase drugs should be continued in the preoperative period, except for the day of surgery as they may interfere with muscle relaxants and enhance bronchial secretions. When oral administration is limited, an equivalent dosage of intravenous neostigmine should be introduced and continued until the patient resumes oral therapy.

12.3.5.2 Mitochondrial Myopathies
These patients may have increased lactate levels during periods of physiological stress. Therefore, preoperative fasting in these patients could be particularly

hazardous. Intravenous isotonic fluid containing dextrose (e.g., 0.9 % sodium chloride with 5 % dextrose) should be started during preoperative fasting period to allow maintenance of normoglycemia, as excessive glycolytic oxidation may increase plasma lactate levels.

12.4   Intraoperative Management

In children with NMDs with decreased pulmonary function, GA should be avoided preferring regional anesthesia whenever possible. If GA is unavoidable, ultrashort-acting drugs, such as propofol and remifentanil, are preferable and succinylcholine must be avoided. Furthermore, administration of volatile anesthetics in myopathic children is usually considered at high risk for life-threatening complications.

12.4.1   Succinylcholine and Halogenated Agents

Four major categories of NMDs (see Table 12.1) should be considered to plan the safest anesthesia strategy: (1) motoneuron diseases, (2) peripheral neuropathies, (3) neuromuscular junction diseases, and (4) muscle diseases.

In *motoneuron* and *peripheral nerve diseases*, the use of halogenated agents is permitted, whereas succinylcholine must be avoided.

In children with *neuromuscular junction disorders*, GA can be performed using halogenated agents.

In *myopathic* children, the use of inhaled anesthetics and succinylcholine is classically considered at high risk for MH or acute rhabdomyolysis. Although only few muscle diseases carry significant risk of MH such as some rare myopathies due to mutation of calcium channels (e.g., ryanodine receptor), "central core myopathies," King–Denborough syndrome, or other rarer conditions, all children with muscle disease carry a risk of rhabdomyolysis. Therefore, it is recommended to avoid the use of succinylcholine and halogenated agents in such children. However, in children with mitochondrial myopathies, halogenated agents can be administered. Some authors agree that faced with a difficult venous access in a patient with myopathy, a brief use of inhalation anesthesia is possible as long as the anesthesiologist is prepared to treat rhabdomyolysis; however, some other authors suggest the use of ketamine in these circumstances. Although i.m. ketamine is used for adult patients, an oral or rectal route is preferred for pediatric patients to avoid unnecessary pain and stress to the child and their family.

12.4.2   Total Intravenous Anesthesia (TIVA)

Whenever inhalation anesthesia must be avoided, GA can be performed using TIVA. However, it should be minded that respiratory and cardiac depression can be induced by intravenous anesthetic agents and opioids. Thus, the dose of these drugs should be carefully titrated to be effective but to avoid excessive respiratory and cardiac depression. Although the effectiveness of target controlled infusion (TCI) of propofol compared with manually controlled infusion remains controversial in adults and in children, some authors reported that careful titration of propofol by TCI enables to evaluate the patient's sensitivity to propofol in subjects with NMDs.

Moreover, despite its well-known limitation in pediatric patients, the use of bispectral index monitor (BIS) may prevent the occurrence of awareness and reduce the risk of drug overdose in children with NMDs.

12.4.3 Nondepolarizing Neuromuscular Blocking Agents (NMB)

In all children with NMDs, nondepolarizing NMB may show prolonged duration of neuromuscular blockade, even with short-acting drugs. Thus, most reports recommend to avoid NMBs whenever possible. However, when NMB are necessary, the dose should be reduced and titrated to effect, neuromuscular function has to be continuously monitored (e.g., using the train-of-four monitoring), and the effect of muscle relaxant should be always antagonized. Nevertheless, anticholinesterase drugs are not recommended because they may lead to hyperkalemia. Therefore, reversal of rocuronium-induced or vecuronium-induced neuromuscular blockade by sugammadex could be beneficial in NMDs to eliminate the risk of postoperative residual muscle paralysis. Finally, the combination of rocuronium and sugammadex could replace the need for succinylcholine in rapid sequence induction in children with NMDs.

12.4.4 Regional Anesthesia

There are potential risks with regional anesthesia in children with preexisting peripheral nervous system diseases. Upton and McComas emphasized that if these patients are exposed to secondary damages such as injuries from needles or catheters, ischemic lesions from vasopressors, or toxicity of a local anesthetic, the probability of neurological damages increases. On the other hand, the use of regional or local anesthesia offers a significant advantage in terms of avoidance of anesthetic drugs and reduction of postoperative respiratory complications for all children with NMDs and mainly in those with reduced pulmonary function. A significant reduction of the required volume of local anesthetic is possible when ultrasound and peripheral nerve stimulator are used for nerve identification. Moreover, the use of ultrasound appeared to reduce the incidence of hematoma formation following vascular puncture. Therefore, regional anesthesia should be warranted whenever possible, including patients with preexisting peripheral nervous system disorders.

12.4.5 Anesthetic Considerations in Specific NMDs

12.4.5.1 Guillain–Barrè Syndrome (GBS)
In patients with GBS, anesthesia may be associated with severe complications due to dysautonomia (i.e., bradycardia, blood pressure swings, and profound hypotension with sedatives). In patients with autonomic dysfunction, a potential sympathetic blockade resulting from regional anesthesia requires careful control of blood pressure. Consequentially, a neuraxial blockade should be cautiously administered to patients with GBS. However, several cases have reported a successful use of epidural and spinal anesthesia in these patients without any case of hemodynamic instability.

12.4.5.2 Myasthenia Gravis (MG)
Factors potentially enhancing neuromuscular blockade should be avoided (e.g., hypothermia, hypokalemia, hypophosphatemia, and several drugs). As local anesthetic agents may block neuromuscular transmission, subarachnoid and epidural anesthesia should be performed using reduced doses and preferably amid local anesthetics, such as bupivacaine and ropivacaine.

Excess of anticholinesterase drugs may produce flaccid muscle paralysis and pupil constriction (cholinergic crisis) in patients with MG. Many patients have a decreased requirement of these drugs in the first 48 h. Thus, intravenous anticholinesterase drugs should be administered slowly and cautiously in the postoperative period. Moreover, meticulous attention to pulmonary toilet is required, particularly since respiratory secretions may be increased by the anticholinesterase drugs. Sugammadex, in combination with neuromuscular monitoring, can be used to reverse rocuronium-induced neuromuscular blockade in patients with MG, thereby avoiding the need for reversal with acetylcholinesterase inhibitors.

12.4.5.3 Dystrophinopathies
Several studies have shown a delayed onset of nondepolarizing muscle relaxants in patients with dystrophinopathies. Therefore, a high dose of rocuronium is needed to shorten the onset time. Reversal of NMB by sugammadex can eliminate the risk of postoperative residual paralysis, even after a high dose of rocuronium.

12.4.5.4 Myotonic Dystrophy
The anesthetic strategy of choice remains uncertain. Whenever possible, peripheral nerve or neuroaxis blockade is preferable. When GA is indicated, extreme care should be taken during all phases of anesthesia. Many authors have proposed the use of halogenated gases in patients with DM1 and DM2, but others consider safer to avoid them. Noteworthy, halogenated agents may induce postoperative shivering which can precipitate myotonia. Moreover, there is an increased sensitivity of DM1 patients against thiopental and propofol. During anesthetic induction, thiopental is relatively contraindicated due to prolonged respiratory depression. Propofol can be successfully used both for induction and maintenance of anesthesia, if the dose is

carefully titrated. In these patients respiratory failure may be caused both by weakness and myotonic reactions. Many factors like hypothermia, postoperative shivering, dyskalemia, mechanical and electrical stimulation, or drugs (i.e., propranolol, succinylcholine, and anticholinesterase agents) can precipitate myotonic contractures. The development of myotonia represents an important problem for anesthesia because, if laryngeal and respiratory muscles are involved, intubation can be difficult or even impossible. Myotonia occurs for an intrinsic change in the muscle and not in the peripheral nerve or neuromuscular junction. Thus, it cannot be abolished by peripheral nerve blockades or neuromuscular blockers. Myotonia may be treated with midazolam; otherwise, the treatment is mainly preventive, avoiding all triggering factors. Consequently, a protocol of safe surgical procedure should be adopted to prevent myotonia. Dyskalemia, triggering drugs, and excessive stress should be avoided, body temperature should be closely monitored to minimize the risk of shivering, and succinylcholine should not be administrated. Careful cardiac monitoring is needed in all DM1 patients, for their high risk of arrhythmic events, which may cause sudden death at any age. Finally, these patients have also a propensity to develop hyperglycemia, dysphagia, and gastroesophageal reflux. Maintaining the torso of the patient elevated in the postoperative period reduces the risks of aspiration.

12.4.5.5 Mitochondrial Myopathies

Mitochondrial myopathies consist of a heterogeneous group of disorders caused by abnormalities in mitochondria leading to muscle weakness, lactic acidosis, and a variable combination of central and/or peripheral nervous system involvement (seizures, hemiparesis, cortical blindness, ophthalmologic abnormalities, hearing loss), bulbar dysfunction with impaired swallowing, cardiac dysfunction, hepatic and renal disease, and defect of insulin secretion. It should be borne in mind that propofol has a mitochondrial depressant effect that can induce lactic acidosis. Moreover, in these patients also other anesthetic agents such as thiopentone, midazolam, halogenated agents, and local anesthetics can cause lactic acidosis interfering with mitochondrial function. Nevertheless, it is noted that all these anesthetic agents have been used with success in patients with mitochondrial myopathies. This suggests that there is no case for avoiding any particular anesthetic agents in these patients. However, caution is required with all anesthetic agents. In particular, it would be seen as pertinent to avoid the prolonged use of propofol for the maintenance of anesthesia. Moreover, lactic acidosis should be prevented with control of excessive stress, maintaining normal serum glucose levels, adequate oxygen balance, stable cardiovascular function, and adequate gas exchange. Finally, the routine perioperative use of lactate-free i.v. fluids in all children with mitochondrial disease undergoing GA is recommended.

12.4.5.6 Glycogenosis Type II (GSDII)

In the infantile form of GSDII, characterized by a significant hypertrophic cardiomyopathy, decreased cardiac output and myocardial ischemia have been observed during anesthesia. In fact, stiffness of the hypertrophied ventricular walls can induce abnormal diastolic relaxation and lead to dynamic left ventricular outflow tract obstruction, elevated left ventricular end-diastolic pressure, and reduced diastolic filling. This condition may precipitate as a consequence of a decrease in systemic vascular resistance, preload, or both eventually induced by anesthetic agents, with an increased risk of intraoperative cardiac arrest.

12.5   Postoperative Management

12.5.1 Pain Control

Adequate pain control is essential to prevent hypoventilation secondary to splinting after thoracic, upper abdominal, and spine surgery.

Intravenous opioids should be titrated to provide adequate analgesia and promote airway clearance minimizing respiratory suppression. This goal is best accomplished with preemptive analgesia and using multiple pharmacological agents. Oral clonidine administered preoperatively has been shown to reduce the requirement for postoperative analgesics. Moreover, i.v. paracetamol, administered alone or in combination with nonsteroidal anti-inflammatory agents (e.g., ketorolac), has been shown to reduce the amount of opiates delivered.

Continuous infusion of opioids via epidural catheters can be used when appropriate to achieve pain control while minimizing respiratory side effects.

Finally, wound infiltration with local anesthetic solutions and continuous infusion of local anesthetic solutions via peripheral nerve block catheters should be offered when appropriate as safer alternatives. Peripheral nerve blocks have been shown to provide postoperative analgesia which is comparable to that obtained with an epidural technique but with less side effects. These neural structures should be localized using ultrasound guidance or nerve stimulation techniques.

In case of hypoventilation after opioid administration, adequate ventilation can be achieved by using NIV or by delaying extubation for 24–48 h. Moreover, MI-E can also be useful when pain prevents the children from coughing spontaneously.

12.5.2 Respiratory Management

Postoperative management should be determined by preoperative respiratory function and the type of surgery performed. Children with normal cough clearance and relatively preserved muscle function are not at increased risk for postoperative complications. On the other hand, children with decreased respiratory muscle strength require close monitoring and aggressive respiratory management.

The application of a protocol based on the combination of NIV with MI-E after extubation for high-risk children with NMDs may provide a clinically important advantage by averting the need for reintubation or tracheotomy and shortening their PICU stay.

NIV as bridge support after extubation should be considered for patients with baseline FVC <50 % of predicted value and should be strongly considered for those with FVC <30 % of predicted value. Postoperatively the use of assisted cough techniques including the use of MI-E must be considered for any teenage with preoperative PCF <270 L/min. These techniques should be adopted before and after extubation. Assisted cough technique is obviously also recommended for patients already using MI-E and NIV preoperatively.

To improve the chance of success, extubation should be delayed until respiratory secretions are well controlled and SpO_2 is normal or baseline in room air.

In patients requiring long-term mechanical ventilation, respiratory support must be continued in the postoperative period.

Oxygen must be applied with caution in children with NMDs because it can correct hypoxemia without treating the underlying cause such as hypercapnia, mucus plugging, and atelectasis. To facilitate appropriate oxygen use, CO_2 levels should be strictly monitored.

References

1. Racca F, Mongini T, Wolfler A et al (2013) Recommendations for Anesthesia and Perioperative management of patients with neuromuscular disorders. Minerva Anestesiol 79:419–433
2. Birnkrant DJ (2009) The American College of Chest Physicians consensus statement on the respiratory and related management of patients with Duchenne muscular dystrophy undergoing anesthesia or sedation. Pediatrics 123(Suppl 4):S242–S244
3. Birnkrant DJ, Panitch HB, Benditt JO, Boitano LJ, Carter ER, Cwik VA et al (2007) American College of Chest Physicians consensus statement on the respiratory and related management of patients with Duchenne muscular dystrophy undergoing anesthesia or sedation. Chest 132(6):1977–1986
4. Bushby K, Finkel R, Birnkrant DJ, Case LE, Clemens PR, Cripe L et al (2010) Diagnosis and management of Duchenne muscular dystrophy, part 2: implementation of multidisciplinary care. Lancet Neurol 9(2):177–189
5. Wang CH, Bonnemann CG, Rutkowski A, Sejersen T, Bellini J, Battista V et al (2010) Consensus statement on standard of care for congenital muscular dystrophies. J Child Neurol 25(12):1559–1581
6. Wang CH, Finkel RS, Bertini ES, Schroth M, Simonds A, Wong B et al (2007) Consensus statement for standard of care in spinal muscular atrophy. J Child Neurol 22(8):1027–1049
7. Gozal D (2000) Pulmonary manifestations of neuromuscular disease with special reference to Duchenne muscular dystrophy and spinal muscular atrophy. Pediatr Pulmonol 29(2):141–150
8. Schmitt HJ, Muenster T (2009) Anesthesia in patients with neuromuscular disorders. Minerva Anestesiol 75(11):632–637
9. Veyckemans F (2010) Can inhalation agents be used in the presence of a child with myopathy? Curr Opin Anaesthesiol 23(3):348–355
10. Wappler F (2010) Anesthesia for patients with a history of malignant hyperthermia. Curr Opin Anaesthesiol 23(3):417–422
11. Gurnaney H, Brown A, Litman RS (2009) Malignant hyperthermia and muscular dystrophies. Anesth Analg 109(4):1043–1048
12. Hayes J, Veyckemans F, Bissonnette B (2008) Duchenne muscular dystrophy: an old anesthesia problem revisited. Paediatr Anaesth 18(2):100–106
13. Klingler W, Lehmann-Horn F, Jurkat-Rott K (2005) Complications of anaesthesia in neuromuscular disorders. Neuromuscul Disord 15(3):195–206

14. Driessen JJ (2008) Neuromuscular and mitochondrial disorders: what is relevant to the anaesthesiologist? Curr Opin Anaesthesiol 21(3):350–355
15. Graham RJ, Athiraman U, Laubach AE, Sethna NF (2009) Anesthesia and perioperative medical management of children with spinal muscular atrophy. Paediatr Anaesth 19(11):1054–1063
16. Birnkrant DJ (2006) New challenges in the management of prolonged survivors of pediatric neuromuscular diseases: a pulmonologist's perspective. Pediatr Pulmonol 41(12):1113–1117
17. Racca F, Del Sorbo L, Mongini T, Vianello A, Ranieri VM (2010) Respiratory management of acute respiratory failure in neuromuscular diseases. Minerva Anestesiol 76(1):51–62
18. Rubino FA (2004) Perioperative management of patients with neurologic disease. Neurol Clin 22(2):V, 261–V, 276
19. Blichfeldt-Lauridsen L, Hansen BD (2012) Anesthesia and myasthenia gravis. Acta Anaesthesiol Scand 56(1):17–22
20. Bach JR, Goncalves MR, Hamdani I, Winck JC (2010) Extubation of patients with neuromuscular weakness: a new management paradigm. Chest 137(5):1033–1039
21. Vianello A, Arcaro G, Braccioni F, Gallan F, Marchi MR, Chizio S et al (2011) Prevention of extubation failure in high-risk patients with neuromuscular disease. J Crit Care 26(5):517–524
22. Bushby K, Finkel R, Birnkrant DJ, Case LE, Clemens PR, Cripe L et al (2010) Diagnosis and management of Duchenne muscular dystrophy, part 1: diagnosis, and pharmacological and psychosocial management. Lancet Neurol 9(1):77–93
23. Hopkins PM (2010) Anaesthesia and the sex-linked dystrophies: between a rock and a hard place. Br J Anaesth 104(4):397–400
24. Muenster T, Mueller C, Forst J, Huber H, Schmitt HJ (2012) Anaesthetic management in patients with Duchenne muscular dystrophy undergoing orthopaedic surgery: a review of 232 cases. Eur J Anaesthesiol 29(10):489–494
25. Salem M, Tainsh RE Jr, Bromberg J, Loriaux DL, Chernow B (1994) Perioperative glucocorticoid coverage. A reassessment 42 years after emergence of a problem. Ann Surg 219(4):416–425
26. Hammond K, Margolin DA, Beck DE, Timmcke AE, Hicks TC, Whitlow CB (2010) Variations in perioperative steroid management among surgical subspecialists. Am Surg 76(12):1363–1367
27. Marik PE, Varon J (2008) Requirement of perioperative stress doses of corticosteroids: a systematic review of the literature. Arch Surg 143(12):1222–1226
28. Yong SL, Marik P, Esposito M, Coulthard P (2009) Supplemental perioperative steroids for surgical patients with adrenal insufficiency. Cochrane Database Syst Rev (4):CD005367
29. Frova G, Guarino A, Petrini F, Merli G, Sorbello M, Baroncini S et al (2006) Recommendations for airway control and difficult airway management in paediatric patients. Minerva Anestesiol 72(9):723–748
30. Keyes LE, Frazee BW, Snoey ER, Simon BC, Christy D (1999) Ultrasound-guided brachial and basilic vein cannulation in emergency department patients with difficult intravenous access. Ann Emerg Med 34(6):711–714
31. Troianos CA, Hartman GS, Glas KE, Skubas NJ, Eberhardt RT, Walker JD et al (2012) Special articles: guidelines for performing ultrasound guided vascular cannulation: recommendations of the American Society of Echocardiography and the Society of Cardiovascular Anesthesiologists. Anesth Analg 114(1):46–72
32. Sofocleous CT, Schur I, Cooper SG, Quintas JC, Brody L, Shelin R (1998) Sonographically guided placement of peripherally inserted central venous catheters: review of 355 procedures. AJR Am J Roentgenol 170(6):1613–1616
33. Sinclair JL, Reed PW (2009) Risk factors for perioperative adverse events in children with myotonic dystrophy. Paediatr Anaesth 19(8):740–747
34. Cardone A, Congedo E, Aceto P, Sicuranza R, Chine E, Caliandro F et al (2007) Perioperative evaluation of myasthenia gravis. Ann Ital Chir 78(5):359–365
35. Dillon FX (2004) Anesthesia issues in the perioperative management of myasthenia gravis. Semin Neurol 24(1):83–94

36. Shipton EA, Prosser DO (2004) Mitochondrial myopathies and anaesthesia. Eur J Anaesthesiol 21(3):173–178
37. Yemen TA, McClain C (2006) Muscular dystrophy, anesthesia and the safety of inhalational agents revisited; again. Paediatr Anaesth 16(2):105–108
38. Malviya S, Voepel-Lewis T, Tait AR, Watcha MF, Sadhasivam S, Friesen RH (2007) Effect of age and sedative agent on the accuracy of bispectral index in detecting depth of sedation in children. Pediatrics 120(3):e461–e470
39. De Boer HD, van Esmond J, Booij LH, Driessen JJ (2009) Reversal of rocuronium-induced profound neuromuscular block by sugammadex in Duchenne muscular dystrophy. Paediatr Anaesth 19(12):1226–1228
40. Unterbuchner C, Fink H, Blobner M (2010) The use of sugammadex in a patient with myasthenia gravis. Anaesthesia 65(3):302–305
41. Walker KJ, McGrattan K, Aas-Eng K, Smith AF (2009) Ultrasound guidance for peripheral nerve blockade. Cochrane Database Syst Rev (4):CD006459
42. Allison KR (2007) Muscular dystrophy versus mitochondrial myopathy: the dilemma of the undiagnosed hypotonic child. Paediatr Anaesth 17(1):1–6

Perioperative Care of Children with a Metabolic Disease

13

Veyckemans Francis and Scholtes Jean-Louis

Metabolic diseases are numerous. They can broadly be divided into three categories depending on their pathophysiology:

- Intoxication by accumulation of a toxic compound that cannot be eliminated: e.g., hyperammonemia in case of urea cycle anomaly
- Lack of energetic resources due to deficiency in their synthesis or use: e.g., lack of aerobic ATP in mitochondrial cytopathies
- Storage of complex molecules: e.g., mucopolysaccharidosis

Some overlap is of course possible: for example, both hypoglycemia and hepatic accumulation of dextrin in case of glycogenosis type III (Cori's disease). Moreover, as a rule, the more important the deficit, the earlier the signs and symptoms of the disorder appear: a mild deficit can thus remain pauci- or asymptomatic for a long period of time or present with signs, for example, neuropsychiatric problems, that do not usually trigger search for a metabolic disorder.

The anesthetic consequences of metabolic diseases vary widely: for example, the main concerns are airway and cardiac related when caring for a child with mucopolysaccharidosis, adequate steroid coverage in case of congenital adrenal hyperplasia, and avoiding increased protein catabolism in the presence of a urea cycle anomaly. Anesthesiologists care for a child with a metabolic disease only for a short but critical period of time, the perioperative period, when many factors can jeopardize its fragile equilibrium. They therefore need the help of the child's caring team to answer the following questions:

V. Francis, MD (✉) • S. Jean-Louis, MD
Anesthesiology, Cliniques universitaires St Luc, Université Catholique de Louvain, Avenue Hippocrate 10-1821, Bruxelles 1200B-1200, Belgium
e-mail: francis.veyckemans@uclouvain.be

© Springer International Publishing Switzerland 2016
M. Astuto, P.M. Ingelmo (eds.), *Perioperative Medicine in Pediatric Anesthesia*,
Anesthesia, Intensive Care and Pain in Neonates and Children,
DOI 10.1007/978-3-319-21960-8_13

- What are the direct consequences of the disease regarding the child's anesthetic management: upper and lower airway, heart, muscle function, neurodevelopmental issues, seizures etc.?
- What is the child's usual treatment and/or diet?
- What could be the effects of some anesthetic drugs on the organs affected by the disease?
- What are the possible effects of the perianesthetic period on the child's metabolic equilibrium: fever, stress, starvation, etc.?
- What intravenous solution should be used as long as the child is unable to follow its usual diet: glucose 5, 10, or 20 % with electrolytes?
- What should be specifically monitored: blood glucose, lactates, or ammonium?
- What have been the child's previous anesthetic experiences?

The first goal of this chapter is to give the reader a frame to help him/her establish an anesthetic plan adapted to the child's known or suspected pathology and its current preoperative status. The second goal is to highlight the importance of developing a "metabolic reflex" when a child presents with an unusual clinical picture in the perioperative period. This will be illustrated with a few examples.

13.1   Sources of Information

It is necessary to check the most recent data about a metabolic disease in order to know its pathophysiology, its usual clinical presentations and outcome, and its treatment, whether curative or symptomatic. This can be done using the paper or electronic literature, for example:

- *Inborn Metabolic Diseases*, 5th edition, by Saudubray, van den Berghe & Walter (Springer, 2012)
- *Genetic Syndromes* by B Bissonnette & B Dalens (McGrawHill, 2005)
- http://www.rarediseases.org/
- http://orpha.net/
- http://orphanaesthesia.eu
- http://ncbi.nlm.nih.gov/Omim/

or, more simply, "googling."

When using Google, it is important to remind that the ranking of the links obtained depends not only on the key word(s) introduced but also on a complex algorithm: the ranking is thus not linked to the quality of the data and each link should be checked (origin, date of update or publication, etc.). Moreover, when considering anesthetic case reports, the information should be interpreted with caution [1] because they generally describe isolated cases, the scientific value of which is relative:

- Either there was no problem: it could be the result of excellent anesthetic care or simply a lucky outcome.

- Or something happened: it is sometimes difficult to determine whether it was associated with the disease or with borderline anesthetic management.
- In addition, the date of publication should be checked: some were published at a time when current equipment (e.g., supraglottic airways) or drugs (e.g., short-acting opiates or muscle relaxants, propofol) were not available yet.

The reviews of large series are therefore the best source of information.

We should also keep in mind that thanks to progress in medicine, the natural history of some diseases has changed: their evolution can be totally or partially controlled by a strict medical treatment (a special diet, e.g., phenylketonuria), by intravenous enzyme replacement therapy (e.g., Gaucher's and Pompe's disease), and/or by organ transplantation (e.g., Hurler's disease) [2, 3]. We currently do not know yet what the evolution of the cured disease and the side effects of its treatment will be, neither what are the possible anesthetic implications of their modified condition.

Last, the parents often know very well their child's disease and can provide the address of useful website specifically dedicated to the disease. And finally, nothing is better than a direct contact with the pediatrician in charge of the child: he/she knows very well both the child and its disease.

13.2 Synthesis of the Informations

The pathophysiology of the disease should be carefully reviewed in the light of anesthetic care. In order to make sure everything has been considered, the authors propose using the NARCO + Age acronym [4] as summarized in Table 13.1. In fact, this

Table 13.1 The NARCO memory tool

Neuromuscular	Any developmental delay?
	muscles: spasticity, contractures, hypotonia?
	Seizures: controlled or not?
	Medical treatment?
Airway	Difficult intubation/ventilation?
	Any risk for regurgitation/inhalation? chronic lung infection?
	Signs of obstructive or central sleep apnea?
Respiratory	Reactive airway?
	Restrictive or obstructive syndrome?
	Chronic lung infection?
Cardiovascular	Dysrhythmia?
	Cardiomyopathy?
Others	Special diet?
	Tolerates fasting?
	Previous anesthesia?
	Psychological issues?
	Communication

Modified from Malviya et al. [4]

system-based approach was originally designed to evaluate the child's anesthetic risk better than the ASA physical status and any other memory jogger can be used such as ABCD with A for airway, B for brain, C for cardiac, and D for drugs, diet, etc.

But the child's age should also be taken into account because, as for any pediatric case, (1) the younger the patient, the higher the risk; (2) young age has its own anatomic, physiologic, and pharmacologic specificities; and (3) because some pathologies become worse with age, for example, mucopolysaccharidosis and mitochondrial cytopathies.

The anesthesiologist should also keep in mind that a child with a metabolic disease remains a child: the "metabolic" tree should not hide the forest! The basic pediatric preoperative evaluation should be undertaken as in any child:

- Personal history: previous anesthesia?
- Allergies?
- Bleeding problem?
- Upper airway: mouth opening? retrognathia? facial asymmetry? midface hypoplasia? loose teeth? snoring during sleep?
- Airway reactivity: recent infection? asthma? passive smoking?
- Difficult venous access?
- Cardiopulmonary examination?

The final anesthetic plan should also be adapted to the procedure for which anesthesia is needed, whether it is an emergency or not, and whether it will occur in an operating room or outside the operating theaters area. It should be borne in mind that an emergency procedure combines the risks of emergency anesthesia (full stomach) with the effects of fever, hypovolemia, and stress on the child's metabolic equilibrium: the child's pediatrician's advice and the availability of a high-dependency bed for the early postoperative period are necessary in this context.

Last but not least, there are psychological issues to consider: as it grows, a child with a metabolic disease becomes a chronic medical patient with its "special needs" and phobias (mask, needle) but also with a critical eye on what is done around him/her. Moreover, compliance with treatment is often a critical issue at the time of adolescence. In short, a child with a metabolic disease is a fragile person and taking care of it, and of its family, needs a mix of science, vigilance, and compassion.

13.3 Example 1: A Urea Cycle Defect

The urea cycle is the succession of six successive enzymatic reactions to transform ammonia, the result of endogenous and exogenous protein catabolism, in urea which can be eliminated in the urine. It occurs only in the hepatocytes [5]. *N*-acetyl glutamate synthetase (NAGS) is one of the three mitochondrial enzyme participating to it. NAGS deficiency is transmitted as an autosomal recessive trait (NAGS gene, 17q21.31) and its prevalence is around 1/70,000. Its clinical signs vary according to the importance of the deficit and thus of the patient's age:

- Neonatal period: difficult feeding, vomiting a few hours after birth, and rapid evolution to hypotonic coma with seizures if not diagnosed and treated.
- Infancy: anorexia, vomiting, and failure to thrive; these children often undergo diagnostic esophagogastroscopies before the definitive diagnosis is established.
- Childhood and adolescence: episode(s) of acute decompensation presenting as a neurologic (encephalopathy, convulsions, ataxia, psychiatric problem), metabolic (coma), or hepatic (cytolysis, Reye-like syndrome) problem precipitated by a stress such as fever, postoperative period, infection, or administration of valproate acid.

The basic principle of the treatment of NAGS is avoiding protein catabolism. The children therefore need a special diet, the protein content of which is carefully adapted to the child's age and decreased in case of infection or stress (e.g., surgery). They often also receive a daily dose of N-carbamyl glutamic acid (30–250 mg/kg/day) according to their blood urea and NH_3 level. Orthotopic liver transplantation can be performed to cure the disease.

Anesthetic implications:

- N: according to the child neurologic status
- A: nothing specific to the disease
- R: nothing specific to the disease
- C: nothing specific to the disease
- O
  - Special diet: a low-protein and hypercaloric diet should be started 1 or 2 days before elective surgery.
  - Preanesthetic fasting time has to be kept as short as possible; a glucose-containing solution with electrolytes should be administered at the beginning of the preanesthesia starving period.
  - Monitoring: NH_3 (nl <50 µmol/L), glycemia.
  - In case of seizures, valproate should not be administered as it inhibits carbamylphosphate transferase, another enzyme of the cycle.
  - There is no specific contraindication to perform a regional block, which is a good way to reduce the patient's perioperative stress response.
  - In case of surgery during or following which blood can enter the digestive tract (e.g., ENT, dental, or gastrointestinal surgery), the gastric content should be aspirated (nasogastric tube) because ingested blood is an important source of exogenous protein.
  - In case of hyperammonemia, the following should be administered in emergency: IV glucose 20 %, Na-benzoate (0.25–0.5 g/kg/day), Na-phenylbutyrate (0.5 g/kg/day), and L-arginine (0.25–0.5 g/kg/day). In case of failure or severe neurologic signs, hemodialysis or peritoneal dialysis should be performed.

13.4   Example 2: A Glycogenosis

In case of glycogenosis type III (also called Cori's or Forbe's disease), the absence of amylo-1, 6-glycosidase impairs complete degradation of glycogen in glucose: both a risk of hypoglycemia and accumulation of dextrin in hepatic and/or muscular cells ensue. Both the liver and the muscles are affected in type A while only muscles cells are affected in form B.

The accumulation of dextrin into the hepatocytes leads to hepatomegaly and progressively to hepatic fibrosis; in some cases, cirrhosis and hepatic adenomas develop during adolescence. These patients are often obese because they require frequent meals to avoid hypoglycemia. Cases of late hypertrophic cardiomyopathy have been described.

Anesthetic implications [6, 7]:

- *N*: sometimes hypotonia in infancy; proximal amyotrophy with elevated CPK in adolescents and adults
- *A*: macroglossia that may be present
- *R*: respiratory comorbidities of obesity, asthma and obstructive sleep apnea
- *C*: echocardiography to rule out cardiomyopathy
- *O*
    - Hepatic function has to be checked; any sign of portal hypertension?
    - Difficult venous access and other comorbidities of obesity.
    - Preanesthetic fasting time has to be kept as short as possible; a glucose-containing solution with electrolytes should be administered at the beginning of the preanesthesia starving period.
    - Monitoring: blood glucose level.
    - Succinylcholine and use of a surgical tourniquet should be best avoided to prevent rhabdomyolysis (fragile muscles).
    - There is no specific contraindication to perform a regional block but ultrasound-guided peripheral nerve blocks could be more tricky to perform because amyotrophy modifies muscular echogenicity.

13.5   A Mitochondrial Cytopathy

The mitochondrion is the main energy provider of the cell and many metabolic reactions occur at least partly into it: metabolism of glucose (tricarboxylic or Krebs cycle), lipids (β-oxidation of fatty acids with the carnitine shuttle system), and protein (urea cycle). In addition, many neurodegenerative diseases (e.g., some forms of Parkinson or Charcot-Marie-Tooth disease) are now known to be caused by defects in what can be called the "maintenance functions" of the mitochondrion. But the term mitochondrial cytopathy refers mainly to pathologies of the respiratory chain or oxidative phosphorylation system, a succession of reactions occurring in the inner membrane of the mitochondrion: it generates an active proton (H+) and a free electron gradient leading to the production of ATP. The five protein complexes involved in the respiratory chain are encoded by genes that are present in the mitochondrial or in the nuclear DNA: their mode of transmission is complex being either maternal or autosomic dominant or recessive. Moreover, their phenotypic expression is highly variable depending on the relative distribution of wild and mutated mitochondria within each cell and on the energetic needs of the tissue wherein they are distributed (threshold effect) [8]. Mitochondrial cytopathies are usually called according to acronyms such as MERFF (myoclonus, epilepsy, ragged red fibers), MELAS (mitochondrial encephalopathy, lactic acidosis, stroke-like episodes), or their discoverer's name (e.g., Leigh or Kearns-Sayre's disease).

A peculiar aspect of the anesthetic care of mitochondrial cytopathies is that many anesthetic agents do interfere in vitro with the respiratory chain. Those data were obtained in vitro on wild mitochondria isolated from tissue: their relevance for clinical practice is thus difficult to define taking into account that almost all anesthetic agents have been used in patients with a mitochondrial cytopathy without observing major clinical effects. However, they should be kept in mind when planning anesthesia, for example:

- Propofol inhibits complexes II and V of the respiratory chain as well as the intramitochondrial transport of free fatty acids by the carnitine system: a continuous infusion of propofol is thus considered as contraindicated because it could induce a propofol infusion syndrome (PRIS) [9]. However small case series have been published showing no untoward effect of a continuous infusion of propofol in patients with a mitochondrial cytopathy provided a glucose-containing solution was associated [10]. Recently a case of neurologic deterioration has been observed after a single dose of propofol given without glucose administration in a girl with MELAS syndrome but her clinical status was deteriorating before anesthesia: it is thus difficult to determine whether her metabolic deterioration would have occurred without propofol [11]. In any case, a glucose-containing solution ($6 \, \mathrm{mg \cdot kg^{-1} \cdot h^{-1}}$) should always be associated with the use of propofol in patients with a known or suspected mitochondrial cytopathy, and their blood lactate level should be monitored if a continuous infusion of propofol is used.
- Barbiturates, etomidate, and ketamine inhibit complex I.
- Nitrous oxide decreases the activity of complex IV which could favor the local synthesis of nitric oxide.
- Halogenated agents act, among others, on the GAS-1 gene which encodes a subunit of complex 1 [12]: it is thus possible that children with a mitochondrial cytopathy are more sensitive to halogenated agents as shown in a series of children with complex I dysfunction who needed less sevoflurane to achieve a BIS level of 60 [13].
- Regarding local anesthetics, lidocaine does not interfere with the respiratory chain but both isomers of bupivacaine inhibit complex I more than ropivacaine [14].

As the mitochondrial cytopathies are all multisystemic and evoluting diseases, the preoperative evaluation of the patient should look at every organ system. Going back to the proposed NARCO memory tool:

- *N*: the patient's neurologic status needs to be carefully evaluated: seizures and their level of control? encephalopathy? amyotrophy? contractures? scoliosis? mental retardation?
    - There is no risk of malignant hyperthermia even though one poorly documented case [15] and an abnormal response to caffeine-halothane contracture test in one adult with a combined mitochondrial and metabolic myopathy [16] have been described: abnormal mitochondria are a frequent finding at histologic examination of diseased muscles and the response to contracture tests can be falsely positive in case of structural muscle disease.
    - There is no risk of anesthesia-induced rhabdomyolysis (AIR) when halogenated agents are used.
    - In case of muscular signs (amyotrophy, contractures, disuse atrophy), succinylcholine should be best avoided to avoid acute rhabdomyolysis.
- *A*: nothing specific to the disease; gastroparesis with delayed gastric emptying can be observed if the gastrointestinal system is involved; this could result in a "full stomach" situation.
- *R*: central and/or obstructive apnea should be looked for. A decreased response to both hypoxia and hypercarbia has been observed in case of Leigh syndrome: preoperative sedation should thus be used with great care if at all [17]. There are signs of obstructive or restrictive pulmonary dysfunction in case of chronic infection (inhalation of saliva or gastric content) and/or scoliosis: pulmonary function tests are usually impossible to perform but measuring SpO_2 on air and percutaneous CO_2 at nighttime can be helpful.
- *C*: ECG and echocardiography to rule out a cardiomyopathy and dysrhythmias or conduction disturbances, respectively.
- *O* [18].
    - Any event increasing the patient's oxygen consumption, such as fever and infection, could deteriorate its neurologic status [11, 19]; in those cases, the indication for surgery and anesthesia should be reevaluated with the whole caring team; in the same way, both preoperative hypo- and hyperthermia, as well as postanesthetic shivering, should be avoided.
    - Liver and kidney function should be checked as well as hemoglobin, platelets, and electrolytes; in case of unexplained hyponatremia/hyperkalemia, subclinical adrenal insufficiency should be suspected.
    - The patient should take its usual treatment (antiepileptics, vitamins, carnitine, CoQ, etc.) up to the day of anesthesia.
    - Preanesthetic fasting time has to be kept as short as possible; a 5–10 % glucose-containing solution with electrolytes should be administered from the beginning of the preanesthesia starving period; it is recommended to avoid any IV fluid solution containing lactates (e.g., Hartmann's solution) even

though the lactate load is actually very low and such solution has been used uneventfully in a series of cases [10]; if the child receives a ketogenic diet to control complex seizures, the neurologist's advice should be asked regarding perioperative fluid content.

– Monitoring: blood glucose and lactate level. The basal blood lactate levels of the patient should be known: it is usually somewhat higher than the upper limit of normal values; to be valid, the venous blood sample on which lactates are measured should be withdrawn without applying a tourniquet; blood glucose should be kept within normal limits because both hypo- and hyperglycemia can be deleterious for the mitochondrial function.

– If a non-depolarizing muscle relaxant is used, neuromuscular function should be carefully monitored because cases of increased sensitivity have been described [20]; moreover, if muscular signs are present, the train-of-four should be obtained before administering the muscle relaxant in order to know the patient's basal value.

– There is no specific contraindication to perform a regional block, and it is a good way to reduce the patient's perioperative stress response; but scoliosis can make a neuraxial block difficult to perform and should be discussed with the parents if demyelinating lesions are present; moreover, some patients present with a paucisymptomatic peripheral neuropathy with a reduction of motor nerve conduction velocity [21]: the possible effects of a regional block on these axonal and/or demyelinating lesions are currently unknown.

13.6 Developing a "Metabolic Disease" Reflex

In Western countries, many metabolic diseases are currently detected at birth via a systematic screening (Guthrie's test). However, some are not detectable in the neonatal period and some children can escape the test for different reasons. Moreover, a partial metabolic disorder can remain asymptomatic for a long time because it is compensated by other metabolic pathways or the patient spontaneously adapted its diet or behavior: for example, patients with a mild form of a urea cycle disorder spontaneously avoid meat because they feel unwell after eating some (hyperammonemia). But the metabolic disorder can suddenly become symptomatic if the patient's fragile metabolic equilibrium is broken following a stressful situation such as fever, starvation, protein catabolism, etc. These are typical encountered during the perioperative period. The anesthesiologist should always think "metabolism" in case of unexplained complication following an apparently uneventful anesthesia such as delayed awakening or behavioral changes.

There are many causes for delayed awakening after anesthesia, such as:

• Hypothermia
• Overdose [22]

Table 13.2 Easily obtained biological signs to detect an acute metabolic disorder

Diabetes mellitus: ↑ or ↓ blood glucose
Mitochondrial cytopathy: ↑ lactates,
Organic acidemia ↑ lactates, ↓ blood glucose
Urea cycle disorder: ↑ NH_4
Hypothyroidism: ↓ blood glucose
Adrenal insufficiency: ↓ blood pressure ↓Na ↓ blood glucose (Cave: asthmatic, child with a transplanted organ)

- Drug interaction [23]
- Cerebral edema whatever its cause: hyponatremic encephalopathy and trauma
- Cerebral ischemia: sickle cell disease, Moyamoya syndrome, etc.
- Cerebral embolism [24]
- Or an asymptomatic cerebral tumor

In the same way, there are many possible causes for postanesthesia behavioral changes: they can be the result of one of the above-mentioned cerebral pathologies or of:

- An idiosyncratic drug reaction [25, 26]
- A hysteric conversion, a diagnosis of exclusion

But they can also be the result of a decompensated metabolic disorder [27, 28]. In those circumstances, the anesthesiologist should not hesitate to obtain a blood sample to check glucose, electrolyte, ammonium, and lactate levels (see Table 13.2) and even to ask for a cerebral CT scan and the advice of a neurologist. This will allow initiate, if necessary, a life-saving symptomatic treatment and the first stage(s) of a diagnostic workup.

Conclusion

The perioperative care of a child with a metabolic disease is a stressful experience for its parents and a clinical, and often pharmacologic, challenge for the anesthesiologist.

A child with a metabolic disease is a fragile person and taking care of it, and of its family, needs a mix of science, vigilance, and compassion, as well as a team approach. After anesthesia, we should not forget the child's future but give the parents a short report on the technique(s) and precautions used as well as some practical issues in order to help colleagues to take care of their child in the future, in elective, as well as in emergency situations.

References

1. Veyckemans F (2012) Case reports: keep a critical eye! Eur J Anaesthesiol 29:559–560
2. Kirkpatrick K, Ellwood J, Walker RWM (2012) Mucopolysaccharidosis type I (Hurler syndrome) and anesthesia: the impact of bone marrow transplantation, enzyme replacement therapy, and fiberoptic intubation on airway management. Paediatr Anaesth 22:745–751
3. Megens JHAM, de Wit M, van Hasselt PM, Boelens JJ, van der Werff DBM, de Graaff JC (2014) Perioperative complications in patients diagnosed with mucopolysaccharidosis and the impact of enzyme replacement therapy followed by hematopoietic stem cell transplantation at early age. Pediatr Anesth 24:521–527
4. Malviya S, Voepel-Lewis T, Chiravuri SD et al (2011) Does an objective system-based approach improve assessment of perioperative risk in children? A preliminary evaluation of the NARCO. Br J Anaesth 106:352–356
5. Dutoit AP, Flick RR, Sprung J, Babovic-Vuksanovic D, Weingarten TN (2010) Anesthetic implications of ornithine transcarbamylase deficiency. Pediatr Anesth 20:666–673
6. Mohart D, Russo P, Tobias JD (2002) Perioperative management of a child with glycogen storage disease type III undergoing cardiopulmonary bypass and repair of an atrial septal defect. Pediatr Anesth 12:649–654
7. Bolton SD, Clark VA, Norman JE (2011) Multidisciplinary management of an obstetric patient with glycogen storage disease type 3. Int J Obstetr Anesth 20:86–89
8. Area-Gomez E, Schon EA (2014) Mitochondrial genetics and disease. J Child Neurol 29:1208–1215
9. Vanlander AV, Jorens PG, Smet J, De Paepe B et al (2012) Inborn oxidative phosphorylation defect as risk factor for propofol infusion syndrome. Acta Anaesthesiol Scand 56:520–525
10. Gurrieri C, Kivela JE, Bojanic K, Gravilova RH, Flick RP, Sprung J, Weingarten TN (2011) Anesthetic considerations in mitochondrial encephalomyopathy, lactic acidosis, and stroke-like episodes syndrome: a case series. Can J Anaesth 58:751–763
11. Mtaweh H, Bayir H, Kochanek PM, Bell MJ (2014) Effect of a single dose of propofol and lack of dextrose administration in a child with mitochondrial disease: a case report. J Child Neurol 29:NP 40–NP 46
12. Kayser E-B, Morgan PG, Sedensky MM (1999) GAS-1: mitochondrial protein controls sensitivity to volatile anesthetics in the nematode *Caenorhabditis elegans*. Anesthesiology 90:545–554
13. Morgan PG, Hoppel CL, Sedensky MM (2002) Mitochondrial defects and anesthetic sensitivity. Anesthesiology 96:1268–1270
14. Sztark F, Magat M, Dabadie P, Mazat JP (1998) Comparison of the effects of bupivacaine and ropivacaine on heart cells mitochondrial bioenergetics. Anesthesiology 88:1340–1349
15. Ohtani Y, Mike T, Ishitsu T et al (1985) A case of malignant hyperthermia with mitochondrial dysfunction. Brain Dev 7:249 (abstract)
16. Fricker RM, Raffelsberger T, Rauch-Shorny S, Finsterer J et al (2002) Positive malignant hyperthermia susceptibility in vitro test in a patient with mitochondrial myopathy and myoadenylate deaminase deficiency. Anesthesiology 97:1635–1637
17. Muravchick S, Levy RJ (2006) Clinical implications of mitochondrial dysfunction. Anesthesiology 105:819–837
18. Niezgoda J, Morgan PG (2013) Anesthetic considerations in patients with mitochondrial defects. Pediatr Anesth 23:785–793
19. Casta A, Quackenbusch EJ, Houck CS, Korson MS (1997) Perioperative white matter degeneration and death in a patient with a defect in mitochondrial oxidative phosphorylation. Anesthesiology 85:420–425
20. Naguib M, El Dawlatly AA, Ashour L et al (1996) Sensitivity to mivacurium in a patient with mitochondrial myopathy. Anesthesiology 84:1506–1509
21. Stickler DE, Valenstein E, Neiberger RE, Perkins LA et al (2005) Peripheral neuropathy in genetic mitochondrial diseases. Pediatr Neurol 34:127–131

22. Barak M, Greenberg Z, Danino J (2011) Delayed awakening following inadvertent high-dose remifentanil infusion in a 13 year old patient. J Clin Anesth 23:322–324
23. Crowe S, McKeating K (2002) Delayed emergence and St John's Wort. Anesthesiology 96:1025–1027
24. Dive AM, Dubois PE, Ide C, Bulpa PA, Broka SM, Installé E (2002) Paradoxical cerebral fat embolism: an unusual cause of persistent unconsciousness after orthopedic surgery. Anesthesiology 96:1029–1031
25. Quraishi SA, Girharry TD, Xu S-G, Orkin FK (2007) Prolonged retrograde amnesia following sedation with propofol in a 12-year-old boy. Pediatr Anesth 17:375–379
26. Saravanakumar K, Venkatesh P, Bromley P (2005) Delayed onset refractory dystonic movements following propofol anesthesia. Pediatr Anesth 15:597–601
27. Neuvonen PT, van den Berg AA (2001) Postoperative coma in a child with carnitine palmitoyltransferase I deficiency. Anesth Analg 92:646–647
28. Bergmann KR, McCabe J, Smith TR, Guillaume DJ, Sarafoglou K, Gupta S (2014) Late-onset ornithine transcarbamylase deficiency: treatment and outcome of hyperammonemia crisis. Pediatrics 133:e1072–e1076

Perioperative Care of Children with OSA 14

Gianluca Bertolizio and Karen Brown

14.1 Introduction

Sleep-disordered breathing (SDB) represents a spectrum of diseases which involves up to 13 % of children and includes snoring, central sleep apnea (CSA), obstructive sleep apnea syndromes, and other sleep-related hypoventilation/hypoxemic conditions [1].

Obstructive sleep apnea (OSA), a disorder of breathing during sleep, is characterized by prolonged partial upper airway obstruction and/or intermittent complete obstruction that disrupts ventilation during sleep and normal sleep patterns [2].

Most of the obstructive respiratory events in children with OSA occur during rapid eye movement (REM) sleep [3], when airways are more vulnerable to collapse [4].

14.1.1 Epidemiology

Adult and pediatric OSA differs. In adults between the ages of 30 and 70 years, OSA affects 20 % of men and 10 % of women.

In children, the prevalence of OSA is 1–6 %, with an equal distribution between boys and girls [2, 5]. The onset usually occurs between 2 and 8 years of age [5], coinciding with lymphadenoid hypertrophy [6]. A second peak is reported during adolescence [7], with boys being more affected than girls [6].

Obstructive apneas have been reported in 36–57 % of infants, with a peak incidence between 2 and 7 weeks of age [8].

G. Bertolizio (✉) • K. Brown
Department of Anesthesia, Montreal Children's Hospital, McGill University,
1001 Boulevard Décarie, Montreal, QC H4A 3J1, Canada
e-mail: gianluca.bertolizio@mcgill.ca

© Springer International Publishing Switzerland 2016
M. Astuto, P.M. Ingelmo (eds.), *Perioperative Medicine in Pediatric Anesthesia*,
Anesthesia, Intensive Care and Pain in Neonates and Children,
DOI 10.1007/978-3-319-21960-8_14

14.1.2 Clinical Presentation

In older children and adolescents, headache, daytime somnolence, and dry mouth are common signs of OSA. Recent data suggest that daytime sleepiness is more common than previously thought [9] and its prevalence may be as high as 35 % [10].

Symptoms of childhood OSA include nightly apneic episodes, nighttime snoring, restless sleep, and daytime sleepiness.

Snoring is reported in 3–14 % of children, whereas witnessed apneas are described in 2–5 % of children younger than 6 years of age [11]. Restlessness, diaphoresis, and parasomnias are also reported.

Infants with OSA may present with mouth breathing, excessive waking, labored breathing, night sweats, and failure to thrive [12]. In infants sleepiness is rarely reported. Prolonged periods of obstructive hypoventilation are often present, especially in the premature infant. In the majority of infants with OSA, craniofacial conditions and adenotonsillar obstruction are identified, whereas obesity is reported only occasionally.

14.1.3 Risk Factors for OSA

OSA and SDB are more common among former preterm infants [13] and in children who reside in disadvantaged neighborhoods [14]. There is a higher incidence of OSA in children of African-American (AA) ethnicity [13, 15]. Furthermore, these children demonstrate more severe oxygen desaturation during obstructive apnea than Latino and Caucasian children [15].

A recent analysis [16] of over 1200 children aged 5–10 years reported that AA ethnicity and prenatal exposure to tobacco smoke were both significantly associated with more severe OSA. Of note, over 90 % of the children with severe OSA were represented by children of AA ethnicity. A limitation of this study was that patients with associated comorbidities and obesity were excluded.

Obesity is also a risk factor for OSA in children, such that the risk of OSA increases by 12 % with each 1 kg/m^2 increment in body mass index (BMI) [9]. However, the BMI does not linearly correlate with the severity of the OSA [17]. The prevalence of OSA among obese children ranges between 22 and 40 % [18, 19].

Asthma is also related to OSA [9]: it usually does not affect baseline saturation, but it may worsen the nadir saturation during REM sleep [20]. Parental history of adenotonsillectomy and tonsillar hypertrophy are also risk factors for OSA [21].

14.1.4 Consequences of OSA

Children with mild SDB have high prevalence of cognitive impairment [9] and learning and behavior problems, with the strongest, most consistent associations for externalizing hyperactive-type behaviors that resemble the attention-deficit/hyperactivity disorder (ADHD) [2].

Children with OSA have autonomic dysregulation and altered baroreflex function [22] and dysregulation of hypothalamus-pituitary-adrenal axis. OSA is associated with a higher incidence of enuresis [9, 23], especially in girls.

Children with OSA have a significant decrease in exercise tolerance that has been attributed to a compromise in cardiac function. In particular, recent data show a reduction of cardiac and stroke volume indexes in children aged 7–12 years with OSA compared to weight-matched healthy subjects [24].

Furthermore, OSA causes endothelial dysfunction [9], systemic [25] and pulmonary [26] hypertension, and left [27, 28] and right [29, 30] ventricular dysfunction. Compared to primary snoring, children with OSA demonstrate a larger left ventricular mass index and a greater relative wall thickness [28] and left ventricular diastolic dysfunction [27]. Compared to age-matched healthy children, patients with OSA have a higher mean pulmonary artery pressure, a shorter ejection time, and a lower myocardial performance index [30].

14.2 Diagnosis of OSA

14.2.1 Physical Exam and Medical History

It is widely held that clinical criteria can be used to diagnose OSA. Snoring, in particular loud snoring, witnessed apnea, mouth breathing, unusual body and head position during sleep are all associated with OSA [31]. During wakefulness, mouth breathing may be present. Daytime sleepiness and tiredness are reported. Both obesity and failure to thrive occur [31]. Table 14.1 lists the signs and symptoms

Table 14.1 Signs and symptoms associated with obstructive sleep apnea in children [32]

History
Frequent snoring (≥ 3 nights/week)
Labored breathing during sleep
Gasps/snoring noises/observed episodes of apnea
Sleep enuresis (especially secondary enuresis) after ≥ 6 months of continence
Sleeping in a seated position or with the neck hyperextended
Cyanosis
Headaches on awakening
Daytime sleepiness
Attention-deficit/hyperactivity disorder
Learning problems
Physical examination
Underweight or overweight
Tonsillar hypertrophy
Adenoidal facies
Micrognathia/retrognathia
High-arched palate
Failure to thrive
Hypertension

Reproduced with permission.

suggestive of OSA reported by the American Academy of Pediatrics (AAP) [32]. In the diagnosis of moderate and severe OSA, the clinical evaluation (history and physical examination) has a poor sensitivity and specificity (59 and 73 %, respectively). Although one study reported a history of snoring every night had a higher sensitivity (91 %) and specificity (75 %) as well as a positive predictive value of 67 % and a negative predictive value of 94 % [33], this study was limited to Asian children and therefore may not be applicable to children of other ethnicities.

Several questionnaires have been developed to aid in the diagnosis of OSA, including the OSA-18 [34] and the Pediatric Sleep Questionnaire (PSQ) [35]. Compared with the gold standard polysomnography (PSG), these detailed questionnaires, often with more than 20 items, have a sensitivity of 78 % and a specificity of 72 % [36]. In a recent study of children with craniofacial disorders, 57 % had positive PSQ, but only 28 % had PSG findings of OSA [37].

It is evident that the accurate diagnosis and stratification of OSA require that clinical evaluation be supplemented with a test [38].

14.2.2 Diagnostics Test

Currently, the gold standard for the diagnosis of OSA is a nocturnal, in-laboratory PSG study [1]. The typical PSG monitoring includes electroencephalography (EEG), chin and anterior tibial electromyography (EMG), bilateral electrooculography, pulse oximetry and photo plethysmography, airflow sensor (nasal pressure transducer, oronasal airflow thermistor, end-tidal capnography), chest and abdominal respiratory inductance plethysmography, body position sensor, microphone, and real-time synchronized video monitoring. Key metrics obtained from PSG are listed in Table 14.2 [1]. Abnormalities of sleep are quantified with the apnea-hypopnea

Table 14.2 Metrics obtained from polysomnography [1]

Respiratory event	Definition
Apnea	Complete cessation of flow (drop of peak signal excursion to ≤ 10 % of the baseline for more than 90 % of the event duration, for ≥ 10 s)
Hypopnea (partial apnea)	Drop of signal by ≥ 30 % of the baseline for at least two breaths and associated with a ≥ 3 % oxygen desaturation by pulse oximetry or an arousal
Respiratory effort-related arousals (RERAs)	Increasing respiratory effort, flattening of the nasal flow waveform, or an elevation in the end-tidal PCO_2, lasting at least two breaths and associated to an arousal from sleep
Hypoventilation	Period of ventilation ≥ 25 % of total sleep time characterized by a $PCO_2 > 50$ mmHg
Apnea-hypopnea index (AHI)	The combined total number of apneas and hypopneas per hour of sleep
Respiratory disturbance index (RDI)	The combined total number of apneas, hypopneas, and RERAs per hour of sleep

Reproduced with permission.

index (AHI), which computes events related to obstruction [39] and various metrics of saturation including the nadir saturation and desaturation index. Hypercarbia is a feature of severe OSA.

Unlike adult OSA, there remains no consensus on the criteria to establish the diagnosis of OSA in children [35].

The following values are considered abnormal: AHI >5 and a nadir or minimum O_2 saturation <92 %. Hypercarbia is defined as a CO_2 50 mmHg >10 % sleep time or a CO_2 45 mmHg >60 % sleep time [40]. Other criteria have also been proposed [41, 42].

14.2.3 Cardiorespiratory Studies

Abbreviated cardiorespiratory studies may be performed at home or at the bedside. These studies limit the recordings to the measurement of oronasal airflow, respiratory inductance plethysmography, body position, snoring sounds, electrocardiography, transthoracic impedance, and pulse oximetry saturation. They correlate well with PSG [43].

14.2.4 Oximetry

The incidence of hypoxemia among children with SDB younger than 3 years is almost 40 %, decreasing by 17 % for each 1-year increase in age [34].

Overnight oximetry, which is potentially more widely available, can be used to evaluate OSA at the bedside and at home [44].

In a population of children referred to sleep laboratories with a high pretest probability of OSA, there is a very high probability (99 %) that an abnormal oximetry will be associated with PSG-proven OSA. However, when applied to the general population where the pretest probability of OSA is lower, the probability that an abnormal oximetry is associated with OSA is lower [45].

Desaturation indices (number of desaturation events >4 % below the baseline saturation) of 2.0, 3.5, and 4.2 correlate with mild, moderate, and severe OSA (AHI >1, AHI >5, and AHI >10, respectively). Each correlation showed high sensitivity (77.7, 83.8, and 89.1 %, respectively) and specificity (88.9, 86.5, and 86.0 %, respectively) [46].

An abnormal oximetry trend study has been defined as at least three clusters of desaturation. The McGill Oximetry Score (MOS) was developed to further stratify the severity of OSA. It identifies three levels of severity (MOS2, MOS3, and MOS4) defined as nadir saturations below 90, 85, and 80 %, respectively. The MOS has been shown to correlate with PSG [47, 48] and may be used as an initial test to evaluate children with SDB [49, 50]. Constantin et al. [34] compared the MOS to the OSA-18 questionnaire. An OSA-18 score of 60 (maximum 126) had very low sensitivity (40 %) but high negative predictive value. Therefore, children with a low OSA-18 score are unlikely to have OSA. This suggests that whereas a careful clinical evaluation may exclude severe OSA, it cannot reliably stratify OSA severity.

14.2.5 Other Studies

Nap studies have also been proposed but results are conflicting. The use of home PSG, respiratory polygraphy, nasal resistance, electrocardiogram-based automated apnea screening, and pulse transit time (PTT) [2, 51] is under investigation. Similarly, audio and videotaping have shown a sensitivity of 94 %, a specificity of 68 %, a positive predictive value of 83 %, and a negative predictive value of 88 %, but they are, like polysomnography, time-consuming to perform or analyze [52].

Radiologic studies (i.e., X-ray) have been also used, but the sensitivity, specificity, and positive and negative predictive values of these tests have yet to be reported [2].

Finally, propofol-induced (and possibly dexmedetomidine-induced) sleep endoscopy [53] and cine MRI [54] have been used to evaluate upper airway dynamics to identify the site of obstruction in children with OSA.

14.2.6 Future Prospective

Several biomarkers, such as chemokines, inflammatory cells, and others, have been investigated as predictors of OSA [9, 51], but their clinical application has yet to be established.

14.3 Anatomical and Physiological Basis of Respiratory Control

14.3.1 Upper Airway Anatomy and Its Relationship with OSA

Infants and children have a small maxilla and a large occiput, which may predispose to airway collapsibility. Within the first year of life, both the maxilla and the cranium will grow and promote the stability of pharyngeal architecture [55].

The upper airway is an "X"-shaped passageway, with the mouth and nose as two distinct entry points, which meet in the pharynx before splitting apart into the larynx and esophagus.

The upper airway contains different anatomical structures, with different growth characteristics. The following section gives an overview of the relative importance of each structure.

14.3.1.1 Nasopharynx

The nose receives support from boney structures and cartilage. Therefore abnormalities of these structures may promote obstruction of the nasal airway [56].

The nasal resistance to airflow spontaneously fluctuates in both adult and children. In adults, nasal obstruction increases the number of apneas and hypopneas [57] and worsens the sleep disturbance [58]. In children, nasal resistance is also affected by body position, increasing in the dependent nostril [59].

In infants, the nasal route of breathing is extremely important as they are preferential nasal breathers [60]. Indeed infants with unrecognized choanal atresia may asphyxiate.

14.3.1.2 Mouth and Pharynx

The oral cavity is limited by the hard and soft palate superiorly and the tongue inferiorly, and it is bounded laterally and anteriorly by the alveolar process. It opens posteriorly into the oropharynx and forms the part of the "X" where the nasal and oral cavities meet.

More inferiorly, the oropharynx continues into the retroglossal region (or "hypopharynx"), which is bounded anteriorly by the tongue and epiglottis, superiorly by the retropalatal oropharynx, inferiorly by the esophagus and larynx, and posteriorly and laterally by the pharyngeal constrictors.

During development, the tonsillar and adenoid tissues grow faster than the surrounding structures, encroaching on the airway and predisposing to pharyngeal obstruction [61].

In normal children, airway closure occurs at the level of soft palate and base of the tongue, whereas in children with SDB, pharyngeal closure occurs at the level of tonsils and adenoids [62].

Children with OSA have shown larger soft palate and bigger tonsils and adenoids, which narrow the retroglossal pharyngeal space [63]. Adenoid size is an important determinant in children between 1 and 12 years.

The tongue plays a critical role in the genesis of OSA. The loss of tongue and neck muscle tone causes the tongue to fall back into the posterior pharynx, often resulting in partial or complete obstruction [64], especially accentuated in mandibular hypoplasia. Furthermore, lingual tonsillar abnormalities can also predispose to airflow obstruction. This is especially important in the child with trisomy 21 [65].

14.3.1.3 Larynx

Below the epiglottis, the upper airway divides into the esophagus, located posteriorly, and the trachea, located anteriorly. Abnormalities of this area are rarely associated with OSA, unless anatomical or neurological abnormalities are present [66].

Redundancy in the arytenoid-aryepiglottic fold area may be associated with OSA [67]. Tracheomalacia has been also implicated in sleep apnea [68].

14.3.2 Neuronal Control of Breathing in Sleep and Airway Collapsibility

Two models have been proposed to describe the airway collapsibility [55]: the anatomical balance model and the neural balance model.

The anatomical balance model [69] considers the upper airway as a tube with a collapsible segment (analogous to the nose, the hypopharynx, and the larynx), surrounded by soft tissue (i.e., tongue) contained in a rigid box (i.e., boney structures). The pressure at which the pharyngeal airway collapses has been investigated. Two pressures have been reported: the critical pressure (Pcrit) and the closing pressure (Pclose). The Pcrit [70] was studied in awake spontaneously breathing children. In contrast, Pclose [62] was determined in paralyzed, anesthetized, apneic patients.

Pharyngeal collapse (Pcrit) occurs when the surrounding pressure is greater than the pressure within the airway segment. If the upstream resistance (nose) is low, as in normal subjects, the downstream (hypopharynx) pressure does not achieve Pcrit and airway patency is determined by the inspiratory pressure.

This model has been successfully applied in wake adults and children to describe the dynamic interaction of neuronal and anatomical components in the genesis of pharyngeal obstruction [70, 71].

In paralyzed and ventilated children, Isono [62] endoscopically evaluated the static changes of pharyngeal cross-sectional area at different pressures and identified the Pclose and the anatomical levels at which the airway collapsed.

In the neural balance model [72], airway patency is determined by the balance between pharyngeal collapsing forces (diaphragm, external intercostal muscles) and pharyngeal dilator muscles (i.e., the genioglossus muscle, which is the major upper airway dilator).

The pharyngeal dilator muscles are regulated by:

1. Consciousness: both sleep and general anesthesia decrease the pharyngeal dilator muscle activity relatively more than the diaphragm and external intercostal muscles, promoting airway collapse.
2. The negative pressure airway reflex.
3. The level of chemical stimuli: pO_2, pCO_2, and pH.

During wakefulness and non-rapid eye movement (NREM) sleep, activation of the pharyngeal dilators during inspiration maintains a patent pharyngeal airway. Transition to sleep results in reduced tone of the pharyngeal dilator and constrictor muscles [73], with a subsequent increase in airway resistance.

The pharyngeal collapsing forces may overcome the dilating forces, creating a subatmospheric (negative) pressure in the pharyngeal airway. Pressure receptors located in the mucosa of the nasopharynx and larynx are stimulated in response to this subatmospheric pressure (negative pressure reflex) [73], activating the pharyngeal dilators to counteract the collapse of the airways [74].

If negative pressure reflex fails, an apnea event occurs, and the subsequent changes in pO_2, pCO_2, and pH may stimulate a ventilatory response and an arousal.

Younes introduced the concept of loop gain (LG), which describes the feedback interaction (loop) between an apnea event, the subsequent increase of pCO_2, and the ventilatory response (gain), which then normalizes the pCO_2 to maintain respiratory homeostasis [75]. If the initial compensatory response overshoots, the resulting hypocarbia will cause a second hypopnea/apnea, which will be more severe than the initial one, and the cycle can perpetuate indefinitely. In normal individuals, this control system is stable (LG is <1). In patients with OSA, the system is unstable (LG >1) [76].

In normal children, the risk of obstruction due to anatomic factors such as small airway size, high nasal resistance, and high chest wall compliance is compensated by an increased ventilatory drive and decreased airway collapsibility [77]. In children with OSA, the neuromotor response to airway collapse has been linked to respiratory afferent cortical processing deficits [78].

14.4   Special Considerations

14.4.1 Infants and Premature Infants

A detailed description of OSA in infants is beyond the scope of this chapter. Interested readers are referred to the excellent review of Katz et al. [79]. Whereas in children high nasal resistance, relative hypoplasia of the mandible and maxilla is an anatomical feature associated with OSA, in infants, laryngomalacia, choanal atresia, cleft palate, and subglottic stenosis are commonly reported [79]. Adenotonsillar hypertrophy may become significant beyond 6 months of age; it is more common among males and preterm or low birth weight infants, and it is associated with high recurrence rate after surgery [80].

In infants, the site of obstruction is palatal or retroglossal, and it increases during neck flexion [79]. In a recent retrospective study [81], premature infants represented the 5.5 % of all surgical patients with SDB. Pulmonary and gastrointestinal comorbidities and airway abnormalities were common (40, 29.8, and 19.3 %, respectively). One third of the patients had abnormal preoperative pulse oximetry.

Polysomnographic criteria for OSA in infants have yet to be established, but OSA should be suspected in any infant with an AHI >2. Furthermore, infants with laryngomalacia and chronic respiratory distress should be evaluated for SDB [79].

In the majority of infants, symptoms of OSA resolve during development [68]. Nonpharmacological management of OSA includes continuous positive airway pressure (CPAP), position therapy, and nasopharyngeal intubation. Surgical options include adenotonsillectomy, supraglottoplasty, lip-tongue adhesion, mandibular distraction, and tracheostomy [79].

14.4.2 The Obese Child

Several factors contribute to OSA in the obese child [82]. Tonsillar or adenoid hypertrophy is reported in 65 % [83]. The adipose tissue, infiltrating the pharyngeal muscles and the surrounding structures [84], may contribute to the airway collapsibility that characterizes OSA. Obesity compromises upper airway patency not only by encroaching on the caliber but also by impairing the function of upper airway muscles. Obesity also decreases the longitudinal tension of the airway and reduces lung compliance and functional residual capacity, all of which promote pharyngeal airway collapse [85].

Severe obesity and OSA are associated with sleep fragmentation and subsequent psychomotor impairment, reduced memory recall, and lower spelling scores [86].

In children, obesity carries higher risk of depression [26], suicide, relationship difficulties, gastroesophageal reflux [87], hepatic diseases, irritable bowel syndrome

[88], metabolic syndrome (note that insulin resistance is present in 30–50 % vs. 4 % in nonobese adolescents) [89], type 2 diabetes mellitus, fatty liver disease [90], hypertension, dyslipidemia, and atherosclerosis [91].

Compared to OSA-matched subjects, obese children showed lower cardiac index volume, stroke volume index, and oxygen consumption at peak exercise capacity [24].

The risk for the metabolic syndrome (insulin resistance, dyslipidemia, hypertension, and obesity) increases with every 0.5-unit increment in BMI z score (odds ratio, 1.55; 95 % CI 1.16–2.08), and it is present in half of the severely obese children (BMI z score >2.5) [89].

A retrospective analysis [92] shows that overweight/obese (BMI >27 kg/m^2) children undergoing adenotonsillectomy are more at risk of desaturation, laryngospasm, and perioperative upper airway obstruction. These children are also admitted more often and hospital stays are longer than healthy children.

Furthermore, adenotonsillectomy has a lower success rate, as residual OSA post-adenotonsillectomy is present in up to 75 % of obese children [83, 93], with an odds ratio for persistent OSA of four compared to normal weight children [42].

14.4.3 Syndromes

Syndromes and medical conditions predisposing to OSA in children and adolescents are summarized in Table 14.3 [94].

If mouth breathing and obesity are combined with poor chin development and long face (adenoidal face), OSA should be suspected [95].

OSA symptoms are common in craniofacial malformations [96]. In a recent study, PSG (AHI >5) was positive in 28 % of children with craniofacial malformations [37]. More than 70 % of patients with syndromic craniosynostosis (Apert, Pfeiffer, and Crouzon) may have OSA (median AHI 12.9), which is severe in most of the cases [96].

These patients frequently require more complex and invasive airway surgery such as tongue reduction or lingular tonsillectomy [97].

Children with trisomy 21 are at high risk of having OSA, and the obstruction may be at several levels in the airway [98, 99]. It has been recently reported that 97 % of these children have abnormal polysomnography, and 59–66 % have moderate to severe OSA [100]. Compared to normally developed children, patients with trisomy 21 show higher MOS and higher EtCO$_2$ at night [101]. At the time of the adenotonsillectomy, children with trisomy 21 may have already developed clinically significant pulmonary hypertension [102].

The Prader-Willi syndrome is a condition that combines anatomical alterations (dimorphisms, including micrognathia) with obesity. Adenotonsillectomy has been proposed to treat the OSA, but it is associated with a higher risk of perioperative complications including delayed emergence, hemorrhage, hypoglycemia, laryngospasm, supplemental oxygen administration, and the need for reintubation [103].

Table 14.3 Syndromes associated with obstructive sleep apnea in children [94]

Craniofacial syndromes associated with significant mandibular or maxillary hypoplasia	Apert syndrome Crouzon syndrome Goldenhar syndrome (hemifacial microsomia) Hallermann-Streiff syndrome Pierre Robin syndrome (Robin sequence) Rubinstein-Taybi syndrome Russell-Silver syndrome Treacher Collins syndrome
Other syndromes featuring prominent craniofacial involvement	Achondroplasia Klippel-Feil syndrome Larsen syndrome Saethre-Chotzen syndrome Stickler syndrome Velocardiofacial syndrome
Conditions associated with macroglossia	Beckwith-Wiedemann syndrome Down syndrome Hypothyroidism Mucopolysaccharide storage disorders (e.g., Hunter, Hurler syndromes)
Conditions associated with anatomic airway obstruction	Adenotonsillar hypertrophy Cleft palate and/or cleft palate repair Choanal atresia or stenosis Fetal warfarin syndrome Laryngotracheomalacia Nasal polyps or septal deviation Pfeiffer syndrome Vascular ring
Neurologic disorders associated with weakness or impaired ventilatory control	Cerebral palsy Cranial neuropathies (e.g., Mobius syndrome, poliomyelitis) Neuromuscular disorders (e.g., Duchenne, myotonic dystrophies) Structural brainstem lesions (e.g., Chiari malformations, syringobulbia)
Conditions characterized by obesity	Morbid obesity/metabolic syndrome Prader-Willi syndrome
Other conditions	Arthrogryposis multiplex congenita Conradi-Hünermann syndrome Gastroesophageal reflux Sickle cell disease

Reproduced with permission.

14.4.4 Central Hypoventilation Syndromes

Congenital central hypoventilation syndrome is a sleep-dependent hypoventilation disorder, which is classically diagnosed at birth but may present late in infancy or even in adulthood (late-onset central hypoventilation syndrome, LOCHS) [104]. It is characterized by an impaired response to hypercapnia and an overnight oxygen saturation trace that differs from the OSA pattern [104]. Mutations of gene PHOX2B have been identified in patients affected by LOCHS. Exposure to anesthesia may result in delayed emergence, which may be confused with opioid hypersensitivity or residual neuromuscular blockade [105]. Postoperative hypoventilation may be the presenting feature.

Rapid-onset obesity with hypothalamic dysfunction (ROHHAD) is another central hypoventilation disorder, which may present in the perioperative period [106]. However, its etiology, pathophysiology, and associated endocrine abnormalities differ from the LOCHS.

14.5 Medical Treatment of OSA

Several studies are investigating medical treatments for OSA in children [107].

Noninvasive positive pressure ventilation (NIV) is extensively used in adults. Increasingly NIV is used to treat infants and children with OSA [108].

Since the settings for NIV systems after surgery may differ from the ones used at home, care must be taken to provide trained staff and monitoring throughout the hospital admission and immediate access to invasive ventilation in the event of respiratory deterioration during the postoperative period [109].

The application of high-flow oxygen nasal cannula, weight loss, and positional therapy (lateral and prone positions versus supine during sleep) are promising therapies in selected OSA patients, but long-term results are inconclusive or unknown [97, 110].

Dental procedures, such as rapid maxillary expansions and oral appliances, may be indicated. Two detailed reviews have been recently published [97, 110].

Since inflammation has been shown to play a pivotal role in tonsil and adenoid hypertrophy [107], immunomodulating drugs such as montelukast may prove useful in the future. Nasal corticosteroids seem to be effective [107, 110] and may be of short-term benefit allowing optimization prior to adenotonsillectomy. Their long-term safety has still to be established [110]. Studies on drugs directed to different biomarkers are under investigation [107].

14.6 Surgical Treatments

The first-line treatment of OSA in children is adenotonsillectomy, which is the most common surgery performed in the United States (annual caseload 500,000).

Adenotonsillectomy has been shown to improve the AHI, quality of life (QOL), behavior, and school performance, regardless of the presence of obesity [83]. Adenoidectomy alone has been shown to reduce airway collapsibility [70].

A recent systematic review analyzed the cardiovascular benefits of adenotonsillectomy [111]. Despite the high heterogeneity of the studies, adenotonsillectomy seemed to have beneficial effects on blood pressure (especially diastolic) and cardiac function [111].

Similarly, a recent study reported a decrease of mean pulmonary pressure, right and left ventricular isovolumetric contraction time length, myocardial performance index values, and an increase of ejection time [30].

Surgical alternatives to adenotonsillectomy have been proposed. In children older than 5 years, partial tonsillectomy has been shown to decrease pain, improve the return to a normal diet, decrease the risk of bleeding, and maintain immunologic function, with minimal risk of regrowth [112].

In fact, residual OSA may occur in 20–40 % [93] of children with severe OSA, depending on AHI threshold criterion to define severe OSA [113]. Obesity, age >7 years, the presence of asthma, a high presurgical AHI [93] and respiratory disturbance index (RDI) [42], AA ethnicity [114], and craniofacial malformation [96] are risk factors for persistent OSA after surgery.

Adenotonsillectomy, however, is not without risks [107, 115, 116]. Hemorrhage, cardiorespiratory events, and medication error are the most common complications (54, 18, and 17 %, respectively) after adenotonsillectomy and are responsible for half of the mortality events [117, 118]. In particular, children may demonstrate a delayed onset of respiratory compromise several hours after surgery [42].

In 3–16-year-old children with mild OSA (AHI between 1 and 5), adenotonsillectomy has been shown to give early relief of symptoms and improvement of QOL compared to conservative clinical observation [119]. However, watchful waiting also showed significant improvements in QOL after 8 months and may be considered as an alternative to adenotonsillectomy.

In a recent retrospective analysis of 126 infants with OSA [120], 86 children underwent a variety of surgical interventions including tonsillectomy, adenoidectomy, and adenotonsillectomy in 35 % of the patients. Comparing these children with those managed with nonsurgical interventions (watchful waiting, antireflux therapy, CPAP), surgical interventions showed a similar success rate at 6 months' follow-up.

A recent large multicenter, single-blind, randomized study, the Childhood Adenotonsillectomy Trial (CHAT) [114], investigated the outcomes of children between 5 and 9 years of age undergoing adenotonsillectomy versus a strategy of watchful waiting. As compared to control, adenotonsillectomy did not improve neurological outcomes (NEPSY attention and executive-function test) at 7 months' follow-up, but children who underwent early adenotonsillectomy had greater behavioral improvement (caregiver and teacher ratings), quality of life (Pediatric Sleep Questionnaire and Pediatric Quality of Life Inventory), and PSG indexes (AHI, change from baseline -1.6 vs. -3.5, $p < 0.001$). Most importantly, PSG findings normalized in 79 % of children in early-adenotonsillectomy group but also in 46 % of watchful waiting group. Of note, 59 % of the obese children (BMI z score >1.65) still manifested severe OSA after surgery (AHI >5).

In children with syndromic craniosynostosis, adenotonsillectomy has been performed to alleviate the symptoms of obstruction, but additional interventions, such as CPAP therapy, mandibular distraction, and tracheostomy, may be required [96].

A recent study [121] compared CPAP with surgical therapy in OSA patients with trisomy 21 and mucopolysaccharidoses. It showed a similar 1-year outcome in terms of PSG, clinical evaluation, Epworth Sleepiness Scale—Children, QOL, and OSA-18 score.

Tongue base suspension and uvulopalatopharyngoplasty, associated or not with adenotonsillectomy, have been applied to selected patients and they may be beneficial. Recently, the European Respiratory Society Task Force has reviewed their clinical application [97]. Finally, tracheotomy is reserved for severe refractory patients [40].

14.7 Anesthesia Management of the Patient with OSA

14.7.1 General Recommendations: The American Society of Anesthesiology Guidelines

The American Society of Anesthesiologists (ASA) recently updated the guidelines for the management of patients with OSA [122]. It must be noted that these guidelines:

1. Do not address patients with central apnea, airways abnormalities (i.e., deviated nasal septum) or obesity not associated with obstructive apnea, and hypersomnolence not secondary to sleep apnea.
2. Do not consider children younger than 1 year.
3. Encourage evaluation of OSA with sleep study. In its absence, the ASA endorses clinical criteria to both diagnose and stratify OSA severity.
4. Recommend that OSA patient to be managed in hospitals that have the facilities to treat postoperative airway complications.
5. Encourage the use of CPAP perioperatively.
6. Recommend a full reversal of neuromuscular blockade.
7. Highlight that OSA patients are at higher risk of respiratory depression secondary to opioids and sedatives.
8. Recommend an accurate assessment of patient in the postoperative period.
9. Encourage a prolonged period of observation. Patients should not be discharged to an unmonitored setting until they are no longer at risk of postoperative respiratory depression. This new recommendation has been introduced in 2014 and highlights the critical role of postoperative monitoring in reducing the risk of respiratory complications.

14.7.2 Anesthesia Management Options

The anesthesiologist should plan the anesthesia based on the severity of the OSA. As mentioned, clinical evaluation with preoperative questionnaires has high negative predictive value but a very low sensitivity [34]. Tait et al. [123] developed a limited five-item questionnaire to identify children with SDB at increased risk for perioperative adverse respiratory events. The study, however, was not designed to stratify the OSA severity, and the respiratory events were restricted to the immediate postoperative period.

Therefore, if sleep study data are not available, the anesthesiologist must assess airway collapsibility clinically. The risk and benefits of premedication should be also carefully weighed in children with severe OSA, since significant airway obstruction and severe oxygen desaturation can occur [124].

The child's response to anesthesia may be informative as it may unmask OSA by inducing skeletal hypotonia simulating conditions during REM sleep. During spontaneous ventilation, the requirement for positive pressure to maintain pharyngeal airway patency, a high apneic threshold for carbon dioxide [125], and a heightened opioid sensitivity are all suggestive of severe OSA and may warrant postoperative admission and extended period of cardiorespiratory monitoring [126].

The use of local anesthesia may also unmask OSA. In children with OSA, the application of local anesthesia results in a relatively greater decrease of pharyngeal cross-sectional area likely from the inhibition of the upper airway dilators [127]. Titration of opioids to the severity of OSA is critical to reduce respiratory complications (see below).

Finally, supplemental oxygen must always be administered carefully in the recovery room as in children with severe OSA, their blunted carbon dioxide responsiveness may render them more dependent on peripheral respiratory drive [125].

14.8   Specific Guidelines for Anesthesia Management of the Children Undergoing Adenotonsillectomy

14.8.1 Recommendations for Adenotonsillectomy: Italian National Program Guidelines, American Academy of Otolaryngology—Head and Neck Surgery Guidelines, and American Association of Pediatrics Guidelines

The 2008 Italian National Program Guidelines [128] state that the decision to perform adenotonsillectomy should be based on clinical evaluation (i.e., loud snoring, low hemoglobin saturation) with or without the use of specific questionnaires. Nocturnal pulse oximetry is recommended as an initial test in children with suspected SDB. PSG is reserved for children with inconclusive pulse oximetry studies [48]. Adenoidectomy alone is not recommended due to the high recurrence of symptoms. Intraoperative morphine is not indicated. Multimodal analgesia with dexamethasone 0.5–1 mg/kg i.v. (max 8 mg), acetaminophen 15 mg/kg p.o. q4 h *around the clock*, and codeine 1 mg/kg p.o. q4 h *pro re nata* are recommended. However, it must be noted that codeine received a black box warning from FDA in 2013 [39].

Short-term antibiotics are also indicated. The guidelines also recommend postoperative admission for children younger than 3 years of age.

The American Academy of Otolaryngology—Head and Neck Surgery recommends PSG before adenotonsillectomy be reserved for children with coexisting diseases, such as obesity, trisomy 21, craniofacial abnormalities, neuromuscular disorders, sickle cell disease, and mucopolysaccharidoses [129]. Importantly, the results of PSG should be communicated to the anesthesiologist prior to the induction of anesthesia. Postoperative admission is recommended for patients younger than 3 years of age and with severe OSA (AHI ≥10 or more obstructive events/h, oxygen saturation nadir <80 %, or both).

The 2012 American Academy of Pediatrics (AAP) [32] recommends adenotonsillectomy as the first-line treatment for children with OSA. Relative contraindications are very small tonsils/adenoids, morbid obesity and small tonsils/adenoids, bleeding disorder refractory to treatment, and a submucous cleft palate. Nocturnal video recording, nocturnal oximetry, daytime nap polysomnography, and ambulatory polysomnography are considered valid alternatives to PSG. The guidelines acknowledge that children may present with chronic rhinorrhea and nasal congestion, even in the absence of viral infections, which makes airway management more challenging. Postoperative admission is recommended for patients younger than 3 years of age and with severe OSA, cardiac diseases due to OSA, failure to thrive, obesity, craniofacial anomalies, neuromuscular disorders, and current respiratory infection. The AAP identifies children with a perioperative nadir saturation <80 % and PCO_2 >60 mmHg or a preoperative AHI >24 are at higher risk for postoperative respiratory complications.

14.8.2 Anesthesia Management Options for Children Undergoing Adenotonsillectomy

Postoperative hospital admission is recommended for children younger than 3 years or in the presence of comorbidity, a bleeding diathesis, excessive distance from a hospital, excessive pain, poor oral intake, postoperative vomiting, and an awake (room air) saturation below 95 %[45].

Elective ICU admission may be considered in case of children less than 24 months with RDI >60 during REM sleep; RDI <60 in REM sleep but associated with coexisting syndrome or significant neuromuscular disease likely may promote airway obstruction, failure to thrive, respiratory compromise, central apnea, complex cyanotic or congenital heart disease [130], or MOS4 [45]. In agreement with AAP practice guidelines, for children with very severe OSA (MOS4) older than 2 years and with no comorbidities, postoperative admission to a monitored setting is an alternative to pediatric intensive care unit [45].

14.8.2.1 Intraoperative Management

There is neither consensus nor randomized controlled trials regarding the anesthesia management in children undergoing adenotonsillectomy for OSA. In the setting of adenotonsillectomy, endotracheal intubation is generally preferred to LMA due to smaller surgical pharyngeal visualization.

Inhalational induction should be carefully used since the decrease in pharyngeal muscle tone and longitudinal tension may unmask the airway collapsibility and require skilled mask airway support. It is therefore mandatory that clinicians perform a careful evaluation of the airway before induction and that advanced airway equipment is immediately available [39]. The application of CPAP through the APL valve may facilitate the ventilation in skilled hands, and the level of CPAP is proportional to the level and the severity of airway collapsibility [55].

Intravenous induction may result in a collapse of the upper airway, making positive pressure ventilation difficult. Insertion of an oral airway usually overcomes the pharyngeal obstruction.

A recent study [131] compared dexmedetomidine-ketamine and sevoflurane-sufentanil undergoing uvulopalatopharyngoplasty. Dexmedetomidine-ketamine showed lower pain score, less emergence delirium/agitation, but longer awake time, higher sedation (Ramsay score), and incidence of desaturation below 95 % in post anesthesia care unit (PACU).

Since OSA patients have demonstrated higher opioid sensitivity [132] and hypoalgesia [133], the intraoperative use of short-acting opioids such as remifentanil may have an advantage in children with severe OSA (MOS 3 and 4). Furthermore the dose of postoperative morphine should be reduced by 50 % and carefully titrated as children with MOS 3 and 4 may require only half of the usual opioid dose [50].

As mentioned in the previous section, infiltration of the pharynx with local anesthesia is discouraged due to the risk of airway collapse. Multimodal analgesia with acetaminophen and intraoperative steroids is advantageous to decrease postoperative pain [115]. The use of nonsteroidal anti-inflammatory drugs in adenotonsillectomy remains under debate [134]. Finally, the routine use of antibiotics is not recommended [115], although postoperative transient bacteremia is common [135].

14.8.2.2 Postoperative Management

Optimization of postoperative management is critical to reduce respiratory events, which may be as high as 60 % after adenotonsillectomy [45].

A recent survey from the Society for Pediatric Anesthesia [136] identified at 16 cases of preventable death/neurological injury within 24 h after surgery, which occurred at home, in PACU, or on the ward [136]. This highlights the need for prolonged postoperative monitoring.

Respiratory complications are common during the first night after surgery, when children with mild and moderate OSA may show a worsening of the symptoms [137]. Patients with preoperative RDI >19 or persistent snoring should undergo PSG follow-up, since they are more at risk of residual OSA [42]. Rhinorrhea, uvular edema, and residual anesthesia may exacerbate postoperative obstruction [130]. Children may also develop postobstructive pulmonary edema in the postoperative period [32]. Finally, dehydration involves 5 % of the patients below 3 years [138].

Conclusions

Pediatric OSA represents a complex disorder with unique pathophysiological features. Understanding the anatomical and physiological basis of airway collapse in children with OSA is crucial to optimize the anesthesia management of these patients. The anesthesiologist must be aware that the stratification of the OSA severity is pivotal to identify patients at high risk for postoperative complication. Furthermore, extended postoperative monitoring and judicious use of narcotics should always be considered in these high-risk patients.

References

1. Berry RB, Budhiraja R, Gottlieb DJ, Gozal D, Iber C, Kapur VK, Marcus CL, Mehra R, Parthasarathy S, Quan SF, Redline S, Strohl KP, Davidson Ward SL, Tangredi MM (2012) Rules for scoring respiratory events in sleep: update of the 2007 AASM Manual for the Scoring of Sleep and Associated Events. Deliberations of the Sleep Apnea Definitions Task Force of the American Academy of Sleep Medicine. J Clin Sleep Med 8(5):597–619. doi:10.5664/jcsm.2172
2. Marcus CL, Brooks LJ, Draper KA, Gozal D, Halbower AC, Jones J, Schechter MS, Ward SD, Sheldon SH, Shiffman RN, Lehmann C, Spruyt K (2012) Diagnosis and management of childhood obstructive sleep apnea syndrome. Pediatrics 130(3):e714–e755. doi:10.1542/peds.2012-1672
3. Goh DY, Galster P, Marcus CL (2000) Sleep architecture and respiratory disturbances in children with obstructive sleep apnea. Am J Respir Crit Care Med 162(2 Pt 1):682–686. doi:10.1164/ajrccm.162.2.9908058
4. Carrera HL, McDonough JM, Gallagher PR, Pinto S, Samuel J, DiFeo N, Marcus CL (2011) Upper airway collapsibility during wakefulness in children with sleep disordered breathing, as determined by the negative expiratory pressure technique. Sleep 34(6):717–724. doi:10.5665/SLEEP.1034
5. Brunetti L, Rana S, Lospalluti ML, Pietrafesa A, Francavilla R, Fanelli M, Armenio L (2001) Prevalence of obstructive sleep apnea syndrome in a cohort of 1,207 children of southern Italy. Chest 120(6):1930–1935
6. Hoban TF (2013) Sleep disorders in children. Continuum (Minneap Minn) 19(1 Sleep Disorders):185–198. doi:10.1212/01.CON.0000427206.75435.0e
7. Erickson BK, Larson DR, St Sauver JL, Meverden RA, Orvidas LJ (2009) Changes in incidence and indications of tonsillectomy and adenotonsillectomy, 1970–2005. Otolaryngol Head Neck Surg 140(6):894–901. doi:10.1016/j.otohns.2009.01.044
8. Kato I, Franco P, Groswasser J, Kelmanson I, Togari H, Kahn A (2000) Frequency of obstructive and mixed sleep apneas in 1,023 infants. Sleep 23(4):487–492
9. Tan HL, Gozal D, Kheirandish-Gozal L (2013) Obstructive sleep apnea in children: a critical update. Nat Sci Sleep 5:109–123. doi:10.2147/NSS.S51907
10. Chervin RD, Weatherly RA, Ruzicka DL, Burns JW, Giordani BJ, Dillon JE, Marcus CL, Garetz SL, Hoban TF, Guire KE (2006) Subjective sleepiness and polysomnographic correlates in children scheduled for adenotonsillectomy vs other surgical care. Sleep 29(4):495–503
11. Castronovo V, Zucconi M, Nosetti L, Marazzini C, Hensley M, Veglia F, Nespoli L, Ferini-Strambi L (2003) Prevalence of habitual snoring and sleep-disordered breathing in preschool-aged children in an Italian community. J Pediatr 142(4):377–382. doi:10.1067/mpd.2003.118
12. Kahn A, Groswasser J, Sottiaux M, Rebuffat E, Franco P (1994) Mechanisms of obstructive sleep apneas in infants. Biol Neonate 65(3–4):235–239
13. Rosen CL, Larkin EK, Kirchner HL, Emancipator JL, Bivins SF, Surovec SA, Martin RJ, Redline S (2003) Prevalence and risk factors for sleep-disordered breathing in 8- to 11-year-old children: association with race and prematurity. J Pediatr 142(4):383–389. doi:10.1067/mpd.2003.28
14. Brouillette RT, Horwood L, Constantin E, Brown K, Ross NA (2011) Childhood sleep apnea and neighborhood disadvantage. J Pediatr 158(5):789–795. doi:10.1016/j.jpeds.2010.10.036, e781
15. Stepanski E, Zayyad A, Nigro C, Lopata M, Basner R (1999) Sleep-disordered breathing in a predominantly African-American pediatric population. J Sleep Res 8(1):65–70
16. Weinstock TG, Rosen CL, Marcus CL, Garetz S, Mitchell RB, Amin R, Paruthi S, Katz E, Arens R, Weng J, Ross K, Chervin RD, Ellenberg S, Wang R, Redline S (2014) Predictors of obstructive sleep apnea severity in adenotonsillectomy candidates. Sleep 37(2):261–269. doi:10.5665/sleep.3394

17. Tripuraneni M, Paruthi S, Armbrecht ES, Mitchell RB (2013) Obstructive sleep apnea in children. Laryngoscope 123(5):1289–1293. doi:10.1002/lary.23844

18. Kaditis AG, Alexopoulos EI, Hatzi F, Karadonta I, Chaidas K, Gourgoulianis K, Zintzaras E, Syrogiannopoulos GA (2008) Adiposity in relation to age as predictor of severity of sleep apnea in children with snoring. Sleep Breath 12(1):25–31. doi:10.1007/s11325-007-0132-z

19. Rudnick EF, Walsh JS, Hampton MC, Mitchell RB (2007) Prevalence and ethnicity of sleep-disordered breathing and obesity in children. Otolaryngol Head Neck Surg 137(6):878–882. doi:10.1016/j.otohns.2007.08.002

20. Gutierrez MJ, Zhu J, Rodriguez-Martinez CE, Nino CL, Nino G (2013) Nocturnal phenotypical features of obstructive sleep apnea (OSA) in asthmatic children. Pediatr Pulmonol 48(6):592–600. doi:10.1002/ppul.22713

21. Alexopoulos EI, Charitos G, Malakasioti G, Varlami V, Gourgoulianis K, Zintzaras E, Kaditis AG (2014) Parental history of adenotonsillectomy is associated with obstructive sleep apnea severity in children with snoring. J Pediatr 164(6):1352–1357. doi:10.1016/j.jpeds.2014.01.021

22. Gozal D, Hakim F, Kheirandish-Gozal L (2013) Chemoreceptors, baroreceptors, and autonomic deregulation in children with obstructive sleep apnea. Respir Physiol Neurobiol 185(1):177–185. doi:10.1016/j.resp.2012.08.019

23. Jeyakumar A, Rahman SI, Armbrecht ES, Mitchell R (2012) The association between sleep-disordered breathing and enuresis in children. Laryngoscope 122(8):1873–1877. doi:10.1002/lary.23323

24. Evans CA, Selvadurai H, Baur LA, Waters KA (2014) Effects of obstructive sleep apnea and obesity on exercise function in children. Sleep 37(6):1103–1110. doi:10.5665/sleep.3770

25. Leung LC, Ng DK, Lau MW, Chan CH, Kwok KL, Chow PY, Cheung JM (2006) Twenty-four-hour ambulatory BP in snoring children with obstructive sleep apnea syndrome. Chest 130(4):1009–1017. doi:10.1378/chest.130.4.1009

26. Sofer S, Weinhouse E, Tal A, Wanderman KL, Margulis G, Leiberman A, Gueron M (1988) Cor pulmonale due to adenoidal or tonsillar hypertrophy or both in children. Noninvasive diagnosis and follow-up. Chest 93(1):119–122

27. Amin RS, Kimball TR, Kalra M, Jeffries JL, Carroll JL, Bean JA, Witt SA, Glascock BJ, Daniels SR (2005) Left ventricular function in children with sleep-disordered breathing. Am J Cardiol 95(6):801–804. doi:10.1016/j.amjcard.2004.11.044

28. Amin RS, Kimball TR, Bean JA, Jeffries JL, Willging JP, Cotton RT, Witt SA, Glascock BJ, Daniels SR (2002) Left ventricular hypertrophy and abnormal ventricular geometry in children and adolescents with obstructive sleep apnea. Am J Respir Crit Care Med 165(10):1395–1399. doi:10.1164/rccm.2105118

29. Tal A, Leiberman A, Margulis G, Sofer S (1988) Ventricular dysfunction in children with obstructive sleep apnea: radionuclide assessment. Pediatr Pulmonol 4(3):139–143

30. Cincin A, Sakalli E, Bakirci EM, Dizman R (2014) Relationship between obstructive sleep apnea-specific symptoms and cardiac function before and after adenotonsillectomy in children with adenotonsillar hypertrophy. Int J Pediatr Otorhinolaryngol 78(8):1281–1287. doi:10.1016/j.ijporl.2014.05.011

31. Bhushan B, Sheldon S, Wang E, Schroeder JW Jr (2014) Clinical indicators that predict the presence of moderate to severe obstructive sleep apnea after adenotonsillectomy in children. Am J Otolaryngol 35(4):487–495. doi:10.1016/j.amjoto.2014.02.010

32. Marcus CL, Brooks LJ, Draper KA, Gozal D, Halbower AC, Jones J, Schechter MS, Sheldon SH, Spruyt K, Ward SD, Lehmann C, Shiffman RN (2012) Diagnosis and management of childhood obstructive sleep apnea syndrome. Pediatrics 130(3):576–584. doi:10.1542/peds.2012-1671

33. Chau KW, Ng DK, Kwok CK, Chow PY, Ho JC (2003) Clinical risk factors for obstructive sleep apnoea in children. Singapore Med J 44(11):570–573

34. Constantin E, Tewfik TL, Brouillette RT (2010) Can the OSA-18 quality-of-life questionnaire detect obstructive sleep apnea in children? Pediatrics 125(1):e162–e168. doi:10.1542/peds.2009-0731

35. Alonso-Alvarez ML, Cordero-Guevara JA, Teran-Santos J, Gonzalez-Martinez M, Jurado-Luque MJ, Corral-Penafiel J, Duran-Cantolla J, Kheirandish-Gozal L, Gozal D (2014) Obstructive sleep apnea in obese community-dwelling children: the NANOS study. Sleep 37(5):943–949. doi:10.5665/sleep.3666
36. Chervin RD, Weatherly RA, Garetz SL, Ruzicka DL, Giordani BJ, Hodges EK, Dillon JE, Guire KE (2007) Pediatric sleep questionnaire: prediction of sleep apnea and outcomes. Arch Otolaryngol Head Neck Surg 133(3):216–222. doi:10.1001/archotol.133.3.216
37. Cielo CM, Silvestre J, Paliga JT, Maguire M, Gallagher PR, Marcus CL, Taylor JA (2014) Utility of screening for obstructive sleep apnea syndrome in children with craniofacial disorders. Plast Reconstr Surg 134(3):434e–441e. doi:10.1097/PRS.0000000000000484
38. Brietzke SE, Katz ES, Roberson DW (2004) Can history and physical examination reliably diagnose pediatric obstructive sleep apnea/hypopnea syndrome? A systematic review of the literature. Otolaryngol Head Neck Surg 131(6):827–832. doi:10.1016/j.otohns.2004.07.002
39. Patino M, Sadhasivam S, Mahmoud M (2013) Obstructive sleep apnoea in children: perioperative considerations. Br J Anaesth 111(Suppl 1):i83–i95. doi:10.1093/bja/aet371
40. Bower CM, Gungor A (2000) Pediatric obstructive sleep apnea syndrome. Otolaryngol Clin North Am 33(1):49–75
41. Kheirandish-Gozal L, Gozal D (2008) The multiple challenges of obstructive sleep apnea in children: diagnosis. Curr Opin Pediatr 20(6):650–653. doi:10.1097/MOP.0b013e328316bdb2
42. Suen JS, Arnold JE, Brooks LJ (1995) Adenotonsillectomy for treatment of obstructive sleep apnea in children. Arch Otolaryngol Head Neck Surg 121(5):525–530
43. Nixon GM, Brouillette RT (2002) Diagnostic techniques for obstructive sleep apnoea: is polysomnography necessary? Paediatr Respir Rev 3(1):18–24
44. Pavone M, Cutrera R, Verrillo E, Salerno T, Soldini S, Brouillette RT (2013) Night-to-night consistency of at-home nocturnal pulse oximetry testing for obstructive sleep apnea in children. Pediatr Pulmonol 48(8):754–760. doi:10.1002/ppul.22685
45. Brown KA (2011) Outcome, risk, and error and the child with obstructive sleep apnea. Paediatr Anaesth 21(7):771–780. doi:10.1111/j.1460-9592.2011.03597.x
46. Tsai CM, Kang CH, Su MC, Lin HC, Huang EY, Chen CC, Hung JC, Niu CK, Liao DL, Yu HR (2013) Usefulness of desaturation index for the assessment of obstructive sleep apnea syndrome in children. Int J Pediatr Otorhinolaryngol 77(8):1286–1290. doi:10.1016/j.ijporl.2013.05.011
47. Nixon GM, Kermack AS, Davis GM, Manoukian JJ, Brown KA, Brouillette RT (2004) Planning adenotonsillectomy in children with obstructive sleep apnea: the role of overnight oximetry. Pediatrics 113(1 Pt 1):e19–e25
48. Brouillette RT, Morielli A, Leimanis A, Waters KA, Luciano R, Ducharme FM (2000) Nocturnal pulse oximetry as an abbreviated testing modality for pediatric obstructive sleep apnea. Pediatrics 105(2):405–412
49. Brown KA, Morin I, Hickey C, Manoukian JJ, Nixon GM, Brouillette RT (2003) Urgent adenotonsillectomy: an analysis of risk factors associated with postoperative respiratory morbidity. Anesthesiology 99(3):586–595
50. Brown KA, Laferriere A, Moss IR (2004) Recurrent hypoxemia in young children with obstructive sleep apnea is associated with reduced opioid requirement for analgesia. Anesthesiology 100(4):806–810; discussion 805A
51. Brockmann PE, Schaefer C, Poets A, Poets CF, Urschitz MS (2013) Diagnosis of obstructive sleep apnea in children: a systematic review. Sleep Med Rev 17(5):331–340. doi:10.1016/j.smrv.2012.08.004
52. Schechter MS (2002) Technical report: diagnosis and management of childhood obstructive sleep apnea syndrome. Pediatrics 109(4):e69
53. Wootten CT, Chinnadurai S, Goudy SL (2014) Beyond adenotonsillectomy: outcomes of sleep endoscopy-directed treatments in pediatric obstructive sleep apnea. Int J Pediatr Otorhinolaryngol 78(7):1158–1162. doi:10.1016/j.ijporl.2014.04.041
54. Shott SR (2011) Evaluation and management of pediatric obstructive sleep apnea beyond tonsillectomy and adenoidectomy. Curr Opin Otolaryngol Head Neck Surg 19(6):449–454. doi:10.1097/MOO.0b013e32834c1728

55. Isono S (2006) Developmental changes of pharyngeal airway patency: implications for pediatric anesthesia. Paediatr Anaesth 16(2):109–122. doi:10.1111/j.1460-9592.2005.01769.x

56. Chen W, Kushida CA (2003) Nasal obstruction in sleep-disordered breathing. Otolaryngol Clin North Am 36(3):437–460

57. Taasan V, Wynne JW, Cassisi N, Block AJ (1981) The effect of nasal packing on sleep-disordered breathing and nocturnal oxygen desaturation. Laryngoscope 91(7):1163–1172

58. Olsen KD, Kern EB, Westbrook PR (1981) Sleep and breathing disturbance secondary to nasal obstruction. Otolaryngol Head Neck Surg 89(5):804–810

59. Haight JS, Cole P (1986) Unilateral nasal resistance and asymmetrical body pressure. J Otolaryngol Suppl 16:1–31

60. Miller MJ, Martin RJ, Carlo WA, Fouke JM, Strohl KP, Fanaroff AA (1985) Oral breathing in newborn infants. J Pediatr 107(3):465–469

61. Jeans WD, Fernando DC, Maw AR, Leighton BC (1981) A longitudinal study of the growth of the nasopharynx and its contents in normal children. Br J Radiol 54(638):117–121

62. Isono S, Shimada A, Utsugi M, Konno A, Nishino T (1998) Comparison of static mechanical properties of the passive pharynx between normal children and children with sleep-disordered breathing. Am J Respir Crit Care Med 157(4 Pt 1):1204–1212. doi:10.1164/ajrccm.157.4.9702042

63. Arens R, McDonough JM, Costarino AT, Mahboubi S, Tayag-Kier CE, Maislin G, Schwab RJ, Pack AI (2001) Magnetic resonance imaging of the upper airway structure of children with obstructive sleep apnea syndrome. Am J Respir Crit Care Med 164(4):698–703. doi:10.1164/ajrccm.164.4.2101127

64. Shorten GD, Opie NJ, Graziotti P, Morris I, Khangure M (1994) Assessment of upper airway anatomy in awake, sedated and anaesthetised patients using magnetic resonance imaging. Anaesth Intensive Care 22(2):165–169

65. Suzuki K, Kawakatsu K, Hattori C, Hattori H, Nishimura Y, Yonekura A, Yagisawa M, Nishimura T (2003) Application of lingual tonsillectomy to sleep apnea syndrome involving lingual tonsils. Acta Otolaryngol Suppl 550:65–71

66. Pinto JA, Kohler R, Wambier H, Gomes LM, Mizoguchi EI, Prestes dos Reis R (2013) Laryngeal pathologies as an etiologic factor of obstructive sleep apnea syndrome in children. Int J Pediatr Otorhinolaryngol 77(4):573–575. doi:10.1016/j.ijporl.2012.12.018

67. Naganuma H, Okamoto M, Woodson BT, Hirose H (2002) Cephalometric and fiberoptic evaluation as a case-selection technique for obstructive sleep apnea syndrome (OSAS). Acta Otolaryngol Suppl 547:57–63

68. Ramgopal S, Kothare SV, Rana M, Singh K, Khatwa U (2014) Obstructive sleep apnea in infancy: a 7-year experience at a pediatric sleep center. Pediatr Pulmonol 49(6):554–560. doi:10.1002/ppul.22867

69. Schwartz AR, Smith PL (2013) CrossTalk proposal: the human upper airway does behave like a Starling resistor during sleep. J Physiol 591(Pt 9):2229–2232. doi:10.1113/jphysiol.2012.250654

70. Marcus CL, McColley SA, Carroll JL, Loughlin GM, Smith PL, Schwartz AR (1994) Upper airway collapsibility in children with obstructive sleep apnea syndrome. J Appl Physiol (1985) 77(2):918–924

71. Schwartz AR, Smith PL, Wise RA, Gold AR, Permutt S (1988) Induction of upper airway occlusion in sleeping individuals with subatmospheric nasal pressure. J Appl Physiol (1985) 64(2):535–542

72. Brouillette RT, Thach BT (1979) A neuromuscular mechanism maintaining extrathoracic airway patency. J Appl Physiol: Respir Environ Exer Physiol 46(4):772–779

73. Horner RL (1996) Motor control of the pharyngeal musculature and implications for the pathogenesis of obstructive sleep apnea. Sleep 19(10):827–853

74. Nishino T (2000) Physiological and pathophysiological implications of upper airway reflexes in humans. Jpn J Physiol 50(1):3–14

75. Younes M (2014) CrossTalk proposal: elevated loop gain is a consequence of obstructive sleep apnoea. J Physiol 592(Pt 14):2899–2901. doi:10.1113/jphysiol.2014.271833

76. Younes M, Ostrowski M, Thompson W, Leslie C, Shewchuk W (2001) Chemical control stability in patients with obstructive sleep apnea. Am J Respir Crit Care Med 163(5):1181–1190. doi:10.1164/ajrccm.163.5.2007013
77. Arens R, Marcus CL (2004) Pathophysiology of upper airway obstruction: a developmental perspective. Sleep 27(5):997–1019
78. Huang J, Marcus CL, Davenport PW, Colrain IM, Gallagher PR, Tapia IE (2013) Respiratory and auditory cortical processing in children with obstructive sleep apnea syndrome. Am J Respir Crit Care Med 188(7):852–857. doi:10.1164/rccm.201307-1257OC
79. Katz ES, Mitchell RB, D'Ambrosio CM (2012) Obstructive sleep apnea in infants. Am J Respir Crit Care Med 185(8):805–816. doi:10.1164/rccm.201108-1455CI
80. Greenfeld M, Tauman R, DeRowe A, Sivan Y (2003) Obstructive sleep apnea syndrome due to adenotonsillar hypertrophy in infants. Int J Pediatr Otorhinolaryngol 67(10):1055–1060
81. Manuel A, Witmans M, El-Hakim H (2013) Children with a history of prematurity presenting with snoring and sleep-disordered breathing: a cross-sectional study. Laryngoscope 123(8):2030–2034. doi:10.1002/lary.23999
82. Gozal D, Kheirandish-Gozal L (2012) Childhood obesity and sleep: relatives, partners, or both? – a critical perspective on the evidence. Ann N Y Acad Sci 1264:135–141. doi:10.1111/j.1749-6632.2012.06723.x
83. Mitchell RB, Boss EF (2009) Pediatric obstructive sleep apnea in obese and normal-weight children: impact of adenotonsillectomy on quality-of-life and behavior. Dev Neuropsychol 34(5):650–661. doi:10.1080/87565640903133657
84. Arens R, Sin S, Nandalike K, Rieder J, Khan UI, Freeman K, Wylie-Rosett J, Lipton ML, Wootton DM, McDonough JM, Shifteh K (2011) Upper airway structure and body fat composition in obese children with obstructive sleep apnea syndrome. Am J Respir Crit Care Med 183(6):782–787. doi:10.1164/rccm.201008-1249OC
85. Canapari CA, Hoppin AG, Kinane TB, Thomas BJ, Torriani M, Katz ES (2011) Relationship between sleep apnea, fat distribution, and insulin resistance in obese children. J Clin Sleep Med 7(3):268–273. doi:10.5664/JCSM.1068
86. Hannon TS, Rofey DL, Ryan CM, Clapper DA, Chakravorty S, Arslanian SA (2012) Relationships among obstructive sleep apnea, anthropometric measures, and neurocognitive functioning in adolescents with severe obesity. J Pediatr 160(5):732–735. doi:10.1016/j.jpeds.2011.10.029
87. Pashankar DS, Corbin Z, Shah SK, Caprio S (2009) Increased prevalence of gastroesophageal reflux symptoms in obese children evaluated in an academic medical center. J Clin Gastroenterol 43(5):410–413. doi:10.1097/MCG.0b013e3181705ce9
88. Teitelbaum JE, Sinha P, Micale M, Yeung S, Jaeger J (2009) Obesity is related to multiple functional abdominal diseases. J Pediatr 154(3):444–446. doi:10.1016/j.jpeds.2008.09.053
89. Weiss R, Dziura J, Burgert TS, Tamborlane WV, Taksali SE, Yeckel CW, Allen K, Lopes M, Savoye M, Morrison J, Sherwin RS, Caprio S (2004) Obesity and the metabolic syndrome in children and adolescents. N Engl J Med 350(23):2362–2374. doi:10.1056/NEJMoa031049
90. Nobili V, Cutrera R, Liccardo D, Pavone M, Devito R, Giorgio V, Verrillo E, Baviera G, Musso G (2014) Obstructive sleep apnea syndrome affects liver histology and inflammatory cell activation in pediatric nonalcoholic fatty liver disease, regardless of obesity/insulin resistance. Am J Respir Crit Care Med 189(1):66–76. doi:10.1164/rccm.201307-1339OC
91. Freedman DS, Mei Z, Srinivasan SR, Berenson GS, Dietz WH (2007) Cardiovascular risk factors and excess adiposity among overweight children and adolescents: the Bogalusa Heart Study. J Pediatr 150(1):12.e12–17.e12. doi:10.1016/j.jpeds.2006.08.042
92. Nafiu OO, Green GE, Walton S, Morris M, Reddy S, Tremper KK (2009) Obesity and risk of peri-operative complications in children presenting for adenotonsillectomy. Int J Pediatr Otorhinolaryngol 73(1):89–95. doi:10.1016/j.ijporl.2008.09.027
93. Bhattacharjee R, Kheirandish-Gozal L, Spruyt K, Mitchell RB, Promchiarak J, Simakajornboon N, Kaditis AG, Splaingard D, Splaingard M, Brooks LJ, Marcus CL, Sin S, Arens R, Verhulst SL, Gozal D (2010) Adenotonsillectomy outcomes in treatment of obstruc-

tive sleep apnea in children: a multicenter retrospective study. Am J Respir Crit Care Med 182(5):676–683. doi:10.1164/rccm.200912-1930OC

94. Hoban TF, Bliwise DL (2007) Ontogeny. In: Kudhida CA (ed) Obstructive sleep apnea: pathophysiology, comorbidities, and consequences, 10th edn. Informa Healthcare USA, New York, pp 39–60

95. Flores-Mir C, Korayem M, Heo G, Witmans M, Major MP, Major PW (2013) Craniofacial morphological characteristics in children with obstructive sleep apnea syndrome: a systematic review and meta-analysis. J Am Dent Assoc 144(3):269–277

96. Zandieh SO, Padwa BL, Katz ES (2013) Adenotonsillectomy for obstructive sleep apnea in children with syndromic craniosynostosis. Plast Reconstr Surg 131(4):847–852. doi:10.1097/PRS.0b013e3182818f3a

97. Randerath WJ, Verbraecken J, Andreas S, Bettega G, Boudewyns A, Hamans E, Jalbert F, Paoli JR, Sanner B, Smith I, Stuck BA, Lacassagne L, Marklund M, Maurer JT, Pepin JL, Valipour A, Verse T, Fietze I (2011) Non-CPAP therapies in obstructive sleep apnoea. Eur Respir J 37(5):1000–1028. doi:10.1183/09031936.00099710

98. Gibson SE, Myer CM 3rd, Strife JL, O'Connor DM (1996) Sleep fluoroscopy for localization of upper airway obstruction in children. Ann Otol Rhinol Laryngol 105(9):678–683

99. Donnelly LF, Surdulescu V, Chini BA, Casper KA, Poe SA, Amin RS (2003) Upper airway motion depicted at cine MR imaging performed during sleep: comparison between young patients with and those without obstructive sleep apnea. Radiology 227(1):239–245. doi:10.1148/radiol.2271020198

100. Austeng ME, Overland B, Kvaerner KJ, Andersson EM, Axelsson S, Abdelnoor M, Akre H (2014) Obstructive sleep apnea in younger school children with Down syndrome. Int J Pediatr Otorhinolaryngol 78(7):1026–1029. doi:10.1016/j.ijporl.2014.03.030

101. Lin SC, Davey MJ, Horne RS, Nixon GM (2014) Screening for obstructive sleep apnea in children with Down syndrome. J Pediatr 165(1):117–122. doi:10.1016/j.jpeds.2014.02.032

102. Eipe N, Lai L, Doherty DR (2009) Severe pulmonary hypertension and adenotonsillectomy in a child with Trisomy-21 and obstructive sleep apnea. Paediatr Anaesth 19(5):548–549. doi:10.1111/j.1460-9592.2009.02936.x

103. Pavone M, Paglietti MG, Petrone A, Crino A, De Vincentiis GC, Cutrera R (2006) Adenotonsillectomy for obstructive sleep apnea in children with Prader-Willi syndrome. Pediatr Pulmonol 41(1):74–79. doi:10.1002/ppul.20334

104. Barratt S, Kendrick AH, Buchanan F, Whittle AT (2007) Central hypoventilation with PHOX2B expansion mutation presenting in adulthood. Thorax 62(10):919–920. doi:10.1136/thx.2006.068908

105. Mahmoud M, Bryan Y, Gunter J, Kreeger RN, Sadhasivam S (2007) Anesthetic implications of undiagnosed late onset central hypoventilation syndrome in a child: from elective tonsillectomy to tracheostomy. Paediatr Anaesth 17(10):1001–1005. doi:10.1111/j.1460-9592.2007.02284.x

106. Chandrakantan A, Poulton TJ (2013) Anesthetic considerations for rapid-onset obesity, hypoventilation, hypothalamic dysfunction, and autonomic dysfunction (ROHHAD) syndrome in children. Paediatr Anaesth 23(1):28–32. doi:10.1111/j.1460-9592.2012.03924.x

107. Kheirandish-Gozal L, Kim J, Goldbart AD, Gozal D (2013) Novel pharmacological approaches for treatment of obstructive sleep apnea in children. Expert Opin Investig Drugs 22(1):71–85. doi:10.1517/13543784.2013.735230

108. Marcus CL, Rosen G, Ward SL, Halbower AC, Sterni L, Lutz J, Stading PJ, Bolduc D, Gordon N (2006) Adherence to and effectiveness of positive airway pressure therapy in children with obstructive sleep apnea. Pediatrics 117(3):e442–e451. doi:10.1542/peds.2005-1634

109. Elliott MW, Confalonieri M, Nava S (2002) Where to perform noninvasive ventilation? Eur Respir J 19(6):1159–1166

110. Tapia IE, Marcus CL (2013) Newer treatment modalities for pediatric obstructive sleep apnea. Paediatr Respir Rev 14(3):199–203. doi:10.1016/j.prrv.2012.05.006

111. Teo DT, Mitchell RB (2013) Systematic review of effects of adenotonsillectomy on cardio-vascular parameters in children with obstructive sleep apnea. Otolaryngol Head Neck Surg 148(1):21–28. doi:10.1177/0194599812463193

112. Zhang Q, Li D, Wang H (2014) Long term outcome of tonsillar regrowth after partial tonsil-lectomy in children with obstructive sleep apnea. Auris Nasus Larynx 41(3):299–302. doi:10.1016/j.anl.2013.12.005

113. Kang KT, Weng WC, Lee CH, Lee PL, Hsu WC (2014) Discrepancy between objective and subjective outcomes after adenotonsillectomy in children with obstructive sleep apnea syndrome. Otolaryngol Head Neck Surg 151(1):150–158. doi:10.1177/0194599814529534

114. Marcus CL, Moore RH, Rosen CL, Giordani B, Garetz SL, Taylor HG, Mitchell RB, Amin R, Katz ES, Arens R, Paruthi S, Muzumdar H, Gozal D, Thomas NH, Ware J, Beebe D, Snyder K, Elden L, Sprecher RC, Willging P, Jones D, Bent JP, Hoban T, Chervin RD, Ellenberg SS, Redline S (2013) A randomized trial of adenotonsillectomy for childhood sleep apnea. N Engl J Med 368(25):2366–2376. doi:10.1056/NEJMoa1215881

115. Baugh RF, Archer SM, Mitchell RB, Rosenfeld RM, Amin R, Burns JJ, Darrow DH, Giordano T, Litman RS, Li KK, Mannix ME, Schwartz RH, Setzen G, Wald ER, Wall E, Sandberg G, Patel MM (2011) Clinical practice guideline: tonsillectomy in children. Otolaryngol Head Neck Surg 144(1 Suppl):S1–S30. doi:10.1177/0194599810389949

116. Brouillette RT (2013) Let's CHAT about adenotonsillectomy. N Engl J Med 368(25):2428–2429. doi:10.1056/NEJMe1305492

117. Stevenson AN, Myer CM 3rd, Shuler MD, Singer PS (2012) Complications and legal out-comes of tonsillectomy malpractice claims. Laryngoscope 122(1):71–74. doi:10.1002/lary.22438

118. Morris LG, Lieberman SM, Reitzen SD, Edelstein DR, Ziff DJ, Katz A, Komisar A (2008) Characteristics and outcomes of malpractice claims after tonsillectomy. Otolaryngol Head Neck Surg 138(3):315–320. doi:10.1016/j.otohns.2007.11.024

119. Volsky PG, Woughter MA, Beydoun HA, Derkay CS, Baldassari CM (2014) Adenotonsillectomy vs observation for management of mild obstructive sleep apnea in chil-dren. Otolaryngol Head Neck Surg 150(1):126–132. doi:10.1177/0194599813509780

120. Leonardis RL, Robison JG, Otteson TD (2013) Evaluating the management of obstructive sleep apnea in neonates and infants. JAMA Otolaryngol Head Neck Surg 139(2):139–146. doi:10.1001/jamaoto.2013.1331

121. Sudarsan SS, Paramasivan VK, Arumugam SV, Murali S, Kameswaran M (2014) Comparison of treatment modalities in syndromic children with obstructive sleep apnea – a randomized cohort study. Int J Pediatr Otorhinolaryngol 78(9):1526–1533. doi:10.1016/j.ijporl.2014.06.027

122. (2014) Practice guidelines for the perioperative management of patients with obstructive sleep apnea: an updated report by the American Society of Anesthesiologists Task Force on Perioperative Management of patients with obstructive sleep apnea. Anesthesiology 120(2):268–286. doi:10.1097/ALN.0000000000000053

123. Tait AR, Voepel-Lewis T, Christensen R, O'Brien LM (2013) The STBUR questionnaire for predicting perioperative respiratory adverse events in children at risk for sleep-disordered breathing. Paediatr Anaesth 23(6):510–516. doi:10.1111/pan.12155

124. Nozaki-Taguchi N, Isono S, Nishino T, Numai T, Taguchi N (1995) Upper airway obstruction during midazolam sedation: modification by nasal CPAP. Can J Anaesth 42(8):685–690. doi:10.1007/BF03012665

125. Strauss SG, Lynn AM, Bratton SL, Nespeca MK (1999) Ventilatory response to CO_2 in chil-dren with obstructive sleep apnea from adenotonsillar hypertrophy. Anesth Analg 89(2):328–332

126. Brown KA, Brouillette RT (2014) The elephant in the room: lethal apnea at home after ade-notonsillectomy. Anesth Analg 118(6):1157–1159. doi:10.1213/ANE.0b013e31829ec1e6

127. Gozal D, Burnside MM (2004) Increased upper airway collapsibility in children with obstructive sleep apnea during wakefulness. Am J Respir Crit Care Med 169(2):163–167. doi:10.1164/rccm.200304-590OC
128. Bellussi L, Busoni P, Camaioni A, Malagola C, Marchisio P, Marletta S, Marolla F, Materia E, Nati G, Pallestrini E, Perletti L, Rinaldi Ceroni A, Romano R, Rumeo A, Sampaolo L, Tempesta F, Vigo A, Villa MP (2008) Appropriatezza e sicurezza degli interventi di tonsillectomia e/o adenoidectomia. Minerva Pediatr 60(5):907–909
129. Roland PS, Rosenfeld RM, Brooks LJ, Friedman NR, Jones J, Kim TW, Kuhar S, Mitchell RB, Seidman MD, Sheldon SH, Jones S, Robertson P (2011) Clinical practice guideline: polysomnography for sleep-disordered breathing prior to tonsillectomy in children. Otolaryngol Head Neck Surg 145(1 Suppl):S1–S15. doi:10.1177/0194599811409837
130. Walker P, Whitehead B, Rowley M (2013) Role of paediatric intensive care following adenotonsillectomy for severe obstructive sleep apnoea: criteria for elective admission. J Laryngol Otol 127(Suppl 1):S26–S29. doi:10.1017/S0022215112001739
131. Cheng X, Huang Y, Zhao Q, Gu E (2014) Comparison of the effects of dexmedetomidine-ketamine and sevoflurane-sufentanil anesthesia in children with obstructive sleep apnea after uvulopalatopharyngoplasty: an observational study. J Anaesthesiol Clin Pharmacol 30(1):31–35. doi:10.4103/0970-9185.125699
132. Rabbitts JA, Groenewald CB, Dietz NM, Morales C, Rasanen J (2010) Perioperative opioid requirements are decreased in hypoxic children living at altitude. Paediatr Anaesth 20(12):1078–1083. doi:10.1111/j.1460-9592.2010.03453.x
133. Doufas AG, Tian L, Padrez KA, Suwanprathes P, Cardell JA, Maecker HT, Panousis P (2013) Experimental pain and opioid analgesia in volunteers at high risk for obstructive sleep apnea. PLoS One 8(1), e54807. doi:10.1371/journal.pone.0054807
134. Lewis SR, Nicholson A, Cardwell ME, Siviter G, Smith AF (2013) Nonsteroidal anti-inflammatory drugs and perioperative bleeding in paediatric tonsillectomy. Cochrane Database Syst Rev (7):CD003591. doi:10.1002/14651858.CD003591.pub3
135. Yildirim I, Okur E, Ciragil P, Aral M, Kilic MA, Gul M (2003) Bacteraemia during tonsillectomy. J Laryngol Otol 117(8):619–623. doi:10.1258/002221503768199951
136. Cote CJ, Posner KL, Domino KB (2014) Death or neurologic injury after tonsillectomy in children with a focus on obstructive sleep apnea: Houston, we have a problem! Anesth Analg 118(6):1276–1283. doi:10.1213/ANE.0b013e318294fc47
137. Nixon GM, Kermack AS, McGregor CD, Davis GM, Manoukian JJ, Brown KA, Brouillette RT (2005) Sleep and breathing on the first night after adenotonsillectomy for obstructive sleep apnea. Pediatr Pulmonol 39(4):332–338. doi:10.1002/ppul.20195
138. Spencer DJ, Jones JE (2012) Complications of adenotonsillectomy in patients younger than 3 years. Arch Otolaryngol Head Neck Surg 138(4):335–339. doi:10.1001/archoto.2012.1

Perioperative Care of Children with Trauma

15

Leonardo Bussolin

Trauma injury remains to be a major cause of death and severe disability in children from 1 to 14 years old.

In pediatric population, traumatic injuries are predominantly blunt, nonpenetrating. This feature results from a number of reasons reported in Fig. 15.1.

Major and lethal pediatric traumas are relatively rare. This aspect makes difficult to accomplish guidelines for the management and treatment of pediatric trauma because most of the publications show small and poor statistically significant populations of patients.

Mortality for traumatic injury presents three peaks:

1. *Immediate*: within the first hour, often upon impact and due to injuries which are incompatible with life (laceration of major intra-thoracic or intra-abdominal vessels, high injury of the cervical spine, rupture of the cardiac chambers, severe brain injury)
2. *Early*: within the first two hours after the traumatic event and secondary to inadequate establishment, stabilization and control of airway, uncontrolled hemorrhage associated with hemodynamic collapse, respiratory failure for pulmonary contusion and hemorrhage or pneumothorax, and intracranial bleeding
3. *Delayed*: for complications occurring during hospitalization (sepsis, progressive respiratory failure, multiorgan failure)

Motor vehicle collisions, pedestrian and bicycle accidents, falls, and burns are the most common causes of injury in children [1].

The essential factors for obtaining successful management of trauma include the quick diagnosis and treatment of primary injuries and the avoidance of secondary

L. Bussolin (✉)
Department of Neuroanesthesia and Neurointensive Care, Pediatric Trauma Center, Pediatric Hospital Meyer, Florence, Italy
e-mail: leonardo.bussolin@meyer.it

© Springer International Publishing Switzerland 2016
M. Astuto, P.M. Ingelmo (eds.), *Perioperative Medicine in Pediatric Anesthesia*,
Anesthesia, Intensive Care and Pain in Neonates and Children,
DOI 10.1007/978-3-319-21960-8_15

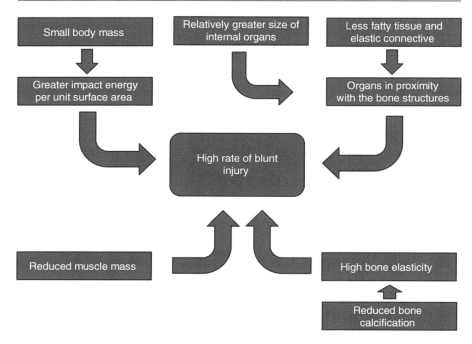

Fig. 15.1 Causes of high rate of blunt injury in children

injury. The term *platinum 30 min (golden hour for adults)*, while not evidence based, refers to an early and critical period in the care of trauma victims, during which the appropriate management may significantly increase patients' survival rate.

Early recognition of primary injuries with rapid control of the airway and replacement of the circulating blood volume remain the cornerstones for a successful resuscitation of the pediatric trauma victim. Secondary injuries, which result from hypoxia and hypotension, are important determinants of morbidity and mortality after trauma, particularly in the presence of head trauma [2].

Pediatric trauma presents significant challenges regarding the anesthetic management, because of the anatomical, physiological, and psychological peculiarities characterizing every step of the development of child that make him a separate individual for each aspect of clinical care. For this reason, successful treatment of the traumatized child requires an accurate knowledge of the anatomical and physiological features that distinguish children from adults. These differences differ as the age increases, with neonates presenting the greatest clinical challenge.

As previously mentioned (Fig. 15.1), children have less fat and more elastic connective tissue with a flexible skeleton placed in close proximity to abdominal and thoracic structures, which can be injured without external lesions.

The larger body surface area to body mass ratio predisposes children to high heat loss than adults, potentially resulting in severe hypothermia.

Children have different physiological response to major trauma compared to adults, since they are able to maintain a near-normal blood pressure until 30–40 % of blood volume is lost. In these situations, the most important monitoring parameters are represented by the increased heart rate and the decreased tissue perfusion, the latter detected by the assessment of capillary refill time. The latter is detected by compressing for 5 s the nail bed, in children, or the sternal region in neonate and infants. The resulting ischemic area (appearing pallid) should return normally perfused within 2 s. A longer capillary refill time indicates a condition of tissue hypoperfusion (Fig. 15.2).

Children may not cope well emotionally in the aftermath of an accident. They need to be managed in a calm, child-friendly environment. The presence of a parent or psychologist in the resuscitation room may help the trauma team by minimizing the injured child's fear and anxieties. It is shown that 25 % of children suffer from post-traumatic stress disorder after a traumatic event [3].

The most challenging anatomical and functional aspects related to pediatric trauma concern the airway and pulmonary function. Children have high oxygen consumption rate, relatively low functional residual capacity, and rapid bradycardic response to hypoxia. They do not tolerate long apneic periods well. Therefore, accurate airway examination is crucial.

The anesthesiologist should be prepared to encounter the following anatomical features of pediatric airway:

- A large protuberant occiput creates the natural flexion of the head in young children. It predisposes the airway to obstruction and requires careful positioning for intubation.
- A small oral cavity, large tongue, the presence of adenoids and tonsils, and occasionally loose deciduous teeth may restrict intraoral manipulation, obstruct visibility with direct laryngoscopy, and create predisposition to easy bleeding.
- The larynx is short and positioned relatively high and more anterior. The epiglottis is often U shaped, long, and floppy. This combination may pose potential difficulties with laryngoscopy, and a short larynx increases the possibility of endobronchial intubation.

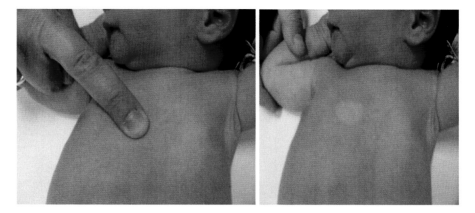

Fig. 15.2 Detection of capillary refill time

- The commonly accepted knowledge that the larynx in infants and children is funnel shaped with the narrowest point of the funnel at the cricoid ring must be revised. Litman et al. [4] demonstrated with magnetic resonance imaging scans that in neonates, infants, and children up to 14 years, the larynx is conical in the transverse dimension with the apex of the cone at the level of the vocal cord and cylindrical in the anteroposterior dimension and does not change throughout development. Subsequently, Dalal et al. [5] confirmed these findings by using video-bronchoscopy imaging.

The role of the anesthesiologist in the management of pediatric trauma extends long before the arrival to the operating room. It includes the emergency department, the radiology suite, the intensive care unit, and the acute pain service. Therefore, pediatric anesthesiologist is involved to provide any or all of these services at any time.

The anesthesiologist may have to take care of traumatized pediatric patients on following occasions:

1. Initial stabilization in the emergency department
2. Sedation and monitoring for imaging
3. Emergency surgical procedures, such as laparotomy or craniotomy
4. After initial stabilization, to perform anesthesia for the fixation of long bone fractures
5. Intensive care unit management
6. Pain control during hospitalization, especially using regional analgesia

For all these reasons, a rapid and well-organized trauma team of an injured child is essential.

15.1   Primary Survey

The main goal of the primary survey is to detect and treat immediate life-threatening conditions, such as bleeding or hypertensive pneumothorax.

In pediatric trauma, the primary survey is classically presented according to ABCDEF sequence with some peculiarities:

A: *a*irway + cervical stabilization
B: *b*reathing + ventilation and oxygenation
C: *c*irculation + hemorrhage control
D: *d*isability
E: exposure
F: *f*amily

The next step of the assessment is not started until the preceding abnormality has been managed and corrected.

Before starting any manipulation of the patient, the level of consciousness must be evaluated by the application of a verbal or slight painful stimulus.

15.1.1 Airway

A number of traumatized patients arrive to the emergency department (ED) already intubated, and therefore, the duty of the anesthesiologist is to evaluate the airway in terms of tube size, cuffed/uncuffed, the presence and magnitude of air leak if uncuffed tube, depth of the tube, breath sounds, ventilation, and oxygenation. Any chest X-ray done in the ED should be reviewed in order to ascertain the correct position of the tracheal tube in mid-trachea and the presence of pneumothorax. If the patient is not intubated, the assessment of the airway must simply determine the ability patency. The mouth is opened to visualize the cavity, and, if the patient is unconscious, the jaw thrust is performed to prevent that the tongue falls back obstructing the upper airways. At the same time, an appropriate-sized cervical collar is chosen and placed (Fig. 15.3). If an appropriate pediatric cervical collar is not available, rolled towels or blankets might be carefully placed on either side of patient's head in young children and infants.

The airway can be obstructed by blood, foreign bodies, teeth, secretions, and vomit in the oropharyngeal space, and any effort should be done to remove or suction them. Throughout the maneuver, the axes of the head, neck, and thorax must be aligned to prevent any dangerous rotation or extension movements of the cervical spine.

15.1.2 Breathing

After step A has been completed, breathing must be assessed. If the patient is spontaneously breathing, then 100 % high-flow oxygen will be administered by a non-rebreathing face mask with a reservoir.

If the child is apneic or is making poor respiratory effort, assisted ventilation is required. When properly performed, bag-valve-mask (BVM) ventilation for a short period of time is as effective as ventilation via an endotracheal tube. Five ventilations must be performed, and of these, at least two must be effective, eventually with

Fig. 15.3 Mouth opening, jaw thrust maneuver, and cervical collar placed

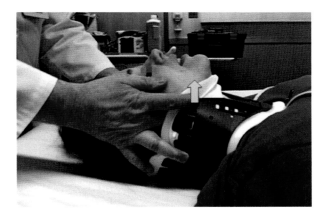

	Size	Weight (kg)
Table 15.1 Sizing of LMA	1	≤ 5
	1.5	5–10
	2	10–20
	2.5	20–30
	3, 4, 5	>30

the aid of an oral airway, if the patient is unconsciousness (considering that inserting an oral airway into a semiconscious child's mouth may cause gagging and vomiting). In traumatized patient, the insertion of the oral airway should be carried out directly (without 180° rotation) with the use of a tongue depressor.

If manual or assisted ventilations by facemask are not effective, endotracheal intubation or insertion of a supraglottic device (laryngeal mask airway (LMA)) has to be performed.

The use of appropriated-sized LMA has been validated even in the prehospital care [6]as an alternative in the case of difficult tracheal intubation.

The sizing of LMA is done on the basis of the weight of the patient (Table 15.1).

If intubation is necessary, a fast assessment of the airway should be made before inducing anesthesia and administration of neuromuscular blocking drug. A plan should be available in the case of a difficult or failed intubation. A video laryngoscope, bronchoscope, or LMA should also be kept handy.

In trauma patient, nasotracheal intubation is contraindicated, especially if an injury of the cranial base is suspected.

The pediatric trauma victims should always be considered as full stomach patients, and rapid sequence induction is preferred as the gold standard for airway management in these patients [7].

In children, the Sellick maneuver may be less effective than in adults, because of the pliability of laryngeal cartilages.

Severely injured children should be intubated with cuffed endotracheal tubes, even in the prehospital settings [8, 9]. The size of the cuffed tube is often determined by *modified Cole formula* (age [years]/4 + 4) for uncuffed tubes, decreased by half-size for cuffed tubes. The cuff should be inflated to get a seal at about 25 cm H_2O of airway pressure.

For neonates, the sizing of tracheal tube is reported in Table 15.2.

The insertion depth of the tracheal tube is calculated by multiplying by three the result of modified Cole formula for uncuffed tubes. The proper position of the tracheal tube must be confirmed by the auscultation of breath sounds and by capnography.

Any destabilization of respiratory parameters (e.g., oxygen desaturation) during ventilation through the tracheal tube should be carefully considered. For this purpose, the acronym *DOPES* is used:

D = dislodgment of the tracheal tube with possible accidental removal or deepening into a bronchus

O = obstruction of the tracheal tube by secretions, vomit, blood, or foreign body

Table 15.2 Sizing of tracheal tube in neonates

Size	Weight (kg)
2.5	<1
3	1–2
3.5	>2

P = pneumothorax
E = equipment (e.g., oxygen line)
S = stomach dilatation following entry of air during the manual ventilation

15.1.2.1 Tension Pneumothorax

Tension pneumothorax occurs when trauma to the chest resulted in wall injury with progressive entry of air that is unable to escape from the pleural space resulting in increased pressure and lung collapse. Since in children the mediastinum is very compliant, it shifts earlier in the course, resulting in decreased venous return and more rapid cardiovascular collapse. This condition leads to a severe condition with dyspnea, hypotension, increased respiratory rate, ipsilateral hyperresonance, and reduced breath sounds. The diagnosis of tension pneumothorax is clinical and not radiological, so the first rule for a correct treatment is to suspect it! Therefore, this life-threatening situation must be promptly treated by urgent needle thoracostomy followed by tube thoracostomy.

15.1.3 Circulation

In children, secondary cardiopulmonary arrest, caused by either respiratory or circulatory failure, is more frequent than primary arrests caused by arrhythmias. The outcome from cardiopulmonary arrest in pediatric patient is poor, and identification of the antecedent stages of cardiac or respiratory failure is a priority, and therefore, effective early intervention may be lifesaving.

The management of *step C* in children presents unique challenges, such as obtaining the cooperativeness of the child for intravenous placement and the potential for psychological trauma, smaller veins, and more subcutaneous fat in children, making both palpating and visualizing veins more difficult. Additional issues include higher likelihood of hypovolemia upon presentation, lower success rates of intravenous insertion by first responders with consequent hematomas, bruises, and nonavailability of these punctured veins for intravenous placement, fractures in the extremity bones, and hypothermia causing peripheral vasoconstriction.

As previously mentioned, a child with normal blood pressure can be in shock. The earliest warning signs that a child is in shock include signs of decreased skin perfusion (capillary refill, temperature, and color), central nervous system perfusion (lethargy, inappropriate response to painful procedures, and lack of recognition of parents), and pulses (tachycardia and the presence or absence of pulses). If hypotension is present with a markedly depressed mental status, the child is in late shock with blood loss up to 40 % of blood volume. Waiting until hypotension is present to begin treating shock is too late.

Obtaining vascular access in a pediatric trauma patient offers unique challenges. These issues include obtaining the cooperativeness of the child for IV placement and the potential for psychological trauma, smaller veins, and more subcutaneous fat in children, making both palpating and visualizing veins more difficult.

Several new devices, such as intraosseous needle systems and techniques such as ultrasonography to cannulate central and peripheral veins, have improved this aspect of pediatric trauma management.

Once shock has been identified and intravenous or intraosseous access has been obtained, resuscitation should be initiated, according to the algorithm shown in Fig. 15.4.

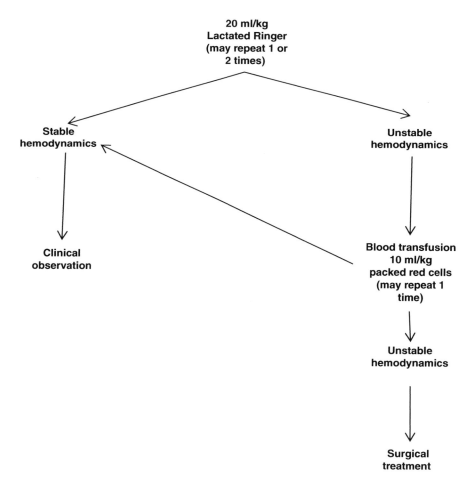

Fig. 15.4 Resuscitation algorithm

15.1.4 Disability

This step involves a quick assessment of neurologic function which must be repeated during the secondary survey to monitor for changes in the child's neurologic status. The level of consciousness is evaluated by the *Glasgow Coma Scale* (GCS) adjusted according to the patient's age (Table 15.3) or by the rapid application of *AVPU* acronym (*A* alert, *V* verbal, *P* pain, *U* unresponsive), considering that P corresponds to GCS ≤ 8.

15.1.5 Exposure

The final passage of primary survey consists in completely undressing the patient and performing the log-roll maneuver, in order to detect any superficial lesion or swelling, while preventing hypothermia and inserting the spinal board (Fig. 15.5).

Table 15.3 Pediatric Glasgow Coma Scale

	>1 year		<1 year	Score
EYE OPENING	Spontaneously		Spontaneously	4
	To verbal command		To shout	3
	To pain		To pain	2
	No response		No response	1
MOTOR RESPONSE	Obeys		Spontaneously	6
	Localizes pain		Localizes pain	5
	Flexion – withdrawal		Flexion – withdrawal	4
	Flexion – abnormal (decorticate rigidity)		Flexion – abnormal (decorticate rigidity)	3
	Extension (decerebrate rigidity)		Extension (decerebrate rigidity)	2
	No response		No response	1
	> 5 years	2–5 years	0–23 months	
VERBAL RESPONSE	Oriented	Appropriate words/phrases	Smiles/coos appropriately	5
	Disoriented/confused	Inappropriate words	Cries and is unconsolable	4
	Inappropriate words	Persistent cries and screams	Persistent inappropriate crying and/or screaming	3
	Incomprehensible sounds	Grunts	Grunts, agitated, and restless	2
	No response	No response	No response	1
TOTAL PEDIATRIC GLASGOW COMA SCORE (3–15)				

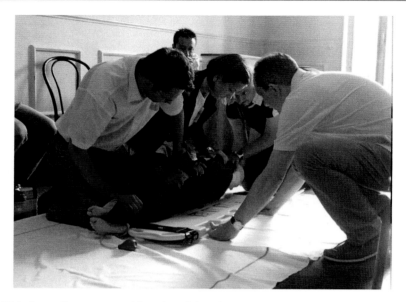

Fig. 15.5 Log-roll maneuver and insertion of the spinal board

15.1.6 Family

The child with trauma, if/when conscious, usually shows a severe distress following related to fear, pain, separation from parents, and the presence of strangers. The appropriate management of traumatized child includes not only the life support but also the psychological support to patient and parents. The aim is to facilitate a good outcome concerning the behavioral and psychological development of the child.

Based on the age of the child, the main goal is to reassure him/her, allowing parents to stay close to him/her.

Even the parents are victims of a severe psychological and emotional trauma. For this reason, it is important that a component of the team establishes an adequate communicative approach with parents, describing the phases of management.

15.2 Preoperative Evaluation and Management

If possible, an accurate history and clinical examination should represent the first step of management before administering anesthesia. However, during emergency, the *AMPLE* acronym may be feasible.

A = allergies
M = medications
P = past medical history

L=last oral intake and last tetanus immunization
E=events related to the injury

Clinical assessment is crucial in pediatric trauma [10]. During emergency, only a rapid evaluation of airway, breathing, and circulation may be possible.

The operating room should be prepared by including age-appropriate equipment, diluting and labeling the medications in age-appropriate doses, raising the ambient temperature to 26 °C for infants and small children, rapid-infusion devices, fluid warmers, and infusion pumps.

Imaging and laboratory testing may be very useful in injured children, but they should not delay emergency procedures. Between all the chest imaging methods, standard anterior-posterior chest X-rays is a cost-effective screening tool that will reveal most of the thoracic abnormalities [11].

Routine laboratory tests such as urinalysis or serum dosages are rarely indicated in pediatric trauma. It is recommended getting blood type, cross matching, and hematocrit even though the patient is hemodynamically stable. Serial hematocrits may help in the monitoring of solid organ injuries [12]. Although coagulopathy is unusually associated with pediatric trauma, PT, PTT, and INR are useful tests in critically injured patients.

15.3   Intraoperative Management

Children with trauma, particularly the smallest, are subject to hypothermia because of their immature thermoregulation, greater body surface area to body mass ratio, and fluid and heat loss from exposed surgical sites; therefore, temperature monitoring is mandatory.

Children with a head injury may require arterial and intracranial pressure monitoring as well as neurophysiologic monitoring during surgery.

The maintenance of anesthesia does not show any specific aspect. No single technique or drug is superior to others [13].

15.4   Intraoperative Fluid Management

As mentioned above, children compensate better hemodynamically in the early stages of injury, and hypotension is a late sign of hemorrhage that may not occur until 30–40 % of the blood volume is lost. The increase of heart rate and capillary refill time should not be overlooked, since children have small blood volumes (Table 15.4), and delay in fluid resuscitation may lead quickly to a significant hypovolemia.

All intravenous fluids should be warmed to 37° to prevent hypothermia.

Resuscitation routinely starts with isotonic crystalloids as the fluid of choice. The end points of fluid resuscitation in children usually include normalization of pulse rate and urine output >1 ml/ kg/h.

Table 15.4 Blood volumes and minimum values of systolic pressure according to age

Age	Blood volume (ml/kg)	Systolic pressure (mmHg)
0–1 month	90	60
1 month – 1 year	80	70
> 1 year	70	70 + 2 x age (years)

The value of diastolic pressure is approximately 2/3 of systolic pressure

The use of hypertonic saline should be considered when trauma is associated with a closed head injury [14] by a starting dose of a bolus of 6.5–10 ml/kg, followed by an infusion of 0.1–1 ml/kg/h.

Hydroxyethyl starch and albumin have also been used in children with no significant adverse effects [15, 16].

Dextrose-containing fluids are usually avoided, because hypotonic solutions may contribute to the development of cerebral edema and also to avoid the risk of hyperglycemia, which is associated with poor neurological outcome in children with a head injury [17].

15.5 Damage Control Strategy (DCS)

Massive hemorrhage in pediatric trauma is a rare event, although not impossible. Most studies concern adults, so that clinical decisions either follow adult protocols or are made according to individual clinical judgment. Deciding on time and volume of blood transfusion may be difficult in children, as well as the optimal ratio of blood components (red blood cells, fresh frozen plasma, platelets). Supplemental use of coagulation factors such as recombinant factor VII and/or cryoprecipitate is advocated if appropriate.

Hemodilution, coagulopathy, acidosis, and transfusion-related complications are associated with excessive crystalloid infusion and administration of blood products.

Coagulopathy, acidosis, and hypothermia represent the so-called lethal triad, and the damage control approach is a strategy for preventing this situation. The main principles of DCS include rapid surgical control of bleeding, permissive modest hypotension that helps preserving the freshly formed thrombus, minimal use of isotonic colloids with the prevention of hemodilution-related complications, and early administration of packed red blood cells in combination with plasma and platelets in a 1:1:1 unit ratio [18].

DCS takes place in three stages (Table 15.5).

15.6 Postoperative Period

Most of the children with major trauma will require monitoring, further stabilization, and continuation of mechanical ventilation in the intensive care unit (ICU) after the initial surgery. Significant fluid shift, acidosis, and soft tissue swelling could be anticipated with massive blood loss and aggressive fluid resuscitation.

Table 15.5 The three stages of damage control

Operating room – damage control surgery
Rapid hemostasis
Control contamination
Temporary abdominal closure
Intensive care – resuscitation
Rewarming
Correct shock – optimize oxygen delivery
Correct coagulopathy
Correct acidosis
Detect abdominal compartment syndrome
Operating room – second-look laparotomy
Definitive repair
Abdominal closure

The decision to perform extubation in the operating room after major trauma must be considered carefully. Successful extubation in patients mechanically ventilated is dependent on cardiovascular stability, normal acid-base balance, presence of intact airway reflexes and ability to clear secretions, an intact central inspiratory drive, ability to exchange gases efficiently, and respiratory muscle strength to meet the work associated with respiratory demand. In pediatric trauma patients, mechanism of injury, such as facial injury, and the absence of an air leak at the time of extubation are the strongest factors predicting post-extubation stridor. Children who cannot be extubated immediately will require transport to the intensive care unit. Before transport, the anesthesiologist should reassess the patient and ensure hemodynamic stability, adequate oxygenation, and functionality of the monitors. Intraoperative monitoring should be continued during transport, and the resuscitation drugs should be immediately available. A detailed report containing history and perioperative events must be given to the intensive care unit team, ensuring the continuity of care and patient safety.

15.7 Sedation and Analgesia

Also for the treatment of postoperative pain, Sedation and analgesia are required for a wide range of procedures in pediatric trauma including painful procedures, such as laceration repair, reduction of bone fractures or joint dislocations, and vascular access, and nonpainful procedures, such as diagnosting imaging (CT, MRI, X-rays). The primary purpose of sedation and analgesia is to provide anxiolysis, control of pain, and movement during the above procedures. Some of these procedures may not require sedation and analgesia and can be managed with nonpharmacological techniques.

The choice of drug and level of sedation should depend on individual needs and whether the procedure is going to be painful or nonpainful. Painful procedures require deeper level of sedation together analgesic, while nonpainful procedures, such as diagnostic imaging, will need minimal to moderate sedation. The medication used for sedation and analgesia includes sedative-hypnotics, analgesics, and/or dissociative agents to relieve anxiety and pain associated with diagnostic and therapeutic procedures in children with injury.

There are two primary methods to relieve anxiety and pain associated with diagnostic and therapeutic procedures in children with injury: inhalational technique with nitrous oxide and/or halogenated agents (sevoflurane) and intravenous technique by using a wide number of drugs, including sedative-hypnotics, analgesics, and/or dissociative agents. Commonly used drugs and their adverse event are shown in Table 15.6 with specific antagonists. Basic pediatric sedation equipment and dosing guide are shown in Fig. 15.6.

15.8   Pain Assessment

Pain evaluation is crucial for an appropriate sedation and analgesia.

Pain assessment in children is challenging, as there is no single tool available for all age groups; hence, age-appropriate pain assessment scales should be used (Table 15.7).

Table 15.6 Pharmacological agents used for sedation and analgesia and antagonists [19]

Drugs and dosage	Clinical effects	Adverse events
Midazolam		
0.5–0.75 mg/kg per os 0.025–0.1 mg/kg i.v. 0.2 mg/kg intranasal	Anxiolysis, amnesia, sedation, hypnotic, anticonvulsant	Hypoventilation, apnea, and paradoxical reactions
Propofol		
1 mg/kg followed by 0,5 mg/kg if necessary	Sedative with rapid onset and brief duration of action	Respiratory depression, apnea, hypotension, and pain on injection
Ketamine		
3–5 mg/kg i.m. 1–2 mg/kg i.v.	Dissociative analgesia and amnesia	Increase in heart rate and blood pressure, increase in exocrine secretion
Fentanyl		
1–2 µg/kg i.v. or intranasal to repeat every 3 min until titration effect	Potent analgesic with no anxiolytic or amnestic effects	Respiratory depression, hypotension, bradycardia
Morphine		
0.2 mg/kg i.v. or 0.3–0.5 mg/kg intranasal	Analgesia	Respiratory depression, nausea, vomiting
Naloxone		
0.1 mg/kg i.v. to repeat every 2 min if necessary	Reversal of respiratory depression by opioids	Shorter effect in reversing long-acting opioids
Flumazenil		
0.02 mg/kg i.v. to repeat every 1 min if necessary	Reversal of clinical effects of benzodiazepines	Shorter effect in reversing long-acting benzodiazepines

Harborview Medical Center – Basic Pediatric Equipment and Dosing Guide

Broselow Color Zone	GRAY			PINK	RED	PURPLE	YELLOW	WHITE	BLUE	ORANGE	GREEN		
Approximate Weight (kg)	3	4	5	6	8	10	13	16	20	26	32	40	45
Approximate Age	Newborn	Newborn	2 mos	4 mos	8 mos	1 yr	2 yr	4 yr	5-6 yr	7-8 yr	9-10 yr	12 yr	13 yr
HR	100-160	100-160	100-160	100-160	100-160	90-150	90-150	80-140	70-120	70-120	70-120	60-100	60-100
RR	30-60	30-60	30-60	30-60	30-60	24-40	24-40	22-34	18-30	18-30	18-30	12-24	12-20
Minimum SBP	40	40	50	60	60	70	70	80	80	80	90	90	90
ETT (uncuffed / cuffed >1 y/o)	3.0/2.5	3.0/2.5	3.5/3.0	3.5/3.0	3.5/3.0	4.0/3.5	4.5/4.0	5.0/4.5	5.5/5.0	6.0/5.5	6.5/6.0	8.5/6.0	7.0/6.5
NG / Foley	5 Fr	5 Fr	5 Fr	5-8 Fr	8 Fr	8-10 Fr	10 Fr	10 Fr	12 Fr	14 Fr	14 Fr	14 Fr	16 Fr
Chest Tube	10-12 Fr	10-12 Fr	10-12 Fr	10-12 Fr	10-12 Fr	16-20 Fr	20-24 Fr	20-24 Fr	24-32 Fr	28-32 Fr	32-36 Fr	36-40 Fr	36-40 Fr
Central Venous Line	3.5-5 Fr UVC		3	3-4	3-4	3-4	3-4	4	4	4-5	4-5	5+	5+
Vent Settings - VT (mL)	24-36	32-48	40-60	48-72	64-96	80-120	104-156	128-192	160-240	208-312	256-384	320-480	360-540
Vent Settings - Rate (BPM)	24-30	24-30	24-30	20-25	20-25	15-25	15-25	15-25	12-20	12-20	12-20	12-16	12-16
C-Collar (Jerome Sizing)	P-0	P-0	P-0	P-0	P-1	P-1	P-1	P-2	P-2	P-2	P-3	use adult collar	
Fluid Bolus (mL)	60	80	100	120	160	200	260	320	400	520	640	800	900
Maintenance Fluids (mL/hr)	12	16	20	28	35	40	45	55	65	70	75	100	115
PRBC (mL) [unit = 350 mL]	30-45**	40-80**	50-75**	60-90	80-120	100-150	130-195	160-240	200-300	280-390	320-480	400-600	450-675
FFP (mL)	30-45	40-60	50-75	60-90	80-120	100-150	130-195	160-240	200-300	280-390	320-480	400-600	450-675
Apheresis Platelets (mL)	15-30	20-40	25-50	30-60	40-80	50-100	65-130	80-160	100-200	130-260	160-320	200-400	225-450
Cryoprecipitate	5-9 mL	6-12 mL	8-15 mL	9-18 mL	12-24 mL	15-30 mL	20-39 mL	24-32 mL	30-60 mL	39-78 mL	6 units	6 units	6 units

** call blood bank (292-6525); consider Pedi-Pak

	PINK	RED	PURPLE	YELLOW	WHITE	BLUE	ORANGE	GREEN					
Acetaminophen PO/PR (mg)	40	40	60	80	80-120	120	160	160-240	240	320	320-400	650	650
Fentanyl IV (mcg)	6-9	8-12	10-15	12-18	16-24	20-30	26-39	16-32	20-40	26-52	32-64	20-40	22-45
Flumazenil IV (mg)	0.03	0.04	0.05	0.06	0.08	0.1	0.13	0.16	0.2	0.2	0.2	0.2	0.2
Glucose IV (mL of D25W)	6 (D10)	8 (D10)	10 (D10)	3-6	4-8	5-10	6-13	8-16	10-20	13-26	16-32	20-40	22-45
Loreazepam IV (mg)	0.15-0.3	0.2-0.4	0.25-0.5	0.3-0.6	0.4-0.8	0.5-1	0.65-1.3	0.8-1.6	1-2	1.3-2.6	1.6-3.2	2-4	2-4
Mannitol IV (gm)	3	4	5	6	8	10	13	16	20	26	32	40	45
Metoclopramide IV (mg)	0.3	0.4	0.5	0.6	0.8	1	1.3	1.6	2	2.6	3.2	4	4.5
Midazolam IV (mg)	0.15-0.3	0.2-0.4	0.25-0.5	0.3-0.6	0.4-0.8	0.5-1	0.65-1.3	0.8-1.6	0.5-1	0.85-1.3	0.8-1.6	0.5-2	0.5-2
Morphine IV (mg)	0.15	0.2	0.25	0.3	0.4-0.8	0.5-1	0.65-1.3	0.8-1.6	1-2	1.3-2.6	1.6-3.2	2-4	2.2-4.5
Naloxone IV (mg)	0.03	0.04	0.05	0.06	0.08	0.1	0.13	0.16	0.2	0.26	0.32	0.4	0.45
Oxycodone PO (mg)	0.15-0.45	0.2-0.6	0.25-0.75	0.3-0.9	0.4-1.2	0.5-1.5	0.65-1.9	0.8-2.4	1-3	1.3-3.9	1.6-4.8	2-6	3-8
Pancuronium/Vecuronium (mg)	0.3	0.4	0.5	0.6	0.8	1	1.3	1.6	2	2.6	3.2	4	4.5
Phenobarbital - IV Load (mg)	60	80	100	120	160	200	260	320	400	520	640	800	900
Phenytoin - IV Load (mg)	45	60	75	90	120	150	195	240	300	390	480	600	675

Fig. 15.6 The Broselow system modified for use at the Pediatric Trauma Center at Harborview Medical Center [19]

Table 15.7 Pain assessment tools in children of different ages

Pain scale	Measurement criteria	Age group
Premature Infant Pain Profile (PIPP)	Assessment of 15 indicators of distress	Neonates and preterm babies
Neonatal Facial Coding System (NFCS)	Assessment of facial actions	Neonates
Face, Legs, Activity, Cry and Consolability (FLACC)	Assessment of distress behaviors in five categories	Children 2 months–7 years
Children's Hospital of Eastern Ontario Pain Scale (CHEOPS)	Assessment of distress behavior in six categories	1–4 years
Faces Pain Scale-Revised (FPS-R)	A series of facial expression illustrating different degrees of discomfort, assigned a numerical score of 1–10	3–5 years
Oucher Scale	Six color photos of a child's face showing different intensities of pain and a numerical scale of scores from 0 (no pain) to 100 (worst pain ever)	7 years or older
Visual analog scale	A line without markers with end points of least or greatest values of intensity of pain	School-age children
Numerical rating scale (NRS)	Variation of VAS. Numbers (0–10 or 0–100) to rate the pain	School-age children

15.9 Conclusion

Trauma is the leading cause of morbidity and mortality in children. Emergency department anesthesiologists are involved in the care of injured children during perioperative treatment. Treatment of the traumatized child requires an accurate knowledge of the anatomical and physiological features that distinguish children from adults.

References

1. Heron M, Hoyert DL, Murphy SL, Xu J, Kochanek KD, Tejada-Vera B (2009) Deaths final data for 2006. Natl Vital Stat Rep 57:1–134
2. Pigula FA, Wald SL, Shackford SR, Vane DW (1993) The effect of hypotension and hypoxia on children with severe head injuries. J Pediatr Surg 28:310–314
3. Schafer I, Barkmann C, Riedesser P, Schulte-Markwort M (2006) Posttraumatic syndromes in children and adolescents after road traffic accidents-a prospective cohort study. Psychopathology 39:159–164
4. Litman RS, Weissend EE, Shibata D, Westesson P-L (2003) Developmental changes of laryngeal dimensions in unparalyzed, sedated children. Anesth Analg 98:41–45
5. Dalal PG, Murray D, Messner AH, Feng A, McAllister J, Molter D (2009) Pediatric laryngeal dimensions: an age-based analysis. Anesth Analg 108:1475–1479
6. Bosch J, de Nooij J, de Visser M, Cannegieter SC, Terpstra NJ, Heringhaus C, Burggraaf J (2014) Prehospital use in emergency patients of a laryngeal mask airway by ambulance paramedics is a safe and effective alternative for endotracheal intubation. Emerg Med J 31:750–753
7. Sagarin MJ, Chiang V, Sakles JC, Barton ED, Wolfe RE, Vissers RJ et al (2002) Rapid sequence intubation for pediatric emergency airway management. Pediatr Emerg Care 18:417–423
8. Clements RS, Steel AG, Bates AT, Mackenzie R (2007) Cuffed endotracheal tube use in paediatric prehospital intubation: challenging the doctrine? Emerg Med J 24:57–58
9. Newth CJ, Rachman B, Patel N, Hammer J (2004) The use of cuffed versus uncuffed endotracheal tubes in pediatric intensive care. J Pediatr 144:333–337
10. Dykes EH (1999) Paediatric trauma. Br J Anaesth 83:130–138
11. Renton J, Kincaid S, Ehrlich PF (2003) Should helical CT scanning of the thoracic cavity replace the conventional chest x-ray as a primary assessment tool in pediatric trauma.? An efficacy and cost analysis. J Pediatr Surg 38:793–797
12. Linzer J (2010) Do routine laboratory tests add to the care of the pediatric trauma patient? Clin Pediatr Emerg Med 11:4
13. Szabo EZ, Luginbuehl I, Bissonnette B (2009) Impact of anesthetic agents on cerebrovascular physiology in children. Paediatr Anaesth 19:108–118
14. Guidelines for the acute medical management of severe traumatic brain injury in infants, children, and adolescent second edition (2012) Pediatr Crit Care Med 13(Suppl 1):S1-S82
15. Sumpelmann R, Kretz FJ, Gabler R, Luntzer R, Baroncini S, Osterkorn D et al (2008) Hydroxyethyl starch 130/0.42/6:1 for perioperative plasma volume replacement in children: preliminary results of a European Prospective Multicenter Observational Postauthorization Safety Study (PASS). Paediatr Anaesth 18:929–933
16. Standl T, Lochbuehler H, Galli C, Reich A, Dietrich G, Hagemann H (2008) HES 130/0.4 (Voluven) or human albumin in children younger than 2 yr undergoing non-cardiac surgery. A prospective, randomized, open label, multicentre trial. Eur J Anaesthesiol 25:437–445
17. Cochran A, Scaife ER, Hansen KW, Downey EC (2003) Hyperglycemia and outcomes from pediatric traumatic brain injury. J Trauma 55:1035–1038
18. Spinella PC, Holcomb JB (2009) Resuscitation and transfusion principles for traumatic hemorrhagic shock. Blood Rev 23:231–240
19. Ramaiah R, Grabinsky A, Bhananker SM (2012) Sedation and analgesia for the pediatric trauma patients. Int J Crit Illn Inj Sci 2(3):156–162

Perioperative Care of Children with Cancer

16

Navi Virk, B. Senbruna, and Jerrold Lerman

16.1 Pediatric Cancer Stats

Cancer is the major cause of pediatric mortality and morbidity. It is the second most common cause of death in children less than 15 years of age [1, 2]. Although the 5-year survival rates exceed 80 %, this leaves chronic and debilitating sequelae for many of these children [3, 4]. The incidence and types of cancer differ with age and differ dramatically from adults (Table 16.1). The pediatric anesthesiologist must be prepared to manage the various conditions associated with cancer patients, as well as the consequences of cancer therapy modalities. Children with cancer can have serious multisystem disease and are prone to various toxicities from chemotherapy and/or radiation therapy and the associated pharmacological treatment.

16.2 Immunomodulatory Effects

Immunosuppression and cancer cell augmentation have been associated with certain anesthetic agents such as ketamine, inhalant anesthetics, and opioids. Propofol and nitrous oxide have been shown to confer less immunosuppression. Regional anesthesia may actually be beneficial in reducing cancer recurrence [5, 6]. Without stronger evidence, at the current time, we cannot recommend a specific anesthetic plan that avoids suppressing the immune system and augmenting cancer.

N. Virk, MD • J. Lerman, MD, FRCPC, FANZCA (✉) • B. Senbruna, MD
University of Rochester, Rochester, NY, USA
e-mail: navvirk@msn.com; jerrold.lerman@gmail.com

© Springer International Publishing Switzerland 2016
M. Astuto, P.M. Ingelmo (eds.), *Perioperative Medicine in Pediatric Anesthesia*,
Anesthesia, Intensive Care and Pain in Neonates and Children,
DOI 10.1007/978-3-319-21960-8_16

Table 16.1 Incidence (%) of pediatric cancer by age

Type of cancer	Age (years)				Overall
	0–4	5–9	10–14	15–19	0–19
Leukemias	36.1	33.4	21.8	12.4	25.2
CNS tumors	16.6	27.7	19.6	9.5	16.7
Lymphomas	3.9	12.9	20.6	25.1	15.5
Carcinomas and epithelial tumors	0.9	2.5	8.9	20.9	9.2
Soft tissue sarcomas	5.6	7.5	9.1	8.0	7.4
Germ cell, trophoblastic, and other gonadal tumors	3.3	2.0	5.3	13.9	7.0
Malignant bone tumors	0.6	4.6	11.3	7.7	5.6
Sympathetic nervous system tumors	14.3	2.7	1.2	0.5	5.4
Renal tumors	9.7	5.4	1.1	0.6	4.4
Retinoblastoma	6.3	0.5	0.1	0.0	2.1
Hepatic tumors	2.2	0.4	0.6	0.6	1.1
Miscellaneous neoplasms[a]	0.5	0.3	0.6	0.8	0.6

[a]Including cardiac tumors

16.2.1 Toxicity of Oncological Therapies

Chemotherapy, radiation therapy, hematopoietic stem cell transplantation (HSCT), and surgical interventions are mainstays of cancer treatment. All of these modalities can significantly affect healthy tissue and lead to multiorgan dysfunction. The toxicities of pharmacologic agents must be understood and recognized by the anesthesiologist in order to optimally manage these children.

16.2.1.1 Chemotherapy

Chemotherapy is one of the cornerstones of cancer treatment. The majority of children with cancer who present for anesthesia are or have been submitted to one or more chemotherapy regimens. These medications can have significant biological effects on a range of organ systems as well as enzyme function. Therefore, the anesthetic must be optimized to address the altered physiology and medication interactions for each child. The greatest concerns pertain to the acute effects of chemotherapy, although occasionally the effects may persist and alter the child's susceptibility to anesthesia years after conclusion of treatment. The effect of chemotherapy on perioperative care is determined by the specific agent, its inherent toxicity, and the cumulative dose. The impact of these agents on cardiorespiratory, hematopoietic, and gastrointestinal systems is most relevant to anesthesia. Table 16.2 provides an overview of chemotherapy agents and their association with organ toxicities.

Cardiotoxicity

Cardiotoxicity can manifest as acute or subacute, chronic, and late-onset pathology. The most common chemotherapy agents that cause cardiotoxicity are anthracyclines (doxorubicin, daunorubicin, and epirubicin), mitoxantrone, cyclophosphamide, bleomycin, 5-fluorouracil, and paclitaxel [7–9].

Anthracyclines and the anthracycline analog, mitoxantrone, impair myocardial contractility that may lead to cardiomyopathy and congestive heart failure, especially if mitoxantrone total does exceeds 140 mg/m^2 [10]. Anthracycline therapy enhances the cardiodepressive effects of anesthesia even in children who have normal resting cardiac function [11]. Dysrhythmias, which develop independent of the dose administered, may be manifested as sinus tachycardia, supraventricular tachycardia, junctional tachycardia, atrioventricular and bundle-branch block, or ventricular tachycardia. Dysrhythmias may occur as early as few hours after the administration of these agents [12, 13]. Forty percent of anthracycline-induced acute toxicity presents as electrocardiographic changes, which include the aforementioned dysrhythmias as well as decreased QRS voltage, and prolongation of the QT interval, which is characteristic of doxorubicin [7, 13]. With the exception of decreased QRS voltage, these changes usually resolve within 1–2 months of the conclusion of therapy. However, sudden death secondary to ventricular fibrillation may occur. Rare cases of subacute cardiotoxicity resulting in acute failure of the left ventricle, pericarditis, or a fatal pericarditis-myocarditis syndrome have been reported particularly in children [14].

Chronic anthracycline cardiotoxicity usually presents as cardiomyopathy. This sequela depends on the cumulative dose administered. The average reported incidence of congestive heart failure is 0.14 % with doses <400 mg/m^2, 7 % with 550 mg/m^2, 15 % with 600 mg/m^2, and 35 % with 700 mg/m^2 total dose of adriamycin [15, 16].

It is important to understand that anthracycline cardiotoxicity can have a late onset. A recent review reported occult ventricular dysfunction, heart failure, and arrhythmias appearing in previously asymptomatic patients more than 1 year after conclusion of anthracycline therapy [17]. Doxorubicin, in particular, can cause subclinical myocardial injury during preadolescent years, which later, during the period of growth spurt, impairs growth of the myocardium. In addition to the total dose of anthracyclines, high-dose radiation to the mediastinum, concurrent cyclophosphamide therapy, extremes of age, prior myocardial injury, hypertension, valvular heart disease, and liver diseases play a significant role in the development of cardiotoxicity.

Table 16.2 Common complications associated with chemotherapeutic agents

System toxicity	Chemotherapeutic agents
Cardiac toxicity	Busulfan, cisplatin, cyclophosphamide, daunorubicin/adriamycin, 5-fluorouracil
Pulmonary toxicity	Methotrexate, bleomycin, busulfan, cyclophosphamide, cytarabine, carmustine
Renal toxicity	Methotrexate, L-asparaginase, carboplatin, ifosfamide, mitomycin-C
Hepatotoxicity	Actinomycin D, methotrexate, androgens, L-asparaginase, busulfan, cisplatin, azathioprine
CNS toxicity	Methotrexate, cisplatin, interferon, hydroxyurea, procarbazine, vincristine
SIADH secretion	Cyclophosphamide, vincristine

Cyclophosphamide is the second agent that can cause myocardial injury. A total dose of cyclophosphamide in excess of 120 mg/kg administered over 2 days can cause severe congestive heart failure, hemorrhagic myocarditis, pericarditis, and necrosis.

Conventional daily oral doses of busulfan may cause endocardial fibrosis that manifests as constrictive cardiomyopathy [18, 19]. In case of preexisting cardiac disease, the use of interferon may exacerbate the disease. Mitomycin may also cause myocardial damage if administered over an extended period of time or in large doses [20]. Paclitaxelin combined with cisplatin has been reported to cause ventricular tachycardia [21].

If any of the aforementioned agents have been used, the child who presents for anesthesia care should undergo a thorough cardiac evaluation that may require echocardiography or nuclear medicine studies. Diastolic dysfunction may present as an early manifestation of anthracycline toxicity. If the left ventricular ejection fraction (LVEF) decreases to less than 45 %, it is considered indicative of anthracycline-induced cardiotoxicity.

The choice of intraoperative monitors should be based on the preoperative symptoms and the specific surgical procedure. Invasive arterial blood pressure monitoring and less commonly central venous catheter or transesophageal echocardiography may be helpful in children with documented cardiac dysfunction. Children who have received anthracycline therapy can develop acute intraoperative left ventricular failure refractory to beta-adrenergic receptor agonists under anesthesia. Amrinone and sulmazole are effective treatments in such cases [22]. Effects of non-anthracycline chemotherapeutic agents on the heart are summarized in Table 16.3.

Pulmonary Toxicity
Children who have cancer often present with pulmonary complications that may be the result of the disease itself or its treatment. Respiratory failure arises secondary to pulmonary metastases or primary lesions, infections, chemotherapy, radiotherapy, and/or extensive surgical pulmonary resections [23]. The mortality rate in these children is as great as 75 % if mechanical ventilation is required [24–26].

Table 16.3 Adverse cardiac effects with non-anthracycline chemotherapeutic agents

Agent	Cardiovascular effect
Cyclophosphamide	Fulminant CHF secondary to hemorrhagic myocarditis
	Acute pericarditis with effusion
	Risk increased with dose > 200 mg/m^2 and anthracycline combination
Bleomycin	Acute pericarditis
5-Fluorouracil	Coronary insufficiency presenting as angina/myocardial infarct due to coronary spasm
Paclitaxel and docetaxel	Asymptomatic bradycardia, severe bradyarrhythmias and tachyarrhythmias including ventricular fibrillation and asystole, conduction disorders, myocardial ischemia and infarction; Overall risk is increased with concomitant cisplatin therapy. Peripheral edema is due to fluid retention (docetaxel)

The primary chemotherapeutic agents that damage the pulmonary system are busulfan, cyclophosphamide, paclitaxel, and bleomycin, the last being the most detrimental of these.

Bleomycin is known to cause six distinct pathologies:

1. Interstitial pneumonitis that can progress to chronic fibrosis
2. Acute hypersensitivity pneumonitis
3. Acute chest pain syndrome
4. Bronchitis obliterans with organizing pneumonia
5. Pulmonary venoocclusive disease
6. Noncardiogenic pulmonary edema

Bleomycin-induced pulmonary toxicity develops 4–10 weeks after therapy with an incidence between 0 and 40 %. Nonlethal pulmonary fibrosis is known to occur in 11–30 % of children with an associated mortality from bleomycin of 2–10 %. As many as 20 % of children with radiological and histological evidence of bleomycin toxicity are symptom-free [27]. Risk factors for bleomycin pulmonary toxicity are old age, cumulative dose >400–450 mg, poor pulmonary reserves, radiotherapy, uremia, greater inspired oxygen concentrations, and concomitantly administered other anticancer drugs.

Bleomycin is believed to cause direct cytotoxicity that involves the production of superoxides and other free radicals. The use of greater concentrations of inspired oxygen augments this process. Although pulmonary injury is thought to develop with cumulative dose >400–450 mg, fetal pulmonary fibrosis has been reported with total doses as low as 50 mg [22]. The fetal injury is believed to occur as type II pneumocytes replace type I pneumocyte in the alveoli. With continuous exposure, type II pneumocytes are replaced by cuboidal epithelium. Further, since effective tissue repair is absent, this leads to the development of fibrosis. The chest X-ray shows bilateral basal and perihilar infiltrates with fibrosis. The clinical picture includes fever, cough, dyspnea, bibasilar rhonchi, and rales. Exertional dyspnea may occur with mild X-ray changes and a normal or low resting PaO_2. Arterial hypoxemia is a common sign of bleomycin toxicity. An increased alveolar-arterial PO_2 gradient and decreased carbon monoxide diffusing capacity (DLCO) are consistent findings in interstitial fibrosis. Pulmonary function testing indicates a restrictive lung pattern. Regression of the injury may occur with immediate cessation of therapy. Steroid therapy has been found to be effective in some cases.

The perioperative inspired oxygen concentration has been a concern in those who received bleomycin therapy. In one report of patients who were treated with bleomycin and who received an intraoperative $FiO_2 > 0.39$, five developed ARDS and subsequently died [28]. In two more recent, larger series, no perioperative pulmonary complications occurred in patients who received bleomycin and who were subsequently exposed to intraoperative $FiO_2 > 0.25$ and >0.41 [29, 30]. A recent, much larger study demonstrated minor pulmonary complications in patients exposed to inspired $FiO_2 > 0.40$ and >0.25, although none progressed to ARDS or died. Instead, meticulous fluid balance, duration of surgery, and postchemotherapy forced vital capacity were recognized as significant predictors of postoperative pulmonary morbidity [31]. In the face of this conflicting evidence, the current recommendations are to minimize the FiO_2 wherever possible to maintain the SpO_2 in excess of 90 % and to use intraoperative PEEP.

During preoperative assessment of patients with pulmonary complications chest X-ray, pulmonary function tests, arterial blood gas analysis, and in some instances DLCO may assist in identifying the severity of the pulmonary dysfunction. In some cases, arterial access may facilitate repetitive intraoperative arterial blood gas analyses. Depending on the preoperative presentation and intraoperative course, postoperative ventilatory support may be anticipated.

Other chemotherapy agents and their adverse pulmonary effects important to anesthesia are listed in Table 16.4.

Hepatorenal Toxicity

The renal system is affected by several chemotherapy agents, the most common and important of which is cisplatin. Approximately 30 % of patients who are treated with cisplatin develop nephrotoxicity, which is the dose-limiting consequence. The most important measure to prevent nephrotoxicity is adequate hydration with forced diuresis. Normal saline is a particularly beneficial fluid to infuse as the large concentration of chloride in the tubules inhibits the hydrolysis of cisplatin [22]. Renal injury stems from coagulation necrosis of proximal and distal renal tubular and collecting duct epithelium that reduces the renal blood flow and glomerular filtration rate (GFR). A single dose of cisplatin of 2 mg/kg or 50–75 mg/m^2 produces nephrotoxicity in 25–30 % of patients [32]. Acute renal failure can occur within 24 h of administration. Chronic decreases in GFR can also occur. The reported decrease in GFR after 16–52 months of cisplatin therapy is 12.5 % [33]. Coadministration of other nephrotoxic drugs, such as aminoglycosides, increases the risk of nephrotoxicity. Newer cisplatin analogs, i.e., carboplatin and oxaliplatin, are less nephrotoxic than cisplatin. Other nephrotoxic agents are listed in Table 16.5.

Table 16.4 Adverse pulmonary effects with non-bleomycin chemotherapy agents

Agent	Incidence (%)	Description
Busulfan	4–10	Pulmonary fibrosis, pulmonary alveolar lipoproteinosis
Cyclophosphamide	<2	Pneumonitis with or without fibrosis
Mitomycin	<10	Similar to bleomycin
Cytosine arabinoside	5–32	Noncardiogenic pulmonary edema with or without pleural effusion
Methotrexate	7	Hypersensitivity pneumonitis or
		Noncardiogenic pulmonary edema or
		Pulmonary fibrosis or
		Pleurisy with acute chest pain

Table 16.5 Adverse nephrotoxic effects with non-cisplatinum chemotherapeutic agents

Agent	Description
Mitomycin	Chronic progressive increase in serum creatinine to microangiopathic hemolytic anemia
Methotrexate	Physical effect because of precipitation of drug within the renal tubules
	NSAIDs reduce excretion of methotrexate and therefore should be avoided [34]
Ifosfamide	Acute tubular necrosis and renal failure

Hepatic injury presents as increased liver enzymes, impaired synthetic function with low protein and coagulation factor synthesis, fatty infiltration of liver, and cholestasis. The cause of the hepatic injury may be due to either the chemotherapy itself or their metabolites. Among these, L-asparaginase and cytarabine are the most common chemotherapeutic agents that induce hepatocellular dysfunction, although cyclophosphamide and mitomycin have been reported to cause dysfunction as well. The resultant hepatic dysfunction can range from mild to very severe, with associated ascites, painful hepatomegaly, and encephalopathy.

Neurotoxicity

Chemotherapy can affect central, peripheral, and autonomic nervous systems. Vincristine is the only known chemotherapeutic agent whose dose is limited by the presence of neurotoxicity. It can affect all aspects of the nervous system. Central nervous system toxicity may be manifested as ophthalmoplegia and facial palsy. Peripheral neuropathy is characterized by depression of deep tendon reflexes and peripheral paresthesia that progresses proximally over the course of chemotherapy. Motor dysfunction and gait disorders can also occur. Autonomic dysfunction may result in orthostatic hypotension, erectile dysfunction, constipation, difficulty in micturition, bladder atony, and more.

About 50 % of those who receive cisplatin treatment develop neurotoxicity that depends on the dose administered and the duration of therapy. It usually presents as peripheral neuropathy in stocking and glove distribution and auditory and visual impairment. A subclinical, unrecognized neuropathy may cause unexpected complications from regional anesthesia. Recently, a diffuse brachial plexopathy was reported after an interscalene block in a patient receiving cisplatin [35]. Therefore, if regional anesthesia is planned, a thorough neurological examination is warranted.

Severe neurologic consequences have occurred after inadvertent intrathecal administration of vincristine. Close to 100 fatal or serious irreversible neurologic injuries have been reported, although the true number of cases is unknown [36].[1] Vincristine is an effective intravenous chemotherapeutic agent for leukemia, lymphoma, Wilms' tumor, neuroblastoma, and other tumors. However when injected intrathecally, it produces either a local motor neuropraxia (resulting in paresis of

---

[1] https://www.ismp.org/newsletters/acutecare/showarticle.aspx?id=58

varying severity) or ascending radiculomyeloencephalopathy, coma, and death. Typically, vincristine is prepared in a syringe for intravenous administration, but when a patient is scheduled for intrathecal chemotherapy, it has been inadvertently given along with or in place of the prescribed intrathecal chemotherapy with disastrous sequelae. Although there is no strategy to prevent the neurologic injury or death once intrathecal vincristine has been given, if the error is identified immediately, then the CSF has been irrigated and flushed with fresh frozen plasma, resulting in para- or tetraparesis and only a 15 % mortality [36]. This contrasts with a 100 % mortality without aggressive treatment with plasma. Since 50 % of vincristine is bound to plasma proteins within 20 min of injection into blood, circulating plasma in the CSF is believed to bind with vincristine, preventing it from destroying the neuronal cytoskeleton and inducing neurologic injury or death. The key strategy to avoid this potentially catastrophic outcome is to never prepare vincristine in a syringe and to always keep vincristine remote from any intrathecal procedures.

Additional neurotoxic chemotherapy agents are listed in Table 16.6.

Hematological Effects

All lines of hematopoiesis can be affected either by the primary malignancy, metastasis to bone marrow, or chemotherapy. A dysfunctional coagulation cascade can prolonged PT and PTT times; increase factor I, V, VIII, IX, XI, and fibrinogen degradation products; reduce platelet life span; and decrease antithrombin III activity. To date, no prospective trials have estimated the minimum platelet count required to prevent bleeding during specific procedures. The empiric recommendation is to maintain the platelet count in excess of 50,000 per microliter during the perioperative period. It is essential to correct any preexisting coagulopathy before commencing surgery.

Anemia is very common in cancer patients. Recommendations differ regarding the transfusion threshold for packed red blood cell (PRBC). Most recommend a hemoglobin threshold of <9 g/dl for transfusion in asymptomatic children, with greater values in symptomatic patients [37]. During perioperative period, the anesthesiologist should closely follow the blood loss and guide the decision to transfuse

Table 16.6 Adverse neurotoxic effects with non-vincristine chemotherapy agents

Agent	Incidence (%)	Description
Cytarabine	15–37	Cerebellar dysfunction, peripheral neuropathy, seizures, encephalopathy, myelopathy, pseudobulbar palsy
Ifosfamide	0–10	Cerebellar dysfunction, hemiparesis, coma, extrapyramidal abnormalities
5-Fluorouracil	0–5	Cerebellar dysfunction, multifocal leukoencephalopathy
Methotrexate	0–2	Meningeal irritation, transient paraparesis, encephalopathy
Paclitaxel	50–70 (high dose)	Peripheral neuropathy, autonomic neuropathy
Procarbazine		Cerebral effects: lethargy, depression to psychosis, peripheral neuropathy

based on age-adjusted estimated allowable blood loss calculations. Immunocompromised children including infants depending on the institutional policy; hematopoietic progenitor cell transplant recipients; those with Hodgkin's disease, leukemia and lymphoma, aplastic anemia with severe lymphocytopenia, and solid organ tumors; those receiving nucleoside analog therapy (i.e., fludarabine); those requiring granulocyte transfusions; and those undergoing intense chemotherapy require irradiated PRBCs. Accordingly, red blood cell transfusions should be planned before surgery in collaboration with the treating oncologist [38].

Most children receiving broad-based chemotherapy will experience immunosuppression. Chemotherapy, by design, targets rapidly dividing cells, including immune system cells. For this reason, these children are more susceptible to infections. Meticulous aseptic techniques are mandatory during all invasive procedures. Wound healing can also be affected by the absence of neutrophils. Nonetheless, children whose WBC exceeds 500/mm^3 generally have uncomplicated surgical wound healing. The effect of chronic anemia on surgical wound healing is minimal [39]. Other factors that complicate wound healing include chemotherapy. The effect of chemotherapy depends on the dose and timing of chemotherapy administration, as well as concurrent radiotherapy.

Myelosuppression caused by chemotherapy is transient and usually resolves within 1–6 weeks after cessation of treatment.

Hormone and Enzyme Production

The most common hormonal disturbance in children treated for cancer is steroid-induced adrenal suppression. The stress response may be blunted for 6 months or greater after therapeutic exogenous corticosteroids. Most children who continue their usual doses of corticosteroids during surgery have appropriate corticosteroid levels and can mount an endogenous stress response [40]. Whether they require a supplemental dose of steroids in the perioperative period remains controversial [41, 42]. The corticotrophin (ACTH) stimulation test is the definitive test to confirm adrenal suppression, but individual testing is labor-intensive, costly, and of limited predictive value. A recent review (with limited power) determined that patients with intact hypothalamic-pituitary axis who are receiving physiologic doses of exogenous steroids more than likely can mount a stress response, whereas those with dysfunction of the hypothalamic-pituitary axis (e.g., Addison's disease) likely cannot mount an endogenous response to steroids and require supplementation [43]. Current practice in most centers favors supplementing children who have taken exogenous steroids in the perioperative period. If a child develops unexplained intraoperative or postoperative hypotension, particularly if it is unresponsive to a fluid bolus and/or pressors, treatment with hydrocortisone (1.5 mg/kg intravenously) is definitely warranted.

Syndrome of inappropriate antidiuretic hormone secretion (SIADH) is best known in association with paraneoplastic syndrome of small cell lung cancer, which is exceedingly rare in children, but it has been associated with other oncologic diseases as well. About 1–2 % of cancer patients develop SIADH. Some drugs, including vasopressin, carbamazepine, oxytocin, vincristine, vinblastine, cyclophosphamide, phenothiazines, tricyclic antidepressant agents, opioids, and monoamine oxidase inhibitors, can also induce SIADH [44]. The diagnostic criteria for SIADH include a serum sodium level <135 mEq/L, plasma osmolality <280 mOsm/kg, urine osmolality >500 mOsm/kg, and urine sodium >20 mEq/L. Patients who develop SIADH can experience malaise, altered mental status, seizures, coma, and occasionally death. Focal neurologic findings can occur in the absence of brain metastases. Acute treatment is indicated if serum sodium concentration is <125 mEq/L. Correction of the hyponatremia should be undertaken slowly, particularly if the hyponatremia has persisted for several days. The increase in serum sodium should be ≤20 mEq/L during the first 48 h of treatment. Children who experience too rapid an increase in the serum concentration of sodium may suffer neurologic insults and central pontine myelinolysis.

Some chemotherapy agents can interfere with several enzyme activities. Alkylating agents such as cyclophosphamide inhibit pseudocholinesterase activity. The effect may persist for 3–4 weeks after the final dose. Accordingly, the use of succinylcholine may cause prolonged muscle paralysis, and a reduction of the dose is indicated in such patients [45]. Procarbazine exerts inhibitory effect on monoamine oxidase. Because of potential synergistic action, barbiturates, antihistaminic, phenothiazines, opioids, and tricyclic antidepressants should be used with caution.

16.2.1.2 Radiation Toxicity

Toxicity from radiation is unavoidable, but children are particularly prone to developing sequelae because of their young age. The duration, dose, and interval of radiation therapy together contribute significantly to the early side effects of the radiation, whereas the dose and age of the child contribute to the late side effects. In general, the sequelae develop in the organ being irradiated, although the singular exception is the development of subsequent solid neoplasms as outlined below [46, 47].

All tissues damaged by radiation are susceptible to inflammation and subsequent fibrosis. For example, radiation to the neck may cause the tissues to stiffen and fibrose, which in turn distort and narrow the airway leading to a potentially difficult airway. Thoracic radiation may affect both the heart and lungs. Cardiac manifestations may include pericarditis, effusions, cardiomyopathy, valvular fibrosis, and conduction abnormalities [48]. To minimize cardiac toxicity, radiation doses are limited to <25–30 Gy. The lungs are particularly at risk for fibrosis. Both fibrosis and interstitial pneumonitis can occur but are more likely to result from chemoradiation combination therapy. In the abdomen, radiation may cause progressive nephrotoxicity at doses exceeding 20 Gy. Gastrointestinal manifestations include malnutrition, chronic enterocolitis, and bowel obstruction. Whole-brain radiation may cause long-term diminution in cognitive function and intelligence quotient, the severity of which depends on the age of onset of the radiation and the magnitude of the dose. The younger the child and the larger the dose, the greater the impact on cognitive function, with learning disabilities and memory loss more prominent than generalized intellectual impairment. Radiation therapy of the sella turcica with doses that exceed 35–40 Gy may cause pituitary dysfunction manifested by isolated hypothyroidism and growth retardation to panhypopituitarism. Finally, both conductive hearing loss and sensorineural hearing loss have been reported after cranial radiation. Other common sequelae of radiation therapy include blistering of the skin and non-melanoma skin cancer, hair loss, nausea, and anemia. Perhaps the most worrisome complication after radiation therapy is the risk of developing a subsequent solid malignant neoplasm. These occur in up to 47 % of children after a 10-year or greater latency period after radiation. The risk of developing a neoplasm that is distinct from the original primary neoplasm increases the younger the child at the time of the radiation exposure and the greater the dose of the radiation. Examples of solid subsequent neoplasms include thyroid, breast, brain, sarcoma, and others.

16.2.2 Anterior Mediastinal Mass (AMM)

Children with AMMs require general anesthesia and/or sedation for a tissue (lymph node) biopsy, CT scan or MRI for diagnosis, or indwelling central line for chemotherapy [49]. Children with these tumors present a significant risk for anesthesia, since cardiac arrest has been reported in the past. Understanding the pathophysiology of the disease enables the clinician to anticipate complications and prepare the anesthetic to avoid them.

Four tissue types comprise most AMMs in children: lymphomas, teratomas, thymomas, and thyroid with lymphomas being the most common, 45 % of AMMs [49]. The most rapidly growing tumor in the anterior mediastinum is the lymphoblastic T-cell lymphoma, a non-Hodgkin's lymphoma, which has a doubling time of only 12–24 h. These children may present with minor findings (e.g., night sweats) that rapidly progress over 1–2 days to life-threatening problems (e.g., orthopnea, superior vena cava syndrome). In children, anesthesia is usually required to delimit the extent of and tumor effects on mediastinal structures in radiology as well as for tissue biopsy and chronic chemotherapy access in the operating room.

The decision to proceed with local, regional, or general anesthesia depends on the age and level of cooperation of the child, the extent of mediastinal organ involvement, and the access of the node or tumor being biopsied or the planned procedure. A multidisciplinary team that includes the surgeon, anesthesiologist, and oncologist should review all radiological and preoperative data before embarking on the surgery.

Preoperatively, all children should have a chest X-ray (anterior-posterior and lateral views) as well as a preoperative echocardiogram. The latter is particularly helpful in determining whether the right atrium, pulmonary artery, pericardium, and pericardial sac are involved with the tumor. Although echocardiographic examinations are performed awake and cannot rule out compression of these structures during anesthesia, they can identify whether the structures may be at risk during anesthesia.

Those children who can tolerate the surgery under local anesthesia and sedation are managed in this manner. However, this is not usually possible in younger children, in children who cannot tolerate local anesthesia and sedation, and in those whose tumor severely compromises the airway and/or pulmonary artery. In such instances, a 12–24 h course of intravenous steroids or limited radiation should be considered and discussed with the oncologists to shrink the tumor to facilitate an anesthetic and reduce the risk of cardiac arrest [50]. The risks associated with administering a brief course of steroids or radiation are infrequent but may include widespread tumor necrosis that may both render the diagnosis of the cell type difficult and possibly trigger tumor lysis syndrome [51]. Some oncologists are reluctant to treat these children with steroids because of the potential difficulty in establishing the tissue diagnosis should extensive tumor necrosis ensue. Establishing the tumor type is critical for determining the treatment regimen for the specific tumor type. Thus, a balance between the oncologist's and anesthesiologist's requirements must be sought.

For most children who require a radiological investigation, tumor biopsy, or chemotherapy access, general anesthesia with spontaneous respiration and avoiding paralysis are the optimal prescription [49]. If the child cannot lie flat, anesthesia can be induced and the trachea intubated with the child positioned in the left lateral decubitus or less desirably, in the sitting position. The trachea should be intubated at induction of anesthesia to ensure a patent airway should it become necessary to turn the child prone to reverse circulatory collapse. Tracheal intubation is performed without muscle relaxation to preserve spontaneous respiration. Spontaneous respiration best preserves the negative intrathoracic pressure gradient to suspend the tumor above the mediastinal structures and avoid pressure on the pulmonary artery and right atrium as well as the tracheobronchial tree. Maintaining spontaneous respiration preserves negative intrathoracic pressures, although simply induction of anesthesia may decrease the magnitude of the negative intrathoracic pressure sufficiently to allow the tumor to press on cardiac vessels. Therefore, one must always monitor the cardiac output (via the capnogram; see below) and be prepared to emergently reestablish circulation. The latter may be achieved by either turning the child prone or applying one towel clip at the sternal notch and one at the xiphoid junction in the anesthetized child and lifting the sternum to restore patency of the cardiac vasculature (usually the pulmonary artery). The capnogram is a very useful monitor to confirm the adequacy of the pulmonary circulation (and cardiac output); the sudden loss of or reduction in the capnogram may herald compression of the pulmonary artery before systemic cardiovascular sequelae occur. Unless the femoral artery and vein have been cannulated before induction of anesthesia, it is exceedingly unlikely that extracorporeal membrane oxygenation could be instituted rapidly enough to restore the circulation in a child who arrests with an AMM.

16.2.3 Airway Lesions

Mucositis and xerostomia are possible sequelae of chemotherapy/radiation therapy developing within weeks of beginning treatment. Mucositis and ulcerative lesions can also occur after hematopoietic stem cell transplant as a part of GVHD. This can result in pseudomembrane formation, supraglottic edema, friability/bleeding, and the potential for aspiration [37]. Irradiation of the neck can lead to fibrosis and airway distortion (subglottic edema, supra and subglottic stenosis, hypoplasia of the jaw, and chondronecrosis of the epiglottis, arytenoids, and trachea) [46]. Concerns for difficult airway, poor LMA seating, and the need for smaller ET tubes may result. For children who received HSCT and required mechanical ventilation, 30 % of intubations were reported to be difficult, most often because of bleeding or edema from mucositis [46].

16.2.4 Neoplasia/Cancer

16.2.4.1 Cardiovascular Effects and Considerations

Although primary cardiac tumors are rare, serious cardiac sequelae may arise from the cardiotoxic nature of oncological pharmacotherapies. Chemotherapeutic agents such as anthracyclines, cyclophosphamide, fluorouracil, alkaloids, and asparaginase are among the commonly utilized cardiotoxic chemotherapies. Their cardiac effects are cumulative with irradiation, leading to recommendations to limit the dose of irradiation to 25–30 Gy whenever it is combined with chemotherapy that is cardiotoxic. Radiation therapy to the thorax can result in pericardial effusions, pericarditis, cardiomyopathy, valvular fibrosis, conduction anomalies, and coronary artery disease [48, 52].

Children treated with anthracyclines and/or chest irradiation should be followed with regular echocardiography, especially if they received anthracycline during infancy, required a dose greater than 240 mg/m^2, or received irradiation greater than 40 Gy alone or greater than 30 Gy coupled with anthracycline therapy [53].

16.2.4.2 Pulmonary Effects and Considerations

Pulmonary neoplasms and resultant chemotherapy can result in many pulmonary complications such as pleural effusions, pulmonary embolus, chylous effusion, AMM, and pulmonary leukostasis, pneumonitis, pulmonary fibrosis, and pulmonary edema. Pneumonitis commonly has a subclinical presentation and is reversible up to the point of radiologic changes [54, 55]. Pulmonary fibrosis frequently occurs during acute treatment but can become manifest months to years after treatment. Children treated with bleomycin are at risk for exacerbation of pulmonary fibrosis and restrictive lung disease with high concentrations of inspired oxygen. There overall risk for pulmonary toxicity with chemotherapy in the children is near 6 %. It increases to 20 % with the addition of radiation therapy and 25 % in those undergoing HSCT [56, 57]. Bleomycin is the most common and best known culprit for pulmonary complications, although there are many other agents that are associated with pulmonary toxicity.

16.2.4.3 Renal Effects and Considerations

Common renal tumors in children include Wilms' tumor, clear cell sarcoma of the kidney, malignant rhabdoid tumor, congenital mesoblastic nephroma, and renal cell carcinoma. Neuroblastoma can infiltrate the kidney leading to obstruction and acute renal failure. Common chemotherapeutic agents that can lead to nephrotoxicity include cisplatin, carboplatin, ifosfamide, cyclophosphamide, and methotrexate. Manifestations of toxicity include Fanconi syndrome (ifosfamide), hypomagnesemia (cisplatin), SIADH, and radiation nephritis. Careful evaluation and management of blood pressure, electrolytes, anemia, and coagulation status is important when treating children with renal dysfunction that was associated with chemotherapy-radiation therapy [37].

16.2.4.4 Hepatic Effects and Considerations

Although rare, primary liver tumors in children include hepatoblastoma, sarcoma, germ cell tumors, and rhabdoid tumors (Table 16.1). Genetic syndromes are associated with up to 20 % of hepatic neoplasms. Beckwith-Wiedemann syndrome is associated with neonatal birth weights greater than 4 kg, macroglossia, and omphalocele [58]. Commonly these infants have exophthalmos, visceromegaly, hyperviscosity syndrome, and hypoglycemia. Careful consideration should be made to the possibility of difficult airway, glucose monitoring, the need for phlebotomy, and the possibility of postoperative airway obstruction.

Chemotherapy and radiation can lead to hepatic toxicity and fibrosis; however, it is usually mild and self-limiting. Sinusoidal obstruction syndrome after HSCT occurs 11–27 % of the time with a high mortality of 19–50 %. Sinusoidal obstruction syndrome is characterized by portal hypertension, liver failure, and subsequent multiorgan failure. For any patients with hepatic dysfunction, it is important to anticipate diminished biotransformation of anesthetic agents and the possibility of coagulopathy.

16.2.4.5 GI Effects and Considerations

Although primary GI tumors are rare, intra-abdominal masses can lead to obstruction (intestinal or biliary), intussusceptions, perforation, and hemorrhage. Chemotherapy toxicity can result in diarrhea, mucositis, neutropenic enterocolitis, stomatitis, anorexia, and malnutrition/dehydration. Anesthetic considerations include aspiration risk, vitamin K deficiency, electrolyte disturbances, and fluid status [37].

16.2.4.6 CNS Effects and Considerations

Common central nervous system neoplasms include astrocytomas, ependymomas, neuroectodermal tumors, and gliomas. Neurotoxicity from chemotherapy is associated with platinum agents, L-asparaginase, ifosfamide, methotrexate, cytarabine, etoposide, vincristine, and cyclosporine A. Irradiation of the brain can lead to neurocognitive delays and leukoencephalopathy. Most tumors require resection and the anesthesiologist should be prepared to manage ICP and treat the possibility of intraoperative seizures [37]. Supplemental steroid therapy may be necessary for those who have received steroids either for their tumor or to decrease the ICP.

16.2.4.7 Endocrine Effects and Considerations

Less than 5 % of childhood cancer includes endocrine tumors (Table 16.1). Gonadal germ cell tumors, thyroid neoplasia, and pituitary masses are the most prevalent endocrine cancers. The main anesthetic concerns involve the use of steroids for cancer treatment and the effects of radiation on hormone secretion.

Adrenal suppression is common in patients receiving glucocorticoid treatment, and stress dose steroids are recommended in any pediatric patient who has received steroid treatment within 1–2 months of surgery. Radiation can result in growth hormone and gonadotropin deficiency in doses as low as 20 Gy. Panhypopituitarism risk increases as the radiation dose rises to approximately 40 Gy [59]. Hypothyroidism can occur 2–4.5 years after radiation in doses up to 20 Gy [60].

16.2.4.8 Hematological Effects and Considerations

Myelosuppression can occur from the effects of the cancer and the chemotherapy. Anemia, thrombocytopenia, and neutropenia are common manifestations in pediatric cancer. Hyperleukocytosis greater than $200,000/mm^3$ can increase blood viscosity and cause leukostasis. Caution must be used to maintain appropriate volume status and avoid excessive transfusion that can exacerbate hyperleukocytosis [61].

Reduction in the treatment dose and the products transfused is standard treatment regimen for myelosuppression. Leukoreduced and irradiated blood products are recommended in immunocompromised patients susceptible to GVHD. Platelet transfusion may be indicated for certain procedures. Recommendations for minor surgical procedures require that platelet counts exceed $20,000/mm^3$. For major invasive procedures, the platelets counts should be in the range of $40,000–50,000/mm^3$. Neurosurgery requires platelet counts of more than $100,000/mm^3$. Bleeding diatheses, which are common in children with ALL and AML, should be readily corrected through leukoreduced FFP transfusion if PT/PTT is increased or there is evidence of surgical bleeding due to coagulopathy [37].

16.2.4.9 Psychiatric Considerations

Neurocognitive and psychiatric changes are often present years after cancer treatment. These can manifest as poor academic performance or emotional trauma. The greatest effects are noted in children undergoing intrathecal methotrexate and cranial irradiation. Demographics, support structures, and the child's involvement in their care regimen are all critical factors in determining the extent of the emotional trauma.

Children should be given the opportunity to assume an active role in their own care. Activities such as pretreatment desensitization, role playing, and discussions with the child about physical and mental expectations are useful to limit the psychiatric stress of cancer therapy and surgical intervention. Posttraumatic stress symptoms are reported in 33–68 % of children undergoing cancer treatment. It is important to have an honest discussion with children about what to expect and the possible outcomes for the treatment and procedures they are undergoing. A preferred anesthetic routine may be established for children undergoing multiple procedures [46].

16.2.5 Tumor Lysis syndrome (TLS)

TLS is caused by tumor cell lysis that results in the release of the cell contents. Tumor cell lysis can be spontaneous or therapy induced (chemotherapy, radiation, glucocorticoids, tamoxifen, or interferons). The greater the tumor cell burden, the more severe the presentation. Although TLS is most commonly associated with non-Hodgkin's lymphoma or acute leukemia, more and more frequently, it is being reported with other tumors. Cairo and Bishop classified TLS either as a laboratory or clinical syndrome [62]. Laboratory TLS requires that two or more of the following metabolic abnormalities occur within 3 days before or up to 7 days after the initiation of therapy: hyperuricemia, hyperkalemia, hyperphosphatemia, and hypocalcemia. In contrast, clinical tumor lysis syndrome is present when laboratory tumor lysis syndrome is accompanied by an increase in plasma creatinine concentration, seizures, cardiac dysrhythmias, or death. Acute renal failure results from the precipitation of urate, xanthine, and phosphate stones in the renal collecting system. Uric acid can induce acute kidney injury not only by intrarenal crystallization but also by crystal-independent mechanisms, such as renal vasoconstriction, impaired autoregulation, decreased renal blood flow, oxidation, and inflammation [63]. Tumor lysis also releases cytokines that cause a systemic inflammatory response syndrome and often multiorgan failure [64]. Calcium phosphate can precipitate throughout the body. Precipitates in the cardiac conducting system can cause serious, possibly fatal dysrhythmias. The risk of TLS is greater in cases of preexisting chronic renal insufficiency, oliguria, dehydration, hypotension, and acidic urine. The mainstay of treatment is hyperhydration with intravenous balanced salt solution (2500–3000 ml/m^2/day in children at the greatest risk for TLS). If the urine output remains poor after achieving an optimal state of hydration, the use of loop diuretics is recommended, with a target urine output of at least 2 ml/kg/h. Urinary alkalinization should be avoided because it increases the solubility of uric acid but decreases the solubility of calcium phosphate, and it is more difficult to correct hyperphosphatemia than hyperuricemia. Control of the serum phosphorus concentration may prevent hypocalcemia, which can lead to life-threatening dysrhythmias and neuromuscular irritability. Asymptomatic hypocalcemia does not require treatment. At the prospect of sudden death due to cardiac dysrhythmias, hyperkalemia remains the most dangerous component of the TLS. Glucose with insulin or beta-agonists can be used as temporizing measures, and calcium gluconate may be used to reduce the risk of dysrhythmia in the acute setting.

When the anesthetic prescription is planned for any child who is undergoing chemotherapy, it is crucial to clarify the risk of developing TLS, its severity, and instituted treatment with the treating oncologist. NOTE: children who present for minor surgical or medical procedures with AMMs have a high incidence of hematopoietic tumors that are untreated. Do NOT administer dexamethasone for postoperative nausea and vomiting until after the biopsy has been taken, and the oncologists have been consulted because a single dose of dexamethasone may precipitate TLS. In fact, a single-dose dexamethasone induced a fatal TLS event in a child with an undiagnosed hematopoietic tumor after adenotonsillectomy [51]. New-onset TLS usually develops 5–7 days after the induction of therapy. Some treatment regimens have reduced risk for TLS than others. It is rare that those with TLS present for anesthesia, but when the occasion arises, one should pay close attention to maintain adequate hydration and measure plasma potassium concentrations frequently (e.g., every 4–6 h).

16.2.6 Retinoic Acid Syndrome

Up to 25 % of those with acute promylocytic leukemia receiving all-trans retinoic acid develop retinoic acid syndrome. It has a 2 % mortality. Retinoic acid syndrome manifests as respiratory distress, pulmonary infiltrates, pericardial effusions, cardiac dysfunction, hypotension, and possibly ARF [37].

16.3   Preoperative Evaluation

Preoperative evaluation and testing for the child with cancer must be tailored to the specific comorbidities and the risks of the individual. Along with a comprehensive history and physical evaluation, a thorough review of the child's medical history and treatment regimen is necessary. Specific interest should be paid to the child who is at risk for anemia, coagulopathy, and electrolyte abnormalities.

Children are at increased risk for anemia if present with a new diagnosis of leukemia/lymphoma and recent chemotherapy/radiation/HSCT and are less than 6 months of age. There is a 20 % incidence of hyperleukocytosis in children with newly diagnosed leukemia. The risk of thrombocytopenia is increased in children who are newly diagnosed with leukemia (75 % incidence), receive chemoradiation, have signs and symptoms of DIC, and who present with splenomegaly [53].

Monitoring coagulation via testing is indicated in those who present with sepsis, vitamin K deficiency, hyperleukocytosis, T-cell ALL, myelomonocytic leukemia, and acute promyelocytic leukemia and have undergone L-asparaginase treatment. If platelet counts are sufficient for the type of surgery required, no further testing is usually indicated.

Common conditions that can lead to electrolyte disturbances include SIADH, hypercalcemia from bone neoplasms or neuroblastoma, dehydration or malnutrition, renal dysfunction, and tumor lysis syndrome.

16.4   Pediatric Cancer Pain

16.4.1 Definition

Pain is a multidimensional phenomenon with sensory, physiological, cognitive, affective, behavioral, and spiritual components. It is the most common discomfort experienced by children with cancer and occurs in almost 89 % of patients in an advanced stage of the disease [65]. Pain affects all aspects of daily life, including physical activities, school attendance, sleep patterns, family interactions, and social relationships and can lead to distress, anxiety, depression, insomnia, and fatigue. Very often, the severity of the pain is underestimated and inadequately treated because of the pediatrician's lack of experience and fear of opioid addiction and depressed respiration.

Pain can be classified according to the pathophysiological mechanism (nociceptive or neuropathic pain), the duration (chronic or acute), the etiology (malignant or nonmalignant), or its anatomic location (somatic or visceral). Most children with cancer suffer from both chronic pain and acute pain. Chronic pain is defined as continuous or recurrent pain that persists beyond the expected normal time of healing, although in children with cancer, it persists secondary to the ongoing disease process. Acute pain has a sudden onset and short duration. It is important to distinguish three different kinds of acute pain: incidental pain, "end of dose" pain, and spontaneous or breakthrough pain. Incidental pain has an identifiable cause such as movement, weight bearing, coughing, and therapeutic procedures. "End of dose" pain occurs when the nadir of the analgesic blood level is less than the minimum effective blood level for analgesia, e.g., toward the end of a dosing interval. This pain may be eliminated by increasing the dose of the long-acting opioid during the maintenance period. Breakthrough pain is characterized by a transient increase in the severity of pain over and above the preexisting baseline level of pain. It has a sudden onset and is severe in intensity and short in duration. Although "rescue" doses of opioids are needed to abate the pain, the likelihood of a positive response is decreased in these children [66]. Approximately 57 % of children with cancer experience breakthrough pain, a pain that may occur multiple times each day. Children 7–12 years of age appear to be at increased risk for breakthrough pain [67]. Breakthrough pain independently contributes to impaired functioning and psychological distress. Children with acute cancer pain have breakthrough pain as a result of progress of the disease or infection at the tumor site, development of tolerance to analgesics, drug interactions, decreasing renal function with the accumulation of nociceptive metabolites (morphine-3-glucuronide or hydromorphone-3-glucuronide), and/or somatization and psychological distress [68].

To tailor appropriate treatment strategies, it is important to distinguish between nociceptive pain and neuropathic pain. Nociceptive pain arises from tissue injury. Activation of nociceptors in either surface tissues (skin, mucosa) or deep tissues such as the bone, joint, muscle, or connective tissue causes somatic pain, and activation of nociceptors located in the viscera causes visceral pain. Neuropathic pain is caused by structural damage and nerve cell dysfunction in the peripheral or central nervous system. It has rarely been studied in infants, children, and adolescents. The main causes of neuropathic pain in cancer patients are nerve injury, nerve entrapment, or external compression by any space-occupying lesion; phantom limb pain; nerve infiltration by cancers; and nerve damage caused by cancer treatment (e.g., chemotherapy, radiation).

16.4.2 Pain Assessment

For optimal pain management, it is essential to establish regular, objective pain level assessment. The pain should be reassessed frequently to evaluate the effectiveness of treatment and to institute modifications if necessary.

There is no single validated tool to measure persistent pain in children; however, several tools are available to assess acute pain in children of different ages. Many pain self-reporting tools can be used in children as young as 3 years. Assessing pain in preverbal children may present a challenge. In such cases, the severity of a child's pain may be best evaluated by parents and/or caregivers who understand their child's behavioral responses to pain.

To improve perioperative pain management in children with oncologic disease who present for repeated surgery, the anesthesia provider should inquire regarding pain management strategies that have been used previously, as well as the efficacy of those treatments.

16.4.3 Pain Treatment

Currently there is limited scientific evidence upon which to base pain management strategies. The WHO and other recommendations are based on low-quality evidence and rely primarily on expert opinions. The principles of pain management include the application of the WHO analgesic ladder, appropriate opioid dose escalation, the use of adjuvant analgesics, and the use of nonpharmacological methods of pain control.

16.4.4 Pharmacological Treatment

The key concepts of pharmacological cancer pain management in children include using a two-step strategy as opposed to three-step ladder in adults, dosing at regular intervals, using the appropriate route of administration, and adapting treatment to the individual child. In the two-step strategy, the severity of pain dictates the choice of analgesic. For mild pain, acetaminophen and/ or nonsteroidal anti-inflammatory agents (e.g., ibuprofen) should be considered as first-line treatments, whereas for moderate to severe pain, an opioid should be the primary intervention. In some situations, however, the first step can be bypassed based on clinical judgment.

16.4.4.1 Acetaminophen

The dose of oral acetaminophen is 10–20 mg/kg, with repeat dosing according to 12.5 mg/kg every 4 h or 15 mg/kg every 6 h IV (2–12 years old and adolescents <50 kg). Acetaminophen is safe in neonates, although its metabolism and elimination are delayed compared with adults. As a result, repeat doses in neonates should be administered at 6 h rather than 4 h intervals. The total dose should not exceed 90–100 mg/kg (PO) or 75 mg/kg (IV) daily as excessive doses can lead to hepatic failure. Hepatic damage has been reported after reduced doses when the usual doses were given to debilitated children, so it is wise to avoid acetaminophen in such cases.

16.4.4.2 Ibuprofen

The dose of oral ibuprofen is 5–10 mg/kg three or four times daily with or after food. The maximum total daily dose is 40 mg/kg/day. Ibuprofen can upset the gastrointestinal tract, impair renal function, and decrease platelet aggregation. In children with mildly impaired renal function, the lowest effective dose of ibuprofen should be used and renal function monitored. Sodium and water retention along with deteriorating renal function are signs of impending renal failure. In moderate to severe renal impairment, and in children younger than 3 months, ibuprofen should not be used. Ibuprofen should also be used with caution in those with impaired hepatic function as there is an increased risk of gastrointestinal bleeding and in those with severe liver disease.

In case of moderate to severe pain, opioids are necessary. Unfortunately, fear and a lack of knowledge about the use of opioids in children often present obstacles to achieving effective pain relief. Morphine is the medicine of choice for the second step in the WHO ladder, although other potent opioids may be considered and made available in order to substitute the opioid because of intolerable side effects. There is insufficient evidence to recommend any alternative to morphine as the opioid of first choice. Selection of alternative opioid analgesics should be guided by considering the safety, availability, cost, and suitability including patient-related factors.

One of the basic and most important principles in managing cancer pain is the administration of analgesics at regular intervals. It is necessary to achieve and maintain steady blood levels of analgesics. Analgesic dosing that is designed on a PRN basis increases the opioid consumption, fails to satisfactorily control pain, and invariably leads to alternating periods of under- and overmedication. Prolonged-release oral formulation, transdermal patches, and intravenous infusions of opioids are widely used to maintain stable analgesic levels. Tables 16.7, 16.8, and 16.9 present the recommended initial doses of opioids according to the child's age. Dosing is titrated to effect with no maximum doses listed. If more than four doses of "rescue" or breakthrough pain medications are needed each day, the background analgesic dose must be increased. The maximum increase in the dose of opioids over 24 h is 50 % in outpatient settings. Experienced prescribers who monitor the children closely can increase the dose up to 100 % over 24 h. To transition from parenteral opioids to oral formulations, it is important to keep the contents of Table 16.10 in mind, although there are few studies in children that address the equivalence of opioid dosing.

The pain management has to be adapted to each child. Opioids, unlike the first-step medications, do not have a maximal (ceiling) dose. Some children require very large doses of opioids. For breakthrough pain, additional morphine (oral

Table 16.7 Doses for opioids in opioid-naive neonates

Medicine	Route of administration	Starting dose
Morphine	IV injection	25–50 mcg/kg every 6 h
	SC injection	
	IV infusion	Initial IV dose 25–50 mcg/kg and then 5–10 mcg/kg/h
Fentanyl	IV injection	1–2 mcg/kg every 2–4 h
	IV infusion	Initial IV dose 1–2 mcg/kg and then 0.2–1 mcg/kg/h

Table 16.8 Doses for opioids in opioid-naive infants (1 month–1 year)

Medicine	Route of administration	Starting dose
Morphine	Oral (immediate release)	80–200 mcg/kg every 4 h
	IV injection	1–6 months: 100 mcg/kg every 6 h
	SC injection	6–12 months: 100 mcg/kg every 4 h (max 2.5 mg / dose)
	IV infusion	1–6 months: initial IV dose: 50 mcg/kg, then: 10–30 mcg/kg/h 6–12 months: initial IV dose: 100–200 mcg/kg, then: 20–30 mcg/kg/h
	SC infusion	1–3 months: 10 mcg/kg/h 3–12 months: 20 mcg/kg/h
Fentanyl	IV injection	1–2 mcg/kg every 2–4 h
	IV infusion	Initial IV dose: 1–2 mcg/kg and then 0.2–1 mcg/kg/h
Oxycodone	Oral (immediate release)	50–125 mcg/kg every 4 h

Table 16.9 Doses for opioids in opioid-naive children (1–12 years)

Medicine	Route of administration	Starting dose
Morphine	Oral (immediate release)	1–2 years: 200–400 mcg/kg every 4 h 2–12 years: 200–500 mcg/kg every 4 h (max 5 mg)
	Oral (prolonged release)	200–800 mcg/kg every 12 h
	IV injection	1–2 years: 100 mcg/kg every 4 h
	SC injection	2–12 years: 100–200 mcg/kg every 4 h (max 2.5 mg)
	IV infusion	Initial IV dose: 100–200 mcg/kg and then 20–30 mcg/kg/h
	SC infusion	20 mcg/kg/h
Fentanyl	IV injection	1–2 mcg/kg, repeated every 30–60 min
	IV infusion	Initial IV dose: 1–2 mcg/kg and then 0.2–1 mcg/kg/h
Hydromorphone	Oral (immediate release)	30–80 mcg/kg every 3–4 h (max 2 mg/dose)
	IV injection or SC injection	15 mcg/kg every 3–6 h
Methadone	Oral (immediate release)	100–200 mcg/kg
	IV injection and SC injection	every 4 h for the first 2–3 doses and then every 6–12 h (max 5 mg/dose initially)
Oxycodone	Oral (immediate release)	125–200 mcg/kg every 4 h (max 5 mg/dose)
	Oral (prolonged release)	5 mg every 12 h

immediate-release formulation, IV injection, or subcutaneous) and fentanyl may be administered as frequently as required. The rescue dose of morphine and other opioids, except fentanyl, is 10 % of the total daily baseline dose. If larger breakthrough doses are required, the regular baseline morphine dose should be increased, guided by the amount of morphine required to control breakthrough pain. Commonly used

Table 16.10 Approximate dose ratios for conversion between parenteral and oral dose formulations

Medicine	Dose ratio (parenteral/oral)
Morphine	1:2–1:3
Hydromorphone	1:2–1:5
Methadone	1:1–1:2

Table 16.11 Usual starting doses for patient-controlled analgesia in children

	Initial bolus until analgesia (mcg/kg)	Continuous infusion (mcg/kg/h)	PCA bolus (mcg/kg)	Lockout time (min)	Maximum hourly dose (mcg/kg/h)
Morphine	100–200	0–20 (max 1000)	10–20 (max 1000)	5–10	60–100
Hydromorphone	2–4	0–4 (max 250)	2–5 (max 250)	5–10	12–20
Fentanyl	0.5–1	0–0.5 (max 50)	0.5–1 (max 50)	5	1.5–2.5

Doses are for children >6 months of age and are capped at 50 kg body weight

opioid regimens include immediate-release oral morphine every 4 h or controlled-release morphine twice daily, plus a PRN dose of 10 % of the 24-h morphine requirement as an hourly fast-release breakthrough pain medication. If the child has IV access, patient-controlled analgesia (PCA) can be administered using a continuous opioid infusion with additional self-administered boluses. If the child is too young or unable to push the PCA demand button, a nurse-controlled analgesia protocol can be introduced (NCA) [67]. Children older than 5 or 6 years are capable of using a PCA. If the PCA bolus dose has to be increased, it should be increased in increments of 50 %, as in the case of the maintenance dose. For usual PCA starting doses, refer to Table 16.11 [68].

16.4.4.3 Morphine

Morphine is available as immediate- and slow-release tablets, oral liquids, granules (to be diluted in water), and injection. Oral long-acting morphine proved to be safe and effective even in the very young patients. Immediate-release morphine is available as oral syrup or tablets and can be easily dosed according to weight. Prolonged-release oral formulations allow for longer dose intervals, therefore improving the patient's compliance by reducing dose frequency. Prolonged-release oral formulations of morphine are administered every 8–12 h but are unsuitable for the treatment of breakthrough pain. Prolonged-release tablets cannot be crushed, chewed, or cut, but prolonged-release granules can replace prolonged-release tablets in such a case.

Immediate-release tablets are used for titrating morphine dosage for the individual child and defining the adequate dose for pain control and can be administered every 4 h. They are also indispensable for the management of episodic or breakthrough pain. Liquid preparations allow for easier dose administration than tablets in infants and small children. Intravenous morphine can be administered either by medical stuff or by patient by PCA or NCA.

Table 16.12 Equianalgesic opioid doses

Opioid agonist	Parenteral dose, IV, SC, IM (mg)	Oral dose (mg)	PO:IV	Duration of action (h)
Morphine	10	30	3:1	3–4
Morphine, long-acting	–	30	–	12
Hydromorphone	1.5	7.5	5:1	2–3
Fentanyl	0.2 mg	–	–	2
Oxycodone	–	15–20	–	3–5
Oxycodone, long-acting	–	20	–	12

The dose in renal impairment should be reduced as follows: mild (GRF 20–50 ml/min or approximate serum creatinine 150–300 micromol/l) to moderate (GFR 10–20 ml/min or serum creatinine 300–700 micromol/l) by 25 %, and severe (GFR <10 ml/min or serum creatinine >700 micromol/l) by 50 % or consider switching to alternative opioid analgesics which have less renal elimination, such as methadone and fentanyl. In hepatic impairment, morphine should be avoided or the dose reduced.

Despite the lack of prospective data, opioid switching or rotation may have a positive impact on managing dose-limiting side effects of, or tolerance to, opioid therapy during cancer pain treatment in children [69]. For equianalgesic doses, refer to Table 16.12.

16.4.4.4   Fentanyl

Fentanyl is a short-acting opioid that can be used by IV infusion or as transdermal patch as maintenance medication or as IV boluses for breakthrough pain. Some suggest using the intranasal route (an off-label use) for breakthrough pain. The nasal mucosa is very well vascularized facilitating rapid absorption and the absorbed fentanyl bypasses first-pass metabolism. The pharmacokinetics of nasal fentanyl are very similar to those of the IV route. However, there are no published studies of transmucosal fentanyl application systems in children. Consequently, these products cannot yet be recommended for use in children with cancer and breakthrough pain.

Initial dosing of IV fentanyl for bolus and infusions is described in Tables 16.7, 16.8, and 16.9.

The dose of fentanyl must be reduced in children with impaired renal function: by 25 % with moderate impairment (glomerular filtration rate (GFR) 10–20 ml/min or serum creatinine 300–700 micromol/L) and by 50 % with severe impairment (GFR <10 ml/min or serum creatinine >700 micromol/L). In the case of impaired hepatic function, fentanyl should be avoided or, at the very least, the dose reduced as coma may be precipitated.

Transdermal fentanyl patch is indicated as a maintenance analgesic in children with chronic pain. In a multicenter study in children, transdermal fentanyl was found to be safe and well tolerated as an alternative to oral opioids [70]. Each transdermal application of fentanyl is designed to be worn for 72 h. The minimal dose delivers 12 mcg/h of fentanyl. The patch should never be cut to adjust the dose of fentanyl. The safety and efficacy of transdermal fentanyl patches in children less than 2 years of

Table 16.13 Dose conversion to transdermal fentanyl patch (Duragesic)

Current opioid	Daily dose (mg/day)			
Oral morphine	60–134	135–224	225–314	315–404
IM or IV morphine	10–22	23–37	38–52	53–67
Oral oxycodone	30–67	67.5–112	112.5–157	157.5–202
Oral hydromorphone	8–17	17.1–28	28.1–39	39.1–51
IV hydromorphone	1.5–3.4	3.5–5.6	5.7–7.9	8–10
Oral methadone	20–44	45–74	75–104	105–134
Recommended transdermal fentanyl patch dose	↓ 25 mcg/ h	↓ 50 mcg/ h	↓ 75 mcg/ h	↓ 100 mcg/ h

age have not been established. To guard against accidental ingestion by children, caution should be exercised when choosing the application site for the transdermal patch. The dose of fentanyl should be reduced with impaired hepatic and renal function (see above). When a transdermal patch is initiated, all around-the-clock opioids should be stopped. The immediate-release morphine equivalent should be available. The dose of the patch dose may be adjusted after 3 days, based on the amount of supplemental opioids required during the previous 48 h, using a ratio of 45 mg/24 h of oral morphine to a 12 mcg/h increase in patch dose. Transdermal fentanyl patch therapy in children who require less than 60 mg/day of oral morphine or an equianalgesic dose of another opioid has not been evaluated in controlled clinical trials. For dose conversion from other opioids to transdermal patch, refer to Table 16.13.

Exposure of the application site and surrounding skin to direct external heat sources such as heating pads or warming blankets may increase the absorption of fentanyl and has resulted in fatal overdose of fentanyl, a respiratory arrest and death. If a child develops a fever or increased core body temperature due to strenuous exertion, they are at risk for increased fentanyl absorption and may require a reduction in the dose of the transdermal fentanyl patch to preclude complications. The application site should be changed as the patch is changed every 72 h.

16.4.4.5 Hydromorphone

Hydromorphone is available as a tablet, an oral liquid, or by injection. Hydromorphone is a potent opioid with substantive differences between oral dosing and intravenous dosing. Extreme caution should be used when converting from one route to another. In converting from parenteral to oral hydromorphone, oral doses may need to be titrated up to 5 times the IV dose. For dosing ranges, refer to Table 16.9.

The dose of hydromorphone should be reduced in children with moderately or severely impaired renal function. Treatment should begin with the smallest dose and titrated according to the child's response. In the case of impaired hepatic function, the initial dose should be reduced with all levels of impaired function.

16.4.4.6 Methadone

Methadone has wide interindividual variability in its pharmacokinetics and thus should only be initiated by practitioners who are experienced with its use. The dose should be titrated during close clinical observation of the child over several days. The dose should initially be titrated like other strong opioids. The dose may need to be reduced by 50 % 2–3 days after the effective dose has been established in order to prevent adverse effects due to methadone accumulation. Thereafter, dosing increases should be undertaken at intervals of 1 week or greater, with a maximum increase of 50 %. For dosing ranges, refer to Table 16.9.

Methadone dose should be reduced or avoided in children with impaired hepatic function. Significant accumulation of methadone is unlikely in children with renal failure, as its elimination occurs primarily via the liver. Nevertheless, in children with severely impaired renal function, the dose should be reduced by 50 % and titrated to effect.

16.4.4.7   Oxycodone
Oxycodone is available in immediate- and prolonged-release oral formulations. The dose in cases of moderately to severely impaired renal function should be reduced. In moderately and severely impaired hepatic function, the dose should be reduced by 50 % or avoided. When converting from oral morphine to oral oxycodone, an initial dose conversion ratio of 1.5:1 is a good starting point. Thereafter, titrate the dose to optimize the level of analgesia. For dosing ranges, refer to Table 16.9.

16.4.4.8   Naloxone
Naloxone is a pure intravenous opioid antagonist that is used to antagonize extreme effects of an opioid overdose. In the opioid-naive neonate, infant, or child, the dose to treat apnea after an opioid is 10 mcg/kg followed by 100 mcg/kg if there is no response. Diagnosis should be reviewed if respiratory function does not improve; further doses may be required if respiratory function deteriorates. Continuous IV infusion may be needed (5–20 mcg/kg/h) and should be adjusted according to response. Smaller doses are required in opioid-tolerant patients: neonate, infant, or child – 1 mcg/kg titrated over time, e.g., every 3 min, until the child is breathing spontaneously and maintaining adequate oxygenation; thereafter, a low-dose IV infusion or intramuscular administration of the same dose that was effective intravenously may be administered to maintain the respiratory rate and level of consciousness until the effect of overdose has resolved. During this period, close monitoring is required. Caution should be exercised to avoid acute withdrawal symptoms. In the case of an opioid overdose caused by renally excreted drugs in children with impaired renal function, extended treatment with a naloxone infusion may be required.

16.4.5 Adjuvant Therapy

Adjuvants have not been widely studied in infants and children. Their use is based on experience in adult pain management, expert opinion, and several case reports. The use of corticosteroids and bisphosphonates is not recommended as adjuvant for pain management in children. The benefits of these medications are unknown and they carry potential for serious side effects.

At present, it is not possible to make a recommendation regarding the use of tricyclic antidepressant and selective serotonin reuptake inhibitors or anticonvulsants (e.g., gabapentin) as adjuvants in the treatment of neuropathic pain in children. The benefits remain unclear.

It is also not possible to make recommendations regarding the benefits and risks of ketamine as an adjuvant to opioids for the management of pain in children. Ketamine is believed to be a useful adjunctive agent; however, there is a paucity of evidence regarding its safety and efficacy in children. In one study, ketamine showed an opioid-sparing effect and improved pain control in children with uncontrolled cancer pain [71].

Based on the available evidence, no recommendation can be made regarding the use of other adjuvants, e.g., benzodiazepines and baclofen, in the management of pain in children with muscle spasm and spasticity.

16.4.6 Nonpharmacological Pain Management

The data on invasive pain management procedures in infants and children are anecdotal, and precise indications on who, when, and how they should receive such treatments remain unclear. Peripheral nerve blocks, catheter-delivered nerve blocks, and epidurals have been reported to be effective in children suffering from advanced stage cancer. Neurolytic nerve blocks can also be considered.

Strong emphasis should be placed on supportive, rehabilitative, and integrative therapies, such as distraction, biofeedback, deep breathing, and self-hypnosis. Education of both family and the child cannot be overestimated.

16.4.7 Post-op Pain in Cancer Patient

Children with cancer can present at any stage of their disease for surgery. If the child is opioid-naive, the pain management strategy is similar to that of other children without cancer. However, if the child has been chronically exposed to opioids before surgery, the dose of perioperative opioids may have to be increased to account for possible resistance to the opioids. Postoperative incidental pain may also require larger doses of opioids than expected. When appropriate, adjuvants like acetaminophen and nonsteroidal anti-inflammatory agents can be used to decrease opioid requirements perioperatively. NMDA receptor antagonists (e.g., ketamine) and magnesium infusions may reduce the dose of opioid required to achieve analgesia in adults chronically exposed to opioids. If the child has been exposed to PCA opioids, the overall dose of opioids may have to be increased substantively after surgery. The increased doses vary depending on the child's resistance to opioids and the surgery performed. If other techniques are used to manage perioperative pain such as epidural or peripheral nerve blocks with or without a catheter, the maintenance dose of opioids should continue to avoid the acute opioid withdrawal.

16.5   Sedation Techniques

Sedation for radiation therapy requires an organized team approach to assure adequate anesthesia for the child with remote and reliable monitoring. These procedures take place in a remote site (radiation oncology) where there is no backup or support. Accordingly, ALL standard anesthetic requirements must be in place before embarking on an anesthetic including appropriate preoperative assessment of the child (fasting) as well as medications, equipment (including resuscitation cart), and recovery personnel. Anesthesia is usually induced in the radiation suite, and once the child is stable, the child is left alone for the brief period of radiation administration while he/she is monitored remotely from the control station. Depending on the site of radiation, there are a number of anesthetic prescriptions that may be used. In all cases, the child must remain still but usually can breathe spontaneously. For children who require a contoured total facemask to pinpoint the radiation beam to the head, the only source for oxygen and monitoring may be nasal prongs. For those who have radiation to anywhere but the head, any airway and anesthetic technique may be used, recognizing that daily serial treatments may be required for up to 60 days. Hence, the least invasive airway management may be preferred.

Several pharmacological options are available to sedate these children, but for the most part, total intravenous anesthesia with propofol is used by many. Other approaches include ketamine, midazolam, and dexmedetomidine infusions. Usually these children have a port or indwelling intravenous access making an intravenous induction facile. A bolus of intravenous propofol, 2 mg/kg, followed by an infusion of 250–300 mcg/kg/min (with larger initial infusion rates for younger infants and those with neurological impairment) should provide immobility while maintaining spontaneous ventilation. If intravenous access was not available, an inhalational induction followed by conversion to the intravenous technique once the child is anesthetized is possible. Standard ASA monitors should include $etCO_2$ via nasal cannula with supplemental oxygen. Proper positioning and padding with foam cushions is important. During the treatment, the children are monitored in a control station adjacent to the radiation suite, and it is paramount that attention is undivided during the anesthetic to ensure adequate oxygenation and ventilation are maintained. With recovery in a room adjacent to the scanner, the child will achieve street readiness for discharge after a brief recovery from the propofol.

16.6   Conclusion

To assure proper preoperative preparation of a cancer patient who is receiving chemotherapy, the following tests, taking in consideration clinical presentation, are suggested: complete blood count, urine analysis, serum electrolytes, fasting blood sugar, serum BUN, pulmonary function tests, arterial blood PaO_2 and $PaCO_2$, serum osmolality, bilirubin, creatinine, amylase, liver function tests, chest X-ray, and ECG. Awareness of the side effects of the various chemotherapeutic agents is prudent for safe and comprehensive anesthesia care.

References

1. Jemal A, Siegal R, Ward E et al (2009) Cancer statistics, 2009. CA Cancer J Clin 59(4):225–249
2. Ries LA, Percy CL, Bunin GR (1999) Introduction. In: Ries LA, Smith MA, Gurney JG et al (eds) Cancer incidence and survival among children and adolescents: Unites States SEER Program 1975–1995. National Cancer Institute SEER Program, Bethesda, p 1. NIH Pub. No. 99–4649 ed
3. Horner MJ, Ries LA, Krapcho M (2009) SEER cancer statistics review, 1975–2006. National Cancer Institute, Bethesda
4. Oeffinger KC, Mertens AC, Sklar CA et al (2006) Chronic health conditions in adult survivors of childhood cancer. N Engl J Med 355(15):1572–1582
5. Heaney A, Buggy DJ (2012) Can anesthetic and analgesic techniques affect cancer recurrence or metastasis? Br J Anaesth 109(Supp 1):i17–i28
6. Tavare AN, Perry NJ, Benzonana LL et al (2012) Cancer recurrence after surgery: direct and indirect effects of anesthetic agents. Int J Cancer 130(6):1237–1250
7. Burrows FA, Hickey PR, Colan S (1985) Perioperative complications in patients with anthracycline chemotherapeutic agents. Can Anaesth Soc J 32:149–157, PubMed: 3986652
8. Lahtinen R, Kuikka J, Nousianinen T et al (1991) Cardiotoxicity of epirubicin and doxorubicin: a double-blind randomized study. Eur J Haematol 46:301–305, PubMed:2044726
9. Lekakis J, Vassilopoulos N, Psichoyiou H et al (1991) Doxorubicin cardiotoxicity detected by indium 111 myosin-specific imaging. Eur J Nucl Med 18:225–226, PubMed: 1645666
10. Weesner KM, Bledsoe M, Chauvenet A et al (1991) Exercise echocardiography in the detection of anthracycline cardiotoxicity. Cancer 68:435–438, PubMed: 2070339
11. Huettemann E, Junker T, Chatzinikolaou KP et al (2004) The influence of anthracycline therapy on cardiac function during anesthesia. Anesth Analg 98:941–947, PubMed: 15041577
12. Steinherz LJ, Steinherz PG, Tan CT et al (1991) Cardiac toxicity 4 to 20 years after completing anthracycline therapy. JAMA 266:1672–1677, PubMed: 1886191
13. Steinberg JS, Cohen AJ, Wasserman AG, Cohen P, Ross AM (1987) Acute arrhythmogenicity of doxorubicin administration. Cancer 60:1213–1218, PubMed: 3621107
14. Bristow MR, Billingham ME, Mason JW, Daniels JR (1978) Clinical spectrum of anthracycline antibiotic cardiotoxicity. Cancer Treat Rep 62:873–879, PubMed: 667861
15. Praga C, Beretta G, Vigo PL, Pollini C, Bonadonna G, Canetta R et al (1979) Adriamycin cardiotoxicity: a survey of 1273 patients. Cancer Treat Rep 63:827–834, PubMed: 455324
16. Von Hoff DD, Layward MW, Basa P, Davis HL Jr, Von Hoff AL, Rozencweig M et al (1979) Risk factors for doxorubicin–induced congestive heart failure. Ann Intern Med 91:710–717, PubMed: 496103
17. Shan K, Lincoff AM, Young JB (1996) Anthracycline-induced cardiotoxicity. Ann Intern Med 125:47–58, PubMed: 8644988
18. Solley GO, Maldonado JE, Gleich GJ et al (1976) Endomyocardiopathy with eosinophilia. Mayo Clin Proc 51:697–708, PubMed: 994551
19. Drzewoski J, Kasznicki J (1992) Cardiotoxicity of antineoplastic drugs. Acta Haematol Pol 23:79–86, PubMed: 1488864
20. Verweij J (1996) Mitomycins. Cancer Chemother Biol Response Modif 6:46–58, PubMed: 8639396
21. Cortes JE, Pazdur R (1995) Docetaxel. J Clin Oncol 13:2643–2655, PubMed: 7595719
22. Gehdoo RP (2009) Anticancer chemotherapy and it's anaesthetic implications (current concepts). Indian J Anaesth 53(1):18–29. PMCID: PMC2900029
23. Varon J (1995) Acute respiratory distress syndrome in the postoperative cancer patient. Cancer Bull 47:38–42
24. Dumont P, Wihim JM, Hentz JG et al (1995) Respiratory complications after surgical treatment of esophageal cancer: a study of 309 patients according to the type of resection. Eur J Cardiothorac Surg 9:539–543, PubMed: 8562096

25. Epner DE, White F, Krasnoff M et al (1996) Outcome of mechanical ventilation for adults with hematologic malignancy. J Invest Med 44:254–260
26. Randle CJ Jr, Frankel LR, Amylon MD (1996) Identifying early predictors of mortality in pediatric patients with acute leukemia and pneumonia. Chest 109:457–461, PubMed: 8620722
27. Waid-Jones M, Coursin DB (1991) Perioperative considerations for patients treated with bleomycin. Chest 99:993–999, PubMed: 1706974
28. Goldiner PL, Schweizer O (1979) The hazards of anesthesia and surgery in Bleomycin-treated patients. Semin Oncol 6:121–124, PubMed: 88070
29. Goldiner PL, Carlon GC, Cvitkovic E, Schweizer O, Howland W (1978) Factors influencing postoperative morbidity and mortality in patients treated with bleomycin. Br Med J 1:1664–1667. PMCID: PMC1605498
30. LaMantia KR, Glick JH, Marshall BE (1984) Supplemental oxygen does not cause respiratory failure in Bleomycin-treated surgical patients. Anesthesiology 60:65–67, PubMed: 6197912
31. Donat SM, Levy DA (1998) Bleomycin associated pulmonary toxicity: is perioperative oxygen restriction necessary? J Urol 160:1347–1352, PubMed: 9751352
32. Madias NE, Harrington JT (1978) Platinum nephrotoxicity. Am J Med 65:307–314, PubMed: 99034
33. Fjeldberg P, Sorensen J, Helkjaer PE (1986) The long term effects of cisplatin on renal function. Cancer 58:2214–2217, PubMed: 3756770
34. Frenia ML, Long KS (1992) Methotrexate and nonsteroidal antiinflammatory drug interactions. Ann Pharmacother 26:234–237, PubMed: 1554938
35. Huettemann E, Sakka SG (2005) Anaesthesia and anti-cancer chemotherapeutic drugs. Curr Opin Anaesthesiol 18:307–314
36. Reddy GK, Brown B, Nanda A (2011) Fatal consequences of a simple mistake: how can a patient be saved from inadvertent intrathecal vincristine? Clin Neurol Neurosurg 113:68–71
37. Latham GJ (2014) Anesthesia for the child with cancer. Anesthesiol Clin 32:185–213
38. Treleaven J, Gennery A, Marsh J et al (2011) Guidelines on the use of irradiated blood components prepared by the British Committee for Standards in Haematology blood transfusion task force. Br J Haematol 152:35–51
39. Schaffer MR, Barbul A (1996) Chemotherapy and wound healing. In: Lefor AT (ed) Surgical problems affecting the patient with cancer. Lippincott-Raven, Philadelphia, pp 305–320
40. Axelrod L. Perioperative management of patients treated with glucocorticoids (2003) Endocrinol Metabol Clin North Am 32:367–383
41. Sabourdin N (2015) Steroids: the evidence. The rationale for perioperative glucocorticoid supplementation for patients under chronic steroid treatment. Curr Anesthesiol Rep 5(2):140–146
42. Garcia JEL, Hill GE, Joshi GP (2013) Perioperative stress dose steroids: is it really necessary? Am Soc Anesthesiol Newsletter 77(11)
43. Marik PE, Varon J (2008) Requirement of perioperative stress doses of corticosteroids: a systematic review of the literature. Arch Surg 143:1222–1226
44. Anderson RJ, Chung HM, Kluge R et al (1985) Hyponatremia: a prospective analysis of its epidemiology and the pathogenetic role of vasopressin. Ann Intern Med 102:164–168, PubMed: 3966753
45. Zsigmond EK, Robins G (1972) The effect of a series of anticancer drugs on plasma cholinesterase activity. Can Anaesth Soc J 19:75–82, PubMed: 4257896
46. Latham GJ, Greenberg RS (2010) Anesthetic considerations for the pediatric oncology patient – part 2: systems-based approach to anesthesia. Pediatr Anesth 20:396–420
47. Landier W, Armenian S, Bhatia S (2015) Late effects of childhood cancer and its treatment. Pediatr Clin North Am 62:275–300
48. Adams MJ, Lipshultz SE, Schwartz C et al (2003) Radiation associated cardiovascular disease: manifestations and management. Semin Radiat Oncol 13(3):346–356
49. Lerman J (2007) Anterior mediastinal masses in children. Semin Anesth Perioper Med Pain 26:133–140

50. Borenstein SH, Gerstle T, Malkin D et al (2000) The effects of pre-biopsy corticosteroid treatment on the diagnosis of mediastinal lymphoma. J Pediatr Surg 35:973–976
51. McDonnell C, Barlow R, Campisi P et al (2008) Fatal peri-operative acute tumour lysis syndrome precipitated by dexamethasone. Anaesthesia 63:652–655
52. Berry GJ, Jorden M (2005) Pathology of radiation and anthracycline cardiotoxicity. Pediatr Blood Cancer 44(7):630–637
53. Latham GJ, Greenberg RS (2010) Anesthetic considerations for the pediatric oncology patient – part 3: pain, cognitive dysfunction, and preoperative evaluation. Pediatr Anaesth 20(6):479–489
54. Abid SH, Malhotra V, Perry MC (2001) Radiation-induced and chemotherapy-induced pulmonary injury. Curr Opin Oncol 13(4):242–248
55. Faroux B, Meyer-Milsztain A, Boccon-Gibod L et al (1994) Cytotoxic drug-induced pulmonary disease in infants and children. Pediatr Pulmonol 18(6):347–355
56. Cerveri I, Fulgoni P, Giorgiani G et al (2001) Lung function abnormalities after bone marrow transplantation in children: has the trend recently changed? Chest 120(6):1900–1906
57. Marras TK, Szalai JP, Chan CK et al (2002) Pulmonary function abnormalities after allogenic marrow transplantation: a systemic review and assessment of an existing predictive instrument. Bone Marrow Transplant 30(9):599–607
58. Litten JB, Tomlinson GE (2008) Liver tumors in children. Oncologist 13(7):812–820
59. Hata M, Ogino I, Aida N et al (2001) Prophylactic cranial irradiation of acute lymphoblastic leukemia in childhood: outcomes of late effects on pituitary function and growth in long-term survivors. Int J Cancer 96(Suppl):117–124
60. Madanat LM, Lahteenmaki PM, Hurme S et al (2008) Hypothyroidism among pediatric cancer patients: a nationwide, registry based study. Int J Cancer 122(8):1868–1872
61. Golub TR, Arceci RJ (2006) Acute myelogenous leukemia. In: Pizzo PA, Poplack DG (eds) Principles and practice of pediatric oncology, 5th edn. Lippincott Williams & Wilkins, Philadelphia, p 591
62. Cairo MS, Bishop M (2004) Tumour lysis syndrome: new therapeutic strategies and classification. Br J Haematol 127:3–11, PubMed: 15384972
63. Shimada M, Johnson RJ, May WS Jr et al (2009) A novel role for uric acid in acute kidney injury associated with tumour lysis syndrome. Nephrol Dial Transplant 24:2960–2964, PubMed: 19581334
64. Nakamura M, Oda S, Sadahiro T et al (2009) The role of hypercytokinemia in the pathophysiology of tumor lysis syndrome (TLS) and the treatment with continuous hemodiafiltration using a polymethylmethacrylate membrane hemofilter (PMMA-CHDF). Transfus Apher Sci 40:41–47, PubMed: 19109071
65. Hechler T, Ruhe AK, Schmidt P et al (2013) Inpatient-based intensive interdisciplinary pain treatment for highly impaired children with severe chronic pain: randomized controlled trial of efficacy and economic effects. Pain (2014) 155:118–128
66. Zeppetella G, O'Doherty CA, Collins S (2000) Prevalence and characteristics of breakthrough pain in cancer patients admitted to a hospice. J Pain Symptom Manage 20:87–92
67. Friedrichsdorf S, Finney D, Bergin M, Stevens M, Collins J (2007) Breakthrough pain in children with cancer. J Pain Symptom Manage 34:209–216
68. Friedrichsdorf SJ, Postier A (2014) Management of breakthrough pain in children with cancer. J Pain Res 7:117–123
69. Drake R, Longworth J, Collins JJ (2004) Opioid rotation in children with cancer. J Palliat Med 7:419–422
70. Finkel JC, Finley A, Greco C, Weisman SJ, Zeltzer L (2005) Transdermal fentanyl in the management of children with chronic sever pain: results from an international study. Cancer 104:2847–2857
71. Finkel JC, Pestieau SR, Quezado ZM (2007) Ketamine as an adjuvant for treatment of cancer pain in children and adolescents. J Pain 8:515–521

Perioperative Care of Children with Cerebral Palsy and Behavioral Problems

17

Martin Jöhr and Thomas M. Berger

17.1   Introduction

Cerebral palsy (CP) is a general term covering a variety of nonprogressive conditions caused by lesions or anomalies of the brain occurring early in development. The incidence in children born at term is 1–2.5 per 1,000 live births in the developed world. The etiology seems to be multifactorial; surprisingly, intrapartum hypoxia is responsible only for a small proportion of CP cases. In the majority of patients, antenatal events seem to be responsible: cerebral malformations, prenatal infections (i.e., toxoplasmosis, rubella, cytomegalovirus, herpes), prenatal strokes, as well as genetic disorders. CP is the final common end point of damage to the central nervous system during early development [1]. CP is probably more common in children born prematurely.

The clinical presentations are highly variable, ranging from subclinical monoplegia with normal intellectual capacity to spastic quadriplegia with severe mental retardation. The motor defects are commonly used for labeling CP: spasticity, dyskinesia, and ataxia [2]. Cognitive function may vary from completely normal, to mild speech difficulties, to severe handicap. Up to 30 % of the patients with CP may suffer from epilepsy. The overall prognosis of these patients is modest: 3 out of 4 patients experience chronic pain, 1 out of 2 have an intellectual disability, 1 out of 3 develop displacement of the hip, 1 out of 3 are unable to walk, 1 out of 4 have behavioral disorders, 1 out of 4 have a bladder control problem, and 1 out of 15 require tube feeding [3].

M. Jöhr (✉)
Pediatric Anesthesia, Department of Anesthesia, Luzerner Kantonsspital, 6000 Luzern 16, Switzerland
e-mail: joehrmartin@bluewin.ch

T.M. Berger
Neonatal and Pediatric Intensive Care Unit, Children's Hospital, 6000 Luzern 16, Switzerland

© Springer International Publishing Switzerland 2016   259
M. Astuto, P.M. Ingelmo (eds.), *Perioperative Medicine in Pediatric Anesthesia*,
Anesthesia, Intensive Care and Pain in Neonates and Children,
DOI 10.1007/978-3-319-21960-8_17

The anesthetic management of patients with CP is not well covered in most pediatric anesthesia textbooks, but it has been summarized in several review articles [4–9].

17.2 Preoperative Evaluation

17.2.1 General Aspects

Developmental delay is common in children with CP, and a thorough assessment of their motor and cognitive deficits is of paramount importance. Normally, the parents or caregivers know the patient and his/her preferences best, and the anesthesiologist should benefit from this knowledge. Some of the key questions concerning severely handicapped children are: what is he/she able to do, how can he/she communicate, which preferences does he/she have, and which are signs of discomfort (Fig. 17.1)? The anesthesiologist should become familiar with all aspects of the patient's life including social aspects: where does the patient live, who is caring for him, and what are the resources of the family [10]? An often underestimated problem is the transition from pediatric to adult care [11]; while a global assessment including all aspects of life is common practice in pediatrics, specialists in adult hospitals tend to focus only on their domain, and important aspects of the patient's care can thus be missed.

17.2.2 Specific Problems

Gastroesophageal reflux is relatively common among patients with CP and associated with an increased risk of pulmonary aspiration. The presence of scoliosis may restrict ventilation (Fig. 17.2), and these patients are also at high risk for pulmonary

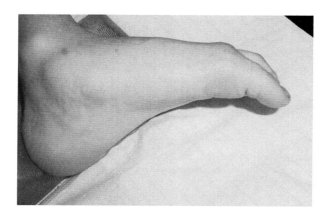

Fig. 17.1 A 14-year-old 25 kg severely disabled boy in severe pain. According to his mother, flexion of the toes is a typical sign of discomfort or pain

complications. Contractures and deformities have to be taken into account because they may significantly limit the possibilities to position the patient. Chronic constipation is common and may lead to rare, but typical, complications, such as superior mesenteric artery syndrome [12]. In addition, many of these patients have cognitive impairments that preclude cooperative behavior even in older children. In adult patients with CP sarcopenia, obesity and sedentary behavior will influence the perioperative course [13]; a lifelong health program is mandatory for these patients [14].

17.2.3 Spasticity

A big challenge in patients with CP is controlling spasticity and avoiding contractures. Pharmacologically, this is often attempted with compounds that modulate motor tone; e.g., benzodiazepines, baclofen, vigabatrin, or tizanidine. All these drugs have the potential to cause drowsiness and dose-dependent sedation.

Baclofen is structurally related to GABA. It can be administered orally or intrathecally. Especially after the first intrathecal trial injections, careful observation of the patient is mandatory [15]. Replacement of pumps is required every 5–7 years, and the pumps have to be refilled at least every 3 months. Baclofen should not be withdrawn abruptly as this can induce acute withdrawal symptoms.

Vigabatrin is primarily used as an antiepileptic agent; it is a GABA analogue that inhibits GABA metabolism.

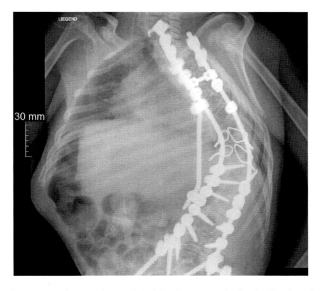

Fig. 17.2 A 15-year-old 12 kg girl scheduled for laparoscopic fundoplication. Positioning is a challenge. The correct position of the endotracheal tube was verified bronchoscopically

Because of its structural similarity with clonidine, *Tizanidine* causes sedation, bradycardia, and hypotension in addition to myorelaxation. It is primarily metabolized by CYP1A2, and blocking this enzyme, e.g., by high doses of ciprofloxacin, may lead to excessive concentrations of tizanidine.

Botulinum toxin (Botox) is injected directly into the muscle and provides functional denervation lasting several months by preventing presynaptic acetylcholine release. In addition, Botox can be used in children with excessive salivation [16] or for controlling bladder detrusor hyperactivity.

Injections into the muscles or into the salivary gland are made under ultrasound control, most often in sedated or anesthetized children. Provided the total dose is restricted, severe adverse events are rare [17]. Reported adverse reactions are mostly related to the sedation procedure and not to the injected compound itself [18].

Neurolytic blocks (also called chemodenervation) are mainly suitable for nerves predominantly consisting of motor fibers, e.g., the obturator nerve in case of adductor spasm [19]. To perform these blocks, skilled anesthesiologists use nerve stimulation and ultrasound to identify nerve location. Today, neurolytic blocks have almost universally been replaced by intramuscular Botox injections. However, selective neurolytic nerve blocks using phenol (5–12 % solutions) may still have a place as they provide relief for a period of 4–8 months [20]. Alcohol may be an alternative to phenol for neurolysis [21].

17.2.4 Epilepsy

Up to 30 % of patients with CP have coexisting epilepsy. Perioperatively, seizure frequency and duration can be increased because factors enhancing seizure activity, such as stress, starvation, sleep deprivation, optical stimulation, and hyperventilation, may be unavoidable. On the other hand, most, if not all, anesthetics protect against convulsive activity [22]. With uninterrupted antiepileptic medication and good clinical care, increased seizure activity should rarely occur [23].

Valproic acid has been associated with severe bleeding complications [24]. The mechanisms involved are only poorly understood, but thrombocytopenia and platelet dysfunction, as well as deficiencies of several coagulation factors, such as fibrinogen, factor XIII, and especially von Willebrand factor type 1, have been implied [25, 26]. Preoperative coagulation tests are suggested for children who are on long-term medication with valproic acid [25]. Another severe complication of valproic acid use is acute pancreatitis [27].

17.3 Perioperative Management

17.3.1 Positioning and Venous Access

Positioning can be very demanding for obvious reasons; often, an inventive spirit is needed. Meticulous padding as well as small adjustments in position of all accessible body parts (e.g., arms, head) is key to avoid pressure sores during prolonged surgery. Severely handicapped children may be at high risk to sustain long bone fractures simply through unskilled positioning.

Venous access can be difficult. In the authors' practice, an inhalational induction is often performed allowing careful selection of the optimal puncture site in a quiet and motionless patient [28]. In the authors' opinion, this can even be justified in patients with a history of reflux [29].

17.3.2 Airway Management

Endotracheal intubation is strongly recommended for children with gastroesophageal reflux and prolonged surgery. On the other hand, for many children with cerebral palsy and no history of reflux, a laryngeal mask airway (LMA) with a gastric access, e.g., LMA Supreme® or LMA ProSeal®, can be a valuable airway tool. In case of scoliosis and severe deformity, optimal positioning for intubation can be challenging, even if the airway itself is normal. Often, the length of the trachea may not be as long as expected for age, and auscultation may not reliably allow identifying bronchial main stem intubation. It is the authors' practice to use fiberoptic control liberally to verify the correct position of the tip of the endotracheal tube.

Intermittent airway obstruction may occur in some patients with CP – even without anesthesia – because of hypotonia of the pharyngeal muscles; the symptoms tend to become worse with increasing age [30] and ultimately may lead to a tracheostomy in some patients. Perioperatively, special attention must be paid to avoid anesthetic overhang or benzodiazepine medication. During mask induction, the skilled practitioner will generally be able to maintain an open airway with jaw thrust and positive airway pressure.

17.3.3 Thermal Homeostasis

Hypothermia is the most common perioperative complication in children with CP [4]. The etiology is probably multifactorial: undoubtedly, the most important factor in its pathogenesis is a reduced metabolic rate ("vita reducta") coupled with exaggerated losses due to exposure of large areas of the body necessary for many orthopedic interventions. In addition, these patients often have very little subcutaneous fat tissue to insulate against heat loss. Finally, it has been speculated that there may be abnormal thermoregulatory mechanisms in patients with a compromised central nervous system.

Forced air systems (e.g., Bair Hugger®) are successfully used to prevent perioperative hypothermia. In addition to an elevated room temperature, the authors use two forced air systems in vulnerable patients: one on which the patient is placed and one that covers the body surface as much as possible. Continuous monitoring of the patient's body temperature using rectal, esophageal, or bladder temperature probes is advisable. With the appropriate use of modern equipment, hypothermia can almost invariably be prevented.

17.3.4 Pharmacodynamics and Pharmacokinetics

Hypnotics: Patients with CP, as well as many other severely handicapped children, seem to be much more sensible to hypnotic agents. Frei et al. reported that the MAC values of halothane are reduced by around 1/3 in children with CP [31]. This is clearly a pharmacodynamic phenomenon: a lower concentration is needed for a certain effect. Similarly, less propofol is needed to reach a target BIS value of 40 [32]. This may also be caused by an altered pharmacodynamic response; however, different pharmacokinetics may also be responsible. Lower BIS values are recorded in children with cerebral palsy while awake, as well as after exposure to different sevoflurane concentrations [33]. Other authors, however, have found similar BIS values before induction among patients with CP when compared with healthy children [34]. The reduced requirement for hypnotic agents seems to be a common phenomenon for most, if not all, severely handicapped children [35]. It is the authors' practice to monitor the hypnotic state with an EEG-based monitor, i.e., bispectral index (BIS®), in all of these patients despite the fact that the validity of these monitors has not been tested extensively in this patient population, and an individual patient may well present with a very low BIS® value before anesthesia induction.

Opioids: Only limited information is available about the sensitivity to opioids in patients with CP. It has been speculated that chronic hypoxia increases the sensitivity to opioids, especially to the respiratory depressant effects of opioids [36]. Children living in high altitude exposed to chronic hypoxic conditions seem to require less opioids after surgery for sufficient pain relief [37]. Typically, increased sensitivity to opioids is discussed in the context of obstructive sleep apnea [38] where it is associated with relevant morbidity and even mortality [39]. There is little doubt that similar phenomena can be found in children with CP; intermittent nocturnal desaturations up-regulate endorphin receptors and enhance sensitivity to opioids [40]. Therefore, careful dosing and adequate monitoring is very important in this patient population.

Neuromuscular blocking agents: Surprisingly, children with CP, despite the fact that they often have a very reduced muscle mass (Fig. 17.3), seem to be resistant to non-depolarizing neuromuscular blocking agents. Clinically, a given dose has a shorter duration of action [41]. This resistance does not appear to be related to concomitant use of antiepileptic medication [42]. Receptor up-regulation seems to be a suitable explanation. This also explains the increased sensitivity to succinylcholine [43]. Hyperkalemia does not seem to be a problem, likely due to a reduced muscular mass [44]. Despite the fact that the airway is usually normal, difficult intubation is reported to be more common in severely handicapped patients; insufficient doses of non-depolarizing neuromuscular blocking agents may be at least in part responsible in some cases. Given the availability of sugammadex, higher doses of rocuronium, which provide excellent intubation conditions, have become an attractive option in patients with CP or other neuromuscular disorders [45].

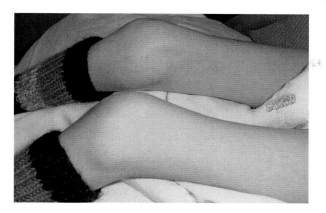

Fig. 17.3 Despite severe muscular hypotrophy, this boy is remarkably resistant to atracurium

17.3.5 Uncooperative Behavior at Induction

The preoperative visit is of paramount importance; patients at risk for a stormy and difficult induction should then be recognized. The parents should be asked about and charts be scrutinized for information concerning previous anesthetics; it is the authors' practice to leave a note in the anesthesia chart on the sedative effects of the premedication and the quality of induction.

Prevention of difficult inductions by using an adequate premedication is of paramount importance. It is the authors' practice to add ketamine to midazolam if relevant uncooperative behavior can be anticipated [46]. Often, a peaceful induction can be achieved by gentle conviction of the patient and parental support. In addition, success is highly dependent on the skill and empathy of the anesthesiologist. Inhalation of nitrous oxide followed by sevoflurane using a flavored mask while the child is in his/her preferred position is a good option. In the authors' institution, an uncooperative child is usually left in his/her hospital bed for induction [47].

The management of uncooperative behavior at induction includes several options: postponing surgery, top-up premedication with ketamine, skilful inhalational or intravenous induction using persuasion, and sometimes gentle physical restraint are all valuable options. The choice of a particular method will depend on the individual practitioner: extensive experience with pediatric patients, appropriate skills, as well as empathy with the child and the parents are key factors for success. Often, only a detailed discussion with the parents can disclose the optimal solution for the individual patient. The authors have induced anesthesia in children sitting on the floor in the corridor in front of the operating theatre refusing to enter it. In one child, refusing to enter the hospital, anesthesia was even induced on the street in front of the hospital. Without doubt, the safest drug under these circumstances is ketamine.

17.3.6 Postoperative Analgesia

In patients with CP, pain is not restricted to the perioperative period but rather a predominant symptom [48]; up to 75 % of young people with CP experience some pain in a typical week [49]. Possibly as a consequence, pain appears to be more difficult to treat in this patient population. A first challenge is to recognize whether the patient is in pain. It is likely that pain is often undertreated in these patients [50]. On the other hand, because of the difficulties to distinguish pain and other causes of agitation, overdosing with oversedation can easily occur.

Whenever possible, regional blocks are probably the most elegant way to provide reliable analgesia in these vulnerable patients; continuous epidural analgesia may be considered after major surgery, especially in conditions where spasms of the muscles of the lower extremities can be expected [51].

17.4 Typical Interventions

17.4.1 Orthopedic Surgery

Major orthopedic surgery is commonly undertaken in children with CP [52]. *Scoliosis surgery* is often extensive involving segments from the high thoracic region down to the sacrum, and pelvic stabilization will assist in sitting. Intraoperative monitoring has become commonplace [53]. Postoperative pain relief is challenging; intrathecal morphine can easily be administered [54], enhances perioperative stability, and thus may reduce blood loss [55]. Epidural catheters, positioned intraoperatively by the surgeons, have also been successfully used [56].

Hip reconstruction involving pelvic and femoral osteotomies is offered even to the most debilitated children with the aim to reduce pain, to facilitate positioning, and even occasionally to allow a sitting position. Palliative surgery, e.g., resection of the femoral head, is nowadays only rarely performed [57]. Postoperative pain relief can be provided through lumbar epidural catheters; in the authors' practice, however, caudal morphine combined with peripheral nerve blocks, e.g., lumbar plexus [58] or femoral and/or sciatic nerve blocks, are often used.

Blood loss can be major. Antifibrinolytic agents, e.g., tranexamic acid, are recommended by most authorities to reduce blood loss [59]; its effectiveness has been specifically shown in cerebral palsy scoliosis too [60]. However, the pediatric data covering other types of surgery are still very limited [61].

Latex allergy seems to be a lesser problem nowadays; nevertheless, all children presenting for repeated surgery are at increased risk (Fig. 17.4) [62]; latex allergy is not caused by spina bifida per se [63].

17.4.2 Fundoplication and Gastrostomy

Nissen fundoplication is considered as the treatment of choice for children with gastroesophageal reflux disease. Laparoscopic Nissen fundoplication is offered

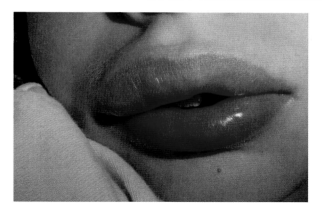

Fig. 17.4 Swelling of the lip after contact with latex gloves in an 8-year-old girl

today as the standard procedure, although the evidence of its superiority over open surgery is limited [64]. The technique involves prolonged pneumoperitoneum with the patient in a head-up position [65]. Ventilation and PEEP have to be adapted to counteract the effects of the elevated intra-abdominal pressure. Pneumothorax can occur by transition of CO_2 from the abdominal cavity to the pleural space through lesions caused by dissection; generally, no specific treatment is required provided that a sufficiently high PEEP level is maintained [66]. Hemodynamic monitoring is crucial; the critical phases are the creation of the pneumoperitoneum as well as its release at the end of surgery. The patients usually develop a transient oliguric state during the period with elevated intra-abdominal pressure [67]; there is some consensus that this does not require aggressive treatment.

Open Nissen fundoplication is a major upper abdominal intervention with relevant morbidity and postoperative pain. In retrospective case series, the use of epidural catheter techniques was associated with a reduced need for postoperative ventilation and fewer complications [68] as well as shorter hospital stays [69].

Gastrostomy is widely accepted as the preferred technique to establish long-term enteral feeding in patients with severe CP. Nowadays, it is performed as a percutaneous endoscopic technique (PEG) in the majority of cases, and a classical open gastrostomy is only rarely done. A preoperative plain x-ray is recommended in all children with scoliosis and suspected distortion of the anatomy [70]. The one-step low-profile percutaneous endoscopic gastrostomy seems to achieve equally good results compared with the classical approach [71]. In children, the procedure is usually performed under general anesthesia. Although the procedure is considered to be minor, and enteral feedings can be restarted within 6 h, pain and discomfort occur commonly and can be considerable. Careful observation of the patient is required, as unintended puncture of other visceral structures, e.g., the colon, can occur. In the authors' practice, an ultrasound-guided subcostal transversus abdominis plane (TAP) block, performed following surgery to avoid distortion of the anatomy, is commonly used for pain control.

Conclusions

Children with CP are vulnerable patients. Intraoperatively, careful positioning, gaining venous access, maintenance of thermal homeostasis, and correct dosing are the most challenging tasks. Postoperatively, the liberal use of regional techniques for pain control is a very attractive concept. Precision and meticulous care is particularly important in these patients to optimize perioperative care and outcome.

References

1. Marret S, Vanhulle C, Laquerriere A (2013) Pathophysiology of cerebral palsy. Handb Clin Neurol 111:169–176
2. Koman LA, Smith BP, Shilt JS (2004) Cerebral palsy. Lancet 363:1619–1631
3. Novak I, Hines M, Goldsmith S et al (2012) Clinical prognostic messages from a systematic review on cerebral palsy. Pediatrics 130:e1285–e1312
4. Wongprasartsuk P, Stevens J (2002) Cerebral palsy and anaesthesia. Paediatr Anaesth 12:296–303
5. Wass CT, Warner ME, Worrell GA et al (2012) Effect of general anesthesia in patients with cerebral palsy at the turn of the new millennium: a population-based study evaluating perioperative outcome and brief overview of anesthetic implications of this coexisting disease. J Child Neurol 27:859–866
6. Nolan J, Chalkiadis GA, Low J et al (2000) Anaesthesia and pain management in cerebral palsy. Anaesthesia 55:32–41
7. Maranhao MV (2005) Anesthesia and cerebral palsy. Rev Bras Anestesiol 55:680–702
8. Theroux MC, Akins RE (2005) Surgery and anesthesia for children who have cerebral palsy. Anesthesiol Clin North America 23:733–743
9. Aker J, Anderson DJ (2007) Update for nurse anesthetists – part 6 – Perioperative care of patients with cerebral palsy. AANA J 75:65–73
10. Parkes J, Caravale B, Marcelli M et al (2011) Parenting stress and children with cerebral palsy: a European cross-sectional survey. Dev Med Child Neurol 53:815–821
11. Brennan LJ, Rolfe PM (2011) Transition from pediatric to adult health services: the perioperative care perspective. Paediatr Anaesth 21:630–635
12. Neuman A, Desai B, Glass D et al (2014) Superior mesenteric artery syndrome in a patient with cerebral palsy. Case Rep Med. doi:10.1155/2014/538289
13. Peterson MD, Gordon PM, Hurvitz EA (2013) Chronic disease risk among adults with cerebral palsy: the role of premature sarcopoenia, obesity and sedentary behaviour. Obes Rev 14:171–182
14. Murphy KP (2010) The adult with cerebral palsy. Orthop Clin North Am 41:595–605
15. Anderson KJ, Farmer JP, Brown K (2002) Reversible coma in children after improper baclofen pump insertion. Paediatr Anaesth 12:454–460
16. Montgomery J, McCusker S, Hendry J et al (2014) Botulinum toxin A for children with salivary control problems. Int J Pediatr Otorhinolaryngol 78:1970–1973
17. Naidu K, Smith K, Sheedy M et al (2010) Systemic adverse events following botulinum toxin A therapy in children with cerebral palsy. Dev Med Child Neurol 52:139–144
18. Papavasiliou AS, Nikaina I, Foska K et al (2013) Safety of botulinum toxin A in children and adolescents with cerebral palsy in a pragmatic setting. Toxins (Basel) 5:524–536
19. Awad EA (1972) Phenol block for control of hip flexor and adductor spasticity. Arch Phys Med Rehabil 53:554–557

20. Viel E, Pellas F, Ripart J et al (2005) Peripheral neurolytic blocks and spasticity (in French). Ann Fr Anesth Reanim 24:667–672
21. Ghai A, Sangwan SS, Hooda S et al (2012) Obturator neurolysis using 65% alcohol for adductor muscle spasticity. Saudi J Anaesth 6:282–284
22. Perks A, Cheema S, Mohanraj R (2012) Anaesthesia and epilepsy. Br J Anaesth 108:562–571
23. Benish SM, Cascino GD, Warner ME et al (2010) Effect of general anesthesia in patients with epilepsy: a population-based study. Epilepsy Behav 17:87–89
24. Cannizzaro E, Albisetti M, Wohlrab G et al (2007) Severe bleeding complications during antiepileptic treatment with valproic acid in children. Neuropediatrics 38:42–45
25. Acharya S, Bussel JB (2000) Hematologic toxicity of sodium valproate. J Pediatr Hematol Oncol 22:62–65
26. Abdallah C (2013) Valproic acid and acquired coagulopathy. Paediatr Anaesth 23:674–675
27. Ozaydin E, Yukselgungor H, Kose G (2008) Acute hemorrhagic pancreatitis due to the use of valproic acid in a child. Eur J Paediatr Neurol 12:141–143
28. Jöhr M, Berger TM (2015) Venous access in children: state of the art. Curr Opin Anaesthesiol 28:314–320
29. Cruvinel MG, Bittencourt PF, Costa JR et al (2004) Residual gastric volume and risk for pulmonary aspiration in children with gastroesophageal reflux. Comparative study. Rev Bras Anestesiol 54:37–42
30. Kontorinis G, Thevasagayam MS, Bateman ND (2013) Airway obstruction in children with cerebral palsy: need for tracheostomy? Int J Pediatr Otorhinolaryngol 77:1647–1650
31. Frei FJ, Haemmerle MH, Brunner R et al (1997) Minimum alveolar concentration for halothane in children with cerebral palsy and severe mental retardation. Anaesthesia 52:1056–1060
32. Saricaoglu F, Celebi N, Celik M et al (2005) The evaluation of propofol dosage for anesthesia induction in children with cerebral palsy with bispectral index (BIS) monitoring. Paediatr Anaesth 15:1048–1052
33. Choudhry DK, Brenn BR (2002) Bispectral index monitoring: a comparison between normal children and children with quadriplegic cerebral palsy. Anesth Analg 95:1582–1585
34. Costa VV, Torres RV, Arci EC et al (2007) Comparison of the bispectral index in awake patients with cerebral palsy. Rev Bras Anestesiol 57:382–390
35. Valkenburg AJ, de Leeuw TG, Tibboel D et al (2009) Lower bispectral index values in children who are intellectually disabled. Anesth Analg 109:1428–1433
36. Moss IR, Brown KA, Laferriere A (2006) Recurrent hypoxia in rats during development increases subsequent respiratory sensitivity to fentanyl. Anesthesiology 105:715–718
37. Rabbitts JA, Groenewald CB, Dietz NM et al (2010) Perioperative opioid requirements are decreased in hypoxic children living at altitude. Paediatr Anaesth 20:1078–1083
38. Brown KA, Laferriere A, Moss IR (2004) Recurrent hypoxemia in young children with obstructive sleep apnea is associated with reduced opioid requirement for analgesia. Anesthesiology 100:806–810
39. Coté CJ, Posner KL, Domino KB (2014) Death or neurologic injury after tonsillectomy in children with a focus on obstructive sleep apnea: Houston, we have a problem! Anesth Analg 118:1276–1283
40. Fitzgerald DA, Follett J, Van Asperen PP (2009) Assessing and managing lung disease and sleep disordered breathing in children with cerebral palsy. Paediatr Respir Rev 10:18–24
41. Moorthy SS, Krishna G, Dierdorf SF (1991) Resistance to vecuronium in patients with cerebral palsy. Anesth Analg 73:275–277
42. Hepaguslar H, Ozzeybek D, Elar Z (1999) The effect of cerebral palsy on the action of vecuronium with or without anticonvulsants. Anaesthesia 54:593–596
43. Theroux MC, Brandom BW, Zagnoev M et al (1994) Dose response of succinylcholine at the adductor pollicis of children with cerebral palsy during propofol and nitrous oxide anesthesia. Anesth Analg 79:761–765

44. Dierdorf SF, McNiece WL, Rao CC et al (1985) Effect of succinylcholine on plasma potassium in children with cerebral palsy. Anesthesiology 62:88–90
45. de Boer HD, van Esmond J, Booij LH et al (2009) Reversal of rocuronium-induced profound neuromuscular block by sugammadex in Duchenne muscular dystrophy. Paediatr Anaesth 19:1226–1228
46. Brunette KE, Anderson BJ, Thomas J et al (2011) Exploring the pharmacokinetics of oral ketamine in children undergoing burns procedures. Paediatr Anaesth 21:653–662
47. Walker H (2009) The child who refuses to undergo anesthesia and surgery – a case scenario-based discussion of the ethical and legal issues. Paediatr Anaesth 19:1017–1021
48. Penner M, Xie WY, Binepal N et al (2013) Characteristics of pain in children and youth with cerebral palsy. Pediatrics 132:e407–e413
49. Parkinson KN, Dickinson HO, Arnaud C et al (2013) Pain in young people aged 13 to 17 years with cerebral palsy: cross-sectional, multicentre European study. Arch Dis Child 98:434–440
50. Ghai B, Makkar JK, Wig J (2008) Postoperative pain assessment in preverbal children and children with cognitive impairment. Paediatr Anaesth 18:462–477
51. Moore RP, Wester T, Sunder R et al (2013) Peri-operative pain management in children with cerebral palsy: comparative efficacy of epidural vs systemic analgesia protocols. Paediatr Anaesth 23:720–725
52. Gibson PR (2004) Anaesthesia for correction of scoliosis in children. Anaesth Intensive Care 32:548–559
53. Glover CD, Carling NP (2014) Neuromonitoring for scoliosis surgery. Anesthesiol Clin 32:101–114
54. Schmitz A, Salgo B, Weiss M (2010) Intrathecal opioid medication for perioperative analgesia in severely handicapped children undergoing spinal operations (in German). Anaesthesist 59:614–620
55. Lesniak AB, Tremblay P, Dalens BJ et al (2013) Intrathecal morphine reduces blood loss during idiopathic scoliosis surgery: retrospective study of 256 pediatric cases. Paediatr Anaesth 23:265–270
56. Saudan S, Habre W, Ceroni D et al (2008) Safety and efficacy of patient controlled epidural analgesia following pediatric spinal surgery. Paediatr Anaesth 18:132–139
57. Boldingh EJ, Bouwhuis CB, van der Heijden-Maessen HC et al (2014) Palliative hip surgery in severe cerebral palsy: a systematic review. J Pediatr Orthop B 23:86–92
58. Dadure C, Bringuier S, Mathieu O et al (2010) Continuous epidural block versus continuous psoas compartment block for postoperative analgesia after major hip or femoral surgery in children: a prospective comparative randomized study (in French). Ann Fr Anesth Reanim 29:610–615
59. Tzortzopoulou A, Cepeda MS, Schumann R et al (2008) Antifibrinolytic agents for reducing blood loss in scoliosis surgery in children. Cochrane Database Syst Rev 3, CD006883
60. Dhawale AA, Shah SA, Sponseller PD et al (2012) Are antifibrinolytics helpful in decreasing blood loss and transfusions during spinal fusion surgery in children with cerebral palsy scoliosis? Spine (Phila Pa 1976) 37:E549–E555
61. Faraoni D, Goobie SM (2014) The efficacy of antifibrinolytic drugs in children undergoing noncardiac surgery: a systematic review of the literature. Anesth Analg 118:628–636
62. Delfico AJ, Dormans JP, Craythorne CB et al (1997) Intraoperative anaphylaxis due to allergy to latex in children who have cerebral palsy: a report of six cases. Dev Med Child Neurol 39:194–197
63. Porri F, Pradal M, Lemiere C et al (1997) Association between latex sensitization and repeated latex exposure in children. Anesthesiology 86:599–602
64. Martin K, Deshaies C, Emil S (2014) Outcomes of pediatric laparoscopic fundoplication: a critical review of the literature. Can J Gastroenterol Hepatol 28:97–102
65. Veyckemans F (2004) Celioscopic surgery in infants and children: the anesthesiologist's point of view. Paediatr Anaesth 14:424–432

66. Joris JL, Chiche JD, Lamy ML (1995) Pneumothorax during laparoscopic fundoplication: diagnosis and treatment with positive end-expiratory pressure. Anesth Analg 81:993–1000
67. Gomez Dammeier BH, Karanik E, Gluer S et al (2005) Anuria during pneumoperitoneum in infants and children: a prospective study. J Pediatr Surg 40:1454–1458
68. McNeely JK, Farber NE, Rusy LM et al (1997) Epidural analgesia improves outcome following pediatric fundoplication. A retrospective analysis. Reg Anesth 22:16–23
69. Wilson GA, Brown JL, Crabbe DG et al (2001) Is epidural analgesia associated with an improved outcome following open Nissen fundoplication? Paediatr Anaesth 11:65–70
70. Pruijsen JM, de Bruin A, Sekema G et al (2013) Abdominal plain film before gastrostomy tube placement to predict success of percutaneous endoscopic procedure. J Pediatr Gastroenterol Nutr 56:186–190
71. Pattamanuch N, Novak I, Loizides A et al (2014) Single-center experience with 1-step low-profile percutaneous endoscopic gastrostomy in children. J Pediatr Gastroenterol Nutr 58:616–620

Perioperative Care of Neonates with Airway Obstruction

18

Pierre Fiset and Sam J. Daniel

18.1 Presentation

Evaluation and treatment of the newborn presenting with airway dysfunction or obstruction demands close collaboration between the anesthesiologist, neonatologist, otolaryngologist, and craniofacial surgeons. Anesthesiologists may be involved in situations of neonatal lifesaving airway rescue, diagnostic processes under GA, or more definitive corrective treatment scenarios. These challenging patients may present with a difficult airway and necessitate the use of specific anesthetic techniques to provide optimal conditions for a precise diagnosis. A comprehensive evaluation of each patient is essential. This review will address most of the major pathologies of the newborn airways with the objective of helping to establish a rational plan for anesthesia.

18.2 Symptoms and Signs

Stridor, apneas, cyanosis, choking on feeding, chronic cough and aspiration, recurrent croup, and failure to thrive are all nonspecific common features of airway obstruction. Tachypnea might be present with intercostal and suprasternal indrawing, which might be intermittent and triggered by feeding, position, or sleep.

P. Fiset, MD, FRCPC (✉)
Department of Anesthesia, Montreal Children's Hospital, MUHC, McGill University, Montreal, QC, Canada
e-mail: pierre.fiset@muhc.mcgill.ca

S.J. Daniel, MD, FRCPC
Department of Pediatric Surgery and Otolaryngology, Montreal Children's Hospital, MUHC, McGill University, Montreal, QC, Canada
e-mail: sam.daniel@mcgill.ca

© Springer International Publishing Switzerland 2016
M. Astuto, P.M. Ingelmo (eds.), *Perioperative Medicine in Pediatric Anesthesia*,
Anesthesia, Intensive Care and Pain in Neonates and Children,
DOI 10.1007/978-3-319-21960-8_18

Some patients present obvious features that immediately suggest a cause for airway obstruction: upper or lower mandibular hypodevelopment, protruding tongue, and facial abnormalities including ear deformities, small mouth opening, and cleft lip/palate.

The context and timing in which symptoms appear is revealing. Whether those start immediately at birth, in the context of prematurity, after an endotracheal intubation or progressively in the first days and weeks of life will suggest different possible etiologies. As part of the initial evaluation of these patients, the significant presence of comorbidities should be kept in mind.

Bedsides flexible fiber-optic endoscopy (FFE) is universally used as an initial and basic exam to help determine the diagnosis and conduct.

18.3   Pathologies of the Upper Airway (Above the Glottis Structures)

The term tongue-based airway obstruction (TBAO) [1] relates to a group of syndromes, pathological presentations, and features that all have in common to cause obstruction of the neonatal airway based on glossoptosis or macroglossia. The Pierre Robin sequence, presenting in a spectrum going form an isolated finding to being associated with a syndrome in 27–82 % of cases, is the most common anomaly of that group. It was originally described as an association of micrognathia, glossoptosis, and obstructive apnea from upper airway obstruction. A good proportion of those patients also have a cleft palate [2].

Treacher Collins and Goldenhar syndromes fall in the TBAO spectrum, as well as different forms of micro- or retrognathia. Treacher Collins syndrome is a rare (1:50,000) genetic disorder involving the development of the first and second branchial arches and limited to the head and neck. Bilateral maxillary, zygomatic, and mandibular hypoplasia is present combined with a small oral aperture, high-arched palate, and temporomandibular joint abnormalities [3]. The incidence of Goldenhar syndrome (hemifacial microsomia) is reported to be between 1:35,000 and 1:56,000. The etiology is unknown, and environmental causes like drug ingestion (vitamin A, tamoxifen, cocaine, retinoic acid) or alcohol use during pregnancy, maternal diabetes, rubella, or influenza may be in cause, but no genetic etiology has yet been identified [4, 5]. The unilateral facial hypodevelopment is accompanied by auricular and ocular defects. Coincident cervical instability and vertebral anomalies are frequent [6].

Macroglossia can be present without an associated mandibular anomaly. In a recent review, it was associated with Beckwith-Wiedemann syndrome [7] in 46 % of cases as well as with trisomy 21 and other chromosomal anomalies, hypothyroidism and vascular and lymphatic malformations. It is an isolated finding in about 15 % of cases [8].

Placing the newborn in prone position, bypassing the obstruction with a nasopharyngeal airway, or maintaining the patency with a CPAP or BiPaP device are all part of the initial treatment of these patients. Some will outgrow their obstruction and avoid surgery, but most of them will be brought to the OR for a systematic evaluation and for a variety of procedures which include mandibular distraction, tongue-lip adhesion, transmandibular K-wiring, subperiosteal release, or tracheostomy [9].

Lesions of the base of the tongue can be present at birth or increase in size in the neonatal period causing immediate or progressive signs of airway obstruction. Possible causes are hemangiomas, teratomas, dermoid cysts, lymphatic or venous malformations, thyroglossal duct, or vallecular cysts. Depending on the size, they can compromise airway visualization by direct laryngoscopy.

Nasal obstruction is another cause of neonatal upper airway obstruction. This can be secondary to choanal atresia, pyriform aperture stenosis, or nasolacrymal duct mucocele [10]. CHARGE syndrome (Coloboma, Heart defect, Atresia choanae, Retarded growth, Genitourinary abnormalities, and Ear anomalies) is the most common diagnosis associated with the condition. Bilateral occlusion is also associated with other syndromes featuring midfacial hypoplasia such as Crouzon, Pfeiffer, Antley-Bixler, or Apert [11]. These associations may contribute to a difficult airway situation. Preoperative FFE is especially useful in this situation for establishing diagnosis and estimating the size, nature, and extent of the lesion. Unilateral choanal atresia is more likely to be isolated, although the presence of associated anomalies should be suspected.

For the anesthesiologist, the common features of the above pathologies are the potential early airway obstruction during induction and the difficulty to visualize the larynx and perform endotracheal intubation.

18.4   Supraglottic and Laryngeal Pathologies

Laryngomalacia is the most common cause of inspiratory stridor in the newborn accounting for 60–70 % of cases. It is frequently classified according to the area of "collapsus" of the larynx [12]. Interestingly, this relates to the fact that the nature and severity of the disease are revealed by the action of air movement on supraglottic structures. Optimal conditions for diagnosis and treatment will be provided in a non-intubated, spontaneously breathing patient. A secondary lesion is present in 63 % of cases, most often tracheomalacia [13]. Gastroesophageal reflux (GERD) is often present, but it remains unclear whether it is the increased negative pressure due the obstruction that causes acid to be drawn up to the level of the larynx or it is the acid reflux that is an independent etiological factor of aggravation. Patients with laryngomalacia needing surgical treatment may have shortened aryepiglottic folds, a retropositioned epiglottis, or a prolapsed/redundant arytenoid mucosa[14].

Laryngeal cleft (LC) is labeled as a rare congenital malformation accounting for 0.5–1.6 % of laryngeal anomalies. Four types are described by Benjamin and Inglis based on the extent of the underdevelopment of the tracheoesophageal septum [15] (Fig. 18.1). It has been traditionally underdiagnosed but is now reported with increasing frequency. The type 1 presents with stridor, feeding difficulties, and recurrent airway infections [16]. Coincidental presence of laryngomalacia may

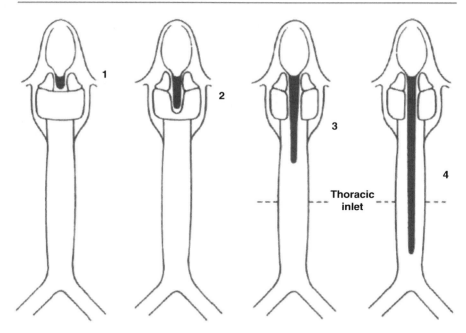

Fig. 18.1 Benjamin's and Inglis' classification of laryngeal clefts. Type 1: Interarythenoid defect, type 2: extending partially into the cricoid cartilage, type 3 complete seperation of the cricoid cartilage extending with possible extension into the tracheoesophageal wall. Type 4: common tracheoesophagus with possible extension to the carinal level (From Pezzettigotta SM et al (2008) Laryngeal Cleft. *Otolaryngol Clin North Am* 41 (2008) 913–933. Used with permission)

mask the diagnosis and contribute to the severity of symptoms. LC is associated with other congenital anomalies, mostly gastrointestinal, more than 50 % of the time [17]. As the proper diagnosis, especially in type 1, is made by probing of the interarytenoid area, suspension laryngoscopy in a non-intubated, spontaneously breathing patient is the anesthetic technique of choice.

Laryngeal webs are rare congenital or acquired malformation in which abnormal fibrous tissue forms anteriorly between two structures within the larynx. They are staged type 1–4 depending on the degree of severity using either Cohen's [18] or Benjamin's [19] classification (Fig. 18.2). They are most frequently congenital, with associated anomalies (mostly cardiac, or deletion of 22q11 chromosome) in 51 % of patients [18], but can be acquired following a surgical procedure, intubation, or infection. Webs can extend from the supra- to the subglottic area. Their definitive treatment is difficult, as vocal cords tend to form fibrosis and granulation tissue following surgery.

Vocal cord paralysis is the second most common cause of inspiratory stridor, accounting for 15–20 % of cases. It can be idiopathic, secondary to central nervous system immaturity, due to a compression of midbrain structures by either a Chiari malformation [20] or any lesion occupying space in the cranium and causing a partial herniation of midbrain structures through the foramen ovale [21]. Unilateral palsy can be seen after head and neck or cardiac surgery. Proper evaluation of the

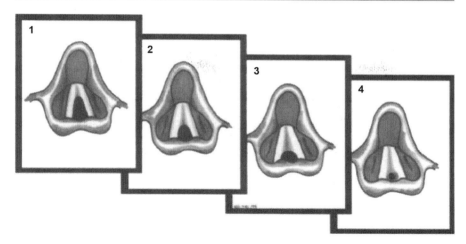

Fig. 18.2 Cohen's and Benjamin's classification of laryngeal webs. Type 1: 35 % or less of the glottis is involved. Type 2: 35–50 %, Type 3: 50–75 %, Type 4: more than 75 % with extension to the subglottic area. In Type 2 and 3, may extend into the subglottis and result in subglottic stenosis. (From *Otolaryngol Clin North Am* 41 (2008) 877–888. Used with permission)

condition is best done without an endotracheal tube in place. These patients may require a tracheostomy.

18.5   Subglottic and Tracheal Pathologies

Subglottic stenosis (SGS) is most frequently caused by endotracheal intubation in the neonatal period. It happens at the level of the cricoid cartilage which is the narrowest point of the pediatric airway. The incidence has decreased in the past 30 years; however, a recent prospective study found that 11.38 % of patients had some degree of stenosis after intubation [22]. Length of intubation and need for additional sedation appeared to be key factors for the development of SGS. The congenital form of SGS is rare, accounting for no more than 10 % of cases. Depending on the severity of the narrowing, these patients will undergo a variety of treatments: observation and repeat examination, balloon dilatation, laser therapy, laryngotracheoplasty, cricoid split, or partial cricotracheal resection. Not infrequently a tracheotomy will be done to insure unobstructed breathing and allow healing after a complex corrective surgery. In the general pediatric population, anesthesiologists should have a high index of suspicion if an infant cannot be intubated with an age-appropriate endotracheal tube. The four-grade Cotton-Myers classification of SGS is based on the relation between the biggest size of endotracheal tube fitting the airway and the expected size of the tube calculated for age [23].

Infantile hemangiomas are the most common benign vascular tumors in children and proliferate rapidly in the first year of life. There seems to be an increased risk of laryngeal hemangioma associated with a "beard" distribution of cutaneous lesions. Left untreated the mortality associated with subglottic hemangiomas can be as high as 50 %. Lesions can be found in any part of the airway where they may extrinsi-cally compromise air entry or grow inside structures, including the trachea. It is a common differential diagnosis in infants presenting with progressive stridor and undergoing diagnostic bronchoscopy. Patients with head and neck hemangiomas should undergo a workup for PHACES (*P*osterior fossa brain malformations, *H*emangiomas of the face, *A*rterial *C*erebrovascular abnormalities, *E*ye abnormali-ties, and *S*ternal defects.). The use of propranolol has been recently reported to have significant effects by decreasing the size of the lesions [24]. For a recent up to date review, see [25]

Tracheomalacia is caused by either the altered structure of the tracheal tissue architecture or by secondary factors like external compression or inflammatory response to various insults. It causes variable degrees of respiratory distress due to the exaggerated collapse of the airway typically during expiration. Bronchoscopic observation during spontaneous ventilation (functional bronchoscopy) is used to evaluate the extent and severity of collapsus; however, there is yet no standardized way to classify the severity. Tracheomalacia might be underdiagnosed in children, some patients being wrongly labeled as asthmatics. Most patients needing more careful follow-up have an associated esophageal atresia or an anomaly of the aortic arch or the supra-aortic vessels causing extrinsic compression [26, 27]. In some instances, an aortopexy will allow decompression of the trachea, but a conservative approach is usually indicated in the first 18 months of age [28]. Extrinsic compres-sion of the tracheal tree can also be caused by a mediastinal mass and a neck mass from tumoral or cystic origin and treated according to the diagnosis.

Congenital distal tracheal stenosis represents only 0.3–1.6 of all laryngotra-cheal lesions and is often accompanied by cardiovascular, gastrointestinal, and pul-monary comorbidities. While patients presenting minimal symptoms can be observed as the stenotic area may grow to a normal size, those having more severe symptoms will undergo surgery. A variety of tracheoplasty techniques may be used: costochondral grafting, resection with end-to-end anastomosis, or slide tra-cheoplasty [29]. Options for anesthetic airway management include intubation with the cuff passed in the stenotic area, selective split endotracheal tube with one side in each mainstem bronchus, selective intubation, bilateral jet ventilation, and cardiopulmonary bypass [30, 31].

18.6   Anesthetic Management

18.6.1 Emergency Airway Rescue

Situations of airway rescue with impending complete obstruction are emergencies during which the anesthesiologist must work in close collaboration with the otolar-yngologist. A variety of airway devices must be available: oro- and nasopharyngeal airways, appropriate sized supraglottic devices [32], various laryngoscope blades of sizes 00 and 0, intubation aids like the family of devices labeled as videolaryngo-scopes, and fiber-optic tracheoscopes. The presence of the otolaryngologist is man-datory in order to establish an emergency surgical airway if needed. Induction of anesthesia should be cautious and progressive. The presence of midfacial deformities or various types of mandibular hypoplasia and macroglossia may impair proper bag and mask ventilation at a very early stage of induction. Inhalational induction probably remains the first choice of many anesthesiologists for induction of anesthesia keeping in mind that the anesthetic administration is more likely to be interrupted while the airway is secured or when the surgeon is working. TIVA with short-acting agents like propofol and remifentanil allows a progressive deepening of anesthetic state, maintenance of spontaneous respiration, and relatively rapid reversal of anesthesia when stopped. An excellent review on the topic has been published by Sims and von Ungern-Sternberg [33].

18.6.2 Anesthesia for Diagnostic and Therapeutic Procedures

Most patients presenting with a symptomatic airway problem will be first evaluated with bedside FFE. Even in an awake patient, a good overall evaluation of the airway down to the level of the glottis can be made, and some pathologies can be identified for further evaluation under anesthesia. Subsequently, patients are brought to the OR for detailed visual characterization of obstructive structures and pathologies, as well as a precise evaluation of the functional mechanics of the airway, ideally and most of the time during spontaneous breathing. Precise evaluation in that context is very challenging for the anesthesiologist as the depth of anesthesia needs to be precisely reached and maintained for the performance of very stimulating procedures like rigid bronchoscopy or airway suspension while spontaneous breathing is maintained. Moreover, during the same diagnostic session, the depth of anesthesia might have to change significantly as the patient may require, for example, deep levels for rigid bronchoscopy followed by very light levels of anesthesia in order to observe the glottis structure behavior in a "sleep-like" state.

A variety of ventilation techniques may be used depending on the context, the nature, and the extent of the obstruction and the level of comfort of the anesthesiologist. In a recent retrospective study on the anesthetic management for subglottic stenosis, Knights et al. found no difference in the outcome between eight different airway management techniques [34].

Extubation of neonatal intensive care patients after prolonged intubation is often made in the operating room because of the significant frequency of immediate reintubation in a sometimes difficult context. In our institution, this is done under general anesthesia and spontaneous breathing with a flexible endoscope in situ to observe the laryngeal area.

Patients with TBAO and pathologies of the upper airway and supraglottic area need careful induction as they might obstruct quite early. Their ability to maintain some airway patency during anesthesia is useful to help determine the need for further intervention, for example, tongue-lip adhesion.

Functional problems like laryngomalacia and tracheomalacia are best evaluated during spontaneous ventilation. Laryngomalacia may exhibit a complex pattern of anterior, posterior, and/or circumferential collapse. Subtle changes in aryepiglottic folds, epiglottic shape, and position of the arytenoid are frequently found in that condition and subject to surgical correction. These are best evaluated during spontaneous breathing without an endotracheal tube in place. Tracheomalacia is classified according to the degree of collapse during spontaneous breathing during rigid bronchoscopy. Anomalies like a Class 1 laryngeal cleft could be missed if an endotracheal tube is in place.

18.6.3 Planning for Postoperative Period

Difficult airway access, surgical interventions, and the use of rigid bronchoscopy with or without suspension are all factors susceptible to induce swelling of respiratory tract structures in the postoperative period. The length of the procedure and extent of surgical trauma will also be considered in deciding if the patient needs to remain intubated or to be observed in a high-acuity area like the intensive or acute care unit. Dexamethasone [35] or l-epinephrine given by aerosol for prevention of post-extubation laryngeal edema is frequently used.

> **Conclusion**
>
> Management of the newborn obstructed airway is one of the most challenging situations in an anesthesiologist's practice. Proper management of these patients requires skillful manipulation of the airway, optimal ventilation techniques, and intimate knowledge of pharmacology. Maintenance of airway patency is complexified by the need of providing conditions that will allow proper evaluation of functional breathing mechanics in order to take optimal surgical decisions.

Bibliography

1. Bookman LB et al (2012) Neonates with tongue-based airway obstruction: a systematic review. Otolaryngol Head Neck Surg 146(1):8–18
2. Cladis F et al (2014) Pierre Robin Sequence: a perioperative review. Anesth Analog 119(2):400–412
3. Hosking J et al (2012) Anesthesia for Treacher Collins syndrome: a review of airway management in 240 pediatric cases. Paediatr Anaesth 22(8):752–758
4. Ashokan CS, Sreenivasan A, Saraswathy GK (2014) Goldenhar syndrome-review with case series. J Clin Diagn Res 8(4):ZD17–ZD19
5. Bogusiak K et al (2014) Treatment strategy in Goldenhar syndrome. J Craniofac Surg 25(1):177–183
6. Healey D, Letts M, Jarvis JG (2002) Cervical spine instability in children with Goldenhar's syndrome. Can J Surg 45(5):341–344
7. Weksberg R, Shuman C, Beckwith JB (2010) Beckwith-Wiedemann syndrome. Eur J Hum Genet 18(1):8–14
8. Prada CE, Zarate YA, Hopkin RJ (2012) Genetic causes of macroglossia: diagnostic approach. Pediatrics 129(2):e431–e437
9. Handley SC et al (2013) Predicting surgical intervention for airway obstruction in micrognathic infants. Otolaryngol Head Neck Surg 148(5):847–851
10. Duval M et al (2007) Respiratory distress secondary to bilateral nasolacrimal duct mucoceles in a newborn. Otolaryngol Head Neck Surg 137(2):353–354
11. Burrow TA et al (2009) Characterization of congenital anomalies in individuals with choanal atresia. Arch Otolaryngol Head Neck Surg 135(6):543–547

12. Olney DR et al (1999) Laryngomalacia and its treatment. Laryngoscope 109(11):1770–1775
13. Adil E, Rager T, Carr M (2012) Location of airway obstruction in term and preterm infants with laryngomalacia. Am J Otolaryngol 33(4):437–440
14. Garritano FG, Carr MM (2014) Characteristics of patients undergoing supraglottoplasty for laryngomalacia. Int J Pediatr Otorhinolaryngol 78(7):1095–1100
15. Benjamin B, Inglis A (1989) Minor congenital laryngeal clefts: diagnosis and classification. Ann Otol Rhinol Laryngol 98(6):417–420
16. van der Doef HP et al (2007) Clinical aspects of type 1 posterior laryngeal clefts: literature review and a report of 31 patients. Laryngoscope 117(5):859–863
17. Rahbar R et al (2006) The presentation and management of laryngeal cleft: a 10-year experience. Arch Otolaryngol Head Neck Surg 132(12):1335–1341
18. Cohen SR (1985) Congenital glottic webs in children. A retrospective review of 51 patients. Ann Otol Rhinol Laryngol Suppl 121:2–16
19. Benjamin B (1983) Chevalier Jackson Lecture. Congenital laryngeal webs. Ann Otol Rhinol Laryngol 92(4 Pt 1):317–326
20. Lyons M, Vlastarakos PV, Nikolopoulos TP (2012) Congenital and acquired developmental problems of the upper airway in newborns and infants. Early Hum Dev 88(12):951–955
21. Alshammari J, Monnier Y, Monnier P (2012) Clinically silent subdural hemorrhage causes bilateral vocal fold paralysis in newborn infant. Int J Pediatr Otorhinolaryngol 76(10):1533–1534
22. Manica D et al (2013) Association between length of intubation and subglottic stenosis in children. Laryngoscope 123(4):1049–1054
23. Myer CM 3rd, O'Connor DM, Cotton RT (1994) Proposed grading system for subglottic stenosis based on endotracheal tube sizes. Ann Otol Rhinol Laryngol 103(4 Pt 1):319–323
24. Leaute-Labreze C et al (2008) Propranolol for severe hemangiomas of infancy. N Engl J Med 358(24):2649–2651
25. Broeks IJ et al (2013) Propranolol treatment in life-threatening airway hemangiomas: a case series and review of literature. Int J Pediatr Otorhinolaryngol 77(11):1791–1800
26. Austin J, Ali T (2003) Tracheomalacia and bronchomalacia in children: pathophysiology, assessment, treatment and anaesthesia management. Paediatr Anaesth 13(1):3–11
27. Kugler C, Stanzel F (2014) Tracheomalacia. Thorac Surg Clin 24(1):51–58
28. Jennings RW et al (2014) Surgical approaches to aortopexy for severe tracheomalacia. J Pediatr Surg 49(1):66–70; discussion 70–71
29. Valencia D et al (2011) Surgical management of distal tracheal stenosis in children. Laryngoscope 121(12):2665–2671
30. Pinsonneault C, Fortier J, Donati F (1999) Tracheal resection and reconstruction. Can J Anaesth 46(5 Pt 1):439–455
31. deLorimier AA et al (1990) Tracheobronchial obstructions in infants and children. Experience with 45 cases. Ann Surg 212(3):277–289
32. Schmolzer GM et al (2013) Supraglottic airway devices during neonatal resuscitation: an historical perspective, systematic review and meta-analysis of available clinical trials. Resuscitation 84(6):722–730
33. Sims C, von Ungern-Sternberg BS (2012) The normal and the challenging pediatric airway. Paediatr Anaesth 22(6):521–526
34. Knights RM et al (2013) Airway management in patients with subglottic stenosis: experience at an academic institution. Anesth Analg 117(6):1352–1354
35. Davis PG, Henderson-Smart DJ (2001) Intravenous dexamethasone for extubation of newborn infants. Cochrane Database Syst Rev (4):CD000308. doi:10.1002/14651858.CD000308

Part IV
Important Techniques for Perioperative Care

Vascular Access in the Perioperative Period

19

Thierry Pirotte

Vascular access is of major importance in the perioperative period. Venous access is a compulsory element during any type of anesthesia and often an inevitable way to initiate treatment in critically ill children. Anesthesiologist and pediatricians, as experts, should master their techniques and have a thorough knowledge of the existing tools that could assist difficult vascular accesses.

Bedside ultrasound examination and real-time needle guidance are the most important progress made over the last decade to facilitate vascular access and reduce complications. A broad range of techniques have been developed far beyond the puncture of the internal jugular vein [1]. The learning curve to apply these techniques in children, and especially in neonates, is not short and should be followed carefully as described in this chapter.

19.1 Ultrasound Guidance

Over the last decade, the importance of perioperative ultrasound (US) became obvious due to the diversity of applications developed in anesthesia: nerve blocks, vascular access, evaluation of the gastric content, or assessment of potential complications (fluid or air in the thoracic or abdominal cavity).

T. Pirotte
Department of Anesthesia, Cliniques universitaires Saint-Luc, Université catholique de Louvain – UCL, Brussels, Belgium
e-mail: t.pirotte@uclouvain.be

© Springer International Publishing Switzerland 2016
M. Astuto, P.M. Ingelmo (eds.), *Perioperative Medicine in Pediatric Anesthesia*,
Anesthesia, Intensive Care and Pain in Neonates and Children,
DOI 10.1007/978-3-319-21960-8_19

19.1.1 Advantages of Ultrasound Guidance

The use of US for vascular access can be divided in US screening, corresponding to an evaluation of the subcutaneous anatomy – or sonoanatomy – and real-time US guidance (USG) of the needle during puncture.

Pre-procedural US screening detects anomalies in vessel size, position, or patency, as well as anomalies of the surrounding structures (hematoma, ganglions, etc.) (Fig. 19.1). If the chosen vessel or insertion site presents too much difficulty, another site is chosen. In comparison with the blind landmark approaches, US techniques detect the difficult puncture before it becomes difficult.

USG of the needle brings the needle tip in the lumen of the vessel without damaging surrounding structures (artery, nerve, pleura), helps the catheterization of the vessel, and, for central venous access, places the needle tip in an optimal position to insert the guide wire (GW) (Fig. 19.2).

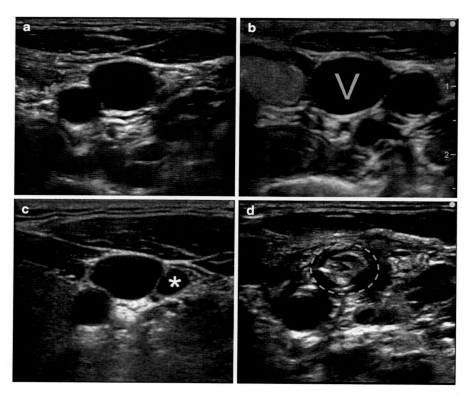

Fig. 19.1 Pre-procedural US screening to detect anatomical variants. (**a**) Normal anatomy, (**b**) abnormal internal jugular vein (*V*) position (median to the carotid artery), (**c**) abnormal surrounding structure (*, ganglion), (**d**) abnormal patency (IJV thrombosis)

Fig. 19.2 Role of ultrasound guidance during vascular puncture. (**a**) (*1*) Guide the needle in the middle of the vein, (*2*) avoid transfixion, (*3*) avoid puncturing surrounding structures, and (**b**) (*4*) catheterize the vessel and place the needle tip in an optimal position to insert the guide wire

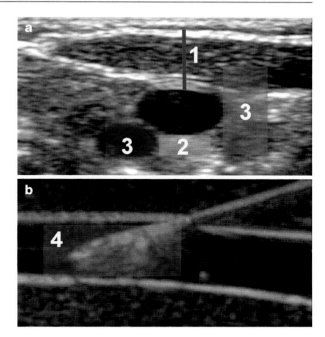

Post-procedural screening is used to confirm the correct migration of the GW and eventually to detect potential life-threatening complications (severe hematoma, pneumothorax, hemopericardium) (Fig. 19.3).

For vascular access, USG has shown an increase in final success rate and in success rate at first attempt and a reduction in complication rate (mainly inadvertent arterial punctures) and in a number of attempts needed to succeed. These factors are extremely important in young children and infants where multiple attempts will lead to potential complications, time consumption, and possible instability (hypothermia, hypotension).

19.1.2 Limitations of Ultrasound Guidance

The availability of the equipment and the learning curve are the two main limitations. The cost of the US machine and the disposable probe covers is consequent but should be balanced with the cost of more complications and sometimes longer procedures with blind landmark techniques. The learning curve is short for US screening but can be much longer for USG and placement of CVC in neonates.

In children, structures are usually superficial offering a nice view of both vessels and needle. The limit of resolution can however be reached in case of very small vessels (radial artery in neonates).

Only few pathological situations, like subcutaneous emphysema, may hamper the use of US.

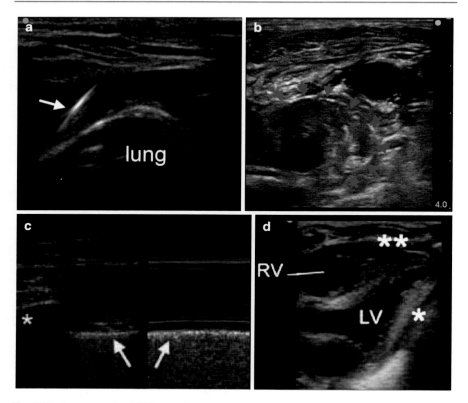

Fig. 19.3 Post-procedural US screening. (**a**) Confirmation of the correct migration of the guide wire (*arrow*) in the brachiocephalic vein. (**b**) Detection of a severe carotid hematoma (*arrows*). (**c**) *Left*: absence of pneumothorax: positive lung sliding sign in 2D-mode (*, rib); *right*: seashore sign in M-mode (*arrow*, pleural line). (**d**) Absence of hemopericardium (*, ** empty spaces; *RV*, *LV* right and left ventricles)

19.1.3 Guidelines for Ultrasound Guidance During Vascular Access

Different societies in different countries and continents do recommend the use of US for vascular access [2–6]. Table 19.1 summarizes their opinion regarding central and peripheral venous access and arterial access. US screening alone can be useful but is evaluated as insufficient and thus not recommended. For some techniques like the subclavian vein puncture, no comparative study is currently found in the literature, making guidelines impossible or very cautious.

19.1.4 Ultrasound Equipment

High-quality US machines are needed to offer sufficient resolution of small vessels and a correct view of the nerves. Doppler and Zoom functions are mandatory to

Table 19.1 Guidelines for ultrasound-guided vascular access in children

	PVA	ART	PICC	IJV	SCV	FEM
NICE – UK – 2002 [2]	n/a	n/a	n/a	+++	+	+
ASA – USA – 2012 [3]	n/a	n/a	n/a	+++	+	+
ASEcho – USA – 2012 [4]	no	+ D	+++	+++	no	+
International – 2012 [5]	+ D	++	+++	+++	+++	+++
SFAR – France – 2014 [6]	+ D	+ D	n/a	+++	no	+++

NICE National Institute for Clinical Excellence, *ASA* American Society of Anesthesiologists, *ASEcho* American Society of Echocardiography, *International* International expert group, *SFAR* French Society of Anesthesia and Reanimation, *PVA* peripheral venous access, *ART* radial artery, *PICC* peripherally inserted central catheters, *IJV* internal jugular vein, *SCV* subclavian vein, *FEM* femoral vein, +++ strong recommendations, ++ recommendation in most cases, + weak recommendations, + D recommendation in expected difficulties, *no* no recommendations, *n/a* not analyzed

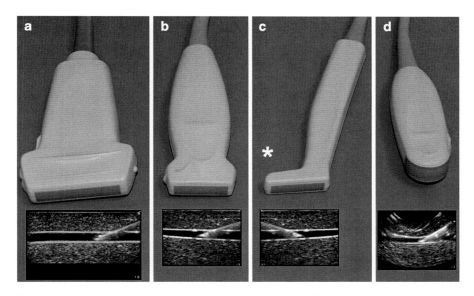

Fig. 19.4 High-frequency probes for vascular access. (**a**) Adult linear, (**b**) linear small footprint, (**c**) linear pediatric "hockey stick" (*, more room for needle handling), (**d**) curvilinear transfontanellar probe (lower resolution and image distortion)

identify thrombosis and to differentiate or puncture very small vessels. Image storage, diffusion, and sharing should be possible to complete the chard of the patient.

High-frequency (>10 MHz) probes are used because of the usual superficiality of the vascular structures in children (Fig. 19.4). Linear probes (giving a rectangular image) are preferred over the curvilinear probes (lower frequency and resolution, distortion of the image). Small-footprint probes (25 mm) are mandatory to treat infants and neonates; they give more room for the placement of the needle (the "hockey stick" probe gives as much space as possible). If the US equipment is

Fig. 19.5 Comparison of
adult and pediatric
equipment in young
children. Adult probes are
limited to US screening
while small-footprint
pediatric probes can be
used for both US screening
and US needle guidance

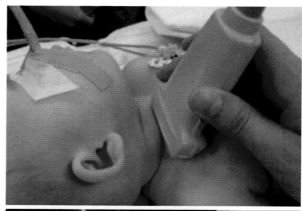

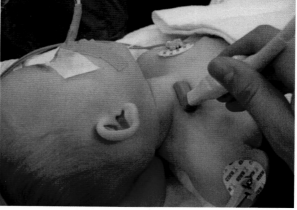

limited to a standard adult linear probe (38 mm footprint) and the child is young, at
least US screening should be used (Fig. 19.5). Sterile US probe covers and sterile
gel are needed and disposed with the US machine.

Recent new developments in US technology are:

- Enhanced needle visualization systems (US beam steering)
- Incorporated teaching course in US machines
- Wireless US probes facilitation sterile handling (Acuson™ – Siemens®)
- GPS needle guidance allowing to predict needle track even before skin puncture
  (eZGuide™ – eZono®)

19.1.5 Puncture Techniques (Fig. 19.6)

Vessels can be visualized by US in two different planes or "views": the short-axis
view or SAX shows a round structure and the long-axis view or LAX a long tubular
structure. Patent vessels are anechoic (black) and thrombosed vessels iso- or hyperechoic (from grey to white). Veins are easily compressible, their size varies with

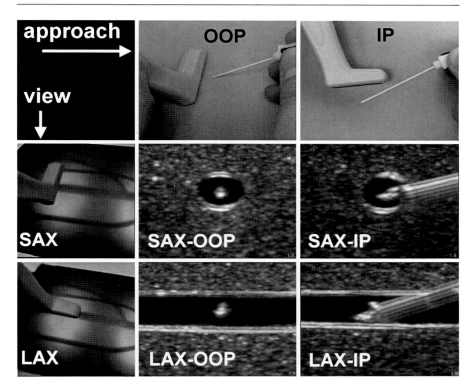

Fig. 19.6 Possible ultrasound-guided puncture techniques for vascular access. By combining two different views of the vessel (*SAX and LAX*) and two different needle approaches (*OOP and IP*), four techniques are formed to puncture vessels

respiration, and they may content valves. Arteries are pulsatile and more difficult to compress.

US needle guidance can be performed with two different needle-to-probe alignments or "approaches": the out-of-plane approach or OOP when the needle is inserted perpendicular to the US beam and is seen as a hyperechoic (white) dot and the in-plane approach or IP when the needle is inserted strictly into and parallel to the US beam and is seen as a hyperechoic (white) line.

With OOP approaches, the vessel is placed in the middle of the screen to lie under the middle part of the probe. The needle is inserted at a distance corresponding to the vessel depth with a flat angle (<45°) to appear in the soft tissues above the vessel (Fig. 19.7). The needle tip is followed by sliding or tilting movements of the probe (Fig. 19.8). Sliding movements, requiring gel on the skin, are used if the site offers enough room for movement. Tilting movements are used if room for probe movement is limited (more frequently in infants and neonates). Probe movements should always precede needle movements because the appearance of the hyperechoic needle tip on the screen is the most obvious pattern recognized by our eyes.

With IP approaches, the probe remains in a stable immobile position while the needle is inserted exactly parallel and under the length of the probe (Fig. 19.9). Perfectly inserted, the needle is seen as a bright hyperechoic line. If the needle

Fig. 19.7 The middle of the screen is the middle of the probe. With OOP needle approaches, placing the vessel exactly in the middle of the screen facilitates the puncture. The needle is inserted with a flat angle (α) under the middle part of the probe to appear above the vessel (*)

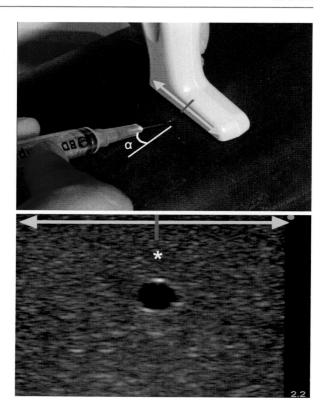

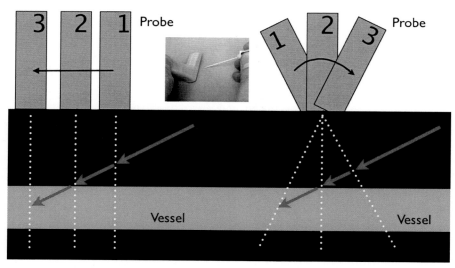

Fig. 19.8 To follow the needle tip during OOP approaches, sliding (*left side*) or tilting (*right side*) movements of the probe are used. Tilting movements more often used in young children when room for probe movement is limited

moves away from this position, it can disappear completely or partially. Needle (or probe) position is corrected to have a constant view of the needle tip and shaft.

Four combinations of vein "views" and needle "approaches" are used in clinical practice depending on the type and size of the vein, the age of the child, and the preference of the operator:

- SAX view with OOP approach: used frequently for peripheral venous and arterial accesses; for jugular, femoral, and axillary access; and for peripherally inserted central catheters (PICCs) insertions.
- SAX view with IP approach: used for the access to the internal jugular vein (IJV) by a posterior approach.
- LAX view with OOP approach: rarely used, only for the infraclavicular access to the subclavian vein in older children.
- LAX view with IP approach: used for the supraclavicular and infraclavicular accesses to the brachiocephalic, subclavian, and axillary veins and can also be used for peripheral accesses when veins are big enough.

19.1.6 Learning Curve

US needle guidance should be trained on gel models, not on patient. Different professional gel models exist that reliably simulate the puncture of small vessels but also the puncture of jugular, femoral, or subclavian veins in children (Fig. 19.10). After "in vitro" training, the first 5–10 punctures should be supervised by an experienced colleague. The variability of the learning curve is important depending on dexterity, three-dimensional orientation, and number of procedures done per week.

19.1.7 Sterile Setting and Ergonomics (Fig. 19.11)

Central venous catheter should be inserted by using maximal barrier precautions including cap, mask, sterile gloves, and gown and large sterile drapes and a long sterile probe cover. Transparent sterile drapes are useful to see the anatomy and the chest movements of the child.

The US machine should be placed in front of the operator allowing an alignment of hands and US scream.

19.2   Peripheral Venous Access

19.2.1 Indications

A peripheral venous access (PVA) is mandatory for every anesthesia. For elective surgeries most children will prefer inhalational induction of anesthesia. The PVA is then placed after the child is asleep but before any manipulation of his airway. The

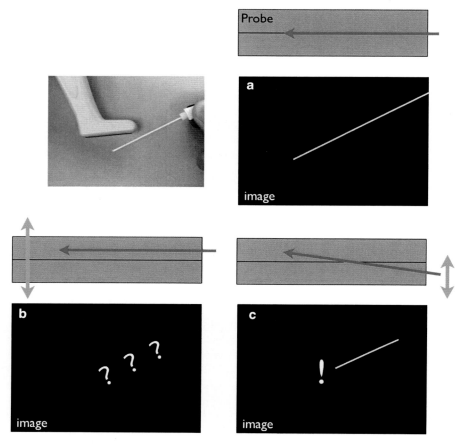

Fig. 19.9 To follow the needle during IP approaches, the needle is precisely inserted parallel and centered under the length of the probe. The needle is seen as an hyperechoic line (**a**). When completely lost, the needle can be retrieved by small sliding movements of the probe (**b**). If the needle disappears partially during its progression, right-to-left movement of the needle will re-center the needle under the probe (**c**)

success rate of PVA in the operation room is high with a success at first attempt between 68 and 80 % and a rate of impossible access less than 0.5 %, which is 10 times lower than the failure rate in the ward (up to 5 %) [7].

The period between induction and the first intravenous access can be critical. Children with a possible difficult PVA should be detected during the preoperative evaluation to allow specific equipment and/or abilities to be prepared for the time of anesthesia [8] (Table 19.2). Allowing children to drink clear fluids 2 h before anesthesia will facilitate the PVA by limiting dehydration. In case a life-threatening condition occurs before the PVA is found (laryngospasm, major bradycardia or cardiac), the intraosseous route should be used without delay (see Intraosseous Route).

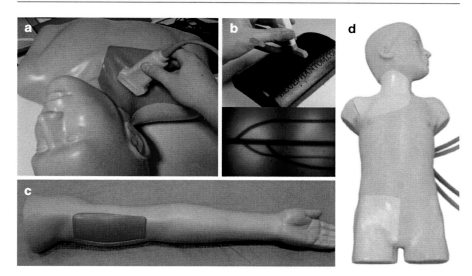

Fig. 19.10 Different gel models used for pediatric vascular access training sessions. (**a**) "Head and torso," (**b**) "pediatric vessels," and (**c**) "PICC insertion arm" from Blue Phantom® and (**d**) "vascular access child" from Simulab®

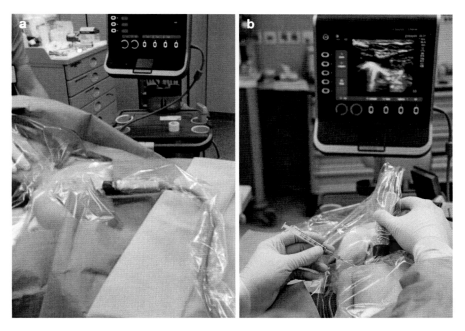

Fig. 19.11 Sterility and ergonomy. (**a**) Long sterile drape and probe covers ensure maximal barrier precautions. (**b**) Hands and US screen are aligned in front of the operator to facilitate handling

Table 19.2 Anticipating a difficult peripheral venous access is of major importance

Difficult PVA	Tips and technologies
Young age (2 months–2 years)	Experience in pediatric and neonatal anesthesia
Former preterm children	Push needle with the thumb (feel the "pop" or
Prolonged illness	"click")
Previous difficult iv access	Fill the cannula with saline (faster venous flashback)
No veins seen or palpated preoperatively	Wet black skin (increase transparency)
Obesity	Warm up the skin
Black skin	Take EMLA® cream off 10 min before puncture
Vasoconstriction	Transillumination
Dehydration	Near-infrared technology
	Ultrasonography
Failed PVA after induction of anesthesia	
Stable conditions: call for help, use advanced technologies (ultrasound), go to a CVA	
Life-threatening condition: call for rapid help, use the intraosseous route	

Experience and advanced technologies are sometimes necessary

PVA peripheral venous access, *CVA* central venous access

In case anesthesia has to be induced intravenously (emergencies, child with a full stomach, risk of malignant hyperthermia, etc.), a technique – or a combination of these techniques – should always be used to reduce pain and possible trauma related to "awake" PVA:

- Application of topical anesthetics: EMLA® cream (lidocaine 2.5 %–prilocaine 2.5 %), Ametop® (tetracaine 4 %), or S-Caine® patch (lidocaine 7 %–tetracaine 7 %) can be used. The last two have the advantage to anesthetize the skin more rapidly (within 20–30 min) but have to be removed also earlier (within 30–45 min). EMLA® cream is applied under an occlusive dressing on two different visible veins 60–90 min before puncture. The maximal application time should never exceed 4 h. Optimal puncture conditions are obtained 5–10 min after wiping the cream of the skin (disappearance of the vasoconstriction induced by the prilocaine). In neonates, EMLA® is limited to 0.5 g with a maximal application time of 1 h.
- Breathing a mixture of O_2 and N_2O (with a fraction of N_2O between 50 and 70 %) for 3–5 min before puncture causes analgesia and some kind of amnesia.
- Hypnosis techniques for school-age children: the Magic Glove, the Magic Pen, the on/off button, or the comfortable location can truly help seriously ill children in case of repeated procedures.
- Infiltration of 0.2–0.5 ml of 1 % lidocaine subcutaneously through an insulin or intradermal needle will offer analgesia after a short massage of the skin. Somewhat painful, this technique is mostly used in adolescents.

19.2.2 The Choice of the Vein

The common challenges to find a PVA are encountered between 2 and 18 months of age (chubby babies) or in case of obesity or multiple previous attempts (blood

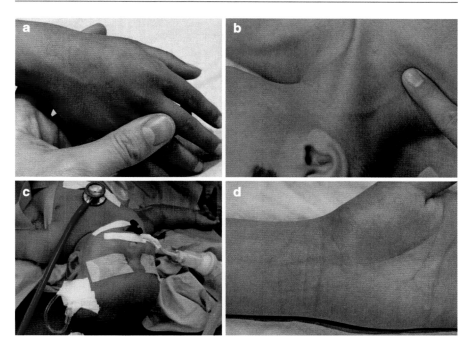

Fig. 19.12 Different peripheral venous accesses used in children. (**a**) Dorsal side of the hand, the first choice; (**b**) external jugular vein, an alternative allowing blood samples (supraclavicular compression); (**c**) epicranial vein, here used during combined hand and foot syndactyly corrections in Ethiopia; (**d**) anterior aspect of the wrist, a last and temporary solution

sample or infusions). The most often used puncture sites are listed below and ranked in order of preference (Fig. 19.12):

- *The hand*: the first choice in the operating room is a nice vein usually seen or discerned at the dorsal side of the hand between the fourth and the fifth metacarpal bones (sometime between the third and the fourth one) [7]. The second vein runs at the radial side of the wrist but is highly mobile in young children and therefore more difficult to puncture.
- *The forearm and the antecubital fossa*: three major veins run along the forearm – the cephalic, the median antecubital, and the basilic vein. Veins at the forearm are difficult to see in young children due to the relatively high fat layer. At the antecubital fossa, veins can be punctured if they are clearly seen or palpated. Veins should be punctured rapidly under the skin and cannulated over a sufficient distance to avoid early dislodgment and delay recognition of extravasation. In difficult cases, USG should be used instead of blind attempts (risk of arterial puncture or medial nerve damage). At the arm level, basilic–brachial and cephalic veins can't be seen or palpated anymore and have to be punctured under USG. At that level, longer catheter – like PICCs or midlines – has to be used to provide a sufficient catheterization length (see Peripherally Inserted Central Catheters).

- *The foot*: the internal saphenous vein runs at the anterior border of the medial malleolus and is rarely absent. Ultrasound guidance can be used in case of a negative palpation. This vein is interesting in case of head and neck surgery when massive blood loss is expected (e.g., craniostenosis). Small veins at the dorsum of the foot or the external saphenous vein can also be cannulated.
- *The scalp*: in neonates, branches of the temporal vein can be prominent on the frontoparietal aspect of the head. Digital compression is used to increase vein size and allow cannulation of a short catheter. Shaving the hair locally helps both puncture and fixation.
- *The neck*: the external jugular vein is seen in the majority of children. Digital compression at the lower end of the vein close to the clavicle increases vein size and prevents the vein from collapsing during inspiration. To gain access, the child is placed head-down with a rolled towel under the shoulders and the head turned away from the puncture site. Ultrasound guidance can be used but is rarely needed. Infusion rate and blood flashback can fluctuate with head position and ventilation. Gentle traction on the skin after catheter fixation usually helps to get a blood sample during surgery (can be used as second PVA for this purpose).
- *The anterior aspect of the wrist*: these tiny and superficial veins are sometimes the only vein seen in a chubby baby or an obese child. These veins are fragile and close to other functionally important structures (artery, nerve, tendons). They represent a last and temporary solution.

19.2.3 Standard Procedure

A rapid evaluation of the four limbs usually detects the most attractive site. A tourniquet is placed at the proximal end of the limb without pinching the skin or interrupting the arterial circulation (presence of distal pulse, no skin whitening). Compression and relaxation of the limb's muscles ("milking") can increase vein filling. In some cases, the vein can only be palpated but not seen. It is advised to start with distal attempts to allow rescue attempts at a more proximal level without risking leaks of infused fluid through prior puncture sites. Black skin is disinfected to increase light reflexion and visualization of superficial veins.

After disinfection, the skin is stretched and the vein immobilized by the nondominant hand. Pushing the needle with the thumb helps to feel the "pop" or "click" when the bevel pierces the wall of the vein. In neonates or hypovolemic children, venous flashback is sometimes not immediate and can take up to 4 s to appear. It is therefore important to wait long enough after having felt the "click." To reduce the risk of future extravasation, only half of the length of the cannula should be used to find the vein, allowing the next half to be catheterized into the vein (Fig. 19.13). Filling the needle with saline can speed up slow blood flows in the needle hub. Once the flashback is recognized, the needle is pushed one or a few millimeters further to allow the cannula (shorter than the needle) to enter the vein. After having confirmed venous flashback into the fully inserted cannula, this one is carefully taped, a few milliliter of saline is injected manually, and the infusion bag is connected.

In case of difficult access (vein not seen, not palpated), specific technique can be used:

- *Transillumination*: by bringing light into the tissues, superficial veins are visualized as black lines in a pink environment. This technique showing the track but not the depth of the vein increases success rate in neonates and children less than 3 years old [9]. Depending on the thickness of the limb, the light-emitting diode (LED) is placed under or at the side of the vein (Veinlite Pedi®, Vein Finder®, Wee Sight®). Short application times should be used to prevent potential burns in neonates.
- *Near-infrared technology*: hemoglobin absorbs more infrared light than the surrounding tissues. Portable devices have been developed to detect superficial veins and project their position in real time (VeinViewer®, AccuVein®). Unfortunately the theoretical thickness of skin analyzed (8 mm) seems overstated. Deep unpalpable veins are currently not detected by these devices (Fig. 19.14). The efficacy of these devices remains thus controversial with a possible benefit for black skin [10, 11].
- *Ultrasound guidance (USG)*: ultrasound allows to detect veins that cannot be seen or palpated. It shows their position, depth, track and patency and can guide the needle into their lumen. Real-time USG reduces the procedure time and the number of attempts needed and increases the success rate in case of difficult PVA [12, 13]. This technique is recommended in these circumstances by different societies [5, 6]. Some experience is needed in young children to bring the needle tip in the lumen of such small vessels. USG is much easier in the operating room after inhalational induction of anesthesia than in the ward when children are awake. The usual sites for USG peripheral access are the ankle with the internal saphenous vein (Fig. 19.15) and the antecubital fossa with the basilic or brachial veins (Fig. 19.16).

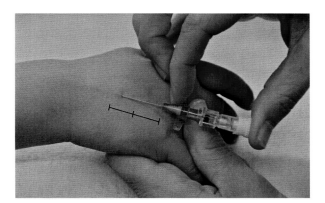

Fig. 19.13 Venous access at the dorsal side of the hand. The left hand stretches the skin to immobilize the vein; the needle is pushed by the thumb to feel the "click." Only half of the needle length is used to find the vein allowing the next half to be catheterized into the vein (reduced risk of extravasation)

Fig. 19.14 Near-infrared technology. Superficial are clearly shown (**a**), but more profound veins are not pointed out (**b**)

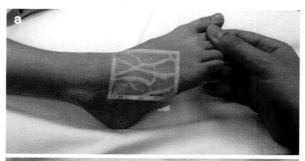

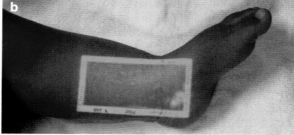

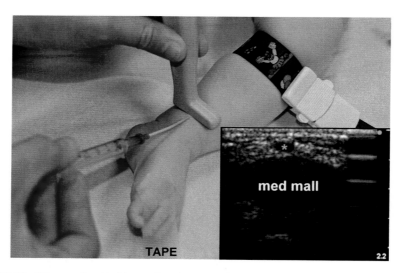

Fig. 19.15 Ultrasound-guided internal saphenous vein puncture. SAX view of the vein, OOP needle approach. The skin of the ankle is stretched by a tape to immobilize the vein. *, vein; *med mall*, medial malleolus

19.2.4 Complications

19.2.4.1 Phlebitis

Phlebitis is caused by mechanical or chemical irritation of the venous endothelium. Contributing factors include the material of the cannula (polyurethane is less phlebogenic than teflon), the nature of the solution (pH, tonicity, and composition), the site of insertion (upper limb less prone to phlebitis), and the duration of catheterization.

19.2.4.2 Extravasation

Depending on the nature, concentration, and volume of fluid injected, extravasation can lead to a temporary swelling, compartment syndrome, necrosis, or even delayed limb deformation. It should be prevented by a careful insertion technique (sufficient length of vein catheterization) and surveillance. In the absence of blood return, correct cannulation of the vein is confirmed by a manual injection of saline or by a free flow of the infusion bag placed at a height of 90 cm and this without any subcutaneous swelling detected.

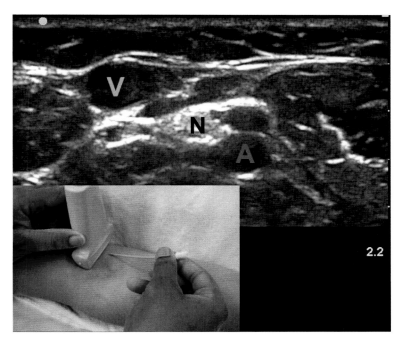

Fig. 19.16 Ultrasound-guided basilic vein puncture at the antecubital fossa. SAX view of the vein, OOP needle approach. Note the proximity of the medial nerve (*N*) and the brachial artery (*A*). *V* basilic vein

19.2.4.3 Injection of a Residual Anesthetic Medication

Medication injected at a distance of the cannula can remain in the infusion tubing if it is not flushed enough. The fact that anesthetic medication (opiates, muscular relaxant) could remain in the tubing even outside the operating room can be dramatic. The next injection through the same infusion site will bring the medication into the bloodstream with dramatic consequences (apnea, muscular relaxation). It is therefore advised to flush every medication with a volume corresponding to twice the volume of both tubing and cannula.

19.2.4.4 Specific Complications

When puncturing vein at *the scalp*, care must be taken to avoid accidental catheterization of a branch of the superficial temporal artery. Skin whitening around the site of insertion after a saline test injection is an early sign. The cannula should be removed immediately and a few minutes of compression applied.

Extravasation or hematoma in *the neck* area can have major (respiratory) consequences. Therefore, a high degree of suspicion should be kept during the (short) use of external jugular vein accesses.

At *the anterior aspect of the wrist*, the medial nerve can be damaged directly by the needle or indirectly by a hematoma.

19.3 Central Venous Access

19.3.1 Indications

The risk of complications related the central venous catheter (CVC) insertions is higher in children than in adults. The benefit/risk balance should therefore be analyzed before every CVC placement. Indications for CVC placement in children are:

- Extensive surgery with potential massive blood loss or hemodynamic instability
- The need to measure the central venous pressure
- Infusion of inotropes
- Infusion of antibiotics or chemotherapy inducing phlebitis (osmolality >500 mOsm, pH <5 or >9)
- Postoperative parenteral nutrition
- Hemodialysis, plasmapheresis
- Neurosurgery is a sitting position (rapid aspiration of air bubbles)
- Lack of peripheral venous access

The experience of the operator and the proper use of USG can, by reducing risks, increase the benefit/risk balance and allow children to access the CVCs for broader indications.

19.3.2 General Aspects

19.3.2.1 Equipment and Technique of Insertion

Skin preparation for CVC placement should be done with chlorhexidine (>0.5 %) with alcohol in children [14]. There is however no consensus for skin disinfection in a neonate younger than 44 gestational weeks. A Seldinger insertion technique is usually used during CVCs insertion: small puncture needle, insertion of a soft metallic guide wire (GW), skin incision, dilation, and introduction of the catheter over the GW. In neonates and infants, the use of a peripheral intravenous (IV) cannula can facilitate the puncture: by having smaller and sharper inner needle tips, they limit depression of the anterior wall of the vein. Whatever the needle used, a syringe should always be connected to increase handling, avoid any blood loss, and prevent air embolism in spontaneous breathing children. In children, it is advised to insert the GW by its J-shaped end. We know however that the diameter of the J-shaped end (close to 4 mm) can exceed the diameter of an infant's veins. Therefore, the soft straight tip can be used with precaution and under some conditions: gentle insertion without any force and ideally under fluoroscopy. Before any dilation or insertion of large-bore catheter, the correct migration of the GW into the chosen vein should be verified by US or fluoroscopy. US is also used to mobilize and redirect the GW in real time if an aberrant migration is detected (Fig. 19.17). Dilators are introduced over the GW till a "click" is felt (passage of the wall of the vein) but not further. If any resistance is felt during dilation, in-and-out movements of the GW are used to detect immediately any unintentional bending of the GW.

CVCs are in polyurethane or silicone and have single or multiple lumens. Catheters should be radiopaque and have centimeter graduations and a distal conical soft end. The size of the CVC depends on the site of insertion and the age/weight of the child (Table 19.3). The diameter of double-lumen (4 F) catheters is large compared to the veins of neonates or preterm infants and should therefore be used only if one lumen is insufficient.

The optimal length of insertion depends on the child (age, weight, length), the approach (site, side, low or high approach), and the mediastinal anatomy (angle and length of the brachiocephalic vein). Some tables and calculation have been made, but the data over left-sided approaches are rare [15]. Whatever the insertion site, verifying the catheter tip position is mandatory.

CVCs are carefully secured to the skin with skin stitches: the goal is to avoid any catheter withdrawal or kinking without damaging the skin (loose skin stitches are used and hard plastic clips avoided) (Fig. 19.18).

19.3.2.2 Complications Common to All Sites

CVC-related complications can be classified in immediate, intermediary, or late complications (Table 19.4). Specific complications linked to the access of the superior or inferior vena cava (SVC or IVC) will develop late.

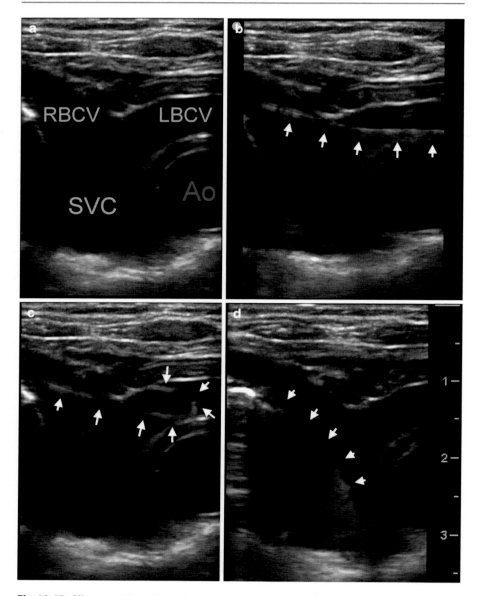

Fig. 19.17 Ultrasound detection and guidance of the guide wire (GW). (**a**) Anatomy before puncture (*RBCV–LBCV* right and left brachiocephalic veins, *SVC* superior vena cava, *Ao* aortic arch). (**b**) Migration of the GW (*arrows*) from the right subclavian to the LBCV. (**c**) Withdrawal of the GW till the J-shaped tip is seen. (**d**) Insertion of the GW downwards in the SVC

Table 19.3   Size of central venous catheters used depending on the weight, age, and vein size

	<1.5 kg	Newborn	6 m–4 years	4–10 years	>10 years
Single-lumen CVC	2 F (22 ga)	3 F (20 ga)	3 F (20 ga)	4 F (18 ga)	5 F (16 ga)
Double-lumen CVC	/[a]	4 F	4 F	5 F	7 F
PICC	1 F (28 ga)	2 F (23 ga)	3 F (vein >3 mm)	4 F (vein >4 mm)	5 F (vein >5 mm)
Umbilical catheters	3.5 F	5 F	/	/	/

Correspondence between French (F) and gauge (ga) are given. Age: m months, y years

[a]Double-lumen 4 F catheters are used in preterm infants only if a single lumen is insufficient

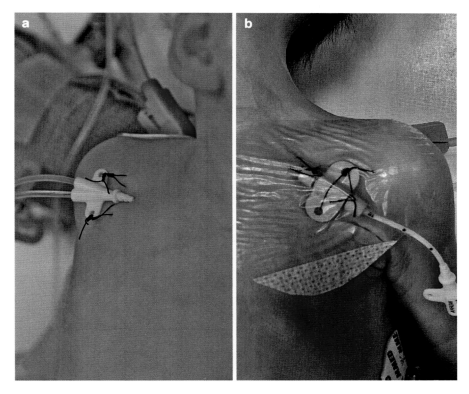

Fig. 19.18   Securing central venous catheters in young children. Loose skin stitches avoid catheter withdrawal without damaging the skin. (**a**) Fully inserted right subclavian catheter. (**b**) Partially inserted left subclavian catheter; the hard plastic clip is not used to avoid excessive pressure on the skin

Table 19.4 Classification of central venous catheter-associated complications

Common complications		
Immediate	**Intermediary**	**Late**
Hemorrhage, hematoma	Tamponade	Catheter occlusion
Arterial puncture	Extravascular fluid infusion	Thrombosis
Arrhythmia		Infection
Extravascular GW migration		Catheter rupture
Air embolism		Arteriovenous fistula
Specific complications		
Access to the SVC	**Access to the IVC**	
Pneumothorax	Peritoneal fluid infusion	
Hemothorax	Perimedullar catheter migration	
Chylothorax	Lower limb ischemia	
	Portal thrombosis[a]	

SVC superior venous cava, *IVG* inferior vena cava, *GW* guide wire
[a]For umbilical catheters

Immediate Complications

Arterial puncture is the most frequent complication. Consequences are hematoma, subsequently difficult or impossible punctures, respiratory difficulties, or development of an *arteriovenous fistula*.

Air embolism occurs mainly at the time of insertion in the spontaneously breathing child.

Extravascular GW migration is more frequent in neonates (fragility of veins and soft tissues) and/or when the GW is inserted by its straight end.

Intermediary Complications

Tamponade can have atypical presentations in children. It should be suspected in case of sudden hemodynamic deterioration after CVC placements.

Vessel perforation and extravascular fluid infusion will have consequences depending on the structure involved, the size of the hole, and the infusion rate. Repeated contact of the catheter against the vessel wall is a risk factor and should be avoided by an optimal catheter tip placement.

Late Complications

Catheter *occlusion* is limited by placing catheters with the lowest number of lumens required at an optimal insertion depth. Lumens are flushed with saline after every blood sample or infusion and between infusion of two incompatible medications. Positive pressure connectors are placed on any lumen that is only intermittently used. CVC occlusion is treated by instillation of alteplase, a recombinant tissue plasminogen activator, during 2 h in the occluded catheter lumen [16]. Alteplase is diluted in a volume of saline corresponding to 110 % of the priming volume of the lumen at the weight-adapted dose of:

- 0.5 mg till 10 kg
- 1 mg from 10 to 30 kg
- 2 mg above 30 kg

The incidence of CVC-related *thrombosis* is probably underestimated because the signs are often subclinical. Risk factors in children are:

- Sepsis
- Intracardiac surgery
- Congenital thrombophilia: protein C, protein S, or antithrombin III deficiency, Factor V Leiden, hyperhomocysteinemia
- Acquired thrombophilia: nephrotic syndrome, varicella, cyanogenic cardiopathy
- Prolonged parenteral nutrition

The usual treatment of CVC-related thrombosis is the removal of the catheter combined with administration of heparin or fibrinolytic drugs. In some cases, the catheter can be left in place to provide local thrombolysis and avoid potential clot dislodgment.

The risk of catheter-related *infection and sepsis* is inversely proportional to gestational age (in neonates) and directly proportional to the duration of catheterization, the use of parenteral nutrition, or mechanical ventilation. Prevention can be divided into an optimal placement (maximal barrier precautions, low number of attempts, and limited duration for placement) and meticulous care for the catheter (sterility, limited manipulations, renewal of dressing, and infusion tubing). Routine change of CVCs after a period of time is not advised if no local or systemic infection signs can be found. Differentiation between catheter infection and contamination is often difficult: peripheral and central blood cultures and catheter tip culture may clarify the diagnostic. If fever persists despite catheter change and antibiotics, endocarditis should be excluded.

Rupture of CVC is rare and almost limited to peripherally inserted central catheters (PICCs): forced attempts to flush blocked lines are a recognized risk. Medially inserted subclavian CVCs can get stuck in the costoclavicular pinch, where repeated respiratory movements can lead to erosion and rupture of the catheter.

19.3.3 Access to the Superior Vena Cava

The placement of peripherally inserted central catheters (PICCs) also aiming for the superior vena cava (SVC) will be discussed in a later paragraph. Any approach in the neck or around the clavicle carries the risk of pleural puncture. The volume of cervicothoracic veins is highly dependent on the respiratory cycle. During the inspiratory phase, especially in spontaneous breathing, the vein collapses and the lung expands, increasing the risks of pneumothorax and lowering the chance of success. It is therefore advised to use USG or to progress with the needle only during the expiratory phase.

To avoid tamponade and reduce the incidence of thrombosis, the catheter tip position in the SVC should be optimal as defined by the cavo-atrial junction. A location method should be used during placement to allow sterile repositioning before catheter fixation. Three methods can be used:

- *Fluoroscopy* is a versatile and widely used tool. It allows real-time guidance of the GW from the insertion point to its central position. In case of hindered GW migration, explanation can be given by the injection of radiopaque agent (phlebography). The optimal tip position is the point just above the right atrium shadow, situated at the thoracic vertebral level T2 or T3, a little lower than the carina. CVCs inserted from the right side can be left in the lower third of the SVC, while those inserted from the left side should be placed lower at the cavo-atrial junction or in the very initial portion of the right atrium in order to have a vertical position parallel to the SVC walls. Any oblique position or contact with the vein walls would increase the risk of perforation. To limit irradiation, guidance of the GW down to the SVC is done by US (Fig. 19.17). Fluoroscopy is only used shortly and with pediatric settings (reduced dose, closed diaphragm, pulsed X-ray impulse) for the final tip position.
- *ECG guidance* is a reliable method for tip position. This method will however be impossible in case of cardiac rhythm disorders or in case of aberrant GW migration.
- *Ultrasonography*: the initial part of the SVC can often be seen in the suprasternal fossa with the usual equipment (high-frequency linear probe). A curvilinear low-frequency probe is on the other hand needed to examine the right atrium or the distal part of the SVC. Cardiac ultrasonography for tip positioning requires thus special equipment, special training, and probably a second operator during placement. This method is not yet validated for accurate CVCs tip positioning.

The presence of a persistent left SVC is observed in 0.3–0.5 % children but can be 10 times more frequent in children with congenital heart defects. When catheterized, the GW or catheter is seen with fluoroscopy at the left side of the vertebral column above the heart shadow (Fig. 19.19).

19.3.3.1 The Internal Jugular Vein

Anatomy and Sonoanatomy

The internal jugular vein (IJV) runs at the latero-vertebral site of the neck, alongside the common carotid artery (CA) in a usual anterolateral position. At its distal end (where valves can be seen), it keeps a superficial track to reach the subclavian vein (SCV) and form the brachiocephalic vein (BCV), while the CA follows a deeper track. At the left side, the thoracic duct drains close to the jugulo-subclavian confluent increasing the risk of complications. US screening studies show that at the level of the cricoid:

- The relationship between IJV and CA is highly variable and unpredictable.
- In neutral position, the IJV overlaps the CA in 25–44 % of the cases and can be found medially in 6 % of the cases. [17]

Fig. 19.19 Presence of a persistent left superior vena cava. The catheter (*arrows*) inserted in the left subclavian vein migrates at the left side of the vertebral column

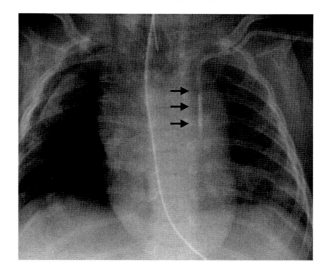

Fig. 19.20 The observed relationship between the internal jugular vein (IJV) (*V*) and the carotid artery (CA) (*A*) depends on the probe position. The vein is seen lateral (*position 1*) or anterior (*position 2*) to the artery. During US screening, the probe follows the curve surface of the neck overestimating the IJV–CA overlapping. To decrease overlapping and facilitate the anterior approach, the probe is held in a more vertical position (1)

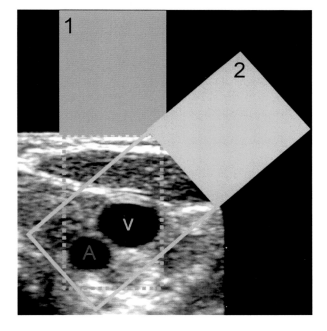

- When the head is progressively turned away from the puncture site and up to 45°, the incidence of overlapping increases even more [18]. These data's should however be read very carefully because the position of the probe in the neck is often not clearly defined and can have a major impact on the ultrasonographic findings, overestimating the real overlap (Fig. 19.20).

- The diameter of the IJV can be increased by Valsalva maneuver, Trendelenburg position, and liver compression. These effects are limited in infants less than 1 year of age where the distance IJV – right atrium – is short and the venous system highly compliant.

For all approaches, the child is placed 15–30° head-down with a rolled towel under the shoulders to increase venous pressure and reduce the risk of air embolism. The head is usually turned 30–45° away to give room for the needed approach. During landmark approaches, the skin over the vessels is stretched cranially by the nondominant hand to increase anteroposterior diameter of the vein and reduce its compressibility. For USG approaches, the skin has to be taped because the non-dominant hand holds the probe [19].

Landmark Approaches

Different "blind" or "landmark-guided" approaches to the IJV can be used in children. However, due to the clear recommendation to use US guidance [2–6] (see Table 19.1), blind approaches should only be used if USG is impossible (no equipment available, insufficient training and experience).

For *anterior approach*, the needle entry site is the convergence of the sternal and clavicular heads of the sternomastoid muscle or in infants halfway between the mastoid and the suprasternal notch. The needle is inserted 30–45° into the skin, just lateral from the carotid pulse, aiming for the ipsilateral nipple. The exploratory needle progresses during expiration with small movements, while negative pressure is created in the syringe.

For *posterior approach*, the needle entry site is on the lateral border of the clavicular head of the sternomastoid muscle, 1–3 cm (depending on age) above the clavicle. The needle is advanced underneath the muscle towards the suprasternal notch. Due to a needle direction towards important surrounding structures, like nerve roots, trachea, and esophagus, this approach is rarely used blindly in young children.

Ultrasound-Guided Approaches

US screening is performed in the neck from the cricoid level to the suprasternal fossa to check the patency of the IJV, the brachiocephalic vein (BCV), and the initial part of the SVC. Any found anomalies will influence the choice of approach (see Fig. 19.1). If the IJV is completely collapsing during inspiration, relative hypovolemia is suspected and administrating an IV fluid bolus and/or increasing the Trendelenburg position may improve the chance to succeed.

For the *anterior approach*, the probe is positioned perpendicular to the neck at the cricoid level (Fig. 19.21). Structure is followed from medial to lateral: trachea, thyroid gland, CA, and IJV (seen in a SAX view) [20]. An OOP approach is used and the needle tip visualized from the skin to its final intraluminal position by sliding or tilting movements of the probe (see Figs. 19.7 and 19.8). In infants and

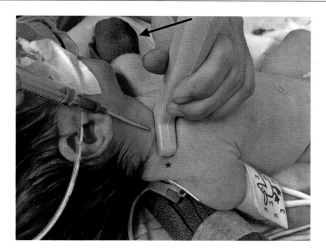

Fig. 19.21 Ultrasound-guided anterior approach of the IJV in infants: SAX view and OOP needle approach. The short neck forces the operator to place the probe above the clavicle and use a tilting movement (*arrow*) to follow the needle tip during its progression. *, needle insertion point for a USG posterior approach (SAX-IP)

neonates, the small size and high mobility of the IJV make punctures, even with US, often difficult. Moreover, the cranial – almost extrathoracic – position of the subclavian artery (SCA) and the lung top (under the distal part of the IJV) increases the risk of arterial or pleural puncture in this population (Fig. 19.22). Accidental arterial punctures during blind anterior approaches of the IJV were probably not only due to carotid but also to subclavian artery punctures. To facilitate GW insertion in these young children, it is interesting to bring the needle tip in the lowest part of the IJV or even in the BCV representing the only veins larger than the J-shaped GW.

For the *posterior approach*, the probe is placed in the same but slightly turned position offering an oblique SAX view of the IJV. The traditional needle approach, towards the suprasternal notch, is used by passing the needle under the length of the probe (IP approach) [1, 21]. This approach is rarely used in young children.

When choosing between anterior or posterior approach, the anatomy of the child (short neck), the operator preference (OOP or IP approach), but also the IJV–CA relationship will play a key role. The posterior approach is interesting when the IJV–CA overlap is important (vein on top of the artery). In that case, the lateromedial needle track reduces the risk of carotid puncture (Fig. 19.23).

Regardless of the approach used, the correct GW migration is checked by US before dilation and insertion of the catheter.

19.3.3.2 Periclavicular Approaches
Central venous catheters can be placed in different veins around the clavicle (Fig. 19.24) [1]:

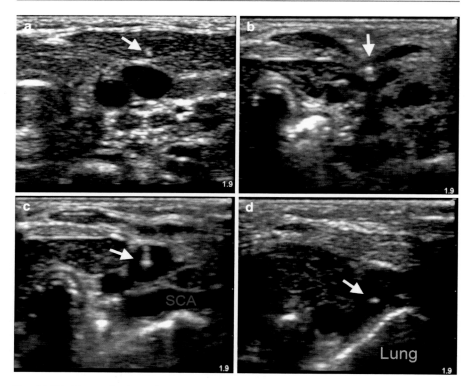

Fig. 19.22 Short-axis view of the right IJV during an anterior OOP approach. (**a**) Needle tip (*arrow*) above the vein; (**b**) needle tip passing the anterior wall; (**c**) needle tip in the IJV lumen above the subclavian artery (*SCA*); (**d**) needle tip brought in the brachiocephalic vein above the lung top to facilitate guide wire insertion

- The brachiocephalic vein (BCV), by a supraclavicular approach
- The subclavian vein (SCV), by an infraclavicular approach or, for its distal part, by the supraclavicular approach
- The axillary vein (AxV), by an infraclavicular transpectoral approach

Each of these approaches has their own advantages and disadvantages and can be applied to all or a certain age category (Table 19.5). The visualization and puncture of these veins are possible and already used for years; however, due to the absence of randomized controlled trials, no recommendations are currently given [2–4, 6]. Only a group of international experts have stated that USG should be used for all the CVC placements in children [5].

From the neck region, the end of the IJV joins with the SCV to form the BCV or innominate vein. The right BCV is shorter and makes a steeper intrathoracic angle compared to the left BCV (Fig. 19.25). The subclavian vessels and BCVs of infants have a more cranial and superficial position compared to children and adults, improving US visualization and puncture. By starting with the well-known SAX

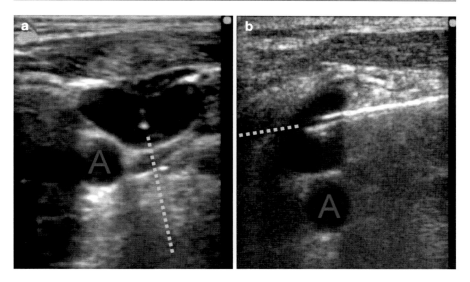

Fig. 19.23 Internal jugular vein (IJV)–carotid artery (CA) relationship is important to chose between anterior or posterior approach of the IJV. With the anterior approach (**a**), the needle track is posterior while it is medial with the posterior approach (**b**). The posterior approach is interesting when there is a major IJV–CA overlap

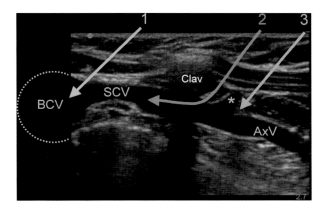

Fig. 19.24 Three possible periclavicular approaches: (*1*) supraclavicular approach of the brachio-cephalic vein (*BCV*), (*2*) infraclavicular approach of the subclavian vein (*SCV*), and (*3*) infracla-vicular approach of the axillary vein (AxV). *Clav*, clavicle; *, cephalic vein

view of the IJV at the cricoid level, the US probe has to slide caudally to the clavicle to see the distal part of the IJV with the subclavian artery (SCA) passing under. When the probe comes in contact with the clavicle, the probe is tilted caudally to have a view of the BCV behind the clavicle. From this position, the probe is rotated slightly with its lateral side towards the axilla to see the SCV (Fig. 19.26). The SCA and the brachial plexus are thus more cranial, separated from the SCV by the ante-rior scalene muscle.

Table 19.5 Comparison between three different periclavicular approaches for CVC placement in children

Approach – Targeted vein	Guidance	Age categories	USG technique	Advantages	Disadvantages
Supraclavicular – brachiocephalic vein	US	All	LAX–IP	Large and open vein Easy puncture	Central approach Exit site ! brachial plexus
Infraclavicular – subclavian vein	US/LM	All[a]	LAX–IP LAX–OOP[a]	Open vein Safe progression Exit site	Shadow clavicle Orientation children/ adolescents[a]
Transpectoral – axillary vein	US	(Children) adolescents	SAX–OOP LAX–IP	Exit site Comfort	Depth Compressibility vein Proximity pleura

US ultrasound, *LM* landmark
[a]The US-guided infraclavicular approach of the subclavian can be more difficult in older children (visualization of the vein, 3D orientation, initial OOP approach)

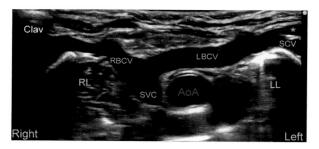

Fig. 19.25 Panoramic view of the major veins leading to the superior vena cava (*SVC*). Note the difference in length and angulation of the right and left brachiocephalic veins (*RBCV–LBCV*). *SCV* subclavian vein, *RL–LL* right and left lungs, *Clav* clavicle, *AoA* aortic arch, * external jugular vein

From the arm, basilic and brachial veins fuse together to form the AxV, which receive the cephalic vein just before its passage under the clavicle. The AxV changes name by passing above the first rib. Above the clavicle, the external jugular vein coming cranially makes a medial turn to become parallel and fuse with the SCV.

Supraclavicular Access to the Brachiocephalic Vein

Although described with landmark approaches, blind punctures of the BCV have never been widely used in children. With US, the BCV is probably the largest vein visible, remaining "open" even in hypovolemic patients. This is a great rescue technique when other techniques have failed, or in cases of expected difficulties (low-weight preterm infants, hypovolemia, and IJV or SCV thrombosis). Used electively in young children, this approach showed excellent results: high success rate even in neonates, extremely low incidence of arterial puncture, and no cases of

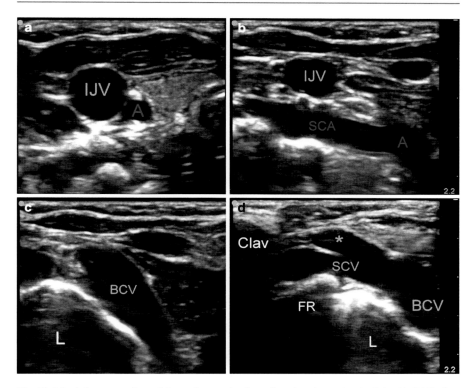

Fig. 19.26 A four-step view of the major cervicothoracic veins above the clavicle. (**a**) SAX view of the internal jugular vein (*IJV*) at the cricoid level. (**b**) Subclavian artery (*SCA*) passing under the distal part of the IJV (probe slided above the clavicle). (**c**) Brachiocephalic vein (*BCV*) (probe tilted cranially above the clavicle). (**d**) Subclavian vein (*SCV*) (probe tilted and rotated towards the axilla above the clavicle). *A* carotid artery, *L* lung top, *FR* first rib, * external jugular vein

pneumothorax [22–24]. Insertion time seems shorten with this technique compared to the USG infraclavicular access of the SCV [25].

Ultrasound-Guided Approach
The child is placed in a slight Trendelenburg position with a rolled towel under the shoulders. The head is turned to the opposite side. The 2-step technique to see the BCV is simple and has a short learning curve: from the cricoid level (IJV), caudal sliding to reach the clavicle followed by tilting of the probe to look behind the clavicle (Fig. 19.26). The degree of cranial tilting of the probe required to see the vein is inversely proportional to the age of the child. The cranial position of the BCV in infants allows their visualization with a limited probe tilting (Fig. 19.27) compared to older children where the probe is tilted a lot, often touching the child's chin (see Fig. 19.30). A strict in-plane (IP) needle approach is used to monitor closely the needle tip progression at any moment (vertical and medial direction towards the mediastinum). The needle should be inserted close to the US probe, not

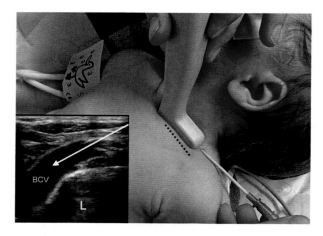

Fig. 19.27 Supraclavicular approach of the brachiocephalic vein (*BCV*). LAX view of the BCV; IP approach above the clavicle (*dotted line*). Tilting the probe is often not necessary in infant due to the cranial position of the vessels. *L* lung top

too lateral in the supraclavicular fossa, to avoid inadvertent subclavian artery or brachial plexus damage.

Infraclavicular Access to the Subclavian Vein

The SCV is a short vein (from 1 cm in neonates to 3–4 cm in adolescents) running from midclavicular to the distal end of the IJV close to the sternoclavicular joint. The direction of the vein is flat behind the clavicle in children and cranial towards the cricoid in infants.

To access the SCV, a rolled towel is placed under the shoulders, the head moderately turned away from the puncture site with the arm along the body, and the table tilted 15–30° head-down. The left SCV is often preferred because it continues into the BCV in a smoother way compared to the right SCV (Fig. 19.25).

Landmark Approach

The puncture site is below the clavicle, in the deltopectoral groove, at the midclavicular level, where the external jugular vein can sometimes be seen on the other side of the clavicle. More lateral approaches increase the risk of subclavian artery puncture and brachial plexus injury. The needle is slightly bent in its middle to make it progress upwards and away from the pleura when passing under the clavicle. The skin is entered 0.5–1 cm below the lower border of the clavicle to avoid any later kinking of the catheter. The exploratory needle is advanced only during expiration to decrease the risk of pleural puncture. When passing under the clavicle, the attached syringe, maintaining a negative pressure, is lowered and the needle directed to:

- The cricoid or the opposite ear lobe in infants less than 6 months
- The midway between the cricoid and the suprasternal notch in infant over 6 months
- The suprasternal notch in children

The needle should never be inserted over a distance superior to the distance from the insertion point to the suprasternal notch. Aspiration of blood can only appear during slow needle withdrawal. If arterial blood is aspirated, SCA puncture is suspected due to too cranial and deep attempts. When inserting the GW, tilting the head towards the puncture side or compressing the end of the IJV prevents catheter malposition in the ipsilateral IJV.

Ultrasound-Guided Approach [26]

The same positioning is used as for the landmark approach, but Trendelenburg position will only be used if needed (small or highly collapsible vein). Head rotation needs sometimes to be increased to allow US probe positioning. Supraclavicular visualization of the SCV is obtained with a 3-step technique from the SAX view of the IJV at the cricoid level: sliding down to the clavicle, tilting cranially, and rotating laterally to the axilla (Fig. 19.26). Pulling the arm downwards flattens the clavicle and increases the visible length of the SCV.

Puncture techniques depend on the age category:

- In infants (Fig. 19.28): the cranial, almost extrathoracic, position of the SCV facilitates US visualization. The end position of the probe showing the SCV will be from the midclavicular to the cricoid. The needle is inserted with an IP approach under the clavicle and strictly under the long axis of the probe. The needle is seen touching and passing under the clavicle. Needle and probe alignment is precisely kept because the US shadow under the clavicle will hinder needle visualization for a short moment. As soon as the needle has passed under the clavicle, its bevel will reappear, allowing US guidance in the lumen of the SCV. With experience and when visualization is good, the needle tip is brought further in the BCV, which is the optimal place to insert the GW. Because the SCV is fixed under the clavicle and doesn't collapse under the pressure of the approaching needle, this technique is found very useful in preterm neonates where IJV punctures are difficult even with USG (Fig. 19.29).
- In children (Fig. 19.30): important tilting of the probe (often touching the child's chin) is often needed to get a view of the SCV. The probe is kept above and parallel to the clavicle (no clavicle or shadowing is seen). The focus is set on the SCV and the initial part of the BCV. The needle insertion point and direction are the same as that for the landmark approach. The bended needle is inserted below the clavicle in order to pass under the US probe with an oblique OOP approach. Once the needle tip (hyperechoic dot) is detected, its cranial progression is stopped to prevent any inadvertent puncture of the SCA and redirected to the suprasternal notch becoming almost an IP approach (needle seen partially in its length). The optimal tip position (centered in the SCV or BCV) is reached before insertion of the GW.

The migration of the GW is always checked by US before dilation and insertion of the catheter. If needed, the guide wire is redirected in real time under USG (see Fig. 19.17). When the GW migrates into the ipsilateral IJV, it can be withdrawn and reinserted after having used the US probe to compress the distal end of the IJV.

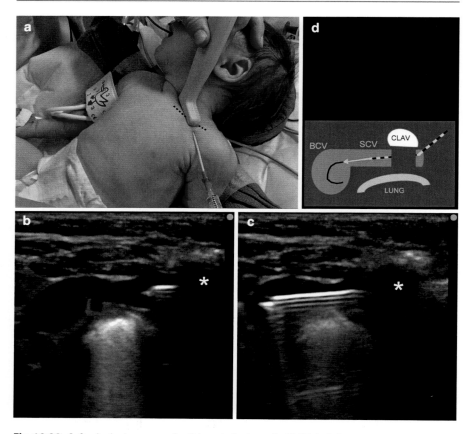

Fig. 19.28 Infraclavicular approach of the subclavian vein (*SCV*) in infants. (**a**) Probe positioned above the clavicle (*dotted line*) with a cranial orientation from midclavicular to the cricoid. The needle is inserted under the clavicle with an IP approach. (**b**, **c**) Needle passing under the clavicle (***), entering the SCV and progressing into the brachiocephalic vein (*BCV*). (**d**) Guide wire insertion is easier when the needle tip is positioned at the BCV

Transpectoral Access to the Axillary Vein

The axillary vein (AxV) and artery are found close to each other in the infraclavicular region. The artery surrounded cranially by the brachial plexus is more cranial and deeper than the vein. The vessels pass deep under the pectoral muscles and cross the clavicle at the midclavicular level.

Only used with USG, this approach is the classic approach for "subclavian accesses" in adults [27]. The difficulty of this technique is that the AxV is deep, close to the pleura, and highly compressible (inspiration or approaching needle). Experienced operators have however shown excellent results in adults. Its use in children is limited and probably only recommended in adolescents. Small needles from PICC insertion sets can be used to reduce depression of the punctured vein. The introducer of these sets allows the insertion of most classic pediatric CVCs.

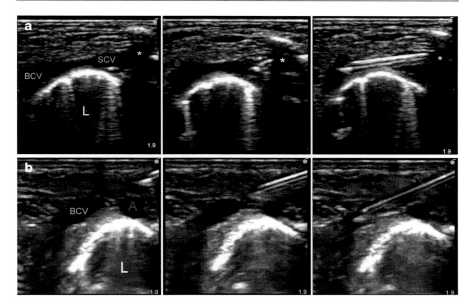

Fig. 19.29 Central venous catheter insertion in preterm neonates (800 g) using two different approaches. Veins are very small: 1.5 mm for the subclavian (*SCV*) and 3 mm for the brachiocephalic vein (*BCV*). (**a**) Infraclavicular approach of the SCV. *, clavicle. (**b**) Supraclavicular approach of the BCV. *A* Subclavian artery. *L* Lung top. Both approaches are in-plane (IP) approaches. In both cases, the needle tip is brought in the BCV to insert the guide wire

Transpectoral approaches, by avoiding any bony contact, are comfortable and can be proposed to older awake children.

Ultrasound-Guided Approaches

Two different approaches can be used depending on the age of the patient and the preference of the operator:

- The OOP approach (Fig. 19.31): a SAX view of the axillary vessels is obtained by placing the probe in sagittal oblique position below the clavicle. The clavicle and its shadow are seen cranially followed by the axillary artery (AxA) and more caudally and superficially the AxV. The cephalic vein is seen merging in the end of the AxV just before passing under the clavicle. The needle progression is followed through the pectoral muscles, entering the AxV by sliding or tilting the probe. This approach has the advantage of a constant view of the artery and pleura and the relative closeness of the insertion site to the clavicle.
- The IP approach (Fig. 19.32): a LAX view of the vein is obtained by placing the probe in an oblique position from the midclavicular to the axilla, the medial part of the probe lying on the clavicle. The vein and artery cannot be seen simultaneously. It is mandatory to differentiate clearly the AxV from the AxA: the vein is more caudal and superficial, it is not pulsating but its diameter changes with

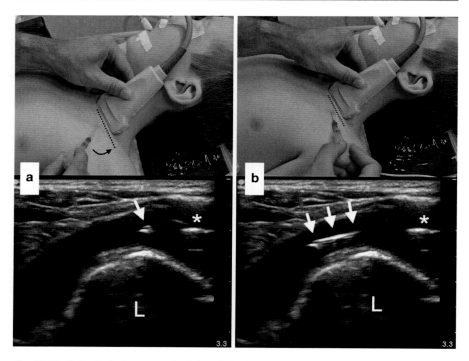

Fig. 19.30 Infraclavicular approach of the subclavian (SCV) in a 10-year-old child. LAX view of the SCV obtained by tilting the probe cranially above the clavicle (*dotted lines*). (**a**) The needle is inserted under the clavicle with an oblique out-of-plane (OOP) approach. When the needle tip is seen as a dot (*white arrow*), the needle is reorientated medially to the sternal notch (*black arrow*). (**b**) By changing needle orientation, the approach becomes almost in-plane (IP), allowing the needle to appear as a line (*white arrows*) progressing in the SCV. *L* lung, * external jugular vein

inspiration, and the cephalic vein merges in its distal portion and valves can be seen in its lumen. Once the vein is identified, the skin is punctured with a strict IP approach. The anterior wall of the vein is compressed and the needle flattened to avoid transfixion. This approach has the advantage of a constant view of the needle tip and shaft and the disadvantage of a more lateral exit site of the catheter, reserving this approach to older children.

Whatever the approach used, it is advised to enter the vein close to its passage under the clavicle because at that point the vein is fixed anteriorly and kept open. The depth and compressibility of the vein combined with the proximity of the pleura force the operator to be careful and already experienced in USG.

19.3.3.3 Complications Associated with SVC Catheterization

Immediate complications are:

- Pneumothorax
- Hemothorax

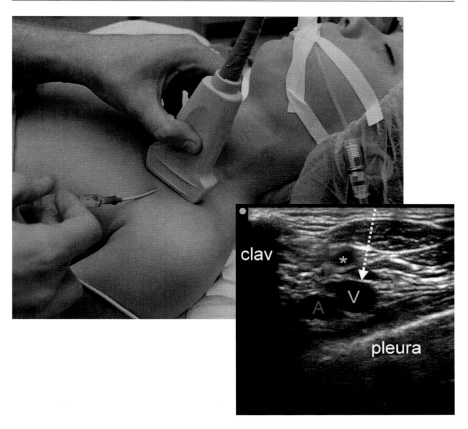

Fig. 19.31 Out-of-plane infraclavicular approach of the axillary vein. SAX view of the vessels obtained under the clavicle. The vein is punctured close to the clavicle (*clav*). *A* axillary artery, *V* axillary vein, * cephalic vein

- Catheter malposition: possible malposition when blood can be aspirated are the thymic, intercostal and azygos veins. The latter, missed on a classic chest X-ray, will require a profile view. Catheters can also migrate in a persistent left SVC (see Fig. 19.19). If no blood can be aspirated, migration in the mediastinum, epidural, or subarachnoid space is possible.

Late complications are:

- Trauma of the thoracic duct (left) or great lymphatic vein (right) leading to yellowish spillage at the insertion point that increases after meals
- Chylothorax, usually caused by venous thrombosis in the area where those lymphatic ducts drain

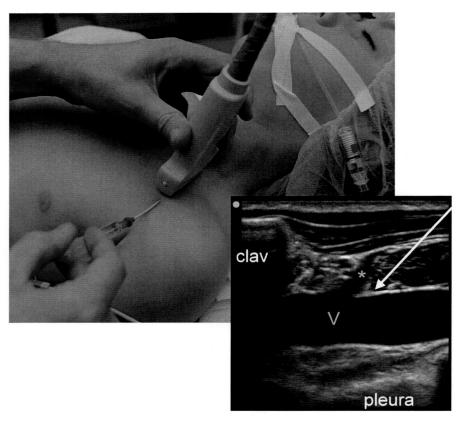

Fig. 19.32 In-plane infraclavicular approach of the axillary vein. LAX view of the axillary vein (*V*) obtained under the clavicle. The vein is punctured close to the clavicle (*clav*) (*arrow*). * cephalic vein

19.3.4 Access to the Inferior Vena Cava

19.3.4.1 The Femoral Vein

The femoral access is useful during reanimation (far from the neck and the chest) but also when other sites are unavailable. In infants and children, the femoral vein (FV) catheterization shows almost the same incidence of infection and mechanical complications as SCV or IJV access. This access is also often used for temporary hemodialysis in young children. Compression in this region is easy in case of venous or arterial hematoma.

Anatomy

The diameter of the FV is around 4 mm at 1 year and 10 mm at the age of nine. The mean diameter of the vein can be increased by using either a reverse Trendelenburg position, a firm compression 1–2 cm above the inguinal ligament, or a combination of them [28]. These maneuvers are also useful to check the patency of femoral and iliac veins.

At the level of the inguinal ligament, US examinations have shown high variability in the position of the FV [29]. Usually medial to the femoral artery (FA), it can be found completely below the artery in some cases. Distally to the inguinal ligament, this overlapping increases even more. External rotation of the hip will reduce this overlapping and bring the vein median to the artery. A small pad can be placed under the buttocks of infants to give a better exposure of the groin.

The ideal position for the catheter tip is at the intervertebral level L4–L5 or maximum L3–L4, at distance of the renal veins implantations. The approximative catheter length for an L3 level is 0.14× the size of the child in cm + 1.49 [30].

Landmark Approach

In a reverse Trendelenburg position, the leg of the child is placed in a straight position with the hip slightly rotated externally. If available, at least US screening should be used to compare both the right and left FV (vein size and importance of FA overlapping). The insertion point is 0.5–1 cm below the inguinal ligament and 0.5 cm medial to the femoral pulse. The needle is inserted with a 30° angle parallel to the femoral pulse in the direction of the umbilicus. Steeper and deeper puncture may injure the coxofemoral articulation.

Ultrasound-Guided Approach

The use of USG for the FV access is recommended in children and infants with strength of recommendation varying from weak to strong [2–6] (see Table 19.1). USG has shown to, at least, reduce the incidence of arterial puncture and often reduce the procedure time and increase the success rate [31].

The probe is placed just below and parallel to the inguinal ligament to obtain a SAX view of the vessels. The image quality is often much lower than in the neck region, especially in young children. Visualization of the FA bifurcation or the cross of the saphenous vein indicates a too distal position of the probe. If the FV is located below the FA, external hip rotation, or even knee flexion (frog-leg position), is tested to find the optimal leg position to reduce vessel overlapping (Fig. 19.33). Abdominal or inguinal compression is performed to test the patency of the femoral and iliac veins (positive if cross section increases). An OOP needle approach is used to enter the vein in its middle (Fig. 19.34). The probe is tilted towards the legs during needle progression to follow the needle tip. Transfixion of the vein can be difficult to avoid in infants. After insertion, the correct GW migration is checked by US before dilation and insertion of the catheter.

19.3.4.2 Complication Associated with IVC Catheterization

These specific complications include:

- Extravasation of fluid in the retroperitoneal cavity.
- Catheter migration in the perimedullar space via the left lumbar and epidural veins. A right FV approach seems to reduce this complication due to the increased angulation between the femoral and lumbar veins on the right side [32]. Only a lateral X-ray can detect this rare complication.

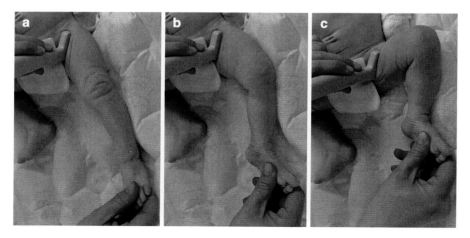

Fig. 19.33 US screening before femoral vein catheterization. The best leg position to reduce vessel overlapping is searched. (**a**) Straight leg position (vein often overlapped by the artery); (**b**) external rotation of the hip (often the optimal position); (**c**) external rotation combined with knee and hip flexion (frog-leg position)

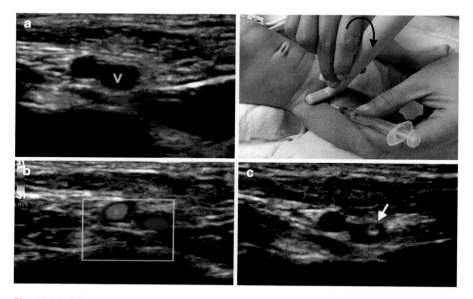

Fig. 19.34 Ultrasound-guided femoral vein puncture. SAX view of the femoral vein (FV) and OOP needle approach. Probe tilting is used to follow the progression of the needle tip (*black arrow*). (**a**) The FV is median to the femoral artery; (**b**) US screening with Doppler function; (**c**) needle (*white arrow*) entering the vein

- Lower limb ischemia: in case of inadvertent FA puncture and complete thrombosis.
- Portal vein thrombosis (see umbilical access).

19.4   Peripherally Inserted Central Catheters

Peripherally inserted central catheters (PICCs) have been used for decades in the neonatal population for intermediate to long-term IV therapy. New materials (low-diameter, high-volume catheters) and improved insertion techniques (USG, micro-introducers) have resulted in PICC now being used for a larger variety of purposes in a broader pediatric population [33]. PICCs are by definition inserted through a peripheral vein (usually in the upper limb) and are positioned with their tip in the lower third of the VCI. Shorter catheters (called midlines) with lengths from 10 to 25 cm can also be used as "improved" peripheral access: their tip, usually in the axillary or subclavian vein, does not reach a central position. These two catheters represent interesting alternatives to avoid repeated peripheral venipunctures (source of significant stress) or the placement of a CVC.

19.4.1 Indications

PICCs are indicated when intermediate- to long-term IV access is needed for medications (antibiotics, chemotherapy), fluid therapy, blood sampling, or parenteral nutrition. Together with the midlines, they complete the available offer of catheter types that can be adapted to the needs of children. When a child needs an IV treatment, there is a reflexion on which is the best catheter for him regarding his venous capital, the type of medication, the length of treatment, and the treatment setting (in the hospital, at home, or both) (Fig. 19.35). midlines can be

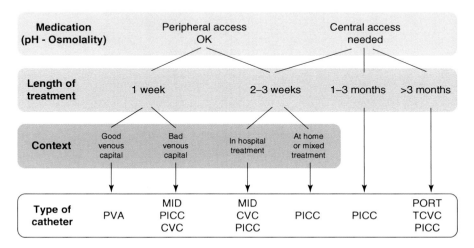

Fig. 19.35 Decision-making tree to find the most appropriate type of catheter needed by the child. Venous capital of the child, type of medications, length of treatment, and treatment setting (in hospital or ambulatory) are important factors. *PVA* peripheral venous access, *MID* midline, *PICC* peripherally inserted central catheter, *CVC* central venous catheter, *PORT* port-a-cath, *TCVC* tunneled CVC

used for up to 3 weeks if the child does not need a central venous access (CVA). PICCs are used if a CVA is needed and/or if the expected length of the treatment exceeds 3 weeks. PICCs are probably the best option for home therapy or if the child alternates in hospital treatments and periods at home. PICCs have therefore shown their value in long-term treatment (up to 1 year) of oncological children [34].

PICCs and midlines are compared to more classic catheters in Table 19.6. Compared to CVCs that usually require GA for insertion, PICCs can often be inserted with light or even no sedation in school-age children. Serious complications described with central approaches, such as severe hematoma, pneumothorax/hemothorax, or air embolism, are extremely rare during PICC insertion. The cost of a PICC catheter is higher than a CVC catheter, but it can be used for a longer period of time and sometimes allows children to continue their treatment at home.

Contraindications for PICC placement are few: local skin damage (infection, burn, radiation), peripheral vein damage (stenosis or thrombosis caused by previous catheter insertion), or central vein damage (stenosis, thrombosis of the ipsilateral SCV or the SVC) may hinder venipuncture or hamper catheter advancement to the correct targeted position. An alternative should be considered in children with chronic renal failure or end-stage renal disease to preserve veins for the formation of an arteriovenous fistula for dialysis. Technical insertion difficulties are more frequent in young children (<2 years/12 kg), and experience will be required in this population.

19.4.2 Catheter Placement

PICC insertions in the forearm or the antecubital fossa by palpation are almost abandoned due to their association with increased incidences of bleeding, phlebitis,

Table 19.6 Comparison between different peripheral and central venous accesses

	PVA	MID	PICC	CVC	PORT or TCVC
Life span	Days	2–3 weeks	Weeks–months	Weeks	Months–years
Necessitate GA or sedation	No	Sometimes	Sometimes	Always	Always
Insertion[a]	Easy	Easy	Easy	Difficult	Difficult
Insertion complications	No	Rare	Rare	Potential	Potential
Systemic complications	No	No	Less frequent	Potential	Potential
Removal	Ward	Ward/home	Ward/home	Ward	Surgery
Cost	+	++	+++	++	++++

PVA peripheral venous access, *MID* midlines, *PICCs* peripherally inserted central catheters, *CVC* central venous catheters, *PORT* port-a-cath, *TCVC* tunneled CVC

[a]Insertion difficulty depends on experience of the operator and age of the child

thrombosis, and discomfort. USG seems mandatory to aim for veins at the arm level and to reach higher success rates.

19.4.2.1 Sedation
The need for sedation will depend on the experience and confidence of the child. Children younger than 6 years will often need some kind of sedation or light general anesthesia (spontaneous breathing with facial or laryngeal masks), while older children (>10 years) often accept placement under local anesthesia. In between, different protocols have been tested alone or combined: midazolam premedication, EMLA® cream application, inhalation of 50 % nitrous oxide, and hypnosis.

19.4.2.2 Vein Selection
Three to four veins can be used for PICC insertion at each arm. Variability is however important and only US screening will help to decide which is the best vein to catheterize (Fig. 19.36). The choices are usually the following:

- n° 1: The basilic vein: superficial, good diameter, straight course
- n° 2: One of the brachial veins: good diameter, straight course to the axillary vein but deeper and close to the nerves and artery
- n° 3: The cephalic vein: superficial, small size, and tortuous course below the clavicle (higher incidence of thrombosis)

19.4.2.3 Catheter Selection
PICCs are made of polyurethane or silicone; the latter is softer and seems to be associated with a lower risk of thrombosis even if the literature remains controversial. The distal end of PICCs can be opened or closed by a valve (Groshong® – Bard). The advantage of a "closed end" is that the valve prevents any reflux of blood in the catheter, reducing the risk of catheter occlusion. The size of the inserted PICC is chosen according to the age of the child and the diameter of the vein. To lower the incidence of thrombosis, only 1/3 of the lumen should be filled by the catheter (Fig. 19.37a):

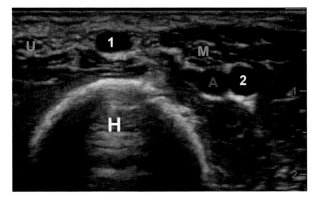

Fig. 19.36 US screening at mid-arm level for the placement of PICCs. The two most appropriate veins are (*1*) the basilic vein and (*2*) one of the brachial veins. *H* humerus, *A* brachial artery, *U* ulnar nerve, *M* medial nerve

Fig. 19.37 Prevention and detection of PICC-related peripheral thrombosis. (**a**) LAX view of the basilic vein after PICC insertion. Sufficient room for blood flow around the catheter reduces the risk of thrombosis. (**b**) LAX view of another basilic vein before puncture. An almost completed thrombosis, due to a previous PICC, is pointed out by the Doppler analyze

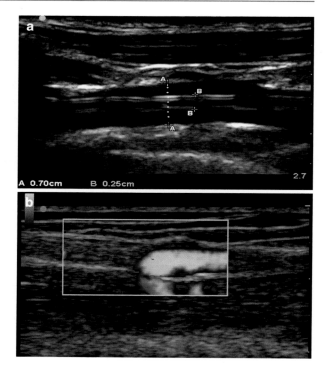

- PICC 1 F: neonates < 1500 g
- PICC 2 F: neonates > 1500 g
- PICC 3 F: age < 6 years and vein > 3 mm
- PICC 4 F: age > 6 years and vein > 4 mm
- PICC 5 F: age > 10 years and vein > 5 mm (5 F = double lumen)

19.4.2.4 Insertion Technique (Fig. 19.38)

The arm of the child is placed in abduction on a table. After placement of a tourniquet, US screening is performed to assess the anatomy of the arm, to chose the best vein (size and accessibility) and the adapted the catheter size. Maximal barrier precautions are applied as for any CVC placement including sterile probe cover and gel for the US equipment. The vein is usually viewed in SAX and punctured with an OOP needle approach. The tip of the tiny needle is followed entering and catheterizing the vein by slow sliding movement of the probe towards the axilla. A guide wire is inserted into the vein (Seldinger technique), a small incision of the skin is made, and the dilator and peel-away introducer are placed. "Open-ended" catheters have to be cut at the appropriate length before insertion. The length is determined by measurement along the course of the vein to the SVC using a tape included in the PICC set. "Close-ended" catheters are introduced and cut distally after confirmation of the tip placement by fluoroscopy. Flexion of the patient's head forwards and towards the ipsilateral shoulder reduces the risk of advancing the catheter into the jugular veins.

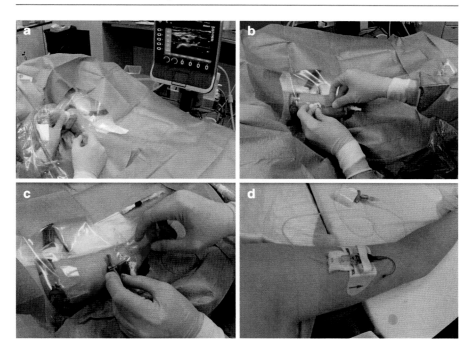

Fig. 19.38 Insertion of a peripherally inserted central catheter on the left arm of a child. (**a**) Sterile dressing and positioning during a USG puncture at mid-arm level (SAX–OOP technique). (**b**) Insertion of the dilator and introducer over the guide wire. (**c**) Insertion of the PICC in the peel-away introducer. (**d**) Fixation by a suture-free StatLock® above the antecubital fossa

19.4.2.5 Catheter Tip Positioning

A non-central placement of the PICC increases the risk of mechanical and thrombotic complications. It is therefore advised to avoid blind insertions and to use either ECG guidance or fluoroscopy. The ideal position is the cavo-atrial junction when the arm is in adduction with the elbow slightly flexed. Fluoroscopy seems to be the easiest and most reliable and versatile tool because it shows the cavo-atrial junction with precision but also helps to direct the PICC from the arm (using phlebography) to the SVC (Fig. 19.39). Irradiation should however be reduced as much as possible in children by using adapted doses and short pulsed emission of X-ray and by closing the diaphragm.

19.4.3 Fixation and Maintenance

PICCs are fixed by a suture-free securing device (StatLock®, BARD) and covered by a transparent dressing. To increase comfort, the fixation should not reach the antecubital fossa and can therefore be placed above the insertion point (Fig. 19.38d). The dressing has to be changed every week and the catheter flushed with 10 ml of

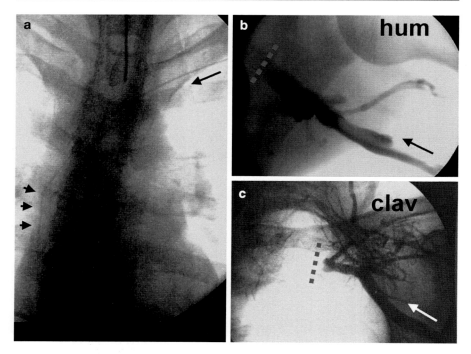

Fig. 19.39 The use of fluoroscopy during PICC insertions. Precise positioning of the catheter tip at the cavo-atrial junction (**a**). Phlebography detecting complete axillary vein thrombosis at the arm (**b**) or infraclavicular level (**c**)

saline every 3 days for "open-ended" catheters and every week for "close-ended" ones. Different waterproof PICC covers exist and allow children to take a shower or a bath or even to go for a swim.

19.4.4 Complications

The overall rates of complications are low in the pediatric population ranging from 1 to 19 per thousand catheter days (TCD), but only 1/3 are serious requiring antibiotic treatment or removal of the PICC. Complication rate increases with patient age <5 years, double-lumen catheters, and multiple daily uses [35].

19.4.4.1 Mechanical Problems

Mechanical complications are rarely life-threatening but may result in the interruption of treatment and need for replacement of the PICC [33]. The most frequent problems are:

- Occlusion of the catheter (0–10 per TCD): caused by a thrombosis, injections of incompatible drugs, or insufficient flushing after blood samples. Careful flushing

with saline or instillation of fibrinolytic agents reduces the incidence of irreversible occlusion to less than 2 per TCD.
- Breakage or leakage (0–2 per TCD): usually due to a forceful attempt to unlock a blocked line with small syringes. PICC should only be flushed with large 10 ml syringes to reduce the injection pressure. Leakage at the catheter exit site can be handled by using a repair kit (new connector), while catheter fracture and embolization within the skin will need a radiologic intervention to retrieve the embolized fragment.
- Accidental dislodgment (0.1–3 per TCD): more frequent in the pediatric population than in the adult or neonatal population.

19.4.4.2 Infection
The PICC-associated infection rate is low (0.2–6.4 per TCD) [33, 36], much lower than for classic CVCs and close to the infection rate of long-term devices (ports and tunneled lines). The risk factors are the length of treatment >21 days, infusion of parenteral nutrition, children with chronic metabolic diseases, and treatment setting (intensive care > in hospital > ambulatory).

19.4.4.3 Thrombosis
PICC-related thromboses are rare and can be divided into peripheral thrombosis (at the arm level) and central thrombosis (as for any CVC) [33, 37]. Peripheral vein thrombosis (incidence 3–4 per TCD) is often asymptomatic but will hinder future catheter placements (Fig. 19.37b). Symptomatic PICC-related central thrombosis is extremely rare (incidence from 0 to 0.2 per TCD).

The specific risk factors are:

- Hematological or oncological disease
- Catheter too large for the vein
- Double-lumen catheter
- Suboptimal, non-central, tip positioning
- History of catheter infection or occlusion
- Long insertion time

19.5 Intraosseous Route

19.5.1 Description

By placing a needle in the medullary cavity, the intraosseous (IO) route gives access to the systemic circulation by an insertion point that is not collapsible or dependent on the volemic status of the child. This access is however an urgent and temporary solution used only if a life-threatening condition occurs when no other venous access could be found (cardiac arrest, polytrauma, major burns). The IO access is rapid and does not usually require general anesthesia compared to CVC placements. It can be used when peripheral access is impossible and waiting for fasting conditions (to place a CVC) represents an excessive risk for the child.

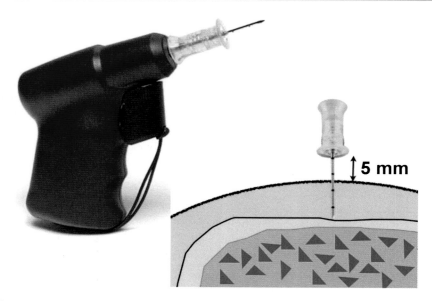

Fig. 19.40 The intraosseous route. The EZ-IO® electric drill is one of the most friendly devices. The needle length is appropriate if the 5 mm mark can still be seen when bone contact occurs

Any medication or fluid can be given by this route. Pharmacokinetics of injected drugs is not known, but the usual posology is advised. Medications are flushed with 5–10 ml of saline. The IO route is used till another (peripheral or central) access is found and usually withdrawn within 24 h.

19.5.2 Perioperative Indications

The IO route is rarely used in the operating room. Different circumstances occurring after inhalational anesthesia should however be considered as indications if no venous access is found rapidly: hemodynamic instability, severe laryngospasm or bleeding compromising the upper airway patency, and impossible venous access in remote location [38]. IO devices should be present in the operating department, their location known by everyone, and anesthesiologists should be trained to use them.

19.5.3 Technique

Three different devices can be used to create an IO route: manually inserted needles (Cook®), air pressure guns (Bone Injection Gun®), and small electric drills (EZ-IO®). A better success rate is found when the drilling machines are used, especially when the operator has almost no experience as most anesthesiologists do [39].

Different sites of insertion can be used in children (distal femur, distal tibia, proximal humerus, iliac crest), but the easiest and safest site for novice operators is the proximal part of the tibia. The insertion point is 1–2 cm (0.5–1 cm in neonates) below and medial to the anterior tibial tuberosity. The needle is pushed through the skin in contact with the bone (at least 5 mm of the needle should remain outside the skin), and the drill is then activated till a loss of resistance is felt (Fig. 19.40). The needle should be firmly fixed into the bone and some blood or bone marrow collected by aspiration. Injection of 5–10 ml of saline should be easy without any sign of extravasation. The needle is firmly fixed and regular inspection of the surrounding skin is performed.

19.5.4 Contraindication

Contraindication for the placement of an IO route can be local (fractured bone, previous IOR (or attempts) in the same bone within 48 h, local infection) or systemic (osteoporosis and osteogenesis imperfecta, right-to-left intracardiac shunt).

19.5.5 Complications

The most frequent complications are extravasation (4–12 %) and needle dislodgment (8–10 %). Severe complications are rare: compartment syndrome (0.6 %) and osteomyelitis (0.5 %) [40]. Fractures were described but are extremely rare, and lesion of the growth plate and fat embolism are theoretical.

19.6   Arterial Access

19.6.1 Indications and Equipment

The placement of an arterial line is indicated in case of surgeries associated with major blood loss or potential hemodynamic instability (when vasoactive drugs are expected to be used), but also if difficult perioperative ventilation is foreseen or postoperative ventilation planned. The most commonly used arteries are the radial and femoral arteries, but other different sites can be used.

Short cannulas (24 G for neonates and 22 G for children) are usually used, but a Seldinger method can be chosen for femoral access in older children.

The needle is inserted through the skin with a flat 20° angle, watching for blood return in its hub. Slow insertion of the cannula prevents vasospasm and arterial trauma.

The cannula is carefully fixed to avoid both accidental removal and kinking at the puncture site.

Tubing and transducer are once more flushed with the heparinized solution just before the connection to the cannula in order to eliminate any bubble of air. A transparent dressing is applied to allow visual inspection of the skin proximal and distal to the entry site to detect early signs of ischemic complications. The heparinized solution should contain 0.5 IU of heparin/ml and be flushed at a constant rate of 1 ml/h.

Blood samplings are performed very slowly to prevent the vessel from collapsing. After each sample, the tubing is flushed gently by hand with a maximal speed of 1 ml over a period of 5 s. Any blanching of the skin should reduce even more the speed of injection.

The arterial line is clearly identified to avoid the accidental intra-arterial injection of any perioperative medication.

19.6.2 The Radial Artery

The forearm of the child is fixed in a stable horizontal position with the wrist taped in light extension (the artery could collapse if excessive extension is applied). The collateral circulation to the hand is checked either by the modified Allen's test or by a US screening confirming the presence of a patent homolateral ulnar artery.

For the *landmark approach*, the pulse is located by pressure on the distal end of the radius and the skin is puncture close to the skin fold of the wrist. A flat approach with an angle of 10–20° is used because of the superficiality of the artery. In small children, the artery is easily transfixed. The access can be gained by slowly withdrawing the cannula without the inner needle till blood flow is obtained and re-inserting it in the arterial lumen.

For the *USG approach*, the radial artery can be followed from the wrist till halfway of the forearm allowing different insertion sites. The distal approach at the wrist is the first choice, but more proximal approaches can be used as rescue techniques. A SAX view of the artery is used because LAX views of small vessels are difficult to obtain and almost impossible to maintain. The artery is punctured with an OOP needle approach (Fig. 19.41). Correct visualization of the radial artery in infants is obtained by using the zoom function (Fig. 19.42). To ensure successful catheterization, the needle tip should be seen progressing into the arterial lumen over a few millimeters by translating the probe slowly cephalad. An experience will be required to apply this technique in neonates and infants. The use of USG increases the success rate at first attempt and reduces finale failure rate [41, 42]. It is therefore at least recommended when a difficult access is suspected or encountered and in case of coagulopathy [4–6].

19.6.3 The Femoral Artery

The positioning of the child is the same as for femoral vein catheterization. External hip rotation, to reduce vessel overlapping, will reduce the risk of arteriovenous fistula creation if the artery is inadvertently transfixed. For infants, a small pad can be placed under their buttocks to give a better exposure of the groin.

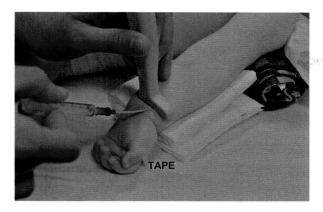

Fig. 19.41 Ultrasound-guided puncture of the radial artery. Arm positioning is of major importance: the forearm is fixed in a stable horizontal position and the wrist taped in extension. SAX view of the artery, OOP needle approach

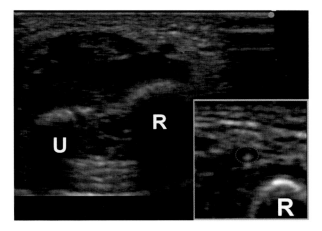

Fig. 19.42 Ultrasound image at the wrist of an infant. The radial artery (*arrow*) is seen in SAX above the radial bone (*R*). Square: the zoom function has to be used to increase visibility of both the artery and needle. The needle tip progresses in the lumen close to the posterior wall. *U* ulnar bone

For the *landmark approach*, the insertion point is situated 0.5–1 cm below the inguinal ligament on top of the femoral pulse. A 45° approach is used and rapidly flattened once arterial blood flashback is found.

For the *USG technique*, the insertion point will be chosen in order to hit the vessel at the level of the common femoral artery (Fig. 19.43). The artery is catheterized over a few millimeters under direct vision. After having inserted the cannula or the guide wire, their correct migration is confirmed by a last US screening. USG seems to increase the first-attempt success rate and decrease the incidence of hematoma by reducing the risk of transfixing the artery. US screening can be used postoperatively to confirm the patency of the femoral artery during the use of the catheter or after withdrawal.

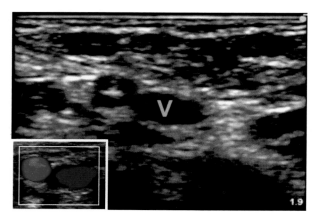

Fig. 19.43 Ultrasound-guided puncture of the femoral artery. SAX view of the femoral vessels, OOP needle approach. The needle tip is seen in the lumen of the artery. *Square* Doppler examination during US screening, *V* femoral vein

19.6.4 Other Arteries

The *ulnar artery* is the largest terminal branch of the brachial artery, but the close proximity of the ulnar nerve could lead to additional complications if USG is not used. Cannulation of the ulnar artery should be avoided when cannulation of the radial artery has already been performed on the same wrist (potential total occlusion of the arterial supply of the hand).

The *posterior tibial artery* runs in the retromalleolar grove posterior to the internal malleolus. It is best palpated with the foot in dorsiflexion.

The *dorsalis pedis artery* runs on the dorsal aspect of the foot, usually between the first two metatarsal bones. It is best palpated with the foot in plantar extension.

The *temporal artery* site is no longer recommended.

The *brachial artery* should be used with caution due to the absence of collateral blood flow at its level and the proximity of the median nerve. USG should therefore be used.

The *axillary artery* is rarely used, and there is some collateral flow at its level, but the artery is surrounded by branches of the brachial plexus, which can be injured by sharp needles.

19.6.5 Complications

The most frequent complication is ischemia. The etiology of ischemia is multiple: vasospasm, thrombosis, and emboli. Ischemic damage is more likely in case of low cardiac output and/or when vasopressors were used. Vasospasm can occur within minutes or hours after insertion. Early signs are pallor, delayed refilling time, and loss or reduced pulse distal to the insertion site. Vasospasm occurs more frequently in neonates and infants. Either injecting a small dose of lidocaine into the catheter or warming the contralateral limb to produce reflex vasodilatation can be used. If no improvement is noticed, the catheter should be removed. The incidence of arterial thrombosis is directly related to the duration of cannulation and is inversely related to the weight of the child. Distal embolization of a thrombus formed in the cannula or proximal embolization of air can occur in case of aggressive flushing. In case of an ischemic complication, local warming, systemic anticoagulation, topical vasodilatation using a nitroglycerine ointment or patch, or a brachial plexus block can be used.

Local infection is rare if the cannula is left in place for less than 4 days. Multiple attempts and technical difficulties increase the risk of infection, reason to use USG in order to reduce the number of attempts. Although there is a theoretical increased risk of contamination for the femoral site due to the proximity of the perineum, the incidence of infection is no greater than for radial catheters.

Other potential complications are nerve damage by the needle or by a compressive hematoma, tendon sheath injury, arteriovenous fistula, and accidental intra-arterial injection of medications.

19.7   Umbilical Access

Umbilical vein and arteries can easily be accessed during the first few days of life. The umbilical cord contains two arteries and one vein buried within Wharton's jelly. The umbilical vein is the recommended emergency access for neonatal resuscitation and can be used as a central venous route for fluid and drugs administration or blood samples. The umbilical artery is used for invasive pressure monitoring and arterial blood gas sampling. Access to the umbilical vessels is done under maximal sterile conditions: the umbilical cord is cut 2 cm above its skin-covered portion, and the stump is gently tied using a tissue lace. Contraindications to umbilical vessel catheterization include omphalocele, gastroschisis, peritonitis, and necrotizing enterocolitis. Umbilical accesses have to be removed before abdominal surgeries. Access to the superior or inferior vena cava is usually achieved in the operating room after induction of anesthesia and just before the surgical act.

19.7.1 The Umbilical Vein

Within the body, the umbilical goes cephalad, enters the liver and divides in the branches: one joins the left branch of the portal vein and the other, called the ductus arteriosus, bypasses the liver and joins the VCI via the suprahepatic veins. The umbilical vein is a wide, thin-walled vessel. Before any insertion, the gaping vessel is cautiously opened and clots removed. The catheter (3.5 F if < 1500 g, 5 F if > 1500 g) is slowly inserted into the upper part of the body. The catheter tip can be placed in a low or a high position. The low position is used for emergency venous access to avoid placement of the catheter in the liver. The distance of insertion varies between

3 cm (preterm) and 5 cm (full term). The ideal tip position is the high position when the catheter is advanced through the ductus venosus into the IVC, just above the diaphragm on the chest X-ray. The insertion length can be estimated according to birth weight (formula: 1.5× kg + 5.5 cm) or by using standardized graphs [43].

19.7.2 The Umbilical Artery

The umbilical arteries turn inferiorly in the abdomen to enter the pelvis and connect with the internal iliac arteries. These vessels are thick walled and usually have a degree of spasm. To be catheterized, they need to be carefully dilated using small forceps. The catheter (3.5 F if < 1200 g, 5 f if > 1200 g) is carefully inserted aiming the lower part of the body. The catheter tip can be placed in a low or a high position. The high position is ideal with the tip in the descending aorta, above the diaphragm at Th7–Th9 level on the X-ray. The insertion length can be calculated according to birth weight (formula: 3× kg + 9 cm) or using standardized graphs [43]. The low position is above the aortic bifurcation and below the renal arteries, corresponding to L3–L4 on the X-ray.

19.7.3 Specific Complications

Some complications are specific to the umbilical access including [44]:

- Infection (omphalitis).
- Thromboembolism with clot: heparin use decreases the incidence of catheter occlusion but not the risk of aortic thrombosis.
- Vessel trauma (perforation and aneurysm formation).
- Blood flow obstruction resulting in enterocolitis or hepatic necrosis.
- Umbilical vein catheter tip malposition: fluid accumulation in different cavities (pleura, pericardium, peritoneum), arrhythmia, hepatic hematoma, and portal vein thrombosis. Portal vein thrombosis can remain asymptomatic for a long period and be revealed only later by a portal hypertension without cirrhosis [45].
- Umbilical artery catheters: systemic hypertension by renal artery obstruction and vasospasm with ischemic complications (lower limbs).

References

1. Pirotte T (2008) Ultrasound-guided vascular access in adults and children: beyond the internal jugular vein. Acta Anaesth Belg 59:157–166
2. NICE (2002) Guidance on the used of ultrasound location devices for placing central venous catheters. Technology appraisal guidance 49. http://www.nice.org.uk/guidance/TA49
3. Rupp SM, Apfelbaum JL, Blitt C et al (2012) Practical guidelines for central venous access: a report by the American society of Anesthesiologist task force on central venous access. Anesthesiology 116:539–573

4. Troianos C, Hartman G, Glas K et al (2012) Guidelines for performing ultrasound guided vascular cannulation: recommendations of the American Society of Echocardiography and the Society of Cardiovascular Anesthesiologists. Anesth Analg 114:46–72
5. Lamperti M, Bodenham AR, Pittiruti M et al (2012) International evidence-based recommendations on ultrasound-guided vascular access. Intensive Care Med 38:1105–1117
6. Zetlaoui P, Bouaziz H, Pierre S et al (2014) Recommandation sur l'utilisation de l'échographie lors de la mise en place des accès vasculaires. French Society of Anesthesia and Reanimation. http://www.sfar.org/article/1209/rfe-recommandations-sur-l-rsquo-utilisation-de-l-rsquo-echographie-lors-de-la-mise-en-place-des-acces-vasculaires. Accessed 10 Apr 2015
7. Cuper NJ, de Graaff JC, van Dijk AT et al (2012) Predictive factors for difficult intravenous cannulation in pediatric patients at a tertiary pediatric hospital. Pediatr Anesth 22:223–229
8. Yen K, Riegert A, Gorelick MH (2008) Derivation of the DIVA score: a clinical prediction rule for the identification of children with difficult intravenous access. Pediatr Emerg Care 24:143–147
9. Hosokawa K, Kato H, Kishi C et al (2010) Transillumination by light-emitting diode facilitates peripheral venous cannulations in infants and small children. Acta Anaesthesiol Scand 54:957–961
10. de Graaff JC, Cuper NJ, Mungra A et al (2013) Near-infrared light to aid peripheral intravenous cannulation in children: a cluster randomised trial of three devices. Anaesthesia 68:835–845
11. van der Woude OC, Cuper NJ, Getrouw C et al (2013) The effectiveness of a near-infrared vascular imaging device to support intravenous cannulation in children with dark skin color: a cluster randomized clinical trial. Anesth Analg 116:1266–1271
12. Benkhadra M, Collignon M, Fournel I et al (2012) Ultrasound guidance allows faster peripheral IV cannulation in children under 3 years of age with difficult venous access: a prospective randomized study. Pediatr Anesth 22:449–454
13. Heinrichs J, Fritze Z, Vandermeer B et al (2013) Ultrasonographically guided peripheral intravenous cannulation of children and adults: a systematic review and meta-analysis. Ann Emerg Med 61:444–454
14. Centers for Disease Control and Prevention (CDC) (2011) Vital signs: central line-associated blood stream infection – United States 201, 2008 and 2009. Morb Mortal Wkly Rep 60:243–248
15. Kim H, Jeong CH, Byon HJ et al (2013) Prediction of the optimal depth of left-sided central venous catheters in children. Anaesthesia 68:1033–1037
16. Choi M, Massicotte P, Marzinotto V et al (2001) The use of alteplase to restore patency of central venous lines in pediatric patients: a cohort study. J Pediatr 139:152–156
17. Roth B, Marciniak B, Engelhardt T et al (2008) Anatomic relationship between the internal jugular vein and the carotid artery in preschool children: an ultrasonographic study. Pediatr Anesth 18:752–756
18. Arai T, Matsuda Y, Koizuka K et al (2009) Rotation of the head might not be recommended for internal jugular puncture in infants and children. Pediatr Anesth 19:844–847
19. Morita M, Sasano H, Azami T et al (2009) A novel skin-traction method is effective for real time ultrasound-guided internal jugular vein catheterization in infants and neonates weighing less than 5 kilograms. Anesth Analg 109:754–759
20. Verghese S, McGill W, Patel R et al (1999) Ultrasound-guided internal jugular vein cannulation in infants: a prospective comparison with the traditional palpation method. Anesthesiology 91:71–77
21. Phelan M, Hagerty D (2009) The oblique view: an alternative approach for ultrasound-guided central line placement. J Emerg Med 37:403–408
22. Rhondali O, Attof R, Combet S et al (2011) Ultrasound-guided subclavian vein cannulation in infants: supraclavicular approach. Pediatr Anesth 21:1136–1141
23. Breschan C, Platzer M, Jost R et al (2011) Consecutive, prospective case series of a new method for ultrasound-guided supraclavicular approach to the brachiocephalic vein in children. Br J Anaesth 106:732–737

24. Breschan C, Platzer M, Jost R et al (2012) Ultrasound-guided supraclavicular cannulation of the brachiocephalic vein in infants: a retrospective analysis of a case series. Pediatr Anesth 22:1062–1067
25. Byon HJ, Lee GW, Lee JH et al (2013) Comparison between ultrasound-guided supraclavicular and infraclavicular approaches for subclavian venous catheterization in children – a randomized trial. Br J Anaesth 111:788–792
26. Pirotte T, Veyckemans F (2007) Ultrasound-guided subclavian vein cannulation in infants and children: a novel approach. Br J Anaesth 98:509–514
27. O'Leary R, Ahmed SM, McLure H et al (2012) Ultrasound-guided infraclavicular axillary vein cannulation: a useful alternative to the internal jugular vein. Br J Anaesth 109:762–768
28. Suk EH, Kim DH, Kil HK et al (2009) Effects of reverse Trendelenburg position and inguinal compression on femoral vein cross-sectional area in infants and young children. Anaesthesia 64:399–402
29. Warkentine FH, Pierce MC, Lorenz D et al (2008) The anatomic relationship of femoral vein to femoral artery in euvolemic pediatric patients by ultrasonography: implication for pediatric femoral central venous access. Acad Emerg Med 15:426–430
30. Shinohara Y, Arai T, Yamashita M (2005) The optimal insertion length of central venous catheter via the femoral route for open heart surgery in infants and children. Pediatr Anesth 15:12–124
31. Aouad MT, Kanazi GE, Abdallah FW et al (2010) Femoral vein cannulation performed by residents: a comparison between ultrasound-guided and landmark technique in infants and children undergoing cardiac surgery. Anesth Analg 111:724–728
32. Bouchut JC, Floret D (2006) Radiographic confirmation following pediatric femoral venous cannulation. Can J Anesth 53:422–423
33. Westergaard B, Classen V, Walther-Larsen S (2013) Peripherally inserted central catheters in infants and children – indications, techniques, complications and clinical recommendations. Acta Anaesthesiol Scand 57:278–287
34. Abedin S, Kapoor G (2008) Peripherally inserted central venous catheters are a good option for prolonged venous access in children with cancer. Pediatr Blood Cancer 51:251–255
35. Barrier A, Williams D, Connely M (2011) Frequency of peripherally inserted central catheter complication in children. Pediatr Infect Dis J 31:519–521
36. Advani S, Reich N, Sengupta A et al (2011) Central line-associated bloodstream infection in hospitalized children with peripherally inserted central venous catheters: extending risk analyzes outside the intensive care unit. Clin Infect Dis 52:1108–1115
37. Dubois J, Rypens F, Garel L et al (2007) Incidence of deep vein thrombosis related to peripherally inserted central catheters in children and adolescents. CMAJ 177:1185–1190
38. Weiss M, Engelhardt T (2012) Cannot cannulate: bonulate! Eur J Anesthesiol 29:257–258
39. Anson JA (2014) Vascular access in resuscitation: is there a role for the intraosseous route? Anesthesiology 120:1015–1031
40. Hallas P, Brabrand M, Folkestad L (2013) Complication with intraosseous access: Scandinavian users' experience. West J Emerg Med 14:440–443
41. Schwemmer U, Arzet HA, Trautner H et al (2006) Ultrasound-guided arterial cannulation in infants improves success rate. Eur J Anaesthesiol 23:476–480
42. Ishii S, Shime N, Shibasaki M et al (2013) Ultrasound-guided radial artery catheterization in infants and small children. Ped Anesth 14:471–473
43. Anderson J, Leonard D, Braner D et al (2008) Umbilical vascular catheterization. N Engl J Med 359, e18
44. Schlesinger AE, Braveman R, DiPietro MA (2003) Neonates and umbilical venous catheter: normal appearance, anomalous positions, complications and potential aids to diagnosis. Am J Roentgenol 180:1147–1153
45. Ji Hye K, Young Seok L, Sang Hee K et al (2001) Does umbilical vein catheterization lead to portal vein thrombosis? Prospective US evaluation in 100 neonates. Radiology 219:645–650

US-Guided Nerve Targets

20

Giorgio Ivani and Valeria Mossetti

There has been a recent increase in the use of regional anesthesia in pediatric patients; this explosive growth, particularly in the use of truncal blocks, can be attributed in part to the refinement of anatomically based ultrasound imaging to facilitate nerve localization. Historically, pediatric regional anesthesia has posed a significant challenge due to the close proximity of nerves to critical structures and the need for limiting the local anesthetic volume below toxic levels in children. Ultrasound guidance, however, allows the visualization of important anatomy and can help overcome many of these traditional obstacles [1].

This technique, in fact, has brought pediatric regional anesthesia to new levels improving the quality of anesthetic blockade with faster onset time, longer duration of blocks, and lower dose of local anesthetics [2].

Although ultrasound may be useful for nerve localization, one of the main benefits is to provide visualization of the dispersion of the local anesthetic within the desired tissue plains. Ultrasound has been shown to provide adequate landmarks for determining the location of nerves in children along with a discriminatory approach to evaluating nerve location and anatomical variations in infants and children. This technology however requires a significant training and skill for its successful implementation.

Ultrasound guidance is therefore strongly recommended when performing peripheral nerve blocks in infants and children [3, 6–8].

This chapter will review a variety of common peripheral nerve and central neuraxial blocks that can be performed using ultrasound guidance in children. We have to emphasize that ultrasound guidance is a relative recent innovation to the field of regional anesthesia; most of the current literature is not evidence based. As a result, much of the data comes from case reports and case series.

G. Ivani (✉) • V. Mossetti (✉)
Anesthesiology and Intensive Care, Regina Margherita Children Hospital, Turin, Italy
e-mail: valeriamossetti@libero.it

© Springer International Publishing Switzerland 2016   341
M. Astuto, P.M. Ingelmo (eds.), *Perioperative Medicine in Pediatric Anesthesia*,
Anesthesia, Intensive Care and Pain in Neonates and Children,
DOI 10.1007/978-3-319-21960-8_20

Our goal is to provide the pediatric anesthesiologist with a comprehensive summary of the relevant sonoanatomy, techniques, and outcomes of ultrasound guidance for peripheral nerve blocks of the extremities and trunk as well as neuraxial blocks in pediatric patients based on currently available literature.

20.1   Ultrasound Equipment

Mobile, usually cart-based, echographs consist primarily of a probe (transducer), a computer that controls the transducer, sends the impulse, receives the echo, and processes the signal, a visualization system, and a storage device for later digital editing and printing (Fig. 20.1a, b). The most important part of the echograph is the transducer which can present different forms depending on its specific use. The important technical specifications are its axial and lateral resolution and the frequency achieved. Resolution is the ability to discern two dots as being distinct from each other on the x and y plane: on the (x) axis – which is parallel to the propagation line of the ultrasonic beam – and on the (y) axis – which is the axis vertical to the ultrasonic beam. Today, due to technological advancement in signal processing software, it is also possible to improve data quality for imaging and to influence the definition: to reduce the phenomenon of signal attenuation, the reflected signals are amplified taking into account the delay with which the signal is received, thus allowing statements as to their depth. Finally, it should be kept in mind that the ultrasonic beam transmitted from the transducer results in the two-dimensional

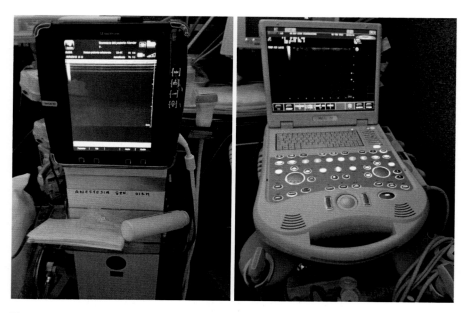

Fig. 20.1   Cart-based echographs

representation of a three-dimensional object. Therefore, recordings from at least two sets of planes are required to be able to reconstruct the object in its original shape [4, 5].

20.2 Minimum Requirements for Regional Anesthesia Ultrasound Equipment

The ultrasound equipment used in regional anesthesia should be transportable. Portable units as well as compact scanner systems mounted on a cart are commercially available.

These should meet at least the following requirements: color Doppler to identify blood vessels and distinguish them from the surrounding tissues, contrast images (gain), and sufficient storage capacity for images and preferably also for films.

For any ultrasound-guided block technique, a sterile preparation of the probe with an adhesive sheet and the block area also using sterile gel is recommended (Fig. 20.2a, b). When a catheter is introduced, it is recommended to completely wrap the probe with a proper sterile cover (Fig. 20.2c).

20.2.1 Ultrasound Probe

Transducer characteristics, such as frequency and shape, determine ultrasound image quality. The transducer frequencies used for peripheral nerve blocks range from 3 to 15 MHz. Linear transducers are most useful for nerve imaging to provide high-resolution images. For superficial structures (e.g., nerves in the interscalene, supraclavicular, and axillary regions), it is ideal to use high-frequency transducers in the range of 10–15 MHz remembering that depth of penetration is often limited to 2–3 cm below the skin surface.

For visualization of deeper structures (e.g., in the infraclavicular and popliteal regions), it may be necessary to use a lower frequency transducer (less than or equal to 7 MHz) because it offers ultrasound penetration of 4–5 cm or more below the skin surface. However, the image resolution is often inferior to that obtained with a higher frequency transducer.

Two types of probes are commonly used in children (Fig. 20.3):

- Linear probes (6–13 MHz): the resulting imagine is square, with good resolution in the near field, but narrow depth; probe frequency is selected according to nerve depth, 7 MHz for structures deeper than 5 cm, 10 MHz for structures between 3 and 5 cm deep, 12 MHz for structures maximally 3 cm deep, and shorter probes such as the Hockey stick probe with a length of 2.5 cm for pediatric use.
- Sector probes (2–5 MHz): the resulting image is trapezoidal, with good resolution and depth, but structures in the near field are poor imaged.

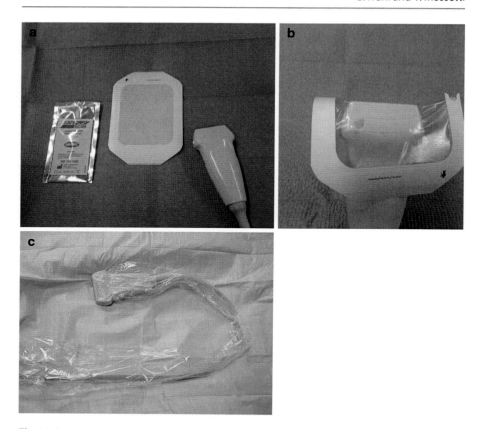

Fig. 20.2 (a) Adhesive sheet, (b) Sterile gel, (c) Sterile cover

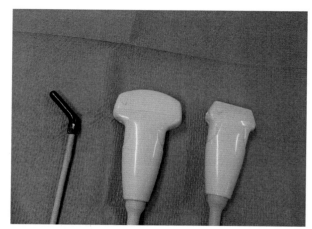

Fig. 20.3 Probes commonly used in children

To correctly perform a nerve block under ultrasound guidance, it is important to proceed as follows:

1. Localize the nerve
2. Move the ultrasound probe
3. Move the block needle

20.2.2 Identification of the Structures in Ultrasonography

The term isoechogenic refers to a structure displayed in an ultrasound image with a certain intensity on a gray scale.

Formations with low echogenicity are called hypoechoic, formations that do not deliver any echo at all are anechoic, and those formations with high echogenicity are called hyperechoic. Normally the echogenicity of an investigated structure corresponds to its type and composition; however, not every anechoic structure is fluid nor must every hyperechoic structure be solid.

The terms shadow cone and acoustic enhancement refer to structures that inhibit the travel of ultrasound, or, respectively, increase its speed. Such situations occur typically in investigations of bone or calcium structures (e.g., gallstones) and formations containing liquid (e.g., liver cysts).

Vessels: their identification is of particular importance because it guides to the neurovascular bundle. Vessels appear hypoechoic; discrimination between arteries and veins and also applying pressure with the probe are possible with color Doppler: veins are compressible while arteries remain pulsatile; gentle pressure is needed because during venous compression, intravenous needle tip placement may be missed.

Muscle: this has a fibrolamellar ultrasonographic appearance with either heterogeneous structures with bandlike hyperechoic intramuscular septae or homogenous structures.

Bones: the cortex of the bone is hyperechoic and the areas behind or deep to the cortex are completely anechoic.

Fatty tissue: hypoechoic.

Tendons, pleura: hyperechoic.

Local anesthetic: direct observation of the spread of local anesthetic during injection is mandatory; local anesthetic solution appears anechoic.

Neuronal structures: every nerve has a particular appearance in ultrasonography with regard to the shape, the echogenicity, and the quantity of connective tissue present between the nerve fibers.

The proximal parts of the brachial plexus appear as hypoechoic round to oval structures; by contrast more peripheral nerve structures appear hyperechoic. In the lower extremity, most of the neural structures appear hyperechoic (Fig. 20.4a, b).

Fig. 20.4 (a) Scanning of the axilla. (b) *A* artery, *N* nerve, *V* vein

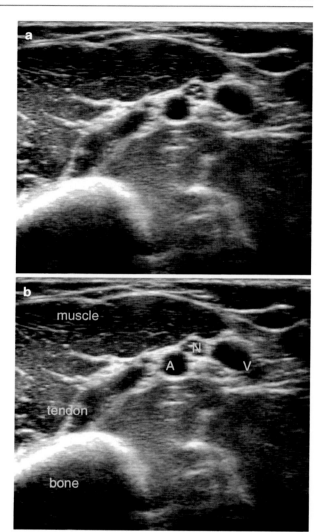

20.2.3 Needle Handling

Proper needle handling skills are required for accurate and smooth needle insertion during ultrasound-guided nerve blocks. If the operator is not ambidextrous and prefers to use the dominant hand to handle the needle and inject local anesthetic, then the operator must choose a proper body location and orientation in relationship to the patient.

There are two ways to align the transducer with the needle:

In plane (IP): The transducer is exactly parallel to the needle. In this case it is possible to see the whole length of the needle and the needle tip. Advantages: Because the needle tip is visualized, it is possible to position it correctly without the risk of injuring nerves or vessels. Disadvantages: Since ultrasound has an extremely narrow beam width, it can be difficult to keep the needle constantly in view (Fig. 20.5a, b).

Out of plane (OOP): The needle and the transducer are perpendicular to each other. In this case it is possible to see the cross section of the needle as a hyperechoic dot, which however can result from any other needle segment and not the tip. Advantages: The needle cross section is easily identified. Disadvantages: One is not sure where the tip of the needle is. This potentially carries the risk of injury to nerves and blood vessels (Fig. 20.6a, b).

20.3   Ultrasound-Guided Regional Anesthetic Techniques

20.3.1 Upper Limb Blocks

Peripheral regional anesthesia is of great utility in children undergoing surgery on the upper extremities. Many approaches to the brachial plexus have been described; in children the most commonly performed and reported brachial plexus blockade is the axillary block. This may be due to the fact that other block sites are situated near critical structures such as the cervical pleura (supraclavicular and infraclavicular) and the spinal cord (interscalene). Introduction of ultrasound imaging will likely greatly increase the performance of brachial plexus blocks in infants and children at locations besides the commonly described axillary approach by allowing for real-time visualization of anatomical structures.

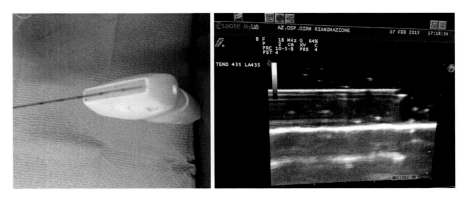

Fig. 20.5 In plane approach

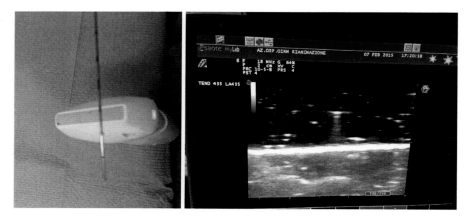

Fig. 20.6 Out of plane approach

Fig. 20.7 *ca* carotid
artery, *jv* jugular vein

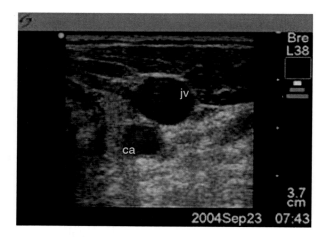

20.3.1.1 Interscalene Approach

The interscalene block is indicated for all upper extremity surgery, but particularly if the shoulder is involved.

Ultrasound imaging allows visualization of the C5, C6, and C7 nerve roots between the anterior and middle scalene muscles. In a transverse oblique plane at the level of the cricoid cartilage and at the posterolateral aspect of the sternocleido-mastoid muscle, the muscle appears as a triangular-shaped structure overlying the internal jugular vein and common carotid artery (Fig. 20.7).

The scalene muscles serve as useful landmarks; the anterior scalene lies deep to the sternocleidomastoid and lateral to the subclavian artery, while the middle and posterior scalenes are located more posterolaterally. The neurovascular (interscalene) sheath appears as a hyperechoic structure within the interscalene groove. The

Fig. 20.8 (a) Scanning of
the interscalene groove.
(b) *SCM*
sternocleidomastoid
muscle, *ASM* anterior
scalene muscle, *MSM*
middle scalene muscle, *VA*
vertebral artery, *arrows*
roots of brachial plexus

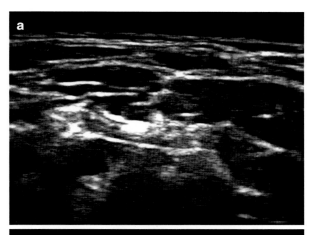

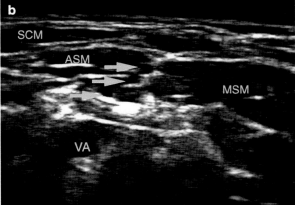

trunks and/or roots of the brachial plexus may be visible as round- or oval-shaped
hypoechoic structures. The roots or trunks lie between the scalenus anterior and the
scalenus medius at this level. The prominent internal jugular (anechoic) lies medially (Fig 20.8a, b).

Interscalenic approach is performed with a high-frequency linear probe; the
transducer position is transverse on neck, 3–4 cm superior to clavicle, over external
jugular vein (Fig. 20.9).

A combined ultrasound-guided nerve stimulating technique may facilitate nerve
localization. Using an in-plane approach and slight redirections to advance the needle close to the brachial plexus, local anesthetic spread around the nerve roots or
trunks may be visualized. Precise needle placement may limit the dose of local
anesthetic required.

The goal, in fact, is local anesthetic spread around superior and middle trunks of
brachial plexus, between anterior and middle scalene muscle (Fig. 20.10).

Fig. 20.9 IP interscalene
approach

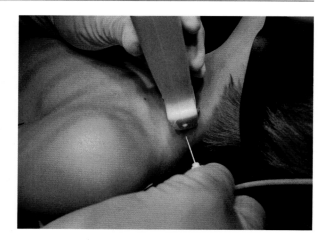

Fig. 20.10 *arrows* roots
of brachial plexus, *yellow
line* needle, blue: local
anesthetic, *red line* spread
of local anesthetic

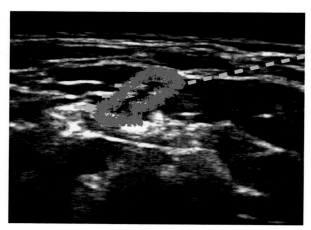

Ultrasound guidance allows multiple injections around the brachial plexus, therefore eliminating the reliance on a single large injection of local anesthetic for block
success as is the case with non-ultrasound-guided techniques. Ability to inject multiple aliquots of local anesthetic also may allow for the reduction in the volume of
local anesthetic required to accomplish the block.

Due to potential adverse effects including pneumothorax, vertebral artery injection, and intrathecal injection, the intrascalene block is not common in pediatrics.
Palpation of the interscalene grove often proves challenging in children under general anesthesia, and as a result, a recent report states that this block is not recommended for any heavily sedated or anesthetized patient. However, the improvements
in nerve localization made possible due to ultrasound guidance have the potential to
increase the use of this block in children [9–11].

20.3.1.2 Supraclavicular Approach

The supraclavicular block is indicated for all upper extremity surgery, but particularly if the shoulder is not involved; in general indications are arm, elbow, forearm, and hand surgery.

It is a popular technique for surgery below the shoulder because the onset and quality of anesthesia are fast and complete.

The proximity of the brachial plexus at this location to the chest cavity and pleura has been of concern to many practitioners; however, ultrasound guidance has resulted in a resurgence of interest in the supraclavicular approach to the brachial plexus. The ability to image the plexus, rib, pleura, and subclavian artery with ultrasound guidance has increased safety due to better monitoring of anatomy and needle placement [12].

The subclavian artery crosses over the first rib between the insertions of the anterior and middle scalene muscles, at approximately the midpoint of the clavicle. The pulsating subclavian artery is readily apparent, whereas the parietal pleura and the first rib can be seen as a linear hyperechoic structure immediately lateral and deep to it, respectively. The rib, as an osseous structure, casts an acoustic shadow, so that the image field deep to the rib appears anechoic or dark. A reverberation artifact often occurs, mimicking a second subclavian artery beneath the rib.

The trunks and divisions of the plexus appear as hypoechoic grapelike clusters laterally and cranially the artery, while a hyperechoic line with dorsal shadowing indicates the first rib (Fig. 20.11).

With a high-frequency probe in the coronal oblique plane, the plexus divisions and/or roots are visible lateral to the subclavian artery (Fig. 20.12). Using an in-plane approach, directing the needle from lateral to medial avoids vascular structures in contact with the plexus.

The goal is local anesthetic spread around brachial plexus, lateral, and superficial to subclavian artery.

This approach lends itself to a continuous catheter technique because nerve structures are close proximity to another.

When compared to other brachial plexus blocks, there is an increased risk of pneumothorax due to the proximity of the lung parenchyma at the level of this block. By using an in-plane approach, ultrasound guidance may reduce this risk by providing clear visibility of the needle shaft and tip, making the supraclavicular approach one of the most reliable and effective blocks of the brachial plexus (Fig. 20.13).

20.3.1.3 Infraclavicular Approach

The indications for the infraclavicular approach to the brachial plexus are arm, elbow, forearm, and hand surgery.

Identification of the arterial pulse on the sonographic image is an easy primary goal in establishing the landmark. The axillary artery and vein are located deep and medial to the cords, with the vein positioned medial and caudal to the artery.

The cords of the infraclavicular portion of the brachial plexus appear hyperechoic and lateral and/or below the subclavian artery; the pleura is hyperechoic and

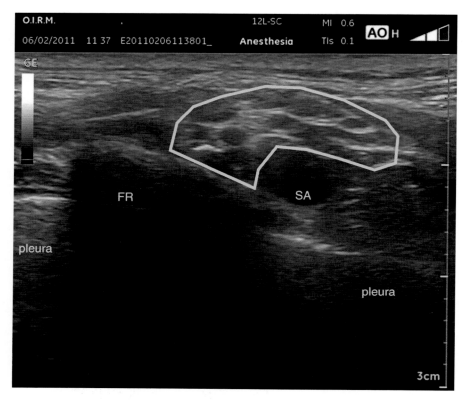

Fig. 20.11 *FR* first rib, *SA* subclavian artery, *yellow line* brachial plexus

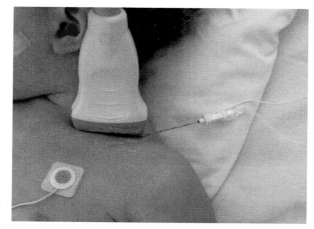

Fig. 20.12 IP suprclavicular
approach

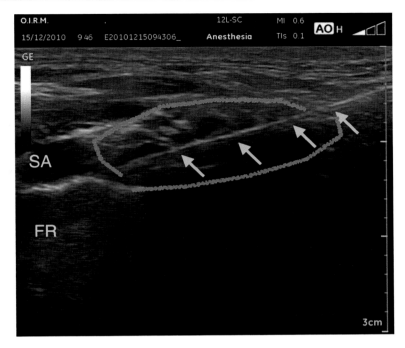

Fig. 20.13 *SA* subclavian artery, *FR* first rib, *Arrows* needle, *red line* spread of local anesthetic

medial. Although all the cords surround the artery, they are not visualized with equal clarity. The lateral cord is most easily viewed and appears as a hyperechoic oval structure. In contrast, the posterior and medial cords may be difficult to visualize, in part because the view may be obstructed by the axillary vasculature; the medial cord lies between the artery and vein while the posterior cord is deep to the artery. The pectoralis major and minor muscles lie superficial to the neurovascular bundle and are separated by a hyperechoic lining (perimysium) (Figs. 20.14 and 20.15).

The block is typically performed with the patient in supine position with the head turned away from the side to be blocked. The arm is abducted to 90° and the elbow flexed.

The probe is positioned immediately medial to the coracoid process of the scapula under the clavicle in a parasagittal plane so that the plexus can be scanned transversely (the marker on the probe is directed toward the patient's head). The transducer is moved in the superior-inferior direction until the artery is identified in cross section. While the plexus lies quite deep in adults, the structure is much more superficial in children, making a higher frequency probe optimal (Fig. 20.16).

The needle is inserted in plane cephalad to the probe and redirected when necessary to ensure optimal spread of the local anesthetic around the cords. The goal is local anesthetic spread around axillary artery; the optimal spread of local anesthetic should be lateral and below the artery, to include the posterior cord (Fig. 20.17).

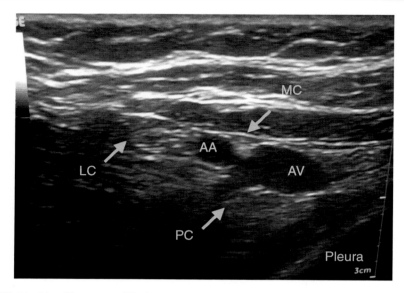

Fig. 20.14 *AA* axillary artery, *AV* axillary vein, *LC* lateral cord, *PC* posterior cord, *MC* medial cord

Fig. 20.15 Color Doppler of the infraclavicular area

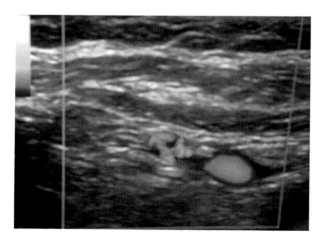

Infraclavicular block is well suited for catheter technique because the musculature of the chest wall helps stabilize the catheter and prevents its dislodgment compared with the more superficial.

The risks of this block are similar to the supraclavicular approach, with the danger of pneumothorax being most serious. Just as with the supraclavicular block, an in-plane needle insertion under ultrasound guidance may minimize the risk by allowing clear visualization of the needle tip and shaft [14, 16]. In

Fig. 20.16 IP
infraclavicular approach

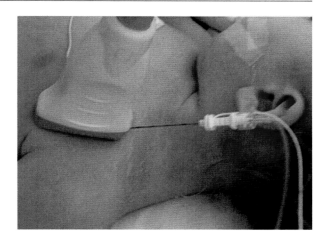

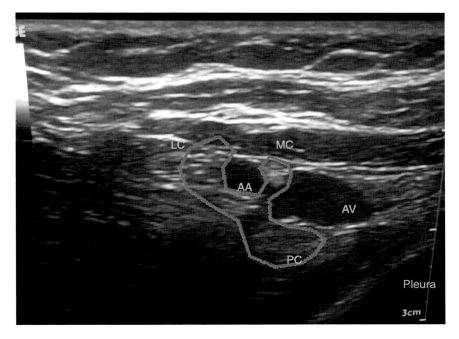

Fig. 20.17 Spread of local anesthetic, *AA* axillary artery, *AV* axillary vein, *LC* lateral cord, *PC* posterior cord, *MC* medial cord

addition, due to the closer proximity of the cervical pleura to the plexus cords medially, a lateral puncture site is recommended [19]. Ultrasound imaging may also be advantageous in avoiding multiple puncture sites and visualizing underdeveloped structures like the coracoid process that may be difficult to palpate in children using "blind" techniques [13, 15, 17].

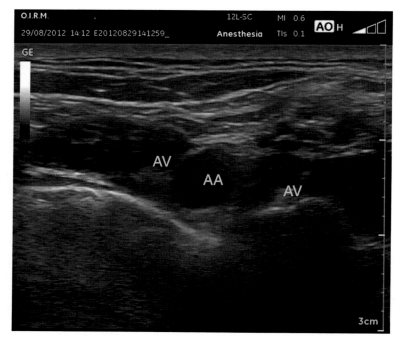

Fig. 20.18 Vascularization of the axilla, *AA* axillary artery, *AV* axillary veins

20.3.1.4 Axillary Approach

The axillary approach to the brachial plexus is the most popular technique for children; it provides analgesia for forearm and hand surgery.

The axillary brachial plexus block requires access to the axilla. Therefore abduction of the arm 90° is an appropriate position that allows for transducer placement and needle advancement. Care should be taken not to overabduct the arm because that may cause discomfort as well as produce tension on the brachial plexus, theoretically making it more vulnerable to needle or injection injury during the block procedure.

The axillary artery is a useful ultrasound landmark and appears as a circular anechoic structure adjacent to the biceps and coracobrachialis muscles. The artery can be associated with one or more axillary veins, often located medially to the artery; color Doppler is also a helpful tool to identify the axillary vasculature (Fig. 20.18). Importantly, an undue pressure with the transducer during imaging may obliterate the veins, rendering veins invisible and prone to puncture with the needle if care is not taken to avoid it (Fig. 20.19). Surrounding the axillary artery are three of the four principal branches of the brachial plexus: the median (superficial and lateral to the artery), the ulnar (superficial and medial to the artery), and the radial (posterior and lateral or medial to the artery) nerves. These are seen as round

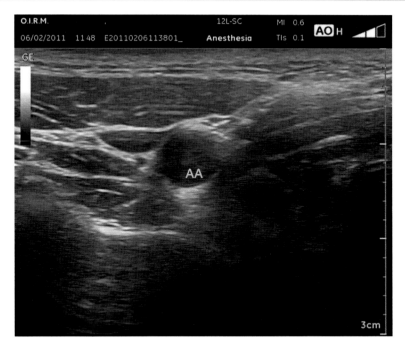

Fig. 20.19   Compression of axillar veins, *AA* axillary artery

hyperechoic structures, and although the previously mentioned locations relative to the artery are frequently encountered, there is considerable anatomical variation from individual to individual.

Three muscles surround the neurovascular bundle: the biceps brachii (lateral and superficial), the wedge-shaped coracobrachialis (lateral and deep), and the triceps brachii (medial and posterior). The fourth principal nerve of the brachial plexus, the musculocutaneous nerve, is found in the fascial layers between biceps and coraco-brachialis muscles, though its location is variable and can be seen within either muscle. It is usually seen as a hypoechoic flattened oval with a bright hyperechoic rim (Fig. 20.20).

A high-frequency linear probe placed perpendicular to the anterior axillary fold provides a short-axis view of the neurovascular bundle with the biceps brachii and coracobrachialis muscles lateral and the triceps brachii medial and deep to the biceps (Fig. 20.21).

An in-plane technique may be used. It is best to use multiple injections with needle redirections to ensure that the local anesthetic surrounds all the terminal nerves of the plexus. Due to the close proximity of the axillary vein and artery, multiple punctures may be necessary to avoid intravascular injection [18] (Figs. 20.22 and 20.23).

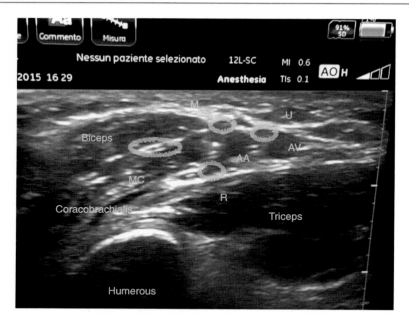

Fig. 20.20 *Yellow circles* nerves, *AA* axillary artery, *AV* axillary vein, *MC* muscolocutaneous nerve, *M* median nerve, *U* ulnar nerve, *R* radial nerve

Fig. 20.21 IP axillar approach

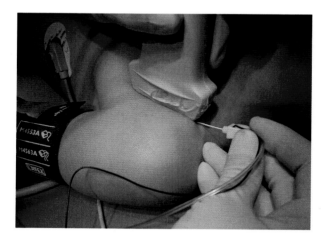

20.3.2 Lower Limb Blocks

20.3.2.1 Femoral Nerve Approach

The femoral nerve originates from nerve roots L2, L3, and L4. Femoral nerve block is an easy block to perform and provides surgical anesthesia and analgesia for the anterior thigh extending to the knee.

The femoral artery is easily visualized and serves as the principle ultrasound landmark. With the probe placed perpendicular to the nerve axis (i.e., coronal oblique) at the level of and parallel to the inguinal crease, the nerve appears lateral

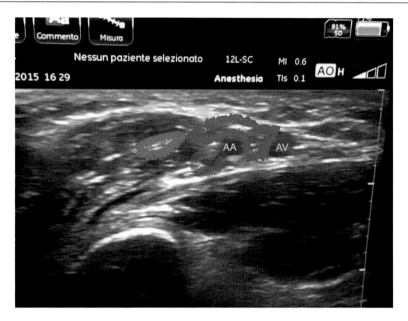

Fig. 20.22 *Red line* spread of local anesthetic. *AA* axillar artery, *AV* axillar vein

Fig. 20.23 Axillar catheter

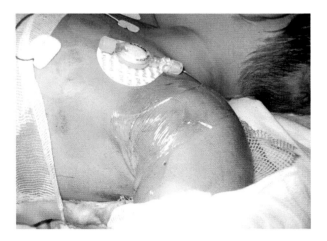

to the large, circular, and anechoic femoral artery. Color Doppler may be helpful to identify the femoral vasculature.

If it is not immediately recognized, sliding the transducer medially and laterally will bring the vessel into view eventually. Immediately lateral to the vessel and deep to the fascia iliaca (separating the nerve from the artery) is the femoral nerve, which is typically hyperechoic and roughly triangular or oval in shape. The nerve is positioned in a sulcus in the iliopsoas muscle underneath the fascia iliaca. Other structures that can be visualized are the femoral vein (medial to the artery) and the fascia lata (superficial in the subcutaneous layer) (Fig. 20.24).

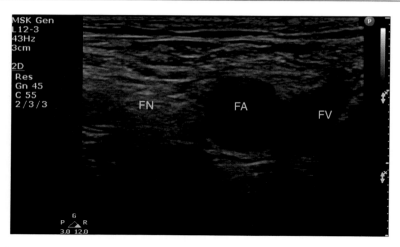

Fig. 20.24 FN: femoral nerve, FA: femoral artery, FV: femoral vein

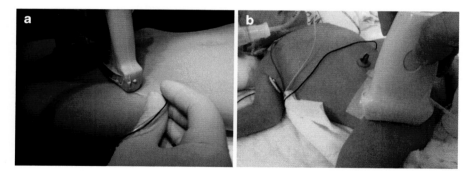

Fig. 20.25 IP femoral approach

The nerve spreads soon after its passage below the inguinal ligament, so that low volumes placed proximally will achieve the best results [20].

Femoral nerve block is performed with a high-frequency linear probe; transducer position is transverse, close to the femoral crease (Fig. 20.25a, b); the needle is inserted using an in-plane approach, so that the needle tip can be visualized as it enters the fascia iliaca (Fig. 20.26). It is important that the needle be placed inside the fascia iliaca compartment. In a study comparing ultrasound guidance to nerve stimulator technique, the nerve was visible in all children studied when the probe was placed parallel and inferior to the inguinal ligament and lateral to the femoral artery. Ultrasound was also used effectively to visualize the needle tip and facilitate needle redirections [21].

Because of the proximity to the relatively large femoral artery, ultrasound may reduce the risk of arterial puncture that often occurs with this block with the use of non-ultrasound techniques. Although there is no direct evidence to prove that ultrasound could reduce this risk, it is the authors' experience that fewer adverse events

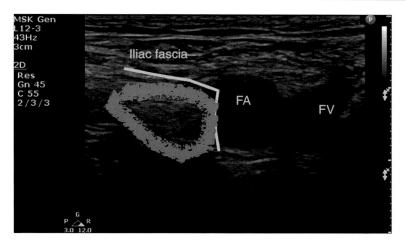

Fig. 20.26   *FA* femoral artery, *FV* femoral vein, *red circle* spread of local anesthetic

occurred when this block was performed under ultrasound guidance. In addition, precise ultrasound imaging of the local anesthetic spread may reduce the need for larger volumes used when injecting blindly.

20.3.2.2 Sciatic Nerve Block

The sciatic nerve is formed by nerve roots L4 to S3 and innervates the posterior thigh and leg below the knee, with the exception of the medial portion. A sciatic block is commonly used for surgical procedures of the foot and ankle, as well as in combination with a femoral nerve block for patients undergoing knee surgery.

As it leaves the pelvis through the greater sciatic foramen, the sciatic nerve can be found inferior to the gluteus maximus muscle. The nerve lies between the ischial tuberosity and the greater trochanter. Curved probes (curvilinear) with moderate-low frequency (e.g., 2–5 MHz) allow deeper ultrasound beam penetration and are often necessary in older children. While the medial aspect of the greater trochanter appears largely hypoechoic, the sciatic nerve is predominantly hyperechoic and is typically elliptical in a short-axis view (Figs. 20.27, 20.28, and 20.29).

The pathway of the sciatic nerve continues through the posterior popliteal fossa before bifurcating to form the common peroneal and tibial nerves. A linear probe transversely oriented in the popliteal crease captures both the tibial and common peroneal nerves located medially and laterally, respectively, to the popliteal vessels. This vasculature, particularly the popliteal artery, serves as useful ultrasound landmarks (color Doppler may be useful). At the popliteal crease, the tibial nerve is found more superficial and most adjacent to the artery. However, as the probe is moved cephalad, the artery becomes deeper and more distant as the tibial nerve moves laterally to join the common peroneal nerve. At and cephalad to the bifurcation, the sciatic nerve appears as a large round to flat-oval hyperechoic structure. The biceps femoris muscle lies superficial to the bifurcating nerves and appears as a large oval-shaped structure with less internal punctuate areas (hyperechoic spots) than the nerves.

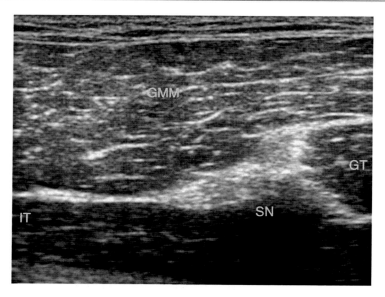

Fig. 20.27 *GMM* gluteus maximus muscle, *GT* greater trochanter, *IT* ischial tuberosity, *SN* sciatic nerve

Fig. 20.28 IP subgluteous approach

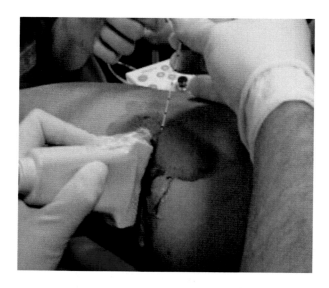

The sciatic nerve is easily located at a midfemoral level and can also be blocked half way up the thigh. In this area the nerve is largely concealed by the biceps femoris and medially slightly by the semimembranosus and semitendinous muscles; underneath lies the adductor magnus. At this level it is quite easy

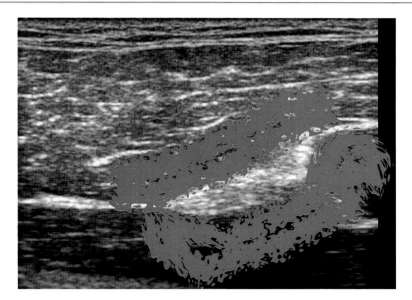

Fig. 20.29 *Red line* local anesthetic spread

to locate the bellies of the two muscles that encompass the nerve: the biceps femoris and the adductor magnus. In this plane the nerve appears as a well-defined, hyperechoic structure that is either triangular or oval in shape. This is an easy block to perform in children under general anesthesia since it can be performed either in the lateral position or in the supine position with elevation of the limb (Figs. 20.30 and 20.31).

Ultrasound imaging can be particularly beneficial when using catheter insertion to confirm the spread of local anesthetic around the nerve (Figs. 20.32, 20.33, 20.34a, b). In addition, ultrasound guidance can be advantageous in instances in which a blind technique is likely to fail. An example of this was described for patients with venous malformations. The use of ultrasound in these patients helped the anesthesiologist avoid vascular puncture during needle placement [22]. Due to the high degree of variability in the division of the sciatic nerve, ultrasound also offers considerable advantages in nerve localization when using the popliteal approach [23, 24].

20.3.2.3 Saphenous Nerve Block

The saphenous nerve is the terminal sensory branch of the femoral nerve. It supplies innervation to the medial aspect of the leg down to the ankle and foot. Blockade of the nerve can be sufficient for superficial procedures in this area; however, it is most useful as a supplement to a sciatic block for foot and ankle procedures that involve the superficial structures in medial territory. The use of ultrasound guidance has improved the success rates of the saphenous blocks, compared with field blocks below the knee and blind transsartorial approaches.

Fig. 20.30 IP midfemoral
approach

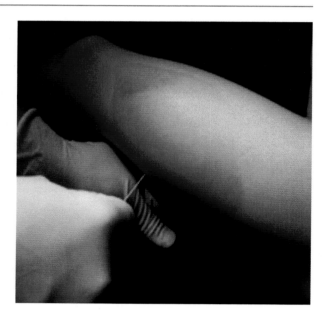

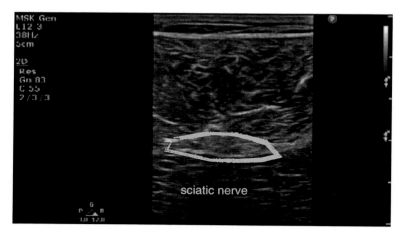

Fig. 20.31 Sciatic nerve at midfemoral level

It is performed with a high-frequency linear probe; transducer position is transverse on anteromedial mid thigh (Fig. 20.35a, b).

The goal is local anesthetic spread lateral to the femoral artery and deep to the sartorius muscle (Fig. 20.36).

Although saphenous nerve is a strictly sensory block, an injection of the local anesthetic in the adductor canal can result in the partial motor block of the vastus medialis. For this reason, caution must be exercised when advising patients regarding the safety of unsupported ambulation after proximal saphenous block.

Fig. 20.32 Sciatic catheter

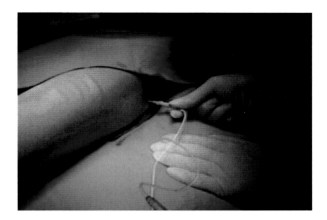

Fig. 20.33 Sciatic catheter in plane with the nerve

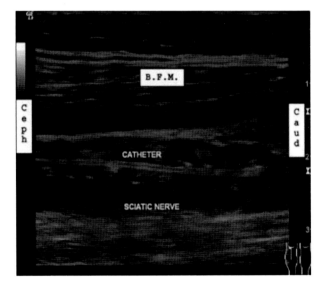

20.3.3 Truncal Blocks

Truncal blocks are becoming a more popular means of providing analgesia for procedures in the umbilical or epigastric regions. The ability to visualize relevant musculature and fascial layers with ultrasound offers an advantage over the more subjective conventional technique of detecting "pops" or "clicks" upon penetration into fascial compartments. This is particularly beneficial in children due to the close proximity of nerve and critical abdominal structures. In addition, visualization of the local anesthetic spread made possible with ultrasonography has the potential to

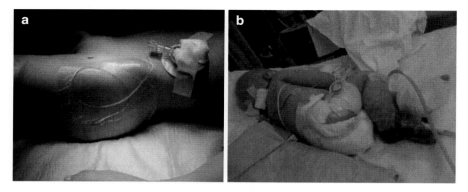

Fig. 20.34 Sciatic catheters

Fig. 20.35 (**a**) *FA* femoral
artery, *SN* sciatic nerve.
(**b**) Colordoppler of the
femoral artery

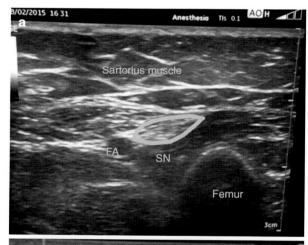

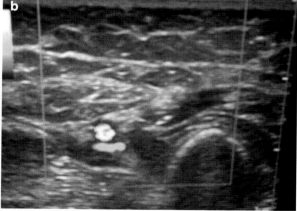

Fig. 20.36 IP saphenous
nerve block

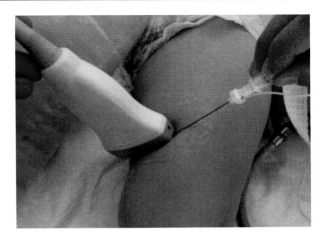

improve success rates and allow for administration of minimal volumes of local anesthetic [25, 26].

20.3.3.1 Ilioinguinal-Iliohypogastric Nerve Block

Both the iliohypogastric (IH) and ilioinguinal (II) nerves arise from L1 and emerge from the upper part of the lateral border of the psoas major muscle. The ilioinguinal nerve is a smaller nerve and courses caudad to the iliohypogastric nerve.

This block provides analgesia for all surgical procedures in the inguinal area.

Blockade of the II and IH nerves is indicated for analgesia following inguinal hernia repair because the nerves provide sensory innervation to the skin of the lower abdominal wall in addition to the upper hip and upper thigh. Because the lateral cutaneous branch of the IH nerve may pierce the internal and external oblique muscles immediately above the iliac crest, it is worthwhile to block the nerves as proximal as possible (i.e., posterior to the anterior superior iliac spine) before the nerve branches (Fig. 20.37).

Ultrasound technique has reduced failure rate and complications (intestinal puncture, pelvic hematoma) compared to techniques based on anatomical landmarks and "fascial click."

The nerves are medial to the anterior superior iliac spine and between the internal oblique and the transverse abdominal muscle. Both nerves appear hyperechoic, with oval shape.

Using a linear probe, it should be placed at the highest point of the iliac crest with the axis facing the umbilicus. This orientation provides a clear view of the relevant muscle layers and nerves (Fig. 20.38). Using an in-plane approach, a needle is inserted toward the ilioinguinal and iliohypogastric nerves (Fig. 20.39).

Both nerves are in close proximity to each other; usually one needle tip position is sufficient for blockade of both nerve (Fig. 20.40).

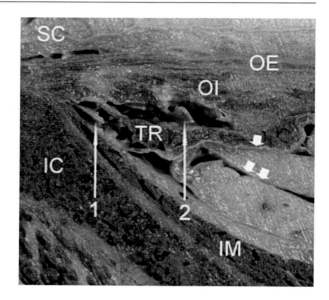

Fig. 20.37 *IC* iliac crest, *OE* external oblique muscle, *OI* internal oblique muscle, *TR* transversus muscle, *1 and 2* ilioinguinal and iliohypogastric nerves

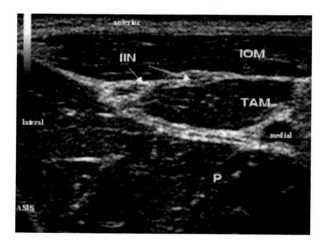

Fig. 20.38 *IOM* internal oblique muscle, *TAM* transversus abdominis muscle, *P* peritoneum, *ASIS* anterior superior iliac spine, *IIN* ilioinguinal and iliohypogastric nerves

    The use of conventional techniques for the ilioinguinal nerve block based on the observance of clicks to determine penetration of the abdominal muscles has a reported success rate of approximately 70 % [27]. Part of the block failure may be attributed to inaccurate nerve localization using traditional landmark-based needle insertion sites and the fascial click method to determine injection. A study by Wientraud et al. used ultrasonography to determine the actual location of local anesthetic distribution when it was injected using traditional methods. The local anesthetic surrounded the nerves in only 14 % of blocks [28]. Thus, the use

Fig. 20.39 IP ilioinguinal/
iliohypogastric nerve block

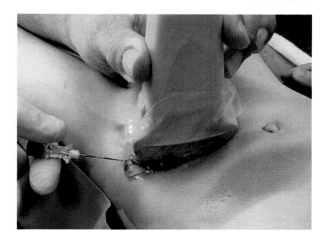

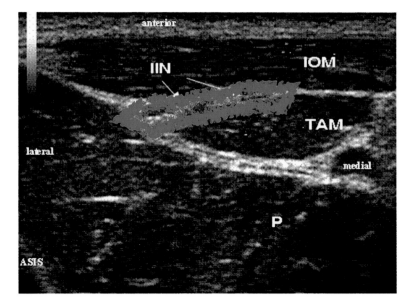

Fig. 20.40 *Red line* spread of local anesthetic

of ultrasound guidance to visualize the plane of nerve localization, needle
trajectory, and local anesthetic dispersion offers significant opportunity for
improvement.

Pharmacodynamic studies have demonstrated the efficacy of lower doses of local
anesthetics for managing postoperative pain in children who received these blocks
under ultrasound guidance. The authors also believe that using lower volumes could

reduce the risk of local anesthetic toxicity [26]. The use of lower volumes of local anesthetic is also supported by a recent pharmacokinetic study that found higher plasma levels of ropivacaine using ultrasound guidance when compared to a single pop technique [29].

20.3.3.2 Rectus Sheath Block

The rectus sheath block is generally used in pediatric surgery for umbilical or epigastric hernia correction and for laparoscopic port insertion. For this purpose the tenth intercostal space nerve in the umbilical region is blocked.

The patient is in supine position. Start by scanning the sonoanatomy of the investigation area (on the left side and on the right side of the umbilicus) to locate the rectus abdominis muscle (Fig. 20.41). Then follow the belly of this muscle to its lateral border; on the outside the aponeuroses of the internal oblique muscle and the transverse muscle can be identified (Fig. 20.42).

The block is performed with a linear high-frequency probe; the probe is positioned on the abdomen near the umbilicus in a tangential plane so that the abdominal muscles can be scanned transversely (the marker on the probe is directed toward the patient's right body side) (Fig. 20.43). The blockade is performed bilaterally. The writers are used to perform this block with the in-plane approach.

Since the tenth intercostal nerve cannot be visualized by ultrasound, the blockade is performed by injecting the local anesthetic between the lateral border of the rectus abdominus muscle and the aponeuroses of the internal oblique muscle and the transverse muscle [26] (Fig. 20.44).

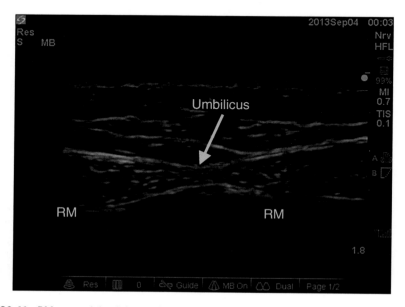

Fig. 20.41 *RM* rectus abdominis muscle

20.3.3.3 Transversus Abdominis Plane Block

The TAP is a potential space located between the internal oblique and the transversus abdominis muscles. The thoracolumbar nerve roots, T8–L1, run in the TAP.

The transversus abdominis plane (TAP) block was first described as a landmark-guided technique involving needle insertion at the triangle of Petit. This is an area bounded by the latissimus dorsi muscle posteriorly, the external oblique muscle

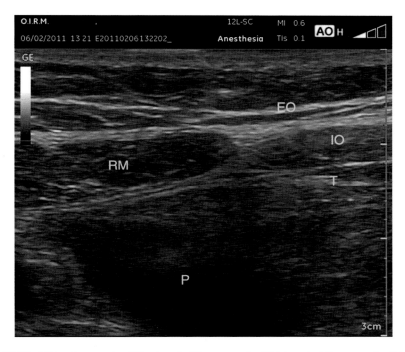

Fig. 20.42 *RM* rectus muscle, *EO* external oblique muscle, *IO* internal oblique muscle, *T* transversus abdominis muscle, *P* peritoneum

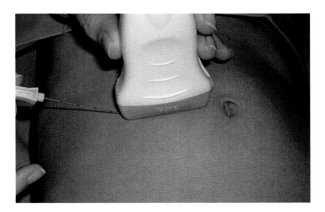

Fig. 20.43 IP rectus sheath block

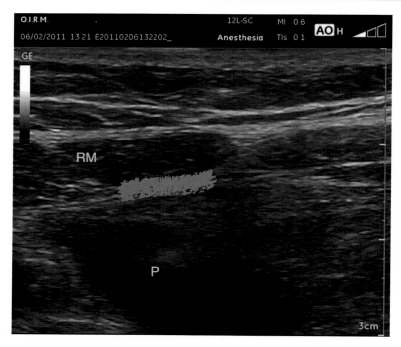

Fig. 20.44 *RM* rectus muscle, *P* peritoneum, *red line* spread of local anesthetic

anteriorly, and the iliac crest inferiorly (the base of the triangle). A needle is inserted perpendicular to all planes, looking for a tactile endpoint of two pops. The first pop indicates penetration of the external oblique fascia and entry into the plane between external and internal oblique muscles; the second pop signifies entry into the TAP plane between internal oblique and transversus abdominis muscles.

It has been shown to provide good postoperative analgesia for a variety of procedures, as well as chronic neuropathic abdominal wall pain [30]. This block is particularly useful when a central neuraxial blockade is contraindicated.

The patient is placed in a supine position and the abdomen is exposed between the costal margin and the iliac crest. A high-frequency linear probe or hockey stick probe is placed on the abdomen lateral to the umbilicus (Fig. 20.45). The probe can be shifted laterally to identify the three layers of the abdominal wall. The 3 muscle layers, external oblique, internal oblique, and transversus abdominis, serve as easily identified landmarks in an ultrasound image. However, there may not be a clear distinction between the individual muscles. The external oblique is most superficial and lies above the internal oblique, followed by the transversus abdominis. Deep to the muscles, the peritoneum appears as a hypoechoic region. The nerves for this block have similar echogenicity when compared to the muscles and travel tangentially to the ultrasound beam axis. As a result, the nerves will not be visualized (Fig. 20.46).

Fig. 20.45 IP TAP block

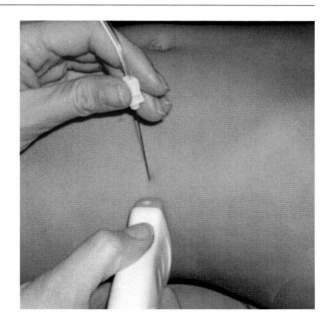

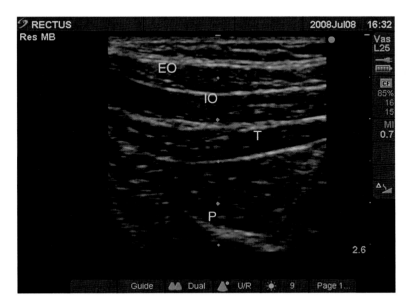

Fig. 20.46 *EO* external oblique muscle, *IO* internal oblique muscle, *T* transverse abdominis muscle, *P* peritoneum

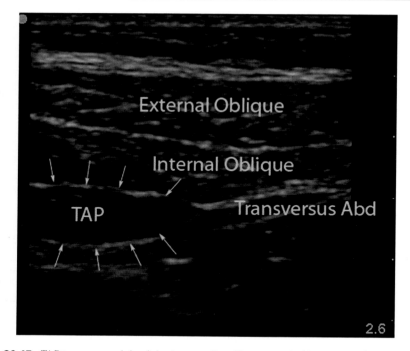

Fig. 20.47 *TAP* transversus abdominis plexus, yellow lines: spread of local anesthetic

Next, a needle is placed at or slightly posterior to the midaxillary line using an in-plane approach. The needle should be inserted into the plane between the internal oblique and the transversus abdominis muscles and the local anesthetic is injected into this potential space. The local anesthetic dispersion will appear as an elliptical opening of the potential space (Fig. 20.47). If this spread is not observed, it is important to hydrodissect with small injections of local anesthetic solution or saline until the exact plane of injection is recognized [31].

20.3.4 Continuous Peripheral Nerve Blocks

Continuous peripheral nerve blocks have been shown to decrease resting and dynamic pain and reduce opiate requirement, side effects, and sleep disturbance after surgery.

The main indications are for procedures associated with significant prolonged postoperative pain, to improve peripheral perfusion after microvascular surgery, in vasospastic disorders involving the limb and for children who have significant painful conditions to allow physical therapy in chronic regional pain syndrome [32].

For catheter placement, ultrasound techniques with needle guidance method are used. The ultrasound image will reveal both the target structures and the needle position; especially designed catheters can be introduced through either a needle or an intravenous cannula.

Continuous catheter placement
There are two common approaches for catheter placement: the in-plane and out-of-plane approaches; in the out-of-plane needle approach, the catheter is ideally positioned for advancement as it exits the tip of the needle parallel to the long axis of the target nerve; insertion using the in-plane needle approach assumes that the catheter can turn 90° upon exiting the tip of the needle to be advanced along the long axis of the nerve.
The ultrasound transducer and cord are covered completely inside a sterile sheath.
The technique of continuous catheter placement follows the same principle as the single-shot injection technique. That is, the procedures for patient positioning, skin preparation and sterilization, and transducer selection are identical.
In general, a 17 G insulated needle is inserted perpendicular to the ultrasound transducer (out-of-plane approach) and advanced to contact the target nerve.
Once the needle is deemed in contact with the target nerve (as indicated by nerve movement and/or nerve stimulation), inject a minimum volume of local anesthetic to distend the perineural space.
Distention of the perineural space will facilitate catheter threading especially in tight spaces, e.g., interscalene groove. A 20 G stimulating or non-stimulating catheter is then inserted 3–5 cm into the perineural space.
The catheter is often inserted without real-time ultrasound guidance unless an assistant is available to hold the ultrasound transducer in place while the principal operator uses one hand to hold the needle and one hand to thread in the catheter.
It is often difficult to visualize the transverse view of the catheter which appears as a hyperechoic dot.
After the needle is withdrawn, real-time assessment of local anesthetic spread is recommended during injection. Circumferential spread indicates that the catheter tip is located in an optimal position. Suboptimal catheter position may be corrected by withdrawing the catheter a short distance before further local anesthetic is injected. Securing catheter can be challenging in a mobile limb; subcutaneous tunneling is an option.

References

1. Giaufre E, Dalens B, Gombert A (1996) Epidemiology and morbidity of régional anesthesia in children: a one year prospective survey of the French-Language Society of Pediatric Anesthesiologists. Anesth Analg 83:904–912
2. Sites BD, Spence BC, Allagher J et al (2008) Regional anesthesia meets ultrasound: a specialty in transition. Acta Anaesthesiol Scand 52(4):456–466
3. Koscielniack-Nielsen ZJ (2008) Ultrasound-guided peripheral nerve blocks: what are the benefits? Acta Anaesthesiol Scand 52(6):727–737
4. Sites BD, Brull R, Chan VW et al (2007) Artifacts and pitfall errors associated with ultrasound-guided regional anesthesia. Part I: understanding the basic principles of ultrasound physics and machine operations. Reg Anesth Pain Med 32(5):412–418
5. Sites BD, Brull R, Chan VW et al (2007) Artifacts and pitfall errors associated with ultrasound-guided regional anesthesia. Part II: a pictorial approach to understanding and avoidance. Reg Anesth Pain Med 32(5):419–433
6. Marhofer P, Schrogendorfer K, Koining H et al (2007) Ultrasonographic guidance improves sensory block and onset time of three-in-one blocks. Anesth Analg 85:854–857
7. Sites BD, Brull R (2006) Ultrasound guidance in peripheral regional anesthesia: philosophy, evidence-based medicine, and techniques. Curr Opin Anaesthesiol 19(6):630–639, Review
8. Grau T (2005) Ultrasonography in the current practice of regional anaesthesia. Best Pract Res Clin Anaesthesiol 19(2):175–200

9. Chan VWS (2003) Applying ultrasound imaging to interscalene brachial plexus block. Reg Anesth Pain Med 28(4):340–343
10. Perlas A, Chan VWS (2004) Ultrasound guided interscalene brachial plexus block. Tech Reg Anesth Pain Manag 8(4):143–148
11. Sinha SK, Abrams JH, Weller RS (2007) Ultrasound-guided interscalene needle placement produces successful anesthesia regardless of motor stimulation above or below 0.5 mA. Anesth Analg 105(3):848–852
12. Chan VWS, Perlas A, Rawson R, Odukoya O (2003) Ultrasound guided supraclavicular brachial plexus block. Anesth Analg 97:1514–1517
13. Dingemans E et al (2007) Neurostimulation in ultrasound-guided infraclavicular block: a prospective randomized trial. Anesth Analg 104:1275
14. Chin KJ, Chan VW, van Geffen GJ (2008) Ultrasound-guided infraclavicular block: the in-plane versus out-of-plane approach. Paediatr Anaesth 18:1279–1280
15. De Jose Maria B, Tielens LK (2004) Vertical infraclavicular brachial plexus block in children: a preliminary study. Paediatr Anaesth 14:931–935
16. De Jose Maria B, Banus E, Navarro EM, Serrano S, Perello M, Marbok M (2004) Ultrasound-guided supraclavicular vs infraclavicular brachial plexus blocks in children. Paediatr Anaesth 18:838–844
17. Bloc S et al (2007) Spread of injectate associated with radial or median nerve-type motor response during infraclavicular brachial-plexus block: an ultrasound evaluation. Reg Anesth Pain Med 32(2):130–135
18. Fleischmann E, Marhofer P, Greher M, Waltl B, Sitzwohl C, Kapral S (2003) Brachial plexus anesthésia in children: latéral infraclavicular vs axillary approach. Paediatr Anaesth 13(2):103–108
19. Greher M, Retzl G, Niel P, Kamolz L, Marhofer P, Kapral S (2002) Ultrasonographic assessment of topographic anatomy in volunteers suggests a modification of the infraclavicular vertical brachial plexus block. Br J Anaesth 88:632–636
20. Casati A et al (2007) Effects of ultrasound guidance on the minimum effective anaesthetic volume required to block the femoral nerve. Br J Anaesth 98(6):823–827
21. Oberndorfer U, Marhofer P, Bösenberg A, Willschke H, Felfernig M, Weintraud M, Kapral S, Kettner SC (2007) Ultrasonographic guidance for sciatic and femoral nerve blocks in children. Br J Anaesth 98(6):797–801
22. van Geffen GJ, Bruhn J, Gielen M (2007) Ultrasound-guided continuous sciatic nerve blocks in two children with venous malformations in the lower limb. Can J Anaesth 54(11):952–953
23. Schwemmer U, Markus CK, Greim CA, Brederlau J, Trautner H, Roewer N (2004) Sonographic imaging of the sciatic nerve and its division in the popliteal fossa in children. Paediatr Anaesth 14(12):1005–1008
24. Domingo-Triadó V et al (2007) Ultrasound guidance for lateral midfemoral sciatic nerve block: a prospective, comparative, randomized study. Anesth Analg 104:1270
25. Willschke H, Marhofer P, Bosenberg A et al (2005) Ultrasonography for ilioinguinal/iliohypogastric nerve blocks in children. Br J Anaesth 95(2):226–230
26. Willschke H, Bosenberg A, Marhofer P et al (2006) Ultrasonography-guided rectus sheath block in paediatric anaesthesia--a new approach to an old technique {dagger}. Br J Anaesth 97:244–249
27. Lim SL, Ng Sb A, Tan GM (2002) Ilioinguinal and iliohypogastric nerve block revisited: single shot versus double shot technique for hernia repair in children. Paediatr Anaesth 12(3):255–260
28. Weintraud M, Marhofer P, Bosenberg A (2008) Ilioinguinal/iliohypogastric blocks in children: where do we administer the local anesthetic without direct visualization? Anesth Analg 106:123–127
29. Weintraud M, Lundblad M, Kottner S (2009) Ultrasound versus landmark-based technique for ilioinguinal/iliohypogastric nerve blockade in children: the implications on plasma levels of ropivacaine. Anesth Analg 108:1488–1492

30. McDonnell JG, O'Donnell B, Curley G, Heffernan A, Power C, Laffey JG (2007) The analgesic efficacy of transversus abdominis plane block after abdominal surgery: a prospective randomized controlled trial. Anesth Analg 104(1):193–197
31. Fredrickson M, Seal P, Houghton J (2008) Early expérience with the transversus abdominis plane block in children. Paediatr Anaesth 18:891–892
32. Fredrickson MJ (2007) Ultrasound-assisted interscalene catheter placement in a child. Anaesth Intensive Care 35:807–808

Noninvasive Hemodynamic and Respiratory Monitoring During the Perioperative Period

Brian Schloss and Joseph D. Tobias

21.1 Introduction

The first public display of the delivery of general anesthesia in the ether dome was quickly followed within 2 years by the first reported case of death related to anesthesia in a child. Despite improvements in medications and preoperative preparation, perioperative morbidity and mortality may still occur [1–4]. Although likely multifactorial in most instances, the incidence of both is increased in younger pediatric patients (neonates and infants) when compared to older pediatric patients, in the presence of comorbid diseases and increased American Society of Anesthesiologists (ASA) status, as well as by a lack of experience or training by the anesthesia provider [5, 6]. Data from the Australian Incident Monitoring Study (AIMS) suggested that 46 % of intraoperative cardiac arrests were thought to be anesthesia related, and of these events, more than half had a preventable factor that could be identified [7].

The incidence of perioperative morbidity and mortality may be modified by several factors, most importantly the presence of personnel with appropriate training in

B. Schloss, MD
Department of Anesthesiology and Pain Medicine, Nationwide Children's Hospital, 700 Children's Drive, Columbus, OH 43205, USA

Department of Anesthesiology and Pain Medicine, The Ohio State University, Columbus, OH, USA

J.D. Tobias, MD (✉)
Department of Anesthesiology and Pain Medicine, Nationwide Children's Hospital, 700 Children's Drive, Columbus, OH 43205, USA

Department of Anesthesiology and Pain Medicine, The Ohio State University, Columbus, OH, USA

Department of Pediatrics, The Ohio State University, Columbus, OH, USA
e-mail: Joseph.Tobias@Nationwidechildrens.org

© Springer International Publishing Switzerland 2016
M. Astuto, P.M. Ingelmo (eds.), *Perioperative Medicine in Pediatric Anesthesia*, Anesthesia, Intensive Care and Pain in Neonates and Children, DOI 10.1007/978-3-319-21960-8_21

the provision of anesthesia to infants and children as well as by the use of standard monitoring and safety devices on the anesthesia machine including continuous electrocardiography, pulse oximetry, end-tidal carbon dioxide ($ETCO_2$), continuous temperature recording, intermittent measurement of blood pressure, an oxygen analyzer, and disconnect or low-pressure alarm of the ventilator/circuit system. The AIMS demonstrated the potential utility of monitoring equipment in early detection of perioperative adverse events. Of 1256 critical incidents, which occurred in association with general anesthesia, 48 % were initially "human detected" by the vigilance of the anesthesia provider, while 52 % were "monitor detected." More than half were detected by either pulse oximetry (27 %) or capnography (24 %) [8, 9]. The remaining events were detected by electrocardiography (19 %), a blood pressure monitoring device (12 %), a low-pressure circuit disconnection alarm (8 %), or an oxygen analyzer (4 %). The percentage of events picked up by pulse oximetry would have increased to 40 % had all of the cases used the modulated pulse tone from the pulse oximeter instead of the tone or "beep" from the electrocardiogram. The pulse oximeter also functioned as a secondary monitor for identifying respiratory events when the primary monitor was either nonfunctional or not in use. These events included circuit disconnects, circuit leaks, esophageal intubation, aspiration, pulmonary edema, endotracheal tube obstruction, failure of oxygen delivery, hypoxic gas mixture, hypoventilation, air embolism, and bronchospasm.

Regardless of the event, these data clearly demonstrate that early detection of critical events is facilitated and that morbidity and mortality can be decreased by adherence to the current guidelines for monitoring during anesthesia. The following chapter discusses current standard for intraoperative monitoring of hemodynamic and respiratory function, the technology available, and its applications during the perioperative period. Additionally, potential new technologies which may allow the continuous, noninvasive measurement of cardiac output, blood pressure, tissue oxygenation, oxygen saturation, and the partial pressure of carbon dioxide ($PaCO_2$) are reviewed and their potential applications in the perioperative period discussed.

21.2   Noninvasive Monitoring of Respiratory Function

A key component of perioperative care involves continuous monitoring of respiratory function. During the intraoperative period, it is generally recommended that this include pulse oximetry, end-tidal carbon dioxide monitoring ($ETCO_2$), and the use of a precordial stethoscope. Given the risk of end-organ damage related to hypoxemia, the general focus of perioperative monitoring remains the detection of changes in oxygenation.

21.2.1 Pulse Oximetry

Although the concept and even early machines were developed in the 1930s and 1940s, the modern generation of pulse oximeters was developed in the 1970s with their widespread introduction into clinical practice in the 1980s. The pulse oximeter generally consists of a light-emitting diode that emits two wavelengths of light (940 and 640 nm) through the tissue. Oxygenated hemoglobin preferentially absorbs light at the higher wavelength (940 nm or infrared spectrum), while unoxygenated hemoglobin absorbs light at the lower wavelength (640 nm or red spectrum) [10]. The detector which collects light after it has traversed the tissue measures the ratio of absorption to determine the oxygen saturation. Plethysmography is used to identify the pulsatile signal, thereby eliminating non-pulsatile venous blood and tissue. The newer generation of pulse oximeters that have been developed over the past 5–10 years has focused on ensuring readings during low flow states, reducing interference from movement, improving accuracy within the lower saturation range (less than 90 %), and measuring variant hemoglobins (carboxyhemoglobin, methemoglobin) through the use of additional wavelengths of light.

In pediatric practice, pulse oximetry must be readily available in any situation where there is a risk of hypoxemia including perioperative care, sedation, the ICU setting, and the emergency department. More recently pulse oximetry has been used not only to identify patients with hypoxemia allowing for earlier therapy but also as a therapeutic decision-making tool as a means of triaging patients and identifying those that may need hospital admission [11–13]. Pulse oximetry has also emerged as a useful monitor during neonatal resuscitation and as a means of screening for congenital heart disease [14]. As skin color has been shown to be an unreliable indicator of oxygenation, pulse oximetry is being used more frequently during resuscitation following delivery [15]. These initiatives have been further pushed by the mounting data showing the deleterious physiologic effects of both hypoxia and hyperoxia [16, 17]. Given these concerns, current guidelines recommend oxygen saturation monitoring in the delivery room for neonates with persistent cyanosis, when assisted ventilation and supplementary oxygen administration are required, or when neonatal resuscitation is anticipated (high-risk deliveries) [18].

Most importantly for perioperative care, pulse oximetry remains an essential monitor during the entire perioperative period and into the postoperative period in patients with significant comorbid conditions or those receiving continuous opioid infusions such as patient-controlled analgesia. These recommendations persist despite the presence of evidence-based medicine which clearly shows a decreased risk of significant morbidity or mortality during the perioperative period [19]. Despite the lack of definitive data during the perioperative period, reviews of adverse events during procedural sedation show the potential impact of inadequate monitoring as a causative or contributing factor [20]. In a review of adverse sedation events derived from the Food and Drug Administration's adverse drug event reporting system, from the US Pharmacopeia, and from a survey of pediatric specialists, the authors investigated 95 adverse events occurring during procedural sedation. Successful outcome of the event and subsequent resuscitation defined as prolonged hospitalization without injury or no harm were associated with the use of pulse oximetry compared with a lack of any documented monitoring.

As with any monitoring device, effective use requires an understanding of the technology and its limitations. Pulse oximetry estimates the percent saturation of

Table 21.1 External and patient-related factors that affect pulse oximetry

Motion artifact
Poor perfusion due to hypothermia or decreased cardiac output
Nail polish and artificial nails
Skin pigmentation
Cardiac arrhythmias
Electromagnetic interference from surgical cautery
Ambient light
Abnormal hemoglobin variants (methemoglobin)
Poor position or application of the probe
Venous pulsation from tricuspid regurgitation
Intravenous dyes (methylene blue)

the hemoglobin and cannot be used as a surrogate measure of the partial pressure of oxygen in the blood (PaO_2). The relationship between PaO_2 and oxygen saturation is affected by many factors including the type of hemoglobin present and the status of the oxyhemoglobin dissociation curve which can be affected by acid-base status, temperature, and 2,3-DPG levels. Pulse oximetry is known to be inaccurate during periods of hypoxemia (saturation less than 85–90 %) and generally reads 98–100 % when the PaO_2 exceeds 100 mmHg, making it ineffective during periods of hyperoxia. Moreover, as the saturation does not change regardless of the hemoglobin concentration, it does not provide information regarding oxygen carrying capacity or oxygen delivery to the tissues, acid-base status, or ventilation [21, 22]. Furthermore, several patient-related or external factors may interfere with its accuracy (Table 21.1), although some of these issues have been addressed to some extent with the newer generation devices. Newer technology has led to the introduction of low-perfusion pulse oximetry that provides accurate readings during low-perfusion states, devices using 6–8 wavelengths of light instead of 2 that can identify abnormal hemoglobin species (carboxyhemoglobin, methemoglobin), improved accuracy at saturation levels less than 90 %, and alternative sites for monitoring (forehead, esophageal) [23–26].

21.2.2 End-Tidal Carbon Dioxide Monitoring

End-tidal carbon dioxide ($ETCO_2$) monitoring or capnography displays the patient's exhaled carbon dioxide concentration continuously during exhalation with the $ETCO_2$ being the peak value before the next breath is initiated. Capnometers estimate $ETCO_2$ through the use of infrared technology such that the concentration of CO_2 in the exhaled gas is measured by the absorption of infrared light by CO_2. Following its introduction into anesthesia practice, it has become the standard of care to continuously monitor $ETCO_2$ whenever general anesthesia is provided. Additionally, the measurement of $ETCO_2$ via infrared or other technology is standard of care whenever endotracheal intubation occurs. When used continuously in the ICU or operating room setting, the technology provides a continuous estimation of the partial pressure of CO_2 ($PaCO_2$) in the blood and serves as a disconnect alarm during mechanical ventilation, monitoring respiratory rate, and providing information regarding pulmonary function via the shape of the capnogram. Abrupt changes in the $ETCO_2$ such as decreases related to increased dead space may alert the clinician to decreased cardiac output or alterations in pulmonary perfusion related to gas or pulmonary embolism. Acute increases in $ETCO_2$ may be the initial sign of malignant hyperthermia or other hypermetabolic states.

The normal capnogram has 3 phases of exhalation and one of inspiration, generally labeled as phases 1–4. Phase 1 is the beginning of exhalation, representing dead space ventilation and therefore having no $ETCO_2$ present. If there is $ETCO_2$ present during phase 1, this is indicative of the rebreathing of exhaled gas, which may be due to inadequate fresh gas flows. Phase 2 is the rapid and steep upslope of the capnogram representing the emptying of alveolar gas with dead space gas. Phase 3 is the plateau phase, which in the normal state should be relatively horizontal. Upsloping of phase 3 of the capnogram indicates obstructive lung disease (asthma, bronchospasm) with differential emptying of alveoli with varying time constants. With the initiation of inspiration, there is an abrupt decrease of the ETCO2 (phase 4) which should return to 0 mmHg.

The $ETCO_2$ generally correlates in a clinically useful fashion with the $PaCO_2$ with the $ETCO_2$ being 2–4 mmHg lower than the $PaCO_2$. This correlation can be used clinically to adjust ventilation techniques both in the operating room and the ICU setting. However, this correlation is dependent on effective matching of ventilation with perfusion, and various technology and patient-related factors may interfere with this accuracy [27–31]. Such issues may be particularly relevant in the practice of pediatric anesthesia where smaller tidal volumes, type of ventilation (continuous versus intermittent flow), and sampling issues can affect the correlation of ET and $PaCO_2$.

Although initially introduced for intraoperative care, capnography has been brought out of the operating room to various clinical arenas. The concern that changes in pulse oximetry may take 60–90 s after the development of apnea in patients receiving supplemental oxygen has led some authorities to recommend the use of continuous $ETCO_2$ monitoring during procedural sedation. While not mandated by all of the current guidelines for procedural sedation, $ETCO_2$ monitoring has been shown to be a beneficial adjunct to monitoring during procedural sedation. While there may be some discrepancy between the $ETCO_2$ value and the $PaCO_2$ especially when monitoring from a nasal cannula, in many cases a direct correlation can be demonstrated [32, 33]. The capnograph provides a continuous and real-time demonstration that air exchange is occurring. If there is upper airway obstruction or central apnea, this is immediately demonstrated as the capnogram extinguishes [34, 35]. Several clinical studies have demonstrated the early identification of respiratory depression using this technology and have clearly indicated its superiority over pulse oximetry in many clinical scenarios in both pediatric and adult patients [36–40]. These data have also been supported by a recent meta-analysis, concluding that episodes of respiratory depression were 17.6 times more likely to be detected by capnography compared with standard monitoring [41]. Owing to the growing evidence, the American Society of Anesthesiologists has amended its standards for basic anesthetic monitoring effective from 2011 to include mandatory $ETCO_2$ monitoring during moderate and deep sedation.

The recent literature and clinical experience clearly demonstrate that capnography is not only effective for confirming ETT placement but may also have an expanded role: the continuous monitoring of tube position in the OR and during transport and monitoring during procedural sedation as a means for providing the immediate identification of apnea or upper airway obstruction. It clearly remains the standard of care for intraoperative monitoring and to document correct endotracheal tube placement wherever endotracheal intubation occurs. Beyond this, it is rapidly becoming the standard of care during procedural sedation especially with the recent revisions of the ASA guidelines. It is also a key monitor in the ICU as a means of rapidly adjusting minute ventilation during mechanical ventilation and for assessing patients with respiratory illnesses. It may provide useful information following endotracheal intubation and during transport as a means of avoiding inadvertent hyperventilation which may be detrimental in patients with traumatic brain injury [42]. More recently, it has been suggested that it can be used to judge the adequacy of resuscitation during cardiac arrest. The depth of chest compression has been shown to correlate with the $ETCO_2$ values [43]. Additionally, higher $ETCO_2$ values during resuscitation have been shown to correlate with a greater chance of return of spontaneous circulation (ROSC). Although initial investigations suggested that an $ETCO_2$ greater than 10 mmHg predicted ROSC, this value has recently been questioned suggesting that the goal $ETCO_2$ during resuscitation should be considered higher, perhaps approaching 25 mmHg [44]. Although $ETCO_2$ was initially applied only in the presence of an ETT, design modifications and the development of new devices allow its application in patients with a native airway during spontaneous ventilation. Given its ability to immediately detect hypercarbia and perhaps respiratory depression, it has been suggested that its use during postoperative period to monitor patients receiving patient-controlled analgesia may lead to the early identification of respiratory depression prior to the development of respiratory arrest thereby improving patient safety [45].

21.2.3 Transcutaneous CO_2 Monitoring

Transcutaneous CO_2 (TC-CO_2) devices can also be used to provide a continuous estimate of $PaCO_2$ in various clinical scenarios. Although introduced for use in the neonatal population where both transcutaneous CO_2 and O_2 monitoring have been used, these devices have also found their way out of the NICU and into the ICU and OR setting as a means of continuously monitoring ventilation. Their use has been driven by concerns of clinical scenarios that affect the accuracy of $ETCO_2$ or limit their use (high-frequency ventilation techniques). In general, these devices apply heat to the skin at 43–45 °C leading to capillary vasodilatation, increasing the transit time of blood through the capillary, resulting in a close approximation of capillary and arterial $PaCO_2$. The vasodilatation of the capillary bed also allows CO_2 to diffuse from the arterial capillary lumen to the membrane of the transcutaneous monitor. Alterations in temperature affect the solubility of CO_2 in blood such that an increase in the temperature increases the partial pressure of CO_2 in the blood and a higher $PaCO_2$ value or a larger gradient between the actual $PaCO_2$ and the $TC\text{-}CO_2$. Additionally, the higher temperature increases the metabolic rate of the tissues, thereby further increasing the $PaCO_2$. These factors are corrected by an internal calibration factor that is used to calculate the $TC\text{-}CO_2$ and thereby makes the TC value an appropriate estimate of the $PaCO_2$. Although used less commonly than $ETCO_2$ devices, these devices have seen increased used in various clinical scenarios in both the OR and the ICU setting. These include conventional and high-frequency mechanical ventilation, in spontaneously breathing patients, during the transport of critically ill patients, and in other clinical scenarios including apnea testing during brain death examination and in the assessment of patients with diabetic ketoacidosis (DKA).

In a cohort of pediatric ICU patients with respiratory failure of various etiologies, ranging in age from 1 to 40 months, 100 simultaneously obtained sets of arterial, transcutaneous, and end-tidal CO_2 values were analyzed [46]. The end-tidal to arterial CO_2 difference was 6.8 ± 5.1 mmHg, while the transcutaneous to arterial CO_2 difference was 2.3 ± 1.3 mmHg, $p < 0.0001$. The absolute difference between the end-tidal and arterial CO_2 was ≤ 4 mmHg in 38 of 100 values, while the absolute difference between the transcutaneous and arterial CO_2 value was ≤ 4 mmHg in 96 of 100 values, $p < 0.0001$. The same investigators demonstrated the improved accuracy and potential application of $TC\text{-}CO_2$ monitoring in an older cohort of patients with respiratory failure who ranged in age from 4 to 16 years of age [47]. A final study evaluated the accuracy of transcutaneous CO_2 monitoring following cardiothoracic surgery in infants and children [48]. Given the potential for various physiologic factors including residual shunt and ventilation-perfusion mismatch which may exist following cardiopulmonary bypass (CPB) and surgery for infants with congenital heart disease, the authors speculated that $ETCO_2$ would be inaccurate in this patient population and of limited benefit for continuous monitoring in the pediatric ICU setting. The study population included 33 consecutive patients following surgery for congenital heart disease. Transcutaneous CO_2 monitoring was initiated if the initial ABG following CPB demonstrated an arterial to end-tidal gradient of 5 mmHg or more. Although the study validated the utility of $TC\text{-}CO_2$ monitoring and its improved accuracy over $ETCO_2$ in this unique patient population, problems with $TC\text{-}CO_2$ monitoring were noted in 3 patients who demonstrated cardiovascular instability and were requiring dopamine at 20 µg/kg/min and epinephrine at 0.3–0.5 µg/kg/min. The cutaneous vasoconstriction induced by these vasopressors impacted the accuracy of $TC\text{-}CO_2$ monitoring. Other reported ICU and OR applications of $TC\text{-}CO_2$ monitoring have included continuous CO2 monitoring during high-frequency ventilation, one-lung ventilation, laparoscopic surgery, apnea testing, and metabolic disturbances where changes in $PaCO_2$ may correlate with acidosis resolution [49–54]. In such settings, $ETCO_2$ may not be feasible due to the ventilation technique or inaccurate due to alterations in pulmonary ventilation-perfusion matching.

Table 21.2 Advantages and disadvantages of transcutaneous and end-tidal devices

	Transcutaneous	End-tidal
Advantages	More accurate than end-tidal in many clinical scenarios Easy to use in both intubated and non-intubated patients Accuracy not affected by pulmonary parenchymal disease, shunt, ventilation-perfusion inequalities, type of ventilator, and low tidal volumes Can be used with high-frequency types of mechanical ventilation	Rapid set-up with no calibration Technically easy to use Confirms intratracheal position of ET tube Provides ventilator disconnect alarm. Capnogram provides information regarding pulmonary function
Disadvantages	More labor intensive than end-tidal devices Requires calibration and placement Must be repositioned every 3–4 h Potential for superficial skin blistering Accuracy affected by decreased perfusion or use of vasoconstricting agents Increasing, but still limited clinical experience outside of the neonatal population	Less accurate than transcutaneous devices in many clinical scenarios Accuracy affected by pulmonary parenchymal disease, shunt, ventilation-perfusion inequalities, type of ventilator, low tidal volumes, and site of sampling Use in non-intubated patients requires specialized sampling device (nasal cannula)

As with all noninvasive monitors, attention to detail regarding specific aspects of $TC\text{-}CO_2$ monitoring is required to ensure the accuracy of the technique. When compared with $ET\text{-}CO_2$ monitoring, $TC\text{-}CO_2$ monitoring requires a longer preparation time including a 5-min calibration period prior to placement and then an additional 5–10 min equilibration period after placement on the patient to allow for an equilibration between the transcutaneous and arterial CO_2 values. The electrode should be recalibrated and placed at another site every 4 h to avoid burns or blistering of the skin when the device is warmed to 45 °C, while newer devices that attach to the ear lobe and are heated to 43 °C have a lower risk of thermal injury and may be left in place for a longer period of time. While various sites (chest or abdomen) have been used in neonates and infants, we prefer the volar aspect of the forearm in adults especially those with obesity. Accuracy may be affected by technical factors related to the monitor itself including trapped air bubbles, improper placement technique, damaged membranes, and inappropriate calibration techniques. Patient-related issues that affect accuracy include variations in skin thickness; the presence of edema, tissue hypoperfusion, and hypothermia; or the administration of medications that result in cutaneous vasoconstriction. When considering these noninvasive monitors of $PaCO_2$, there are advantages and disadvantages to both (Table 21.2). Given their different clinical utilities, perhaps they should be considered as complimentary rather than competing devices.

21.2.4 Acoustic Impedance Monitoring

The latest addition to the respiratory armamentarium is the rainbow acoustic monitoring (RAM, Masimo Corporation, Irvine, California). RAM technology provides continuous, noninvasive monitoring of respiration rate using an innovative adhesive sensor with an integrated acoustic transducer that is externally applied to the patient's neck. The patented technology, known as Signal Extraction Technology (SET®), separates and processes the respiratory signal to display continuous acoustic respiration rate. Preliminary studies have suggested that this technology is responsive to changes in respiratory rate and is superior to capnography in detecting respiratory pauses. Its use of noninvasive adhesive sensors that are applied externally to the lateral aspect of the patient's neck may be more easily tolerated than ETCO$_2$ capturing devices. In a study comparing acoustic monitoring with capnography in 33 adults in the post-anesthesia care unit following general anesthesia, the acoustic monitor and capnometer both reliably monitored ventilatory rate, while the acoustic monitor more sensitively identified pauses in ventilation [55]. Although the acoustic monitor was statistically more accurate and more precise than capnography, the clinical differences were modest without proven clinical significance. The authors concluded that acoustic monitoring may provide an effective and convenient means of monitoring ventilatory rate in postsurgical patients. Other studies have demonstrated that respiratory rate monitoring with the acoustic monitor correlates well with that monitored by capnography and that the device is better tolerated than other devices such as a facemask for capnography (Capnomask) [56, 57]. Its preliminary validation and success in these areas have led to its use in the pediatric population for perioperative monitoring and in the adult population outside of the operating room [58–60]. While all of these preliminary studies have suggested that it is better tolerated than capnography by mask or nasal cannula, other advantages over capnography have yet to be determined. Further work is needed to delineate its role in perioperative and postoperative respiratory monitoring.

21.3   Noninvasive Monitoring of Hemodynamic Function

Along with respiratory monitoring (oxygen saturation and ETCO$_2$), the monitoring of cardiovascular parameters and hemodynamic function remains an integral component of standard perioperative monitoring. Although blood pressure monitoring remains a required component of perioperative care, it fails to provide us with even more essential information regarding cardiovascular performance including cardiac output, systemic tissue oxygen delivery, and tissue oxygenation. While these monitors are not considered essential for perioperative care, there remains great interest in the technology that would allow us to noninvasively monitor these parameters.

21.3.1 Cardiac Output Monitoring

The ability to measure cardiac output (CO) at the bedside became a reality in the 1970s, courtesy of the pulmonary artery catheter (PAC) developed by Drs. Swan and Ganz [61]. While the use of a PAC has failed to decrease mortality, there continues to be great interest in CO measurement in the operating room and beyond with the hopes of identifying parameters, which, when altered, will improve outcome [62]. This is evidenced by a Cochrane Database review which concluded that optimizing CO in a goal-directed fashion reduces hospital stay, as well as complications such as respiratory failure, renal impairment, and wound infection [63].

The PAC measures CO by way of the thermodilution technique. Using the thermodilution method, an injectate is administered centrally (right atrium) and a downstream (pulmonary artery) temperature change is measured. The magnitude of the change and its rapidity are directly related to CO. Using a variation of the "Stewart-Hamilton" indicator dilution equation, CO is calculated [62]. Although this method was introduced over 40 years ago, it generally remains accepted as the most accurate method of measuring CO at the bedside. Precision errors as low as 13 % have been reported with the use of PACs in animal models [64]. To eliminate the need for repeated injections which provide only intermittent measures of CO, a PAC was developed with a coil which sits in the right atrium that warms to slightly greater than body temperature, thereby warming the blood and eliminating the need for intermittent injection. Despite their accuracy, PAC use has fallen out of favor with many clinicians given their invasive nature, which may mitigate any clinical advantage their CO measurements bring. In addition, the size of PACs precludes their use in small children, while intracardiac shunts mitigate the accuracy of thermodilution measures of CO, thereby making it even less common among pediatric clinicians.

Transpulmonary thermodilution (TPTD) is another method of CO measurement, which is similar to the PAC. An injectate is administered centrally and a downstream temperature change is measured. However, the technique eliminates some of the invasiveness of the procedure as the distal measurement is measured in the femoral artery rather than the pulmonary artery. This method is likely equivalent in accuracy to the PAC, although it remains an invasive option, requiring the use of specialized central venous and femoral artery catheters [65]. While thermodilution remains the clinical gold standard in CO measurement, it is invasive and often impractical. Given the theoretical benefit of optimizing CO in the perioperative period, newer and less invasive methods of CO measurement are being developed and evaluated.

Doppler techniques offer a noninvasive alternative for the measurement of CO. These monitors are based on the Doppler effect, which states that the change in frequency of a reflected ultrasound signal is proportional to the speed of the reflecting object (blood flow) [66]. These changes in frequency can then be used to calculate velocity and ultimately quantify stroke volume and hence CP. Transthoracic and transesophageal echocardiography use Doppler ultrasound to accurately measure CO; however, they require specialized training and their regular use in the operating room is not feasible [67]. More practical approaches involve esophageal and transcutaneous (suprasternal) Doppler probes. Esophageal Doppler monitors (EDM) are a particularly attractive option in the operative room given its relative ease of placement and lack of interference with most surgical fields. For this reason, it is far more common than suprasternal probes. An EDM simply involves a probe, which is placed in the esophagus and is connected to an analyzer. The probe sends and receives ultrasound signals to the descending aorta, while the analyzer interprets the frequency changes, calculating velocity, which is then used to determine CO. However, up to one third of CO is diverted away from the aorta prior to the point of measurement by an EDM. Additionally, the aortic cross-sectional area is needed to calculate CO based on the measured velocity. These factors are estimated by the analyzer using the patient's age, weight, and height. Given these limitations, it is not surprising that the absolute values of EDM-measured CO are not interchangeable with the gold standard of thermodilution [68]. However, EDM does consistently show high correlations with thermodilution reference methods. This suggests that EDM may still be useful in the perioperative period by accurately tracking acute changes in CO.

The pulse contour analysis technique involves calculation of cardiac performance based on an arterial waveform tracing. This process necessitates the placement of an arterial catheter and often involves a specialized transducer, which accompanies the signal analyzer. Pulse contour analysis monitors can be categorized as calibrated and non-calibrated varieties. The available calibrated pulse contour monitors use either TPTD or lithium dilution to measure cardiac output [68]. Uncalibrated devices derive CO purely from waveform analysis without input from the other forms of CO measurement. The accuracy of pulse contour analysis remains in question given their significantly smaller body of literature compared with thermodilution and Doppler techniques. With this in mind, the studies suggest that calibrated pulse contour monitors are more accurate when compared to their uncalibrated counterparts. In addition, both types have decreased accuracy during periods of hemodynamic instability [69–73].

Thoracic electrical bioimpedance (TEB) is a completely noninvasive method of monitoring CO, requiring the placement of several electrodes on the external surface of the thorax. This method assumes that resistance to electrical flow is directly related to blood volume within the thorax so that changes in this resistance are used to calculate changes in the intrathoracic blood volume and hence CO. The electrodes are both transmitters and receivers of electrical current, constantly measuring changes in amplitude. The amplitude changes are caused by changes in thoracic fluid volume and ultimately related to descending aortic blood flow. An electrocardiogram measures ventricular ejection time, and the amount of amplitude change during ventricular ejection time is directly proportional to stroke volume. Unfortunately, TEB is prone to errors secondary to pulmonary edema, electrical interference, patient movement, and skin temperature. As such, TEB has shown poor correlation with clinical reference standards [74–76].

Bioreactance is a similar technique, which was developed in an effort to improve on the inaccuracies of TEB. Bioreactance refers to the "phase shift" of voltage, which occurs specifically during pulsatile blood flow. Given the fact that pulsatile flow in the thorax is predominantly taking place in the aorta, bioreactance is able to more accurately measure cardiac output without interference from thoracic fluid (pulmonary edema). Validation studies suggest that bioreactance is far more accurate than TEB when compared with thermodilution [77–79]. However, more research is needed before it can be recommended for routine use.

In conclusion, thermodilution techniques remain the clinical gold standard for cardiac output monitoring. The invasiveness of thermodilution techniques remains their primary drawback; however, no technology to date has proven itself to be superior. Doppler-based techniques, specifically transesophageal Doppler, provide a noninvasive alternative with accuracy that is similar, though not superior, to thermodilution. Calibrated pulse contour analysis is superior to its uncalibrated pulse contour analysis, though both tend to suffer during periods of hemodynamic instability. Bioreactance is completely noninvasive and shows promising accuracy in comparison to thermodilution. It is, however, a relatively newer technology when compared to thermodilution and Doppler counterparts. More research is needed before meaningful conclusions can be made regarding the clinical utility of bioreactance, while bioimpedance monitors have shown poor accuracy and cannot be recommended for clinical use.

21.3.2 Electrocardiogram Monitoring

Continuous monitoring of the electrocardiogram (ECG) remains one of the standard intraoperative monitors during the provision of anesthesia care. Although arrhythmias are uncommon outside of the pediatric cardiac anesthesia arena, bradycardia may occur due to the administration of volatile anesthetic agents (halothane or sevoflurane), hypoxemia, hypothermia, and alterations in intracranial pressure or from the oculocardiac or trigeminocardiac reflex. Although the negative chronotropic effect is less with sevoflurane when compared to halothane, bradycardia may still occur, thereby making continuous ECG monitoring mandatory regardless of the duration of the anesthetic or sedation event [80]. While many of these bradycardic responses are self-limiting, treatment may be required when the heart rate fails to respond to initial therapies such as release of surgical traction or a decrease in the volatile agent concentration. In most clinical scenarios for the pediatric population, a 3-lead ECG is used with the demonstration of lead II to facilitate the identification of P wave morphology and arrhythmia analysis. In adult patients and in specific pediatric patients, a 5-lead ECG is used to facilitate ischemia detection.

Other applications for ECG monitoring include identification of potentially lethal electrolyte disturbances including hyperkalemia, rare instances of prolonged QT syndrome (congenital, acquired, or drug induced), and monitoring for inadvertent systemic injection of local anesthetic agents. Over the years, there has been a dramatic increase in the use of regional anesthesia in infants and children, which has resulted in the increased administration of local anesthetic agents in the age group. Given its prolonged duration of action, the long-acting agent, bupivacaine, is frequently used. As it is relatively cardiotoxic when compared with other agents, a means of identifying inadvertent intravascular or systemic injection is mandatory. To accomplish this, a small amount of epinephrine is generally added to the solution as a test dose [81]. Although this was proposed to result in an increase in heart rate with a high sensitivity, subsequent work demonstrated that when anesthetized with a volatile anesthetic agent, the sensitivity of a heart rate increase was less than expected and not adequate to ensure the safety of the technique. [82–84] By using the T wave, systolic BP, and HR criteria, the positive response rate to an epinephrine test (0.1 mL/kg of a 1:200,000 solution or 0.5 µg/kg) was 100, 95, and 71 %, respectively, during sevoflurane anesthesia and 90, 71, and 71 % during halothane anesthesia [85].

21.3.3 Near-Infrared Spectroscopy

Near-infrared spectroscopy (NIRS) uses infrared light, a technique similar to pulse oximetry, to noninvasively estimate brain tissue oxygenation by measuring the absorption of the light by tissue chromophores (hemoglobin and cytochrome aa_3). Pulsatile flow is not required and therefore the device works during CPB and other non-pulsatile states such as cardiopulmonary bypass. Based on the relative absorption of the infrared light at various wavelengths, the specific concentration of the hemoglobin species can be determined using a modification of the Beer-Lambert law [86]. There are two basic types of NIRS monitors: a saturation monitor that measures the difference absorption between oxygenated and unoxygenated hemoglobin and a concentration monitor that measures the concentration of oxygenated and reduced hemoglobin and the relative redox state of cytochrome aa_3. The saturation monitor is the one used most commonly in clinical practice and the ones that are currently commercially available for widespread clinical use. To improve the ease of use, instead of providing the specific concentrations of oxygenated and unoxygenated hemoglobin, the NIRS monitors provide a single numeric value known as cerebral oxygenation (rSO_2). Cerebral oxygenation monitoring is initiated by placing a self-adhesive probe over the patient's forehead. Infrared light is directed into the cranium from a light source, and two sensors placed at fixed distances from the light source measure the light after it has passed through extracranial tissue (proximal sensor) or both extracranial and intracranial tissues (distal sensor).

Clinical evidence supports the correlation of the NIRS number (rSO_2) with cerebral blood flow (CBF) and oxygenation as changes in rSO_2 easily correlate with clinical changes that alter CBF such as blood pressure, $PaCO_2$, and systemic oxygenation. During CPB, rSO_2 increases during cooling, with improvements in cardiac output and oxygen delivery. Cerebral oxygenation (rSO_2) decreases exponentially and in a predictable and reproducible fashion during deep hypothermic cardiac arrest. Clearly the rSO_2 decreases rapidly during periods of hypoxemia, hypocarbia, hypoperfusion, or cardiac arrest. In fact, the rSO_2 has been shown to be an earlier and more sensitive indicator of hypoxemia than pulse oximetry [87, 88]. Furthermore, anecdotal experience supports its ability to identify problems related to cannula positioning during CPB. To date, NIRS monitoring has found the greatest use during cardiac surgery in both the adult and the pediatric population. There is accumulating evidence in the adult population which suggests that monitoring rSO_2 and acting on changes may alter outcome; however, additional studies are needed to validate these findings in the pediatric population [89–91]. More recent work has demonstrated the use of the NIRS to determine the autoregulatory threshold, demonstrating it to be widely altered in critically ill patients and also suggesting that maintenance of blood pressure within the autoregulatory limits alters outcome [92].

Despite its potential utility, one must also recognize the limitations of cerebral oxygenation monitoring using rSO_2. Unlike pulse oximetry, there is generally no "normal value" that can be assigned to rSO_2. Studies in the pediatric population have demonstrated a wide variation in the baseline values in patients without clinical signs of cerebral hypoxemia. Our clinical experience demonstrates similar variability depending on the age of the patient, underlying type of congenital heart disease, and perhaps head circumference and depth of penetration of the near-infrared light. Although the development of neonatal and pediatric probes has overcome some of these issues, NIRS should be regarded as a trend monitor with the need for additional prospective trials to demonstrate which values constitute true cerebral hypoxemia and the risk of subsequent neurologic damage. It is likely that adverse outcomes relate not only to the nadir of the rSO_2 but also to the duration of time spent at low values (the area under the curve). The current literature suggests that values less than 40 % or an absolute decrease of 20 % (a decrease from an rSO_2 value of 64–44 %) from baseline values should alert the clinician to the need for interventions to reverse potential cerebral hypoxemia. These interventions may include changing head position, verifying appropriate cannulation placement or increasing pump flow during CPB, allowing the $PaCO_2$ to increase, and increasing oxygen delivery (increasing cardiac output, increasing systemic oxygen saturation, or increasing hemoglobin). If the above measures fail to increase rSO_2, based on the clinical scenario, therapeutic maneuvers to decrease the cerebral metabolic rate for oxygen may be indicated.

21.3.4 Blood Pressure Monitor

Blood pressure (BP) monitoring in the perioperative period is an obvious necessity. Fluctuations in hemodynamics are common secondary to anesthetic medications, surgically induced nociception, fluid shifts, and blood loss. Blood pressure is most commonly measured with a noninvasive, oscillometric blood pressure (NIBP) cuff during this period. However, certain clinical scenarios involving wide BP swings or significant blood loss dictate the use of an arterial cannula. The advantage of an arterial cannula is its continuous monitoring capability and the ability to draw frequent blood samples for laboratory evaluation. While the arterial cannula is both reliable and accurate, its advantages are mitigated by its invasive nature, which can lead to complications such as arterial occlusion, distal ischemia, bleeding, infection, and unintended injection of medications. However, such complications are rare and infrequently seen especially when short-term monitoring is used intraoperatively. More importantly, there may be situations in which an arterial cannula cannot be placed due to patient-related issues or positioning. Furthermore, the need for an arterial cannula may not have been anticipated prior to the onset of rapid blood loss or acute hemodynamic instability. For these reasons, there remains interest in technology which offers beat-to-beat BP monitoring in a noninvasive fashion.

The most common technique of continuously and noninvasively monitoring BP was first described by Jan Peñàz in 1973 [93]. Peñàz, a physiologist, described a technique referred to as "vascular unloading" which employs the use of an inflatable finger cuff and a distal infrared plethysmograph. The plethysmograph is used to estimate the blood volume in the finger, while the cuff attempts to maintain that blood volume at a constant within the finger. The two aspects of the monitor are in a constant feedback loop as the cuff pressure varies with systole and diastole. This information is then incorporated into a formula which displays a waveform mimicking an invasive arterial tracing. Modern monitors using variations of Peñàz technique also incorporate NIBP readings to help calibrate the formula. Although generally accurate, there are limitations associated with this technique. Fluctuations in temperature, vascular disease, and the use of vasoactive agents can interfere with proper readings [94]. Also, as with NIBP devices, the accuracy varies based on cuff size. Despite these limitations, the technology behind this device is now commercially available. The preliminary clinical data suggests that this may be a promising technique in the adult and older pediatric population [95, 96].

Another technique for noninvasive continuous blood pressure monitoring is known as arterial tonometry [97]. This method requires a peripheral artery of a large diameter which is adjacent to a bony structure. The radial artery is the most common choice. A tonometer with a pressure sensor is placed over the artery, and pressure is applied until the artery is compressed, but not totally occluded. It is believed that the pressure between the skin overlaying the artery and the tonometer is a good approximation of arterial intraluminal pressure. The pressure fluctuations at the skin are then transmitted into a real-time arterial pressure tracing. While the tonometry method offers the advantage of a more proximal measurement, one of the major drawbacks is its reliance on calibration from an NIBP cuff. The tonometry module must assume that an oscillometric BP measurement is completely accurate, which can create a significant degree of error. It has also been reported that there is a wide variation in the oscillometric readings among the different devices from various manufacturers [98]. Additionally, there can be some difficulty in properly placing a tonometer directly over the intended artery. For these reasons, tonometry-based noninvasive blood pressure monitors have not gained widespread popularity and clinical use.

Pulse transit time is another technique which may have promise for future continuous noninvasive blood pressure monitoring [99]. This method measures the difference in propagation time of pulsatile blood at two separate peripheral sites. The ECG waveform can be used to detect the beginning of a pulse wave, while the actual distal pulse is detected at two separate sites using plethysmographic waveforms. These time variations can then be related to systolic blood pressure. The technique is also cuffless which removes the errors that are common with cuffed methods. Presently, there is no commercial monitor available that uses the pulse transit time technique. A recent meta-analysis by Kim et al. examining commercially available noninvasive blood pressure monitors concluded that the accuracy and precision of these devices is larger than has been deemed acceptable by the Association for the Advancement of Medical Instrumentation [100]. To put this conclusion into perspective, the meta-analysis stated that if a systolic arterial pressure is measured to be 100 mmHg using an arterial catheter, the systolic pressure measured by a commercially available noninvasive monitor could range from 74 to 123 mmHg. While these devices have shown great promise for future use, they will likely require additional improvements in accuracy before they find a significant foothold in modern perioperative care.

Conclusions

The years have seen improvements in both the pharmacology and technology of anesthesia, which have resulted in a decrease in the risks of perioperative morbidity and mortality. Many of these advancements have been linked with the introduction of standard monitoring during perioperative care to include a continuous ECG display, pulse oximetry, end-tidal CO_2, temperature, and intermittent BP. Additional devices have been introduced for both respiratory and hemodynamic monitoring, which may fill in some of the deficiencies of the currently used monitor. These newer devices offer options for transcutaneous CO_2 monitoring, NIRS, and continuous noninvasive BP or CO monitoring. However, prior to their widespread acceptance and integration into perioperative care, evidence-based medicine demonstrating their impact on outcome is needed. Furthermore, the technology behind some of these devices falls short of the accuracy required for clinical decision making. However, we hold firmly to the knowledge that the early detection of critical events has been shown to decrease morbidity and mortality. As such, the search continues for monitors that will supplement the current perioperative armamentarium.

References

1. Rackow H, Salintire E, Green L (1961) Frequency of cardiac arrest associated with anesthesia in infants and children. Pediatrics 28:697–704
2. Morray JP (2002) Anesthesia-related cardiac arrest in children. Anesth Clin North Am 20:1–28
3. Morray JP, Geiduschek J, Ramamoorthy C et al (2000) Anesthesia-related cardiac arrest in children: initial findings of the POCA registry. Anesthesiology 93:6–14
4. Bhanaker SM, Ramamoorthy C, Geiduschek JM et al (2007) Anesthesia-related cardiac arrest in children: update from the Pediatric Perioperative Cardiac Arrest Registry. Anesth Analg 105:344–350
5. Tiret L, Nicoche Y, Hatton F et al (1988) Complications related to anesthesia in infants and children. A prospective survey of 40,240 anesthetics. Br J Anaesth 61:263–269

6. Flick RP, Sprung J, Harrison TE et al (2007) Perioperative cardiac arrests in children between 1988 and 2005 at a tertiary referral center. Anesthesiology 106:226–237

7. Morgan CA, Webb RK, Cockings J, Williamson JA (1993) The Australian Incident Monitoring Study. Cardiac arrest: an analysis of 2000 incident reports. Anaesth Intensive Care 21:626–637

8. Runciman WB, Webb RK, Barker L, Currie M (1993) The Australian Incident Monitoring Study. The pulse oximeter: applications and limitations - an analysis of 2000 incident reports. Anaesth Intensive Care 21:543–550

9. Webb RK, Van der Walt JH, Runciman RB et al (1993) The Australian Incident Monitoring Study. Which monitor? An analysis of 2000 incident reports. Anaesth Intensive Care 21:529–542

10. Aoyagi T (2003) Pulse oximetry: its invention, theory, and future. J Anesth 17:259–266

11. Coté CJ (2012) American Academy of Pediatrics sedation guidelines: are we there yet? Arch Pediatr Adolesc Med 166:1067–1069

12. Mansbach JM, Clark S, Christopher NV et al (2008) Prospective multicenter study of bronchiolitis: predicting safe discharges from the emergency department. Pediatrics 121:680–688

13. Mallory MD, Shay DK, Garrett J, Bordley WC (2003) Bronchiolitis management preferences and the influence of pulse oximetry and respiratory rate on the decision to admit. Pediatrics 111:e45–e51

14. Mahle WT, Newburger JW, Matherne GP et al (2009) American Heart Association, Congenital Heart Defects Committee of the Council on Cardiovascular Disease in the Young, Council on Cardiovascular Nursing, and Interdisciplinary Council on Quality of Care and Outcomes Research; American Academy of Pediatrics, Section on Cardiology and Cardiac Surgery. Committee on Fetus and Newborn. Role of pulse oximetry in examining newborns for congenital heart disease: a scientific statement from the AHA and AAP Pediatrics. Circulation 124:823–836

15. O'Donnell CP, Kamlin CO, Davis PG, Carlin JB, Morley CJ (2007) Clinical assessment of infant colour at delivery. Arch Dis Child Fetal Neonatal Ed 92:F465–F467

16. Wyckoff MH (2013) Neonatal resuscitation guidelines versus the reality of the delivery room. J Pediatr 163:1542–1543

17. Vento M, Saugstad OD (2010) Oxygen as a therapeutic agent in neonatology: a comprehensive approach. Semin Fetal Neonatal Med 15:185–188

18. Kattwinkel J, Perlman JM, Aziz K et al (2010) American Heart Association. Neonatal resuscitation: 2010 American Heart Association Guidelines for cardiopulmonary resuscitation and emergency cardiovascular care. Pediatrics 126:e1400–e1413

19. Shah A, Shelley KH (2013) Is pulse oximetry an essential tool or just another distraction? The role of the pulse oximeter in modern anesthesia care. J Clin Monit Comput 27:235–242

20. Coté CJ, Notterman DA, Karl HW, Weinberg JA, McCloskey C (2000) Adverse sedation events in pediatrics: a critical incident analysis of contributing factors. Pediatrics 105:805–814

21. Toffaletti J, Zijlstra WG (2007) Misconceptions in reporting oxygen saturation. Anesth Analg 105(6 suppl):S5–S9

22. Zijlstra WG (2005) Clinical assessment of oxygen transport-related quantities. Clin Chem 51:291–292

23. Aoyagi T, Fuse M, Kobayashi N, Machida K, Miyasaka K (2007) Multiwavelength pulse oximetry: theory for the future. Anesth Analg 105(6 suppl):S53–S58

24. Agashe GS, Coakley J, Mannheimer PD (2006) Forehead pulse oximetry: headband use helps alleviate false low readings likely related to venous pulsation artifact. Anesthesiology 105:1111–1116

25. Berkenbosch JW, Tobias JD (2006) Comparison of a new forehead reflectance pulse oximeter with a conventional digit sensor in pediatric patients. Respir Care 51:726–731

26. Zaouter C, Zavorsky GS (2012) The measurement of carboxyhemoglobin and methemoglobin using a non-invasive pulse CO-oximeter. Respir Physiol Neurobiol 182:88–92

27. Pansard JL, Cholley B, Devilliers C et al (1992) Variation in the arterial to end-tidal CO_2 tension differences during anesthesia in the "kidney rest" lateral decubitus position. Anesth Analg 75:506–510
28. Grenier B, Verchere E, Meslie A et al (1999) Capnography monitoring during neurosurgery: reliability in relation to various intraoperative positions. Anesthesiology 88:43–48
29. Short JA, Paris ST, Booker BD et al (2001) Arterial to end-tidal carbon dioxide tension difference in children with congenital heart disease. Br J Anaesth 86:349–353
30. Burrows FA (1989) Physiologic dead space, venous admixture and the arterial to end-tidal carbon dioxide difference in infants and children undergoing cardiac surgery. Anesthesiology 70:219–225
31. Badgwell JM, Heavener JE, May WS et al (1987) End-tidal PCO_2 monitoring in infants and children ventilated with either a partial rebreathing or non-rebreathing circuit. Anesthesiology 66:405–410
32. Tobias JD, Flanagan JF, Wheeler TJ, Garrett JS, Burney C (1994) Noninvasive monitoring of end-tidal CO_2 via nasal cannulas in spontaneously breathing children during the perioperative period. Crit Care Med 22:1805–1808
33. Flanagan JF, Garrett JS, McDuffee A, Tobias JD (1995) Noninvasive monitoring of end-tidal carbon dioxide tension via nasal cannulas in spontaneously breathing children with profound hypocarbia. Crit Care Med 23:1140–1142
34. Tobias JD (1999) End-tidal carbon dioxide monitoring during sedation with a combination of midazolam and ketamine for children undergoing painful, invasive procedures. Pediatr Emerg Care 15:173–175
35. Tobias JD, Kavanaugh-McHugh A (1995) Oximetry and capnography during sedation for transesophageal echocardiography: useful information to determine the etiology of cardiorespiratory arrest. Clin Pediatr 34:565–566
36. Hart LS, Berns SD, Houck CS et al (1997) The value of end-tidal CO_2 monitoring when comparing three methods of conscious sedation for children undergoing painful procedures in the emergency department. Pediatr Emerg Care 13:189–193
37. Lightdale JR, Goldmann DA, Feldman HA, Newburg AR, DiNardo JA, Fox VL (2006) Microstream capnography improves patient monitoring during moderate sedation: a randomized, controlled trial. Pediatrics 117:e1170–e1178
38. Cacho G, Pérez-Calle JL, Barbado A, Lledó JL, Ojea R, Fernández-Rodríguez CM (2010) Capnography is superior to pulse oximetry for the detection of respiratory depression during colonoscopy. Rev Esp Enferm Dig 102:86–89
39. Burton JH, Harrah JD, Germann CA, Dillon DC (2006) Does end-tidal carbon dioxide monitoring detect respiratory events prior to current sedation monitoring practices? Acad Emerg Med 13:500–504
40. Deitch K, Miner J, Chudnofsky CR, Dominici P, Latta D (2010) Does end tidal CO_2 monitoring during emergency department procedural sedation and analgesia with propofol decrease the incidence of hypoxic events? A randomized, controlled trial. Ann Emerg Med 55:258–264
41. Waugh JB, Epps CA, Khodneva YA (2011) Capnography enhances surveillance of respiratory events during procedural sedation: a meta-analysis. J Clin Anesth 23:189–196
42. Tobias JD, Garrett J, Lynch A (1996) Alterations of end-tidal CO_2 during the intra-hospital transport of children. Pediatr Emerg Care 12:249–251
43. Sheak KR, Wiebe DJ, Leary M et al (2015) Quantitative relationship between end-tidal carbon dioxide and CPR quality during both in-hospital and out-of-hospital cardiac arrest. Resuscitation 89:149–154
44. Hartmann SM, Farris RW, Di Gennaro JL, Roberts JS (2015) Systematic review and meta-analysis of end-tidal carbon dioxide values associated with return of spontaneous circulation during cardiopulmonary resuscitation. J Intensive Care Med (in press)

45. Overdyk F, Carter R, Maddox R et al (2007) Continuous oximetry/capnometry monitoring reveals frequent desaturation and bradypnea during patient controlled analgesia. Anesth Analg 105:412–418
46. Tobias JD, Meyer DJ (1997) Non-invasive monitoring of carbon dioxide during respiratory failure in toddlers and infants: end-tidal versus transcutaneous carbon dioxide. Anesth Analg 85:55–58
47. Berkenbosch JW, Lam J, Burd RS, Tobias JD (2001) Noninvasive monitoring of carbon dioxide during mechanical ventilation in older children: end-tidal versus transcutaneous techniques. Anesth Analg 92:1427–1431
48. Tobias JD, Wilson WR Jr, Meyer DJ (1999) Transcutaneous monitoring of carbon dioxide tension after cardiothoracic surgery in infants and children. Anesth Analg 88:531–534
49. Berkenbosch JW, Tobias JD (2002) Transcutaneous carbon dioxide monitoring during high-frequency oscillatory ventilation in infants and children. Crit Care Med 30:1024–1027
50. Tobias JD (2001) Transcutaneous carbon dioxide measurement during apnea testing in pediatric patients. J Intensive Care Med 16:76–78
51. McBride ME, Berkenbosch JW, Tobias JD (2004) Transcutaneous carbon dioxide monitoring during diabetic ketoacidosis in children and adolescents. Paediatr Anaesth 14:167–171
52. Cox P, Tobias JD (2007) Non-invasive monitoring of $PaCO_2$ during one-lung ventilation and minimal access surgery in adults: end-tidal versus transcutaneous techniques. J Min Access Surg 3:8–13
53. Nosovitch M, Johnson JO, Tobias JD (2002) Non-invasive intraoperative monitoring of carbon dioxide in children: end-tidal versus transcutaneous techniques. Paediatr Anaesth 12:48–52
54. Griffin J, Terry BE, Burton RK, Ray TL, Keller BP, Landrum AL, Johnson JO, Tobias JD (2003) Non-invasive carbon dioxide monitoring during general anesthesia in obese adults: end-tidal versus transcutaneous techniques. Br J Anaesth 91:498–501
55. Ramsay MA, Usman M, Lagow E, Mendoza M, Untalan E, De Vol E (2013) The accuracy, precision and reliability of measuring ventilatory rate and detecting ventilatory pause by rainbow acoustic monitoring and capnometry. Anesth Analg 117:69–75
56. Frasca D, Geraud L, Charriere JM, Debaene B, Mimoz O (2015) Comparison of acoustic and impedance methods with mask capnometry to assess respiration rate in obese patients recovering from general anaesthesia. Anaesthesia 70:26–31
57. Mimoz O, Benard T, Gaucher A, Frasca D, Debaene B (2012) Accuracy of respiratory rate monitoring using a non-invasive acoustic method after general anaesthesia. Br J Anaesth 108:872–875
58. Guechi Y, Pichot A, Frasca D, Rayeh-Pelardy F, Lardeur JY, Mimoz O (2015) Assessment of noninvasive acoustic respiration rate monitoring in patients admitted to an Emergency Department for drug or alcoholic poisoning. J Clin Monit Comput (in press)
59. Autet LM, Frasca D, Pinsard M, Cancel A, Rousseau L, Debaene B, Mimoz O (2014) Evaluation of acoustic respiration rate monitoring after extubation in intensive care unit patients. Br J Anaesth 113:195–197
60. Patino M, Redford DT, Quigley TW, Mahmoud M, Kurth CD, Szmuk P (2013) Accuracy of acoustic respiration rate monitoring in pediatric patients. Paediatr Anaesth 23:1166–1173
61. Swan HJ, Ganz W, Forrester J et al (1970) Catheterization of the heart in man with use of a flow-directed balloon-tipped catheter. N Engl J Med 283:447–451
62. Harvey S, Harrison DA, Singer M et al (2005) PAC-Man study collaboration: assessment of the clinical effectiveness of pulmonary artery catheters in management of patients in intensive care (PAC-Man): a randomised controlled trial. Lancet 366:472–477
63. Grocott MP, Dushianthan A, Hamilton MA et al (2013) Perioperative increase in global blood flow to explicit defined goals and outcomes following surgery. Br J Anaesth 111:535–548
64. Yang XX, Critchley LA, Joynt GM (2011) Determination of the precision error of the pulmonary artery thermodilution catheter using an in vitro continuous flow test rig. Anesth Analg 112:70–77

65. Pauli C, Fakler U, Genz T et al (2002) Cardiac output determination in children: equivalence of the transpulmonary thermodilution method to the direct Fick principle. Intensive Care Med 28:947–952
66. Singer M (2009) Oesophageal Doppler. Curr Opin Crit Care 15:244–248
67. Schuster AH, Nanda NC (1984) Doppler echocardiographic measurement of cardiac output: comparison with a non-golden standard. Am J Cardiol 53:257–259
68. Linton RA, Young LE, Marlin DJ et al (2000) Cardiac output measured by lithium dilution, thermodilution, and transesophageal Doppler echocardiography in anesthetized horses. Am J Vet Res 61:731–737
69. Johansson A, Chew M (2007) Reliability of continuous pulse contour cardiac output measurement during hemodynamic instability. J Clin Monit Comput 21:237–242
70. Bein B, Meybohm P, Cavus E et al (2007) The reliability of pulse contourderived cardiac output during hemorrhage and after vasopressor administration. Anesth Analg 105:107–113
71. Zöllner C, Haller M, Weis M et al (2000) Beat-to-beat measurement of cardiac output by intravascular pulse contour analysis: a prospective criterion standard study in patients after cardiac surgery. J Cardiothorac Vasc Anesth 14:125–129
72. Krejci V, Vannucci A, Abbas A et al (2010) Comparison of calibrated and uncalibrated arterial pressure-based cardiac output monitors during orthotopic liver transplantation. Liver Transpl 16:773–782
73. Hadian M, Kim HK, Severyn DA et al (2010) Cross-comparison of cardiac output trending accuracy of LiDCO, PiCCO, FloTrac and pulmonary artery catheters. Crit Care 14:R212
74. Marik PE, Pendelton JE, Smith R (1997) A comparison of hemodynamic parameters derived from transthoracic electrical bioimpedance with those parameters obtained by thermodilution and ventricular angiography. Crit Care Med 25:1545–1550
75. Critchley LA, Calcroft RM, Tan PY et al (2000) The effect of lung injury and excessive lung fluid, on impedance cardiac output measurements, in the critically ill. Intensive Care Med 26:679–685
76. Kamath SA, Drazner MH, Tasissa G et al (2009) Correlation of impedance cardiography with invasive hemodynamic measurements in patients with advanced heart failure: the bioimpedance CardioGraphy (BIG) substudy of the evaluation study of congestive heart failure and Pulmonary Artery catheterization effectiveness (ESCAPE) trial. Am Heart J 158:217–223
77. Keren H, Burkhoff D, Squara P (2007) Evaluation of a noninvasive continuous cardiac output monitoring system based on thoracic Bioreactance. Am J Physiol 293:H583–H589
78. Raval NY, Squara P, Cleman M et al (2008) Multicenter evaluation of noninvasive cardiac output measurement by bioreactance technique. J Clin Monit Comput 22:113–119
79. Squara P, Denjean D, Estagnasie P et al (2007) Noninvasive cardiac output monitoring (NICOM): a clinical validation. Intensive Care Med 33:1191–1194
80. Kraemer FW, Stricker PA, Gurnaney HG, McClung H, Meador MR, Sussman E, Burgess BJ, Ciampa B, Mendelsohn J, Rehman MA, Watcha MF (2010) Bradycardia during induction of anesthesia with sevoflurane in children with Down syndrome. Anesth Analg 111:1259–1263
81. Tobias JD (2001) Caudal epidural block: a review of test dosing and recognition of systemic injection in children. Anesth Analg 93:1156–1161
82. Desparmet J, Mateo J, Ecoffey C, Mazoit X (1990) Efficacy of an epidural test dose in children anesthetized with halothane. Anesthesiology 72(2):249–251
83. Varghese E, Deepak KM, Chowdary KV (2009) Epinephrine test dose in children: is it interpretable on ECG monitor? Paediatr Anaesth 19:1090–1095
84. Tanaka M, Nishikawa T (2002) Does the choice of electrocardiography lead affect the efficacy of the T-wave criterion for detecting intravascular injection of an epinephrine test dose? Anesth Analg 95:1408–1411
85. Kozek-Langenecker SA, Marhofer P, Jonas K, Macik T, Urak G, Semsroth M (2000) Cardiovascular criteria for epidural test dosing in sevoflurane- and halothane-anesthetized children. Anesth Analg 90:579–583

86. Tobias JD (2006) Cerebral oxygenation monitoring: near infrared spectroscopy. Expert Rev Med Devices 3:235–243
87. Ullman N, Anas NG, Izaguirre E, Haugen W, Ortiz H, Arguello O, Nickerson B, Mink RB (2014) Usefulness of cerebral NIRS in detecting the effects of pediatric sleep apnea. Pediatr Pulmonol 49:1036–1042
88. Tobias JD (2008) Cerebral oximetry monitoring with near infrared spectroscopy detects alterations in oxygenation before pulse oximetry. J Intensive Care Med 23:384–388
89. Casati A, Fanelli G, Pietropaoli P et al (2005) Continuous monitoring of cerebral oxygen saturation in elderly patients undergoing major abdominal surgery minimizes brain exposure to potential hypoxia. Anesth Analg 101:740–747
90. Murkin JM (2009) NIRS: a standard of care for CPB vs. an evolving standard for selective cerebral perfusion? J Extra Corpor Technol 41:P11–P14
91. Murkin JM, Adams SJ, Novick RJ, Quantz M, Bainbridge D, Iglesias I, Cleland A, Schaefer B, Irwin B, Fox S (2007) Monitoring brain oxygen saturation during coronary bypass surgery: a randomized, prospective study. Anesth Analg 104:51–58
92. Ono M, Brady K, Easley RB, Brown C, Kraut M, Gottesman RF, Hogue CW Jr (2014) Duration and magnitude of blood pressure below cerebral autoregulation threshold during cardiopulmonary bypass is associated with major morbidity and operative mortality. J Thorac Cardiovasc Surg 147:483–489
93. Peňáz J (1973) Photoelectric measurement of blood pressure, volume and flow in the finger. Digest of the 10th international conference on medical and biological engineering, Dresden
94. Imholz BP, Wieling W, van Montfrans GA, Wesseling KH (1998) Fifteen years' experience with finger arterial pressure monitoring: assessment of the technology. Cardiovasc Res 38:605–616
95. Tobias JD, McKee C, Herz D, Teich S, Sohner P, Rice J, Barry N, Michalsky M (2014) Accuracy of the CNAP™ monitor, a noninvasive continuous blood pressure device, in providing beat-to-beat blood pressure measurements during bariatric surgery in severely obese adolescents and young adults. J Anesth 28:861–865
96. Kako H, Corridore M, Rice J, Tobias JD (2013) Accuracy of the CNAP™ monitor, a noninvasive continuous blood pressure device, in providing beat-to-beat blood pressure readings in pediatric patients weighing 20–40 kilograms. Paediatr Anaesth 23:989–993
97. Drzewieck GM, Meblin J, Noordergraaf A (1983) Arterial tonometry: review and analysis. J Biomech 2:141–152
98. Hansen S, Staber M (2006) Oscillometric blood pressure measurement used for calibration of the arterial tonometry method contributes significantly to error. Eur J Anaesthesiol 23:781–787
99. Drzewiecki GM, Melbin J, Noordergraaf A (1983) Arterial tonometry: review and analysis. J Biomech 16:141–152
100. Kim SH, Lilot M, Sidhu KS, Rinehart J, Yu Z, Canales C, Cannesson M (2014) Accuracy and precision of continuous noninvasive arterial pressure monitoring compared with invasive arterial pressure: a systematic review and meta-analysis. Anesthesiology 120:1080–1097

Part V

Early and Long Term Consequences of Anesthesia and Surgery

Negative Behaviour After Surgery

22

Marta Somaini and Pablo M. Ingelmo

22.1 Emergence Delirium, Emergence Agitation and Postoperative Pain

Smessaert et al. [57] introduced the concept of 'mode of recovery', describing the different types of behaviours whilst consciousness is being regained following anaesthesia and surgery. They described three models of recovery: patients who made a tranquil and uneventful recovery; patients with moderate degree of restlessness; and patients markedly delirious and uncooperative, requiring special care and restraint. Eckenhoff et al. [21] described the incidence and the aetiology of post-anaesthetic excitement, studying more than 14,000 patients in recovery room. They defined as having 'emergence excitement' patients who were crying, sobbing, thrashing about and disoriented upon awakening from general anaesthesia. The latter entity of this syndrome was considered emergence delirium (ED).

Since the early 1960s, the terms emergence delirium (ED), emergence agitation (EA), 'emergence excitement' and 'maladaptive postoperative behaviour' were often used as synonymous without a clear consensus on definition [4, 48, 65]. Recently, Bortone et al. [8] introduced the term early postoperative negative behaviour (e-PONB) that collectively includes different unsettle behaviours after awakening and differentiates early phase from later postoperative behavioural changes.

The more relevant components of e-PONB have been identified as pain, ED and EA [4, 8]. Up to 80 % of children undergoing general anaesthesia can experience

M. Somaini, MD (✉)
Department of Anaesthesia and Intensive Care, Niguarda Ca' Granda Hospital,
Milan-Bicocca University, Milan, Italy
e-mail: ma.somaini@gmail.com

P.M. Ingelmo, MD
Department of Anesthesia, Montreal Children's Hospital, MUHC, McGill University
Montreal, QC, Canada
e-mail: pablo.ingelmo@mcgill.ca

© Springer International Publishing Switzerland 2016
M. Astuto, P.M. Ingelmo (eds.), *Perioperative Medicine in Pediatric Anesthesia,*
Anesthesia, Intensive Care and Pain in Neonates and Children,
DOI 10.1007/978-3-319-21960-8_22

e-PONB depending on clinical setting and on the perioperative management [18, 48, 58].

The standard diagnostic criteria for delirium (Diagnostic and Statistical Manual of Mental Disorders, Fifth Edition – DSM-V) are disturbances in attention and awareness (reduced ability to direct, focus, sustain and shift attention) associated with change in cognition (disorientation, language disturbance) and perceptual disturbance. Sickic and Lerman [56] defined ED as 'a mental disturbance during the recovery from general anaesthesia consisting of hallucinations, delusions and confusion manifested by moaning, restlessness, involuntary physical activity, and thrashing about in bed'.

The most frequently quoted incidence of ED in young children is probably 20 % [5, 48, 65]. ED occurs during the first 20 min after spontaneous awakening [29, 65]. The onset of this behaviour is almost always within 5 min after awakening and lasts for about 10–15 min, is self-limiting in almost all cases and never restarts in the same child [8, 28].

EA is a state of restlessness and mental distress and not all children that have EA have delirium. A child may be agitated for numerous reasons including pain, hunger or fear because of the absence of a primary caregiver or unfamiliar surroundings. 'Agitation' can be used as a general term that encompasses all of these states, but it should be avoided on publications that specifically discuss the ED phenomenon [5, 48, 65].

22.2   Consequences of e-PONB

Children with e-PONB are at risk of self-injury or accidental removal of IV catheters and drainages. It usually requires extra nursing care and eventually supplemental sedative or analgesic drugs. Also, an unsettle behaviour reduces parental and caregivers' satisfaction [48, 63, 66]. Long-term psychological implications of e-PONB are unclear, but it has been demonstrated that children who show ED whilst emerging from anaesthesia have a higher risk of developing separation anxiety, apathy, sleep and eating disorders weeks after surgery [24, 37, 59]. Children with e-PONB could also present nightmares, waking up crying, temper tantrums or more serious behavioural changes such as the new-onset enuresis [20, 31]. Kain et al. reported that up to 60 % of children between 1 and 7 years old undergoing elective outpatient procedures develop negative behaviours on the first day after surgery. The negative behaviour could persist up to 2 weeks after surgery [31]. The prevalence of at least one negative behaviour in children from 6 to 12 years ranged from a maximum of 80 % (95 % CI 71–90 %) in the first day after surgery 1 to a minimum of 43 % (95%CI 31–56 %) 6 months after elective adenotonsillectomy surgery [5, 60].

Postoperative pain may be a significant contributing factor to EA when assessing the cause of a child's behaviour upon emergence. Inadequate pain relief may cause EA, particularly after short surgical procedures [19, 23, 26]. However, recent publications suggested that ED and postoperative pain are independent behaviours with different trend over the first 30 min after spontaneous awakening from general anaesthesia [8, 12]. It is important to distinguish ED from pain, since the aetiology and management are likely to be different [5, 48, 58]. A wrong diagnosis can lead to the treatment of self-limiting behaviour (ED) and/or to the under-treatment or delayed treatment of postoperative pain.

22.3 Risk Factors

In 1960, Smessaert et al. described two main factors associated to ED. The first one was related to the intraoperative period (anaesthesia management, cyclopropane more than ether or barbiturates) and to the surgical procedures (peripheral surgery is less frequently associated to ED than intrathoracic or intra-abdominal surgery). The second one was the individual characteristics of the patient (e.g. sex, age and temperament), and they hypothesized that the behaviour during emergence from surgical anaesthesia was primarily influenced by the patient's personality structure. They did not consider pain as an essential factor causing delirium [57]. More recently, e-PONB was associated with the type of anaesthesia; the surgical setting; the child's age, experience and temperament; the preoperative anxiety; and the parental presence during awakening and with the postoperative pain [18, 22].

22.3.1 Age and Gender

Since from 1960s, it was described that the incidence of e-PONB is higher in childhood and decreases with age [21]. However, more information provided by recent literature could not support the inverse relationship between age and incidence of e-PONB. Different development stages are characterized by different psychological development. For example, it is unlikely that infants experience separation anxiety, which is very common in small children between one and three 3 years old. Children in preschool respond positively to distraction, and older children/adolescents want to be part in the decision-making process as mechanisms to decrease anxiety [5, 50]. Gender seems to do not affect the incidence of e-PONB. But some authors report that ED occurs more frequently in male preschool children [18]. As consequence, the use of age-specific tools may help on a more accurate evaluation, prevention and treatment of e-PONB.

22.3.2 Parents and Culture

Ethnicity, language and cultural values could influence the report of negative behaviour changes. Spanish-speaking Hispanic parents reported lower incidence of negative behavioural changes compared to English-speaking White parents. Stoicism is a common cultural value within Hispanic families, and as a consequence, they tend not to report e-PONB [25].

22.3.3 Preoperative Anxiety

Preoperative anxiety is an independent predictor for postoperative negative behaviours. Kain et al. described the strong correlation between preoperative anxiety and postoperative negative behaviour in young children undergoing general anaesthesia. The risk of postoperative negative behaviour changes is up to 3.5-fold greater in children who experienced preoperative anxiety [32, 34, 35].

The identification of anxiety traits before surgery may help to improve the perioperative management and prevent e-PONB. Clinical and laboratory parameters (i.e. heart rate and blood pressure, plasma cortisol concentrations) have been considered to assess anxiety, but these values had low validity and reliability [5]. The modified Yale preoperative anxiety scale (m-YPAS) is a validated and reliable tool, but too complex to be use in a normal busy clinical practice [32].

The induction compliance checklist (ICC) was validated for use during inhalation induction of anaesthesia [33]. Beringer et al. developed the Paediatric Anaesthesia Behaviour (PAB) score, to quantify the level of anxiety during induction of anaesthesia. The PAB score identifies children who are distressed during induction of anaesthesia. They described three behavioural scenarios where children could be described as:

1. Happy – calm and controlled. Compliant with induction
2. Sad – tearful and/or withdrawn but compliant with induction
3. Mad – loud vocal resistance (screaming or shouting) and/or physical resistance to induction requiring physical restraint by staff and/or parents

There was significant correlation between the PAB score and the ICC and m-YPAS. A high PAB score during induction was associated with increased incidence and intensity of e-PONB in PACU and with the development of behavioural changes after discharge home [6].

22.3.4 Surgery

The relationship between the type of surgery and the incidence e-PONB is unclear. Some authors reported that ear, nose and throat surgery, ophthalmologic procedures [3], genitourinary surgery [43] and surgical procedures in admitted patients [47] were associated with increased risk of postoperative behavioural changes. On the contrary, several studies excluded the increase risk of postoperative negative behaviour in association with the type of surgery [5].

22.3.5 Inhalation Anaesthesia

Sevoflurane and desflurane, agents with low blood/gas solubility, were associated with higher incidence of ED and EA when compared with halothane [3, 17, 69].

The faster clearance of sevoflurane and desflurane in the central nervous system may explain the high incidence of ED after volatile anaesthesia. This hypothesis has been supported by the increased incidence of postoperative agitation since the introduction of fast-acting volatile agents. The late emergence of cognitive function compared to other brain functions, such as audition and locomotion, has been considered the cause of the confusion state [18]. In support of this theory, Bong et al. recently found that the only significant predictor for ED is the time taken to awake from general anaesthesia. With every minute increase in wake-up time, the odds of ED had been reduced by 7 % [7]. Recently, the biphasic effect of sevoflurane has been described as possible contributing factor to the genesis of ED in young children [5]. This drug potentiates GABA alfa-receptor-mediated inhibitory postsynaptic currents at high concentrations and blocks these currents at low concentrations [53].

When compared sevoflurane and desflurane anaesthesia on postoperative behaviour, the incidence of ED varied between 10 and 55 %. However, in most of the studies on the argument, there is no consensus on definition, and the incidence and magnitude of the postoperative behaviours were measured with not validated scales to assess ED [11, 12, 64, 68]. Welborn et al. reported 55 % of ED after desflurane compared with 10 % in the sevoflurane group, in children undergoing ENT surgery [68]. Cohen assessed the postoperative behaviour of preschool children undergoing adenotonsillectomy, using a three-point scale (calm, agitated but consolable, very agitated and inconsolable). There were no significant differences on the incidence of EA between children receiving sevoflurane (18 %) or desflurane (24 %) [41]. As well, Valley et al. found a 33 % overall incidence of ED without significant differences between children receiving sevoflurane or desflurane [64].

Locatelli et al. investigated the incidence of ED, using the PAED. One in four children undergoing sub-umbilical surgery with sevoflurane or desflurane and effective regional anaesthesia had ED. They found no differences on incidence of ED between sevoflurane and desflurane anaesthesia. However, ED had a longer duration in children receiving sevoflurane anaesthesia [46].

22.3.6 Propofol

The incidence and intensity of ED after propofol anaesthesia were significantly lower than volatile anaesthetics. The incidence of ED in children undergoing eye examinations with sevoflurane group was 38 % compared to 0 % for propofol group [27]. Maintenance with propofol significantly reduces the risk of EA (RR 0.35, 95 % CI 0.25–0.51) when compared with sevoflurane anaesthesia even when children in propofol groups received sevoflurane induction [15]. Similar results were obtained when compared to children receiving only sevoflurane or propofol maintenance (RR 0.59, 95 % CI 0.46–0.76) [9, 13, 14, 15, 62].

Different authors investigated the effect of single bolus of propofol at induction or at the end of the surgery on EA incidence during sevoflurane anaesthesia. Propofol 2 or 3 mg/kg at induction did not reduce the incidence and severity of EA. Instead, children receiving propofol 1 mg/kg at the end of sevoflurane anaesthesia showed reduce risk of EA (RR 0.58, 95 % CI 0.38–0.89) [15]. Recently, Costi el at reported that transition to propofol 3 mg/kg for 3 min at the end of sevoflurane anaesthesia reduces the incidence and severity of EA. [16]

22.4 Tools to Recognize and Quantify e-PONB

The recognition of pain, ED and EA in the recovery room is clinically relevant, as different condition should receive different management [4, 8, 48, 65]. Young children who are unable to verbalize pain, anxiety, discomfort, fear, hunger or thirst may manifest all these different conditions with similar behaviours. Moreover, it is possible to observe significant behaviours (pain, ED and EA) overlap during the first minutes after awakening [58]. The lack of 'gold standard' to identify ED and the impossibility of using self-report pain scales during awaken makes the differentiation between the major components of e-PONB extremely difficult.

Several observational scales were developed to measure EA, pain and ED in young children. EA is frequently described using three to five categories [67]. The most common EA scales (Watcha, Cravero, Aono, etc.) have not been psychometrically tested and include behaviours such as crying, inconsolability and lack of cooperation. Substantially, these scores describe a generic agitation state, but they are unable to discriminate between different aetiologies neither to identify ED [48]. ED should not be diagnosed only on the basis of crying and consolability, and then the scales measuring EA should be only used to identify generically agitated children.

In 2004, Sikich and Lerman developed the Pediatric Anesthesia Emergence Delirium (PAED) scale, the only tool validated to assess ED in young children [56]. The PAED scale includes five items: 'Eye contact', 'Purposeful actions', 'Awareness of the surroundings', 'Restlessness' and 'Inconsolability' (Table 22.1). The items evaluating consciousness ('Eye contact' and 'Awareness of the surroundings') and cognition ('Purposeful actions') are domains included in the definition of delirium reported by the Diagnostic and Statistical Manual of Mental Disorders IV and V. Instead, 'Restlessness' and 'Inconsolability' reflect disturbance in psychomotor behaviour and emotion. They can also be an expression of pain, stress, anxiety or apprehension. The PAED scale has some limitations. First, the items have objective criteria, but the score for each one is influenced by subjectivity. Second, as described by the same authors, the last two items could reflect both pain-linked and ED-linked behaviours. Third, there is no consensus about the cut-off used to identify ED (from ≥ 10 to ≥ 16 depending on the author [48].

Locatelli et al. divided the PAED scales in a delirium-specific score (ED1 – 'Eye contact' and 'Awareness of the surroundings' and 'Purposeful actions') and in non-specific delirium score (ED2 – 'Restlessness' and 'Inconsolability'). In their study, ED1 (≥ 9 points in 'Eye contact' and 'Awareness of the surroundings' and 'Purposeful actions') was highly correlated with ED episodes in young children undergoing

Table 22.1 FLACC scale [52]

Face, Legs, Activity, Cry, Consolability scale
Face
0. No particular expression/smile, eye contact and interest in surroundings
1. Occasional grimace or frown, withdrawn, disinterested, worried look to face, eyebrows lowered, eyes partially closed, cheeks raised, mouth pursed
2. Frequent to constant frown, clenched jaw, quivering chin, deep furrows on forehead, eyes closed, mouth opened, deep lines around nose/lips
Legs
0. Normal position or relaxed
1. Uneasy, restless, tense, increased tone, rigidity, intermittent flexion/extension of limbs
2. Kicking or legs drawn up, hypertonicity, exaggerated flexion/extension of limbs, tremors
Activity
0. Lying quietly, normal position, moves easily and freely
1. Squirming, shifting back and forth, tense, hesitant to move, guarding, pressure on body part
2. Arched, rigid, or jerking, fixed position, rocking, side to side head movement, rubbing of body part
Cry
0. No cry/moan (awake or asleep)
1. Moans or whimpers, occasional cries, sighs, occasional complaint
2. Crying steadily, screams, sobs, moans, grunts, frequent complaints
Consolability
0. Calm, content, relaxed, does not require consoling
1. Reassured by occasional touching, hugging or 'talking to' distractible
2. Difficult to console or comfort

Table 22.2 PAED scale (Pediatric Anesthesia Emergence Delirium scale) [9]

	Not at all	Just a little	Quite a bit	Very much	Extremely
Child makes eye contact with the caregiver	4	3	2	1	0
Child's actions are purposeful	4	3	2	1	0
Child is aware of his/her surroundings	4	3	2	1	0
Child is restless	0	1	2	3	4
Child is inconsolable	0	1	2	3	4

sub-umbilical surgery with effective caudal block. Moreover, the incidence of ED1 recognized ED cases (sensitivity 93 %) and non-ED cases (specificity 94 %). In contrast, ED2 correctly identified non-ED cases (specificity 95 %), but was not reliable in identifying ED cases (sensitivity 34 %) [46].

The descriptors used in some EA scales and in the PAED scale may overlap with those used by pain evaluation tools like the Face, Legs, Activity, Cry, Consolability (FLACC) scale (Table 22.2) [48]. The FLACC scale is a reliable observational score to assess pain in young children. It was validated to assess postoperative pain in fully awake children, observing the child over 5 min and recording the worse behaviour of each item [51].

The PAED scale and the FLACC scales overlap three criteria: 'Inconsolability', 'Purposeful actions' and 'Restlessness'. High scores on restlessness and inconsolability items, even associated with low scores on ED-specific items, may produce a false-positive diagnosis of ED [48]. On the other hand, if evaluated with FLACC scale, facial expression in combination with inconsolability and motor restlessness may diagnose pain instead of ED.

The categories 'No eye contact' and 'No awareness of surroundings' are unique to the PAED scale and considered as the most important items for ED identification [46, 48, 56]. The association of 'No eye contact' and 'No awareness of surroundings' is strongly correlated to ED episodes with 99 % sensitivity and 63 % specificity during the first 15 min after awakening. The association of 'Abnormal facial expression', 'Crying' and 'Inconsolability' demonstrates 93 % sensitivity and 82 % specificity to detect pain during the early postoperative period [28].

22.5   Prevention and Treatment

The treatment of e-PONB should be ideally preventive. Pharmacologic and non-pharmacologic strategies are largely investigated.

22.5.1 Non-pharmacologic Approach

The strong correlation between preoperative anxiety and postoperative behavioural supported the use of pharmacological and non-pharmacological preventive strategies. Different strategies to decrease preoperative anxiety have been proposed. They include decrease sensory stimuli during induction of anaesthesia, distraction and hypnosis, clown therapy, children and parents preparation with movies, videos or interactive book [72]. The efficacy of parental presence during induction in reducing anxiety in children is still controversial [30, 36, 44, 49]. The perioperative information and distraction reduce the perioperative anxiety, salivary cortisol concentrations and postoperative morphine consumption in children [70].

Kain et al. evaluated the ADVANCE strategy (anxiety-reduction, distraction, video modelling and education, adding parents, no excessive reassurance, coaching and exposure/shaping) for family preparation [38]. Informed parents are involved in the distraction of their own child before and during the induction of anaesthesia. This programme decreases preoperative anxiety of children and the incidence of ED. Moreover, it was more effective than premedication with midazolam on ED prevention [18].

Recently, Seiden et al. compared the tablet-based interactive distraction (TBID) method with midazolam premedication in children undergoing ambulatory surgery. TBID method reduced perioperative anxiety, incidence of ED and the discharge time and increased parental satisfaction [55].

22.5.2 Pharmacologic Approach

22.5.2.1 Midazolam

Midazolam is the most common used drug to prevent and treat preoperative anxiolysis [34, 35]. However, the efficacy of midazolam on preventing e-PONB or its long-term sequels is controversial. Few studies supported the use of midazolam premedication to prevent EA [11, 12, 42, 43]. Other studies reported no effect on e-PONB [11, 12, 15, 18]. Recently, Chuo et al. showed that intravenous midazolam 0.03 mg/kg just before the end of surgery decreases the incidence of EA in children undergoing elective strabismus surgery. They suggested that premedication midazolam is unable to reduce e-PONB because its effect may not last enough in longer procedures [10].

22.5.2.2 Alpha2-Adrenergic Agonists

There is strong evidence that intravenous clonidine or dexmetomidine reduced the incidence of postoperative e-PONB (overall summary odds ratio 0.28, 95 % CI 0.19–0.40) [10]. It should be consider that most of these studies investigated EA, and not specifically ED, and no studies investigate the effect on long-term behaviour changes. The administration of alpha2-adrenergic agonists prolongs the time in recovery room, but this finding seems to be clinically irrelevant [54].

Mikawa et al. found that 4 mcg/kg clonidine premedication is more effective on reduce EA when compared with clonidine 2 mcg/kg, midazolam 0.5 mg/kg, diazepam 0.4 mg/kg or placebo [52]. Yao et al. demonstrated that intranasal dexmedetomidine premedication (1–2 mcg/kg) significantly reduces incidence and severity of ED in children aged 3–7 years undergoing general anaesthesia [71].

The mechanism of alpha2-adrenergic agonist on e-PONB is unclear. Some authors hypothized that clonidine reduces the noradrenaline content in adrenergic areas of the brain increased by all the inhaled anaesthetics [61].

22.5.2.3 Intravenous Anaesthesia with Propofol

The combination of a propofol infusion and nitrous oxide with an effective regional block or a low dose of opioid represents the best strategy for the prevention of e-PONB [5, 8]. Propofol, either as a single bolus at the end of surgery or as an infusion, has been shown to decrease the incidence of ED after sevoflurane anaesthesia [40, 41].

22.5.2.4 Pain Management

Inadequate pain control remains a potential contributor of e-PONB analgesia and is considered the first act to prevent negative behaviour changes after awakening [1, 2, 5, 11, 12, 39–41].

Caudal block and loco-regional anaesthesia had been showed to reduce the risk of EA [2, 39]. As well nonsteroidal anti-inflammatory drug administration decreases the incidence of e-PONB. Intraoperative fentanyl showed an overall decrease in risk of EA (RR 0.37, 95 % CI 0.27–0.50) ($I^2 = 54$ %) [26, 15]. The incidence of EA and pain but not ED can be reduced by fentanyl, but not clonidine, before surgery in children undergoing lower abdominal surgery with sevoflurane without affecting awakening and discharge from PACU. Whilst this strategy may reduce both EA and pain after awakening, it was also associated with a higher incidence of PONV the day after surgery [8].

The mechanisms of action of opioids on the prevention of e-PONB are unclear. Fentanyl inhibits neurons of the hypocretin-orexin system in the hypothalamus, which regulate arousal and maintenance of the awake state [45].

22.5.3 When and How to Treat e-PONB?

Clinicians should consider treating e-PONB according to the severity and duration of the symptoms and concerns over the safety of the child [5]. However, there is no evidence that if left untreated the ED episodes have any sequelae in young children.

Clinicians should consider two aims during e-PONB management: protect the child from self-injury and second provide a quiet setting where the child can recover. The parental presence in recovery room does not affect the incidence of ED. Heath providers in PACU should explain the phenomenon and reassure parents that ED is self-limiting and their child will return to his/her normal behaviour [5].

If clinicians consider treating e-PONB, they first need to define if the negative behaviour is the expression of ED, pain or both. If it is clearly an ED episodes (PAED score ≥10 or the association of 'No eye contact' and 'No awareness of surroundings'), a small bolus of propofol (0.5–1 mg/kg) should be enough to control the child. If the origin of the distressing behaviours is difficult to understand, fentanyl (1–1.5 mcg/kg) should be the first option as it is possible to control pain and ED [17, 18].

Conclusion

e-PONB significantly affects the awakening of young children. The recognition of the different components of e-PONB is clinically relevant but remains a challenge, even for expert nurses and doctors. Prevention of preoperative anxiety, propofol anaesthesia, associated with adequate analgesia and an accurate assessment during early period after awakening remain the main tools for the prevention of e-PONB.

References

1. Aouad MT, Nasr VG (2005) Emergence agitation in children: an update. Curr Opin Anaesthesiol 18(6):614–619
2. Aouad MT, Kanazi GE, Siddik-Sayyid SM et al (2005) Preoperative caudal block prevents emergence agitation in children following sevoflurane anesthesia. Acta Anaesthesiol Scand 49:300–304

3. Aouad MT, Yazbeck-Karam VG, Nasr VG et al (2007) A single dose of propofol at the end of surgery for the prevention of emergence agitation in children undergoing strabismus surgery during sevoflurane anesthesia. Anesthesiology 107(5):733–738

4. Bajwa SA, Costi D, Cyna AM (2010) A comparison of emergence delirium scales following general anesthesia in children. Pediatr Anesth 20:704–711

5. Banchs RJ, Lerman J (2014) Preoperative anxiety management, emergence delirium, and postoperative behavior. Anesthesiol Clin 32(1):1–23

6. Beringer RM, Greenwood R, Kilpatrick N (2010) Development and validation of the Pediatric Anesthesia Behavior score – an objective measure of behavior during induction of anesthesia. Paediatr Anaesth 24(2):196–200

7. Bong CL, Lim E, Allen JC et al (2015) A comparison of single-dose dexmedetomidine or propofol on the incidence of emergence delirium in children undergoing general anaesthesia for magnetic resonance imaging. Anaesthesia 70(4):393–399

8. Bortone L, Bertolizio G, Engelhardt T et al (2014) The effect of fentanyl and clonidine on early postoperative negative behavior in children: a double-blind placebo controlled trial. Paediatr Anaesth 24(6):614–619

9. Bryan YF, Hoke LK, Taghon TA et al (2009) A randomized trial comparing sevoflurane and propofol in children undergoing MRI scans. Paediatr Anesth 19(7):672–681

10. Chuo EJ, Yoon SZ, Cho JE et al (2014) Comparison of the effect of 0.03 and 0.05 mg/kg midazolam with placebo on prevention of emergence agitation in children having strabismus surgery. Anesthiology 120(6):1354–1361

11. Cohen IT et al (2002) Propofol or midazolam does no reduce emergence delirium in pediatric patients. Paediatr Anesth 12:604–609

12. Cohen IT, Finkel JC, Hannallah RS et al (2002) The effect of fentanyl on the emergence characteristics after desflurane or sevoflurane anesthesia in children. Anesth Analg 94(5):1178–1181

13. Cohen IT, Finkel JC, Hannallah RS et al (2003) Rapid emergence does not explain agitation following sevoflurane anaesthesia in infants and children: a comparison with propofol. Paediatr Anesth 13(1):63–67

14. Cohen IT, Finkel JC, Hannallah RS et al (2004) Clinical and biochemical effects of propofol EDTA vs sevoflurane in healthy infants and young children. Paediatr Anesth 14(2):135–142

15. Costi D, Cyna AM, Ahmed S et al (2014) Effects of sevoflurane versus other general anaesthesia on emergence agitation in children. Cochrane Database Syst Rev;(9):CD007084

16. Costi D, Ellwood J, Wallace A et al (2015) Transition to propofol after sevoflurane anesthesia to prevent emergence agitation: a randomized controlled trial. Paediatr Anaesth 25(5):517–523. doi:10.1111/pan.12617

17. Dahmani S, Stany I, Brasher C et al (2010) Pharmacological prevention of sevoflurane- and desflurane-related emergence agitation in children: a meta-analysis of published studies. Br J Anaesth 104(2):216–223

18. Dahmani S, Delivet H, Hilly J (2014) Emergence delirium in children: an update. Curr Opin Anaesthesiol 27(3):309–315

19. Davis PJ, Greenberg JA, Gendelman M et al (1999) Recovery characteristics of sevoflurane and halothane in preschool-aged children undergoing bilateral myringotomy and pressure equalization tube insertion. Anesth Analg 88:34–38

20. Eckenhoff JE (1958) Relationship of anesthesia to postoperative personality changes in children. Am J Dis Child 86:587–591

21. Eckenhoff JE, Kneale DH, Dripps RD (1961) The incidence and etiology of postanesthetic excitement. A clinical survey. Anesthesiology 22:667–673

22. Faulk DJ, Twite MD, Zuk J et al (2010) Hypnotic depth and the incidence of emergence agitation and negative postoperative behavioral changes. Paediatr Anaesth 20(1):72–81

23. Finkel JC, Cohen IT, Hannallah RS et al (2001) The effect of intranasal fentanyl on the emergence characteristics after sevoflurane anesthesia in children undergoing surgery for bilateral myringotomy tube placement. Anesth Analg 92:1164–1168

24. Fortier MA, Del Rosario AM, Rosenbaum A et al (2010) Beyond pain: predictors of postoperative maladaptive behavior change in children. Paediatr Anaesth 20(5):445–453
25. Fortier MA, Tan ET, Mayes LC et al (2013) Ethnicity and parental report of postoperative behavioral changes in children. Paediatr Anaesth 23(5):422–428
26. Galinkin JL, Fazi LM, Cuy RM et al (2000) Use of intranasal fentanyl in children undergoing myringotomy and tube placement during halothane and sevoflurane anesthesia. Anesthesiology 93(6):1378–1383
27. Gupta A, Stierer T, Zuckerman R et al (2004) Comparison of recovery profile after ambulatory anesthesia with propofol, isoflurane, sevoflurane and desflurane: a systematic review. Anesth Analg 98(3):632–641
28. Ingelmo PM, Somaini M, Marzorati C et al (2013) A comparison of observational scales to assess pain and Emergence Delirium in recovery. In: Poster presented on the ASA congress A3115 – San Francisco, USA Oct 2013
29. Johr M (2002) Postanaesthesia excitation. Paediatr Anaesth 12:293–295
30. Kain ZN (1995) Parental presence during induction of anaesthesia. Paediatr Anaesth 5:209–212
31. Kain ZN, Mayes LC, O'Connor TZ et al (1996) Preoperative anxiety in children, predictors and outcomes. Arch Pediatr Adolesc Med 150:1238–1245
32. Kain ZN, Mayes LC, Cicchetti DV et al (1997) The Yale Preoperative Anxiety Scale: how does it compare with a "gold standard"? Anesth Analg 85:783–788
33. Kain ZN, Mayes LC, Wang SM et al (1998) Parental presence during induction of anesthesia versus sedative premedication: which intervention is more effective? Anesthesiology 89:1147–1156
34. Kain ZN, Mayes LC, Wang SM et al (1999) Postoperative behavioral outcomes in children: effects of sedative premedication. Anesthesiology 90:758–765
35. Kain ZN, Wang SM, Mayes LC et al (1999) Distress during the induction of anesthesia and postoperative behavioral outcomes. Anesth Analg 88:1042–1047
36. Kain ZN, Mayes LC, Wang SM et al (2000) Parental presence and a sedative premedicant for children undergoing surgery: a hierarchical study. Anesthesiology 92:939–946
37. Kain ZN, Caldwell-Andrews AA, Weinberg ME et al (2005) Sevoflurane versus halothane: postoperative maladaptive behavioral changes: a randomized, controlled trial. Anesthesiology 102(4):720–726
38. Kain ZN, Caldwell-Andrews AA, Mayes LC et al (2007) Family-centered preparation for surgery improves perioperative outcomes in children: a randomized controlled trial. Anesthesiology 106:65–74
39. Kim HS, Kim CS, Kim SD et al (2011) Fascia iliaca compartment block reduces emergence agitation by providing effective analgesic properties in children. J Clin Anesth 23(2):119–123
40. Kim MS, Moon BE, Kim H et al (2013) Comparison of propofol and fentanyl administered at the end of anaesthesia for prevention of emergence agitation after sevoflurane anaesthesia in children. Br J Anaesth 110(2):274–280
41. Kim D, Doo AR, Lim H et al (2013) Effect of ketorolac on the prevention of emergence agitation in children after sevoflurane anesthesia. Korean J Anesthesiol 64(3):240–245
42. Ko YP, Huang CJ, Hung YC et al (2001) Premedication with low-dose oral midazolam reduces the incidence and severity of emergence agitation in pediatric patients following sevoflurane anesthesia. Acta Anaesthesiol Sin 39(4):169–177
43. Lapin SL, Auden SM, Goldsmith LJ et al (1999) Effects of sevoflurane anaesthesia on recovery in children: a comparison with halothane. Paediatr Anaesth 9(4):299–304
44. Lardner DR, Dick BD, Psych R et al (2010) The effects of parental presence in the postanesthetic care unit on children's postoperative behavior: a prospective, randomized, controlled study. Anesth Analg 110:1102–1108
45. Li Y, van den Pol AN (2008) Mu-opioid receptor-mediated depression of the hypothalamic hypocretin/orexin arousal system. J Neurosci: Off J Soc Neurosci 28(11):2814–2819

46. Locatelli BG, Ingelmo PM, Emre S et al (2013) Emergence delirium in children: a comparison of sevoflurane and desflurane anesthesia using the Paediatric Anesthesia Emergence Delirium scale. Paediatr Anaesth 23(4):301–308
47. Lumley MA, Melamed BG, Abeles LA (1993) Predicting children's presurgical anxiety and subsequent behavior changes. J Pediatr Psychol 18:481–497
48. Malarbi S, Stargatt R, Howard K et al (2011) Characterizing the behavior of children emerging with delirium from general anesthesia. Paediatr Anaesth 21(9):942–950
49. Margolis JO, Ginsberg B, Dear GL et al (1998) Paediatric preoperative teaching: effects at induction and postoperatively. Paediatr Anaesth 8:17–23
50. McGraw T (1994) Preparing children for the operating room: psychological issues. Can J Anaesth 41:1094–1103
51. Merkel S, Voepel-Lewis T, Shayevitz JR et al (1997) The FLACC: a behavioral scale for scoring postoperative pain in young children. Pediatr Nurs 23(3):293–297
52. Mikawa K, Nishina K, Shiga M (2002) Prevention of sevoflurane-induced agitation with oral clonidine premedication. Anesth Analg 94(6):1675–1676
53. Olsen RW, Yang J, King RG et al (1986) Barbiturate and benzodiazepine modulation of GABA receptor binding and function. Life Sci 39:1969–1976
54. Pickard A, Davies P, Birnie K et al (2014) Systematic review and meta-analysis of the effect of intraoperative α-adrenergic agonists on postoperative behaviour in children. Br J Anaesth 112(6):982–990
55. Seiden SC, McMullan S, Sequera-Ramos L et al (2014) Tablet-based Interactive Distraction (TBID) vs oral Midazolam to minimize perioperative anxiety in pediatric patients: a noninferiority randomized trial. Paediatr Anaesth 24(12):1217–1223
56. Sikich N, Lerman J (2004) Development and psychometric evaluation of the pediatric anesthesia emergence delirium scale. Anesthesiology 100(5):1138–1145
57. Smessaert A, Schehr CA, Artusio JF (1960) Observations in the immediate postanaesthesia period. II Mode of recovery. Br J Anaesth 32:181–185
58. Somaini M, Sahillioğlu E, Marzorati C et al (2015) Emergence delirium, pain or both? a challenge for clinicians. Paediatr Anaesth 25(5):524–529
59. Stargatt R, Davidson AJ, Huang GH et al (2006) A cohort study of the incidence and risk factors for negative behavior changes in children after general anesthesia. Paediatr Anaesth 16(8):846–859
60. Stipic SS, Carev M, Kardum G et al (2015) Are postoperative behavioural changes after adenotonsillectomy in children influenced by the type of anaesthesia?: A prospective, randomised clinical study. Eur J Anaesthesiol 32(5):311–319
61. Tesoro S, Mezzetti D, Marchesini L et al (2005) Clonidine treatment for agitation in children after sevoflurane anesthesia. Anesth Analg 101:1619–1622
62. Uezono S, Goto T, Terui K et al (2000) Emergence agitation after sevoflurane versus propofol in pediatric patients. Anesth Analg 91(3):563–566
63. Uezono S, Goto T, Terui K et al (2002) Emergence agitation after sevoflurane versus propofol in pediatric patients. Anesth Analg 91(3):563–566
64. Valley RD, Freid EB, Bailey AG et al (2003) Tracheal extubation of deeply anesthetized pediatric patients: a comparison of desflurane and sevoflurane. Anesth Analg 96:1320–1324
65. Vlajkovic GP, Sindjelic RP (2007) Emergence delirium in children: many questions, few answers. Anesth Analg 104(1):84–91
66. Voepel-Lewis T, Malviya S, Tait AR (2003) A prospective cohort study of emergence agitation in the pediatric postanesthesia care unit. Anesth Analg 96:1625–1630
67. Watcha MF, Ramirez-Ruiz M, White PF et al (1992) Perioperative effects of oral ketorolac and acetaminophen in children undergoing bilateral myringotomy. Can J Anaesth 39:649–654
68. Welborn LG, Hannallah RS, Norden JM et al (1996) Comparison of emergence and recovery characteristics of sevoflurane, desflurane, and halothane in pediatric ambulatory patients. Anesth Analg 83:917–920

69. Wells LT, Rasch DK (1999) Emergence "delirium" after sevoflurane anesthesia: a paranoid delusion? Anesth Analg 88(6):1308–1310
70. Wennstrom B, Tornhage CJ, Nasic S et al (2011) The perioperative dialogue reduces postoperative stress in children undergoing day surgery as confirmed by salivary cortisol. Paediatr Anaesth 21:1058–1065
71. Yao Y, Qian B, Lin Y et al (2015) Intranasal dexmedetomidine premedication reduces minimum alveolar concentration of sevoflurane for laryngeal mask insertion and emergence delirium in children: a prospective, randomized, double-blind, placebo-controlled trial. Paediatr Anaesth 25(5):492–498
72. Yip P, Middleton P, Cyna AM et al (2009) Nonpharmacological interventions for assisting the induction of anaesthesia in children. Cochrane Database Syst Rev CD006447

Acute Pain Management and Prevention 23

Sylvain Tosetti

23.1 Introduction

Evaluation, management, and relief of pain are fundamental human rights, whatever the age of the patient [1]. Postoperative pain could be better understood if we consider its multiple components: sensorial, affective, behavioural, and cognitive.

Cutaneous sensory receptors appear as early as 7 weeks of gestation, and the spread all over cutaneous surfaces is complete around 20 weeks of gestation. The pain perception mediators and the thalamo-cortical connections are functional since the 24th week of gestation. The release of cortisol, endorphins, and norepinephrine by the 24th week of gestation suggests conscious suffering [2]. The remodelling process of nociceptor units during gestation includes an increase amount of receptors [3] resulting in low activation thresholds. The descending inhibitory system is not completely functional after birth as infants are prone to long-lasting hyperalgesia [4] due to central sensitization [5].

The subjective and emotional components are predominant and indissociable; moreover, the ability to verbalize painful experience (pattern, intensity, and location) is a key step in evaluation and then transmission of information to parents and healthcare workers. Pain assessment, not surprisingly, is one of the major challenges in paediatric pain especially in neonates, preverbal children, or patient with cognitive impairment.

Despite considerable educational efforts and the publication of pain management guidelines [6, 7], moderate to severe pain still remains an actual problem both in the hospital setting and at home [8, 9]. The challenge is to provide "safe effective pain management comprehensively to all children whatever the procedure, clinical

S. Tosetti, MD
Anaesthesia Department, The Montreal Children's Hospital, Montreal, QC, Canada
e-mail: sylvain.tosetti@mail.mcgill.ca; sylvain.tosetti@chuv.ch

© Springer International Publishing Switzerland 2016
M. Astuto, P.M. Ingelmo (eds.), *Perioperative Medicine in Pediatric Anesthesia*,
Anesthesia, Intensive Care and Pain in Neonates and Children,
DOI 10.1007/978-3-319-21960-8_23

setting, developmental state or comorbidities" [10]. Moreover, postoperative analgesia is not just to eliminate pain but improve surgical outcomes and prevent chronicity
allowing rapid return to normal activity levels [11] and overall quality of life [12].

23.2 Assessment of Pain

Appropriate management of pain in children depends on valid and reliable assessments and measurements, and pain should be considered as the "fifth vital sign".
The essence of pain measurement in the postoperative setting is to provide an intensity value useful to make practical decisions and to guide the therapeutic plan. The
use of self-report tools, the gold standard in postoperative pain evaluation, is not
feasible in infants, young children, and children with cognitive disabilities. Different
observational/behavioural scales have validated to measure acute and procedural
pain in infants and children that can't rate their own pain experience. Table 23.1
resumes the most commonly used tools in different ages and clinical situation.

The child's parents are essential members of the treatment team. In the day hospital clinical setting, they are the sole dispenser of analgesic medication once back
home. Dedicated pain assessment tools have been developed for parental postoperative pain management, like the Parents' Postoperative Pain Measure (PPPM).
Unfortunately, even with such tools and correct assessment of pain condition, parents still give few analgesics medications, mainly due to fear of pain medication's
adverse effects [13, 14].

Children with special needs remain a vulnerable population at risk of poor pain
control after surgery. The underpinning condition often compromises their ability to

Table 23.1 Examples of pain assessment tools depending on the age and/or situation

Age	Self-report scale	Hetero-evaluation scale
Premature and infants	n/a	PIPP-R,COMFORT
Before 3 years	n/a	FLACC
After 5–6 years	Faces, Poker Chips, NRS, VAS	FLACC, CHEOPS
Situation		
PACU/ward	VAS, Faces, Poker Chips, NRS	FLACC, CHEOPS
PICU/NICU	VAS, Faces, Poker Chips, NRS	FLACC, CHEOPS, COMFORT
Children with special needs	n/a	m-FLACC, NCCPC-PV
At home	VAS, NRS (if >5–6 years)	PPMP (>2 years)

Adapted from PedIMMPACT [21]
n/a not adapted, *COMFORT, PIPP-R* Premature Infant Pain Profile-Revised [19], *VAS* visual analog scale, *NRS* numerical rating scale, *(m-)FLACC* (modified-)Face, Legs, Activity, Cry,
Consolability, *CHEOPS* Children's Hospital Of Eastern Ontario Pain Scale, *NCCPC-PV* Non-
communicating Children's Pain Checklist-Postoperative Version [20], *PPPM* Parents' Postoperative
Pain Measure

express pain. The parents of children with cognitive impairment usually develop unique abilities for the assessment of their child level of discomfort and pain [15, 16].

The use of hemodynamic parameters has not been standardized to assess the effectiveness of analgesia and hence may be prone to imprecise evaluation and decision management in the perioperative setting. However, new technologies like the Analgesia Nociception Index (ANI) and the Pupillary Reflex Dilatation (PRD) deserve a special attention as alternatives for nociception assessment during surgery. Both ANI and PRD monitor the balance between sympathetic and parasympathetic activities, either through heart rate variability or pupillary diameter evolution in response to a noxious stimulus. These technologies were used to evaluate the effectiveness of nerve block [17] and remifentanil [18] in children undergoing sevoflurane anaesthesia.

23.3   Multimodal Analgesia

The timing of the antinociceptive intervention [22] seems to be less important than the modality and duration [23, 24]. Preventive analgesia focuses on attenuating the perioperative noxious stimuli and aims to diminish perioperative pain and analgesic requirements during and after the surgical period. The key point is a judicious use of multimodal strategies, targeting different pathways of pain signalling, enhancement, or perpetuation. This may also reduce the short-term morbidity (urinary retention, constipation, nausea and vomiting, respiratory depression, etc.) as well as some long-term consequences of the acute nociceptive stimulus like the chronic postsurgical pain [25].

23.4   Control of Acute Pain

23.4.1 Opioid Analgesics (Table 23.2)

Opioids are an essential tool for the prevention and treatment of moderate to severe pain in children. Due to its efficacy and versatility, they have a central role in multimodal analgesia.

Whenever feasible, the oral administration should be preferred in the postoperative setting. The administration on an as-needed basis (PRN: pro re nata) may provide less clinical disponibility than on a regular basis (ATC: around the clock) or continuous infusion.

The adverse effects associated to the use of opioids varies from nausea and vomiting, pruritus or constipation to more serious like opioid-induced respiratory depression (OIRD) and opioid withdrawal after prolonged use. Opioid-naive neonates and infants are at more risk of OIRD reducing doses and increasing the administration intervals increases the opioid safety margin in those populations [26, 27]. The concomitant use of non-opioid analgesics and regional analgesia techniques further reduces opioid-related risks. An alternative management to common

Table 23.2 Examples of dosing for currently used opioids and their routes of administration

Opioid	Route	Age group	Dose/interval
Morphine	PO	Infants and children	100–250 µg/kg q3–4H
	IV bolus	Preterm neonate Full-term neonate Infants and children	25–50 µg/kg q3–4H 50–100 µg/kg q3H
	IV infusion	Preterm neonate Full-term neonate Infants and children	2–5 µg/kg/h 5–10 µg/kg/h 15–30 µg/kg/h
Hydromorphone	PO	Infants and children	40–80 µg/kg q4H
	IV bolus		10–20 µg/kg q3–4H
	IV infusion		3–5 µg /kg/h
Fentanyl	IV bolus	Infants and children	0.5–1 µg/kg q1–2H
	IV infusion		0.5–2 µg/kg/h
	IN		1–2 µg/kg q1–2H
Sufentanil[a]	IV bolus	Infants and children	0.1–1 µg/kg
	IV infusion		0.1–2 µg/kg/h
	IN aerosol		1–2 µg/kg
Remifentanil[a]	IV bolus	Infants and children	1–2 µg/kg
	IV infusion		0.1–1 µg/kg/h[b]
Methadone	IV bolus	Infants and children	0.05–0.1 mg/kg
Nalbuphine	IV bolus	Infants and children	0.1–0.2 mg/kg
Tramadol	IV or PO start dose	Infants and children	1–2 mg/kg q6H (max 400 mg/day)

Adapted from the *Acute Pain Guidelines of the Montreal Children's Hospital*
PO per os (orally), *IV* intravenous, *PR* per rectum (rectally), *IM* intramuscular, *IN* intranasal, *q* every, *H or h* hour, *m* minutes
[a]Administration limited to acute care setting
[b]Higher infusion rates may be used for a limited time duration (possible link to opioid-induced hyperalgesia)

opioid-induced side effects is the use of naloxone at low dose as a continuous IV infusion [28].

23.4.1.1 Morphine

Morphine is a very versatile molecule, dispensable through various routes, of which PO and IV are the most used in hospitalized patients. The hydrophilic properties of morphine allow longer duration of analgesia compared to more lipophilic opioids.

The total body clearance of morphine represents 80 % of the adult range 6 months after birth and 96 % by 1 year of age [29]. Morphine undergoes hepatic metabolism and then renal excretion. Infants and premature neonates may display a large range of elimination half-life due to immaturity of the glucuronidation mechanism. Half-life may vary from 9 ± 3 h in premature neonates, 6.5 ± 2.8 h in term neonates, to 2.0 ± 1.8 h in infants and children [26, 27, 30].

23.4.1.2 Fentanyl
Fentanyl is frequently used for acute pain prevention and management during surgery. It also offers benefits in patients with renal failure or in those at risk of histamine release. Its high lipid solubility promotes fast IV or IN onset with peak of action of less than 5 min or 15 min, respectively. New dispersion formulation like oral transmucosal fentanyl citrate (OTFC) may be interesting for moderately painful procedures of short duration, when IV access is not in place or not desirable [31].

Fentanyl is commonly used as continuous infusion in PICU and NICU. Premature babies and infants are at risk of accumulation due to a reduced plasmatic clearance [32].

23.4.1.3 Sufentanil
Sufentanil is eight to ten times more potent than fentanyl. The clearance of sufentanil in normal children is twice that in adolescents; thus a greater maintenance regimen is necessary. In opposition to fentanyl, sufentanil presents less accumulation over time during continuous infusion, thus offering stable plasmatic levels with shorter half-life and less postoperative respiratory depression. Its lipophilic properties promote residual analgesia and diminished postoperative agitation in PACU.

Another advantage is its versatility of use through different routes, like intranasal. A single IN dose as premedication may cover analgesia for short and moderately painful procedures, for example, myringotomies, dressing changes, or tubes removal [33], with the combined advantage of providing preprocedural anxiolysis and sedation.

23.4.1.4 Remifentanil
Remifentanil is rapidly metabolized in the plasma by nonspecific esterases and does not accumulate with prolonged infusions [34]. Those properties allow high titratability and make remifentanil a useful molecule for short procedures with minimal post-procedural pain, like cardiac catheterization or biopsies. One drawback is the potential induction of acute opioid tolerance (AOI) and opioid-induced hyperalgesia (OIH) [35] precluding its use during a prolonged time and/or at high dose. Infusion rates between 0.1 and 0.3 mcg/kg/min seem not to induce AOI or OIH [35].

23.4.1.5 Oxycodone
Oxycodone is 1.5–2 times more potent than oral morphine and is provided in short-acting and long-lasting PO formulation. The metabolism in patients older than 6 months shows stable values and clearance 50 % higher than adults [36, 37]. Onset, peak, and duration of action are similar to those of oral morphine, thus rendering oxycodone a valid option for opioid rotation in the context of opioid-induced hyperalgesia or due to adverse effects.

23.4.1.6 Hydromorphone

Hydromorphone is commonly used in the paediatric population due to its renal elimination as an inactive metabolite and lack of histamine release [38, 39]. It is five to seven times more potent than morphine with similar onset and duration of action. Common routes of administration are IV, PO, or epidural. Hydromorphone is also a popular second-choice molecule when opioid rotation is needed. PCA mode is convenient; however one should be careful with conversion calculation and the risk of errors with small boluses.

23.4.1.7 Methadone

Methadone has been safely used for postoperative pain in children [40], burns [41], or trauma [42], by IV or PO routes. It is also frequently used for opioid rotation and treatment of opioid withdrawal syndrome due to its NMDA receptor antagonist properties [43]. The longer duration of action could represent a double-edged sword, as side effects related to over dosage would last longer. The administration of methadone in opioid-naive patient should only be initiated in a hospital setting, paying close attention to side effects and various drug interactions.

Methadone is considered a second-line opioid for acute pain management; however it could be used as a single bolus co-analgesic for procedures that are relatively painful in the first 24 h [44] like orchidopexy, as weaning from regional anaesthesia or in the context of surgery with high nociceptive impact like spinal surgery.

23.4.1.8 Nalbuphine

Nalbuphine is an agonist-antagonist semi-synthetic opioid with pharmacological potency comparable to morphine, usually indicated in procedures with minimal to moderate pain intensity. Because of its κ-receptor agonist and μ-receptor antagonist properties, the risk of respiratory depression associated with μ-receptor is prevented. The effect on the κ-receptor reduced the incidence of emergence agitation in PACU [45]. Nalbuphine has minimal effect on bowel or bladder function, characteristics of interest in ambulatory surgery. On the other hand, nalbuphine has a ceiling effect above 0.4 mg/kg, and the induced sedation may trigger upper airway obstruction.

23.4.1.9 Tramadol

Tramadol is a weak μ-opioid receptor agonist and a monoaminergic (MAO) reuptake inhibitor [46, 47]. It is derived from codeine and metabolized in the liver through the CYP2D pathway [48]. Its MAO properties may play a role in minimizing the μ side effects like constipation and especially respiratory depression [49]. This makes tramadol an alternative option in children with known risk factor for OIRD, like obstructive sleep apnoea [50]. It was associated with a similar incidence of postoperative nausea and vomiting as morphine. It has a similar safety profile either in patients with neuropathic pain and with nociceptive pain [51].

The recommended IV dose is 1 mg/kg and 100 mg is approximately equivalent to 10 mg of morphine [52, 53]. It has been effectively used by mouth, IV, IM, caudal/epidural, or local infiltration [54] as well as topical application during tonsillectomy [55]. Tramadol/acetaminophen combination is a convenient analgesic post-tonsillectomy pain control, especially at home. One consideration to rise is the theoretical risk of hypoglycemia in predisposed patients and serotoninergic syndrome with the concomitant use of selective serotonin re-uptake inhibitors.

23.4.1.10 PCA, NCA, and PARCA (Table 23.3)

The patient-controlled analgesia (PCA) gives autonomy to patients over their pain control and positively influences the latter through patient's empowerment [56]. It is a safe alternative for pain management in children of 6 years old and older. PCA implies the understanding of the concept, the ability to self-evaluate pain, and the capacity of activate the dosing device. It is also useful in hospital "frequent flyer" children younger than 6 years of age with closer monitoring from the acute pain team.

Table 23.3 Example of PCA/NCA/PARCA

Drug	Bolus dose (µg/kg)	Lockout time (minutes)	Basal infusion (µg/kg/h)	1 h limit (µg / kg/h)
Children >6 years and appropriate developmental/motor state				
Morphine PCA	10–30	6–15	0–4–20[c]	100–400
Morphine + ketamine PCA (1:1)	10–30	6–15	0–4–20	100 - 400
Hydromorphone PCA[a]	2–6	6–15	0–1–5	20–80
Fentanyl PCA[b]	0.2–0.5	6–8	0–0.1–0.5	2–5
Morphine NCA				
Preterm neonates	4	30	0–2–4	50
Term neonates Infants <2 months	20	20	0–4–10	100
Ward: children >2 months	50	15	0–10–20	100–400
Morphine PARCA				
Preterm neonates	n/a	n/a	n/a	n/a
Term neonates Infants < 2 months	n/a	n/a	n/a	n/a
Ward: children >2 months	50	15	0–10–20	100–400
Hydromorphone NCA[a]				
Preterm neonates	1	30	0–0.5–1	10
Term neonates Infants <2 months	4	20	0–1–2	20
Ward: children >2 months	6–10	15	0–1–5	50–100
Fentanyl NCA[b]				
Ward: Children >2 months	0.2–1	15–30	0–0.1–0.5	2–5

Adapted from *APS guidelines of the Acute Pain Service of the Montreal Children's Hospital and of the Mother and Child Hospital Lyon*
PARCA parent-controlled analgesia, *n/a* non-applicable
[a]First line for morphine allergy; first line for renal failure; second line for morphine side effects
[b]First line for renal failure; second line for morphine side effects
[c]0–4–20=either no basal infusion or between 4 and 20 µg/kg/h

Younger children or those unable to manipulate the machine (with special needs or physical restraint) benefit from proxy-controlled analgesia, usually the nurse in charge of the patient or a parent. A recent survey of 252 American centres [57] showed that the vast majority of centres (96 %) would provide PCA but has proxy-controlled analgesia (nurse or parent) in only 38 %. Indeed, this latter technique provides excellent pain relief for children unable to use it by themselves but may create some safety challenges given the subjectivity of the proxy, bypassing the inherent safety features of analgesics dispensed by the patient itself. The main concern is a slightly augmented incidence of respiratory depression [58], easily detected by proper monitoring and treatment without major consequences. Parent-/nurse-controlled analgesia for children with developmental delay is efficient and safe but implies a reinforced monitoring, strict education of the proxy, and clear, written, instruction [59].

The standard monitoring includes oxygen saturation and respiratory rate. More advanced measurements like continuous capnography or breathing sounds through a microphone placed on the neck may further augment safety and prevent oversedation.

The use of a background continuous infusion is controversial. The aim is to improve analgesia through an increase of the plasmatic levels of opioids, especially during night-time, when patient uses PCA less. The increased risk of respiratory adverse events may not justify the potential analgesic advantages.

An acute pain team, informed proxy or nursing staff, and an adequate monitoring increase the safety independently of the modality (PCA, NCA, or PARCA) or the risk of the patient (opioid tolerant, neonates, OSA, etc.)

23.4.2 Non-opioid Analgesics (Table 23.4)

Non-opioid analgesics could be indicated as a single therapy for mild pain and as adjuvants for moderate to severe pain [60]. The combination of more than one non-opioid analgesic may potentiate their respective efficacy and has shown significant opioid-sparing effects [61]. The early use of non-opioid analgesic adjuvants is associated with reduced risk of serious postoperative opioid adverse events (OAE) [62].

23.4.2.1 Acetaminophen (Paracetamol)

Acetaminophen is a common co-analgesic medication in children. The multiple routes of administration allow an easy adaptation to the patient's needs. The intravenous route gives more reliable plasmatic levels, bioavailability, and a slightly faster onset time over rectal or oral routes [63].

Acetaminophen exerts its analgesic effects through the inhibition or prostaglandin release, as a cannabinoid ligand, enhancing inhibitory descending pathways by serotoninergic interactions [64]. The administration of acetaminophen is safe in neonates as far as doses are lowered by 50 % taking in account the longer half-life (up to 7 h).

Table 23.4 Examples dosing of non-opioid analgesics and routes of administration

Drug	Age group	Route/dose/interval	Max. daily dose
Acetaminophen (paracetamol)	Term infants and children:	PO: 10–15 mg/kg q4–6H PR: 20–40 mg/kg q6H	Children <100 mg/kg/day Infants 75 mg/kg/day
	Neonates <32 wPCA Neonates >32 wPCA	PO/PR: 10–15 mg/kg PO/PR: 15–20 mg/kg	Neonates <32 w. 40 mg/kg/day neonates >32 w. 60 mg/kg/day
IV paracetamol (propacetamol)	Term neonates Infants and children	7.5 mg/kg q6H 12.5 mg/kg q6H	30 mg/kg/day max 3.75 g/day
Ibuprofen	Children Term neonates[a]	PO/PR: 5–10 mg/kg q6–8H PO: 5 mg/kg q12–24H	<40 mg/kg/day <30 mg/kg
Ketorolac	Children[a]	IV: 0.5 mg/kg q6–8H	<2 mg/kg/day <5 consecutive days
Sucrose	Preterm neonates Term neonates	PO 24 % solution: 0.5 ml 1 ml	Doses shouldn't exceed 10/day
Dexamethasone	All ages	IV: 0.1–0.15 mg/kg	Single bolus

wPCA weeks post conceptional age, *q* every, *H* hour
[a]Should be used cautiously <6 months of age and reassessed daily

23.4.2.2 NSAIDs

NSAIDs analgesic effects are mediated by the inhibition of COX-1 and COX-2 activity. As a group, they inhibit the biosynthesis of prostaglandins with the subsequent reduction of excitatory amino acids [65]. Due to its opioid-sparing effects, NSAIDS are effective for the reduction of opioid-induced adverse effects [61, 66]. NSAIDS are useful for the prevention of pain rebound during weaning from regional analgesia. Parents should be taught to give NSAIDS (and acetaminophen) before wearing off a regional block [67].

Inadequate pain relief has been associated with the fear of opioids' adverse effects at home. The association of oral ibuprofen 10 mg/kg every 8 h and oral acetaminophen 10–15 mg/kg every 6 h provided similar analgesia than PO morphine, with less respiratory adverse effects in children undergoing tonsillectomy [68]. It is possible that with adequate information, parents would have a better adherence to the postoperative pain programmes with non-opioid-based analgesic plan.

Ketorolac is commonly used intravenously, and more recently, the intranasal route has also been described [69]. Even if it has been safely used in infants, the lower age limit is still under debate. The administration of ketorolac 0.5 mg/kg every 6–8 h was associated with a 17 % incidence of bleeding events (fresh blood in tubes, surgical wound or intra-abdominal bleeding, blood-positive stools) in small infants (average 21 days) [70].

Ketorolac use in infants should be limited to specific cases only for a limited period with close monitoring of renal function and bleeding events. Ketorolac has been also contraindicated in children undergoing tonsillectomy due to the increase risk of postoperative bleeding; however a single postoperative dose lowers PACU pain scores.

23.4.2.3 Dexamethasone
Dexamethasone is frequently used for the prevention of postoperative nausea and vomiting and to enhance postoperative analgesia after adenotonsillectomy. A single dose of 0.15 mg/kg during surgery has been associated with a significant opioid-sparing effects [71].

23.4.2.4 Ketamine
Ketamine, an NMDA receptor antagonist, is used during the perioperative period as adjuvant for postoperative analgesia and to prevent opioid-induced hyperalgesia in the context of major surgery with expected high postoperative opioid requirements [72]. A Cochrane review showed reduced postoperative morphine requirements and opioid side effects (PONV) [73], but preventive properties and infusion regime need to be studied in children as no definitive conclusion has been drawn yet [74]. Even if the usual ratio of morphine/ketamine is 1:1, the optimal ketamine dose as an adjunct in PCA has not yet been determined.

23.4.2.5 Clonidine/Dexmedetomidine
Clonidine and dexmedetomidine are both α-2 central agonists with sedative and analgesic properties. Dexmedetomidine has been associated with the reduction of postoperative analgesic requirements and reduction in opioid-related adverse effects after adenotonsillectomy [75].

23.4.2.6 Sucrose
Sucrose 24 % is known to trigger the release of endorphins that contribute to pain control [76]. Sucking with or without sucrose seems to provide the same effect on pain reduction [77].

23.4.2.7 Gabapentinoids
Gabapentinoids (gabapentin and pregabalin) are α-2-δ modulators with demonstrated analgesic activity and opioid-sparing properties in paediatric scoliosis surgery. Preoperative administration 30 min before surgery (10–15 mg/kg, max 600 mg) seems efficient, followed by a dose every 8 h, for 2–4 weeks [78].

23.4.2.8 Lidocaine Infusion
Lidocaine as intravenous infusion has demonstrated analgesic and opioid-sparing properties in adults (bolus 1.5 mg/kg, followed by 1.5 mg/kg/h). Currently, there are no paediatric data except a case report of a terminally ill child successfully treated [79] with an infusion of up to 3 mg/kg/h, without toxic adverse events.

23.4.3 Regional Anaesthesia

Regional anaesthesia, as part of a multimodal analgesia regimen, could be considered the standard of perioperative care for various procedures in children. The use of regional analgesia reduces the peri- and postsurgical stress [80], prevents postoperative pain, and allows significant reduction on opioid consumption and opioid-related adverse events [81–84]. Regional anaesthesia in children is a safe practice in experienced and well-trained hands [85–87], even when performed asleep [88]. The use of ultrasound guidance has improved the safety and efficacy of most peripheral blocks [81].

The timing of block administration (before or after the surgical procedure), the type (central or peripheral), and the modality (single shot, continuous, PCA) vary depending on the type of surgery, the conditions of the patient (hospitalized or ambulatory), and the training of the caregiver.

Epidural blocks represent the most common regional analgesia technique used for pain prevention and treatment. Neuraxial techniques are effective and safe [87], with a rate of severe complications for caudal anaesthesia as low as 0.03–0.005 % [85]. Nevertheless, some catastrophic complications have been described following epidural placement [89] promoting the search for alternatives to central blockade [90, 91].

Current evidence strongly supports the use of peripheral regional anaesthetic techniques in children. Generally speaking, single-shot blocks could be used for the majority of ambulatory procedures, providing analgesia for the first 6–12 h.

Ultrasound guidance has improved the visibility of targets and allowed real-time needle tracking, thus reducing the amount of blind needle paths. Interfascial spread of local anaesthetics (LAs) allows injection from certain distance of the nerve bundles. The needle is being placed between two fascias, allowing the spread of the solution towards the target, without needle repositioning. This concept, already used in blocks like obturator, pectoralis block (PEC 1 + 2), and transversus abdominis plane block (TAP), can be extended to almost every nerve that courses in between two fascias, like the saphenous and mid-thigh (between sartorius and vastus lateralis) and the median nerve at the forearm (between flexor digitorum superficialis and profundus), etc.

Continuous peripheral nerve blocks (CPNBs) are indicated in procedures associated with significant pain for more than 24–48 h [23, 25]. Nowadays, more complex surgical procedures are performed on an outpatient basis or with shorter hospital stay, and the use of CPNBs has been extended after hospital discharge [92]. Recently large case series of children undergoing orthopaedic surgery demonstrated the safety and efficacy of that technique [93]. The use of CPNBs in the ambulatory setting demands careful preparation and follow-up including troubleshooting protocol for complications, inadequate analgesia, and/or catheter removal. The logistic of those services could be too complicated for small-volume facilities.

The continuous infusion is the most common delivery mode of LAs through a peripheral or a central catheter. Similar to PCA or PARCA, adequately chosen proxies and children may benefit from the patient-/proxy-controlled nerve analgesia (PCNA) or from the patient-/proxy-controlled epidural analgesia (PCEA) [94, 95].

Children, especially neonates and infants, require a careful selection of the type and dosing of LAs to avoid systemic toxicity [83]. L-enantiomers like ropivacaine and levobupivacaine have safer toxicity profile than bupivacaine [96]. Bupivacaine combined with epinephrine and injected at low concentration is still widely used but should be avoided for continuous infusions.

Description of block techniques goes beyond the scope of this chapter [96, 97]. Table 23.5 describes common regional blocks and dosing regimens used in paediatrics and Table 23.6 some suggested LA doses, volumes, and infusion protocols.

The use of adjuncts to LA solutions prolongs the duration of action of single-shot blocks and the efficacy of continuous infusion [98, 99] (Table 23.7).

Table 23.5 Common regional blocks in paediatrics and examples of dosing regimens

Peripheral blocks		
Level	Site	Ropivacaine 0.2 % (2.5–3 mg/kg)[a]

Upper limb	Brachial plexus:
	  Interscalene
	  Supra-/infra-clavicular
	  Axillar
		0.2–0.3 ml/kg (max 15–20 ml)

	Median nerve (elbow, forearm)	0.1 ml/kg/nerve (max 5–6 ml)[b]
	Radial nerve (elbow, forearm)	
	Ulnar nerve (elbow, forearm)	
Hand	Wrist (median, radial, ulnar)	0.05–0.1 ml/kg/nerve (max 2–3 ml)[b]
	Digital blocks	

Lower limb	Sacral plexus:
	  Sub-gluteal
	  Anterior mid-femoral
	  Popliteal (lateral approach)
		0.2–0.5 ml/kg (max 20–25 ml)

	Lumbar plexus: Lumbar (paravertebral) Femoral Saphenous (mid-thigh)	Lumbar 0.2–0.5 ml/kg (max 20 ml) Femoral and saphenous 0.2–0.4 ml/kg (max 15–20 ml)
	Fascia iliaca	0.2–0.3 ml/kg (max 15 ml)
	Obturator	0.1 ml/kg/nerve (max 5 ml)
	Lateral femoral cutaneous	
Foot	Ankle (tibial, saphenous, peroneal)	0.1 ml/kg/nerve (max 5 ml)[b]
	Toe blocks (ring approach)	
Thorax	PEC blocks 1 + 2	0.2–0.3 ml/kg/site (max 15–20 ml)
	Intercostal	0.05–0.1 ml/kg/rib (max 2–3 ml)
	Paravertebral	0.1 ml/kg/space (max 5 ml/space)[c]

Table 23.5 (continued)

Peripheral blocks		
Abdomen	TAP subcostal or lateral	0.2–0.3 ml/kg/side (max 15 ml/side)
	Quadratus lumborum	
	Paravertebral lumbar	
	Umbilical	0.1 ml/kg/nerve (max 5 ml)
	Ilio-inguinal, ilio-hypogastric	0.1–0.2 ml/kg (max 10 ml[d])
Genitalia	Penile	0.1 ml/kg/side (max 2.5 ml/side)
	Pudendal	0.1–0.2 ml/kg (max 10 ml)
Head and neck	Scalp blocks	0.05–0.1 ml/kg/nerve (max 2 ml/nerve)
	Peri-orbital (supra/infra)	
	Peri-auricular (greater/lesser auricular)	
	Maxillary	0.1–0.2 ml/kg/side (max 10 ml)

PEC pectoralis block 1 + 2, *TAP* transversus abdominis plane block, *LA* local aesthetic
[a]Alternatively levobupivacaine 0.25 % or dilute bupivacaine at 0.125–0.175 %
[b]The solution doesn't need to spread all over the nerve
[c]Could be injected at one space to facilitate the insertion of a catheter
[d]Higher volume augments the risk of spread to the femoral nerve

Table 23.6 Examples of infusion guidelines of local anaesthetics and adjuncts

Molecule	Solution	Limits
Ropivacaine	0.1–0.2 %	0.2 mg/kg/h <1 month 0.3 mg/kg/h <6 months 0.4 mg/kg/h >6 months
Fentanyl	1–2 µg/ml	1–2 µg/kg/h
Sufentanil	0.1–0.2 µg/ml	0.1–0.2 µg/kg/h
Clonidine	1 µg/ml	0.5–1 µg/kg/h
PCEA/PCNA (>5–6 years of age)	Ropivacaine 0.1–0.2 %	0.1 mg/kg/h + bolus 0.1 mg/kg, lockout 10 min
PACEA/NCEA (>1 year of age)	Ropivacaine 0.1–0.2 %	0.2 mg/kg/h + bolus 0.1 mg/kg, lockout 30 min

Adapted from *APS Guidelines Mother and Child Hospital Lyon*
PCEA patient-controlled epidural analgesia, *PCNA* patient-controlled nerve analgesia, *PACEA* parent-controlled epidural analgesia, *NCEA* nurse-controlled epidural analgesia

23.4.4 Non-pharmacological Management of Pain and Anxiety

Anxiety and other psychological factors have significant impact on pain intensity and analgesic requirements. There is growing evidence supporting the benefits of family centred non-pharmacological techniques during the perioperative period [100].

Many strategies have been described, including videogames or tablet-based distraction [101], clown doctors, child life specialists, and family-based preparation [102]. Children, especially under the age of 8 years, display a vivid imagination and caregivers can take clinical advantage of the "magical thinking" and the potent effect of the context-induced placebo analgesia [103].

Table 23.7 Common adjuncts to nerve blocks and examples of dosing regimens

Molecule	Site of injection	Suggested dosing
Morphine[a]	Epidural (caudal, lumbar, or thoracic)	30–50 µg/kg q12–24H
	Intrathecal	3–5 µg/kg (single shot)
Clonidine[b]	Epidural (co-administration)	1–2 µg/kg (single shot)
	Peripheral (intravenous co-injection[c])	1–2 µg/kg (single shot)
	Adjunct to continuous infusion of LAs	0.5–1 µg/kg/h
Dexamethasone	Intravenous co-injection[c]	0.1–0.15 mg/kg (usually single shot, up to q8H)

q every, *H* hours, *LAs* local anaesthetics
[a]Mandatory respiratory monitoring
[b]For children >1 year old
[c]Intravenous co-injection displays the same efficacy as perinervous injection

Hypnosis is increasingly being recognized as an effective technique for pain control in the perioperative period. Patients receiving hypnosis present significantly reduced anxiety level and shortened hospital stay after surgery [104].

23.5 Time to Procedures Specific Strategies?

Paediatric anaesthesia societies have proposed general guidelines for perioperative pain management [6]. Few specific pharmacological or non-pharmacological interventions could be used as a sole strategy. There are currently no specific procedure-related guidelines, as presented by the PROSPECT project (www.postoppain.org) in adults [105]. This could be due to the fact that most of the efforts were directed to evaluate specific analgesic methodologies and few studied procedure-specific solutions. The current heterogeneity of outcomes and methodologies in paediatric studies precludes an adequate comparison between techniques and development of robust procedure-specific guidelines [106].

23.6 Analgesia at Home

Most surgical procedures are nowadays performed on an ambulatory regime. Discharge information and parental education about pain evaluation, analgesic plan, and rescue medication management are of paramount importance. Not unusually parents are reluctant to provide rescue medication [9, 107] due to a variety of factors and misconceptions. A detailed analgesic plan should be part of the postoperative surgical indications: it should include the doses, timing, and a plan B in case of inadequate analgesia or adverse effects. Whenever possible, the timing of medication should fit the child/family activity, for example, synchronizing medication during meal times, at bedtime, etc. [108].

Conclusions

Efficient pain relief is of paramount importance in the perioperative care of infants and children. Postoperative pain in children presents specific physiological, anatomical, psychological, and pharmacological challenges. The analgesic modalities and routes of administration should be adapted to the age, unique anatomy, developmental status, and physiology. A dedicated acute pain service (APS) team best provides postoperative pain management, especially in the context of more complex techniques during admission. Multimodal perioperative pain management is a key concept for postoperative pain prevention and treatment. Opioids are the preferred medication for severe pain. They should be associated with non-opioid medications, regional anaesthesia/analgesia, and non-pharmacological strategies. Future research should focus on clinical outcomes other than pain when evaluating paediatric procedure-specific techniques.

References

1. Walco GA, Cassidy RC, Schechter NL (1994) Pain, hurt, and harm. The ethics of pain control in infants and children. N Engl J Med 331:541–544
2. Bartocci M, Bergqvist LL, Lagercrantz H et al (2006) Pain activates cortical areas in the preterm newborn brain. Pain 122:109–117
3. Fitzgerald M, Walker SM (2009) Infant pain management: a developmental neurobiological approach. Nat Clin Pract Neurol 5:35–50
4. Fitzgerald M, Beggs S (2001) The neurobiology of pain: developmental aspects. Neuroscientist 7:246–257
5. Beggs S, Currie G, Salter MW et al (2012) Priming of adult pain responses by neonatal pain experience: maintenance by central neuroimmune activity. Brain 135:404–417
6. APAGBI (2012) Good practice in postoperative and procedural pain management 2nd Edition, 2012. Paediatr Anaesth 22:1–79
7. Physicians T.R.A.C.O. (2006) Guidelines statement: management of procedure-related pain in children and adolescents. J Paediatr Child Health 42:1–29
8. Groenewald CB, Rabbitts JA, Schroeder DR et al (2012) Prevalence of moderate-severe pain in hospitalized children. Paediatr Anaesth 22:661–668
9. Hegarty M, Calder A, Davies K et al (2013) Does take-home analgesia improve postoperative pain after elective day case surgery? A comparison of hospital vs parent-supplied analgesia. Paediatr Anaesth 23:385–389
10. Morton NS (2012) The pain-free ward: myth or reality. Paediatr Anaesth 22:527–529
11. Chidambaran V, Sadhasivam S (2012) Pediatric acute and surgical pain management: recent advances and future perspectives. Int Anesthesiol Clin 50:66–82
12. Walker SM (2014) Overview of neurodevelopment and pain research, possible treatment targets. Best Pract Res Clin Rheumatol 28:213–228
13. Rony RY, Fortier MA, Chorney JM et al (2010) Parental postoperative pain management: attitudes, assessment, and management. Pediatrics 125:1372–1378
14. von Baeyer CL, Chambers CT, Eakins DM (2001) Development of a 10-item short form of the parents' postoperative pain measure: the PPPM-SF. J Pain 12:401–406
15. Carter B, McArthur E, Cunliffe M (2002) Dealing with uncertainty: parental assessment of pain in their children with profound special needs. J Adv Nurs 38:449–457
16. Khin Hla T, Hegarty M, Russel P et al (2014) Perception of pediatric pain: a comparison of postoperative pain assessments between child, parent, nurse, and independent observer. Paediatr Anaesth 24:1127–1131

17. Migeon A, Desgranges FP, Chassard D et al (2013) Pupillary reflex dilatation and analgesia nociception index monitoring to assess the effectiveness of regional anesthesia in children anesthetised with sevoflurane. Paediatr Anaesth 23:1160–1165

18. Sabourdin N, Arnaout M, Louvet N et al (2013) Pain monitoring in anesthetized children: first assessment of skin conductance and analgesia-nociception index at different infusion rates of remifentanil. Paediatr Anaesth 23:149–155

19. Stevens BJ, Gibbins S, Yamada J et al (2014) The premature infant pain profile-revised (PIPP-R). Initial validation and feasibility. Clin J Pain 30:238–243

20. Breau LM, Finley GA, McGrath PJ et al (2000) Validation of the non-communicating children's pain checklist–postoperative version. Anesthesiology 96:528–535

21. McGrath PJ, Walco GA, Turk DC et al (2008) Core outcome domains and measures for pediatric acute and chronic/recurrent pain clinical trials: PedIMMPACT recommendations. J Pain 9:771–783

22. Brennan TJ, Taylor BK (2000) Analgesic treatment before incision compared with treatment after incision provides no improvement on postoperative pain relief. J Pain 1:96–98

23. Pogatzki-Zahn E, Zahn PK (2006) From preemptive to preventive analgesia. Curr Opin Anaesthesiol 19:551–555

24. Shipton EA (2014) The transition of acute postoperative pain to chronic pain: part 2 – Limiting the transition. Trends Anaesth Crit Care 4:71–75

25. Gilron I, Kehlet H (2014) Prevention of chronic pain after surgery: new insights for future research and patient care. Can J Anaesth 61:101–111

26. Kart T, Christrup LL, Rasmussen M (1997) Recommended use of morphine in neonates, infants and children based on a literature review: part 1 – pharmacokinetics. Paediatr Anaesth 7:5–11

27. Kart T, Christrup LL, Rasmussen M (1997) Recommended use of morphine in neonates, infants and children based on a literature review: Part 2--Clinical use. Paediatr Anaesth 7:93–101

28. Maxwell LG, Kaufmann SC, Blitzer S et al (2005) The effects of a small-dose naloxone infusion on opioid-induced side effects and analgesia in children and adolescents treated with intravenous patient-controlled analgesia: a double-blind, prospective, randomized, controlled study. Anesth Analg 100:953–958

29. Bouwmeester NJ, Anderson BJ, Tibboel D et al (2004) Developmental pharmacokinetics of morphine and its metabolites in neonates, infants and young children. Br J Anaesth 92:208–217

30. Saarenmaa E, Neuvonen PJ, Rosenberg P et al (2000) Morphine clearance and effects in newborn infants in relation to gestational age. Clin Pharmacol Ther 68:160–166

31. Robert R, Brack A, Blakeney P et al (2003) A double-blind study of the analgesic efficacy of oral transmucosal fentanyl citrate and oral morphine in pediatric patients undergoing burn dressing change and tubbing. J Burn Care Rehabil 24:351–355

32. Collins C, Koren G, Crean P et al (1985) Fentanyl pharmacokinetics and hemodynamic effects in preterm infants during ligation of patent ductus arteriosus. Anesth Analg 64:1078–1080

33. Nielsen BN, Friis SM, Romsing J et al (2014) Intranasal sufentanil/ketamine analgesia in children. Paediatr Anaesth 24:170–180

34. Ross AK, Davis PJ, Dear GL et al (2001) Pharmacokinetics of remifentanil in anesthetized pediatric patients undergoing elective surgery or diagnostic procedures. Anesth Analg 93:1393–1401

35. Kim SH, Stoicea N, Soghomonyan S et al (2014) Intraoperative use of remifentanil and opioid induced hyperalgesia/acute opioid tolerance: systematic review. Front Pharmacol. doi:10.3389/fphar.2014.00108

36. Pokela ML, Anttila E, Seppala T et al (2005) Marked variation in oxycodone pharmacokinetics in infants. Paediatr Anaesth 15:560–565

37. Olkkola KT, Hamunen K, Seppala T et al (1994) Pharmacokinetics and ventilatory effects of intravenous oxycodone in postoperative children. Br J Clin Pharmacol 38:71–76

38. Zernikow B, Michel E, Craig F et al (2009) Pediatric palliative care: use of opioids for the management of pain. Paediatr Drugs 11:129–151
39. Babul N, Darke AC, Hain H (1995) Hydromorphone and metabolite pharmacokinetics in children. J Pain Symptom Manage 10:335–337
40. Berde CB, Beyer JE, Bournaki MC et al (1991) Comparison of morphine and methadone for prevention of postoperative pain in 3- to 7-year-old children. J Pediatr 119:136–141
41. Williams PI, Sarginson RE, Ratcliffe JM (1998) Use of methadone in the morphine-tolerant burned paediatric patient. Br J Anaesth 80:92–95
42. Shir Y, Shenkman Z, Shavelson V et al (1998) Oral methadone for the treatment of severe pain in hospitalized children: a report of five cases. Clin J Pain 14:350–353
43. Siddappa R, Fletcher JE, Heard AM et al (2003) Methadone dosage for prevention of opioid withdrawal in children. Paediatr Anaesth 13:805–810
44. Gerbershagen HJ, Aduckathil S, van Wijck AJ et al (2013) Pain intensity on the first day after surgery. Anesthesiology 118:934–944
45. Schultz-Machata AM, Becke K, Weiss M (2014) Nalbuphine in pediatric anesthesia (article in German). Anaesthesist 63:135–143
46. Marzuillo P, Calligaris L, Barbi E (2014) Tramadol can selectively manage moderate pain in children following European advice limiting codeine use. Acta Paediatr 103:1110–1116
47. Saudan S, Habre W (2007) Pharmacokinetics of tramadol in children. Ann Fr Anesth Reanim 26:560–563
48. Anderson BJ, Palmer GM (2006) Recent developments in the pharmacological management of pain in children. Curr Opin Anaesthesiol 19:285–292
49. Hullett BJ, Chambers NA, Pascoe EM et al (2006) Tramadol vs morphine during adenotonsillectomy for obstructive sleep apnea in children. Paediatr Anaesth 16:648–653
50. Kosarac B, Fox AA, Collard CD (2009) Effect of genetic factors on opioid action. Curr Opin Anaesthesiol 22:476–482
51. Lundeberg S (2015) Pain in children – are we accomplishing the optimal pain treatment? Paediatr Anaesth 25:83–92
52. Ali SM, Shahrbano S, Ulhaq TS (2008) Tramadol for pain relief in children undergoing adenotonsillectomy: a comparison with dextromethorphan. Laryngoscope 118:1547–1549
53. Bozkurt P (2005) Use of tramadol in children. Paediatr Anaesth 15:1041–1047
54. Numanoglu KV, Ayoglu H, Er DT (2014) Efficacy of tramadol as a preincisional infiltration anesthetic in children undergoing inguinal hernia repair: a prospective randomized study. Ther Clin Risk Manag 10:753–758
55. Akbay BK, Yildizbas S, Guclu E et al (2010) Analgesic efficacy of topical tramadol in the control of postoperative pain in children after tonsillectomy. J Anesth 24:705–708
56. McDonald AJ, Cooper MG (2001) Patient-controlled analgesia: an appropriate method of pain control in children. Paediatr Drugs 3:273–284
57. Nelson KL, Yaster M, Kost-Byerly S et al (2010) A national survey of American Pediatric Anesthesiologists: patient-controlled analgesia and other intravenous opioid therapies in pediatric acute pain management. Anesth Analg 110:754–760
58. Monitto CL, Greenberg RS, Kost-Byerly S et al (2000) Safety and efficacy of parent-/nurse-controlled analgesia in patients less than six years of age. Anesth Analg 91:573–579
59. Howard RF, Lloyd-Thomas A, Thomas M et al (2010) Nurse-controlled analgesia (NCA) following major surgery in 10,000 patients in a children's hospital. Paediatr Anaesth 20:126–134
60. Dahl JB, Nielsen RV, Wetterslev J et al (2014) Post-operative analgesic effects of paracetamol, NSAIDs, glucocorticoids, gabapentinoids and their combinations: a topical review. Acta Anaesthesiol Scand 58:1165–1181
61. Wong I, St John-Green C, Walker SM (2013) Opioid-sparing effects of perioperative paracetamol and nonsteroidal anti-inflammatory drugs (NSAIDs) in children. Paediatr Anaesth 23:475–495
62. Voepel-Lewis T, Wagner D, Burke C et al (2013) Early adjuvant use of nonopioids associated with reduced odds of serious postoperative opioid adverse events and need for rescue in children. Paediatr Anaesth 23:162–169

63. Schultz-Machata AM, Weiss M, Becke K (2014) What's new in pediatric acute pain therapy? Curr Opin Anaesthesiol 27:316–322
64. Anderson BJ (2008) Paracetamol (Acetaminophen): mechanisms of action. Paediatr Anaesth 18:915–921
65. Choi SS, Lee JK, Suh HW (2001) Antinociceptive profiles of aspirin and acetaminophen in formalin, substance P and glutamate pain models. Brain Res 921:233–239
66. Michelet D, Andreu-Gallien J, Bensalah T et al (2012) A meta-analysis of the use of nonsteroidal antiinflammatory drugs for pediatric postoperative pain. Anesth Analg 114:393–406
67. Williams BA, Bottegal MT, Kentor ML et al (2007) Rebound pain scores as a function of femoral nerve block duration after anterior cruciate ligament reconstruction: retrospective analysis of a prospective, randomized clinical trial. Reg Anesth Pain Med 32:186–192
68. Kelly LE, Sommer DD, Ramakrishna J et al (2014) Morphine or ibuprofen for post-tonsillectomy analgesia: a randomized trial. Pediatrics 135:307–313
69. Boyer KC, McDonald P, Zoetis T (2010) A novel formulation of ketorolac tromethamine for intranasal administration: preclinical safety evaluation. Int J Toxicol 29:467–478
70. Dawkins TN, Barclay CA, Gardiner RL et al (2009) Safety of intravenous use of ketorolac in infants following cardiothoracic surgery. Cardiol Young 19:105–108
71. Hermans V, De Pooter F, De Groote F et al (2012) Effect of dexamethasone on nausea, vomiting, and pain in paediatric tonsillectomy. Br J Anaesth 109:427–431
72. Lavand'homme P (2011) The progression from acute to chronic pain. Curr Opin Anaesthesiol 24:545–550
73. Bell RF, Dahl JB, Moore RA et al (2006) Perioperative ketamine for acute postoperative pain. Cochrane Database Syst Rev 25:1–42
74. Dahmani S, Michelet D, Annack PS et al (2011) Ketamine for perioperative pain management in children: a meta-analysis of published studies. Paediatr Anaesth 21:636–652
75. He XY, Cao JP, Shi XY et al (2013) Dexmedetomidine versus morphine or fentanyl in the management of children after tonsillectomy and adenoidectomy: a meta-analysis of randomized controlled trials. Ann Otol Rhinol Laryngol 122:114–120
76. Holsti L, Grunau RE (2002) Considerations for using sucrose to reduce procedural pain in preterm infants. Pediatrics 125:1042–1047
77. Stevens B, Yamada J, Beyene J et al (2005) Consistent management of repeated procedural pain with sucrose in preterm neonates: is it effective and safe for repeated use over time? Clin J Pain 21:543–548
78. Mayell A, Srinivasan I, Campbell F et al (2014) Analgesic effects of gabapentin after scoliosis surgery in children: a randomized controlled trial. Paediatr Anaesth 24:1239–1244
79. Massey GV, Pedigo S, Dunn NL et al (2002) Continuous lidocaine infusion for the relief of refractory malignant pain in a terminally ill pediatric cancer patient. J Pediatr Hematol Oncol 24:566–568
80. Bosenberg AT, Johr M, Wolf AR (2011) Pro con debate: the use of regional vs systemic analgesia for neonatal surgery. Paediatr Anaesth 21:1247–1258
81. Marhofer P, Ivani G, Suresh S et al (2012) Everyday regional anesthesia in children. Paediatr Anaesth 22:995–1001
82. Marhofer P, Lonnqvist PA (2014) The use of ultrasound-guided regional anaesthetic techniques in neonates and young infants. Acta Anaesthesiol Scand 58:1049–1060
83. Gunter JB (2002) Benefit and risks of local anesthetics in infants and children. Pediatr Drugs 4:649–672
84. Goeller JK, Bhalla T, Tobias JD et al (2014) Combined use of neuraxial and general anesthesia during major abdominal procedures in neonates and infants. Paediatr Anaesth 24:553–560
85. Suresh S, Long J, Birmingham PK et al (2015) Are caudal blocks for pain control safe in children? An analysis of 18,650 caudal blocks from the Pediatric Regional Anesthesia Network (PRAN) database. Anesth Analg 120:151–156
86. Long JB, Birmingham PK, De Oliveira GS Jr et al (2014) Transversus abdominis plane block in children: a multicenter safety analysis of 1994 cases from the PRAN (Pediatric Regional Anesthesia Network) database. Anesth Analg 119:395–399

87. Ecoffey C, Lacroix F, Giaufré E et al (2010) Epidemiology and morbidity of regional anesthesia in children: a follow-up one-year prospective survey of the French-Language Society of Paediatric Anaesthesiologists (ADARPEF). Paediatr Anaesth 20:1061–1069
88. Taenzer AH, Walker BJ, Bosenberg AT et al (2014) Asleep versus awake: does it matter? Pediatric regional block complications by patient state: a report from the Pediatric Regional Anesthesia Network. Reg Anesth Pain Med 39:279–283
89. Allison CE, Aronson DC, Geukers VG et al (2008) Paraplegia after thoracotomy under combined general and epidural anesthesia in a child. Paediatr Anaesth 18:539–542
90. Oliver JA, Oliver LA (2013) Beyond the caudal: truncal blocks an alternative option for analgesia in pediatric surgical patients. Curr Opin Anaesthesiol 26:644–651
91. Bhalla T, Sawardekar A, Dewhirst E et al (2013) Ultrasound-guided trunk and core blocks in infants and children. J Anesth 27:109–123
92. Dadure C, Capdevila X (2012) Peripheral catheter techniques. Paediatr Anaesth 22:93–101
93. Gurnaney H, Kraemer FW, Maxwell L et al (2014) Ambulatory continuous peripheral nerve blocks in children and adolescents: a longitudinal 8-year single center study. Anesth Analg 118:621–627
94. Birmingham PK, Wheeler M, Suresh S et al (2003) Patient-controlled epidural analgesia in children: can they do it? Anesth Analg 96:686–691
95. Birmingham PK, Suresh S, Ambrosy A et al (2009) Parent-assisted or nurse-assisted epidural analgesia: is this feasible in pediatric patients? Paediatr Anaesth 19:1084–1089
96. Ivani G, Mossetti V (2008) Regional anesthesia for postoperative pain control in children: focus on continuous central and perineural infusions. Paediatr Drugs 10:107–114
97. Astuto ME (2013) Pediatric anesthesia, intensive care and pain: standardization in clinical practice. Springer-Verlag, Italia, pp 113–144
98. Lonnqvist PA (2015) Adjuncts should always be used in pediatric regional anesthesia. Paediatr Anaesth 25:100–106
99. Bailard NS, Ortiz J, Flores RA (2014) Additives to local anesthetics for peripheral nerve blocks: evidence, limitations, and recommendations. Am J Health Syst Pharm 71:373–385
100. Power NM, Howard RF, Wade AM et al (2012) Pain and behaviour changes in children following surgery. Arch Dis Child 97:879–884
101. André C, Tosetti S, Desgranges FP et al (2014) Gestion de l'anxiété pré-opératoire en pédiatrie: étude randomisée comparant une tablette éléctronique au Midazolam. Ann Fr Anesth Reanim 33:A93–A94
102. Fortier MA, Blount RL, Wang SM et al (2011) Analysing a family-centred preoperative intervention programme: a dismantling approach. Br J Anaesth 106:713–718
103. Krummenacher P, Kossowsky J, Schwarz C et al (2014) Expectancy-induced placebo analgesia in children and the role of magical thinking. J Pain 15:1282–1293
104. Kuttner L (2012) Pediatric hypnosis: pre-, peri-, and post-anesthesia. Paediatr Anaesth 22:573–577
105. Joshi GP, Schug SA, Kehlet H (2014) Procedure-specific pain management and outcome strategies. Best Pract Res Clin Anaesthesiol 28:191–201
106. Di Pede A, Morini F, Lombardi MH et al (2014) Comparison of regional vs. systemic analgesia for post-thoracotomy care in infants. Paediatr Anaesth 24:569–573
107. Dorkham MC, Chalkiadis GA, von Ungern Sternberg BS et al (2014) Effective postoperative pain management in children after ambulatory surgery, with a focus on tonsillectomy: barriers and possible solutions. Paediatr Anaesth 24:239–248
108. MacLaren Chorney J, Twycross A, Mifflin K et al (2014) Can we improve parents' management of their children's postoperative pain at home? Pain Res Manag 19:115–123

Long-Term Consequences of Anesthesia (and Surgery) on the Infant Brain

24

Tom Giedsing Hansen

24.1 Introduction

Very few issues (if any) within pediatric anesthesia have caused so much concern and emotional gravity than the fact that the past roughly 15 years, a plethora of animal studies have uniformly shown that exposure to most of the currently used anesthetics possibly during a vulnerable period of brain development (i.e., brain growth spurt or peak of synaptogenesis) may lead to neurodegeneration (particularly apoptosis) and abnormal synaptic development [1–4]. Importantly, the observed morphological abnormalities are associated with functional deficits in learning and behavior later in life [5]. Initial studies were mainly performed in immature rodent pups, but more recent studies have included nonhuman primates (rhesus monkeys) [6–8]. Given the number of neonates, infants, and young children anesthetized annually worldwide, these findings could have significant public health implications. Both gamma-aminobutyric acid (GABA) agonists (e.g., inhalational anesthetics, propofol, benzodiazepines) and n-methyl-d-aspartate (NMDA) antagonists (e.g., ketamine and nitrous oxide) are implicated [3, 4]. Although results from animal studies using opioids, α-2 receptor agonists, and xenon are less overwhelming – and in some cases/circumstances have indicated that these agents may in fact possess neuroprotective properties – they are generally inconclusive.

Translating these animal studies into a human clinical context is difficult. How do various developmental stages of brain development in animal models translate into humans? The anesthetic techniques and managements used in the majority of

T.G. Hansen, MD, PhD (✉)
Department of Anesthesiology and Intensive Care – Pediatric Section,
Odense University Hospital, Odense DK-5000, Denmark

Institute of Clinical Research – Anesthesiology, University of Southern Denmark,
Odense DK-5000, Denmark
e-mail: tomghansen@dadlnet.dk

© Springer International Publishing Switzerland 2016
M. Astuto, P.M. Ingelmo (eds.), *Perioperative Medicine in Pediatric Anesthesia*,
Anesthesia, Intensive Care and Pain in Neonates and Children,
DOI 10.1007/978-3-319-21960-8_24

animal (rodent) studies are extremely different to normal clinical practice, for example, the use of supra-clinical doses and long duration of exposure to anesthetic drugs sometimes resulting in excessively high mortality (20–80 %). Additionally, the use of multiparameter monitoring and control of airway and respiration are difficult (or even impossible) due to the small size of the neonatal animals, which also precludes repeated blood gas and glucose measurements due to small circulating blood volumes [3]. This may be of utmost importance. A recent animal study by Wu et al. compared the effects of mechanical ventilation and spontaneous breathing on outcome in 14-day-old rats exposed to isoflurane and sevoflurane. Compared with mechanical ventilated rats, spontaneous breathing rats had significantly higher mortality, neuroapoptosis, and impaired neurocognitive outcome [9].

24.2 Limitations of Animal or Preclinical Data

The initial animal studies on anesthesia-related neurotoxicity and the developing brain were never driven by any clear or well-defined associations between general anesthesia and subsequent specific neurocognitive deficits in humans or the applicability to clinical care of human infants. Additionally, many inherent factors limit the applicability of animal-derived data to humans. More specifically, ontogenic differences in neurodevelopment between humans and animals that may impact outcome are largely unknown. Factors regarding the administration of anesthesia and study design, for example, differences in anesthetic drug potency between human and animals, lack of surgical stress, differences in monitoring and correction of physiologic, metabolic, and biochemical aberrations induced by anesthetic drugs and surgery, use of excessively high doses of anesthetics for a long period of time, and use of agents that are rarely used in modern clinical practice (such as ketamine, isoflurane, and nitrous oxide), may complicate matters [1]. Furthermore, there is a lack of systematic evidence for the clinical benefits of animal research in general and animal neuroscience in particular [10].

24.3 Normal Development of Human Brain

Morphology and function of the brain is not a static process but rather a complex, continuous, and lifelong process. Immediately after birth, the brain is about 25 % of its adult size and unevenly matured [3, 4]. The brain stem and spinal cord are relatively well developed, whereas the limbic system and cerebral cortex are still immature. Despite being produced before birth, the cortical neurons are poorly connected, and most synapses are produced after birth during a peak synaptogenesis where the rate of cortical synapse formation is estimated to be two million new synapses per second. At the age of 2 years, the cerebral cortex comprises more than 100 trillion synapses. The newborn brain contains little myelin, and myelination appears to be virtually an "automatic or innate" process in that its sequence succession is very predictable, and it appears that severe malnutrition is the only single individual environmental factor known to impact myelination. Sensory afferent stimuli before and after birth differentiate the function of neurons and neural pathways, ensuring neuroplasticity of the CNS [3, 4]. However, this plasticity may be a two-edged sword in that it implies that on one hand young children's brains are more open to learning and enriching influences on the other they may also be more vulnerable and susceptible to environmental changes. Selection and formation of active neural circuits (pruning) occurs throughout life but is much more common in early childhood. This initial excess of neurons and synapses is followed by significant neuronal death and decline in synapses. This normal and DNA-programmed cell death or apoptosis is necessary to ensure normal CNS morphology and function. It is an intimate and integral part of normal brain development and maintenance. The net result is that <50 % of neurons survive into adult life. Any interference with this normal apoptotic process may have detrimental effects to the central nervous system. All commonly used anesthetics have been shown in preclinical studies to markedly increase neuroapoptosis. However, several other studies have subsequently also documented acute neuronal cell loss, altered dendritic architecture, reduced synaptic density, destabilization of the cytoskeleton, and cell cycle abnormalities following exposure to all commonly used general anesthetics [3, 4]. For obvious reasons, it remains to be proven whether similar anesthesia-induced neurodegeneration occurs in human clinical settings.

24.4 Human Studies

Relative to the magnitude of animal investigations, the number of human studies is relatively limited. The majority of these are listed in the reference list and have recently been reviewed in details elsewhere [11, 12], where more detailed information about these studies can be obtained. Fortunately, all these studies have been inconclusive, that is, it has been very difficult to show whether this animal phenomenon has a human corollary [13–26]. In the following, the most important issues related to the human studies are presented.

24.5 Relevant Human Outcome Measure

It remains to be determined how anesthesia-related neurotoxicity (if it exists) will reveal itself in humans. Contrary to babies with, for example, fetal alcohol syndrome or babies born to mothers on certain antiepileptic drugs in whom distinctive mental and physical defects are well described, any detrimental effect associated with anesthetic exposure in infancy must be of a minor nature [3]. Otherwise, it would be easy to demonstrate and it would most likely have been suspected many years ago. Therefore, the following questions are of utmost importance: what is a meaningful outcome measure and when and how do we best measure it? Should we search for developmental disorders in preschool, learning disabilities (LD) in elementary school, social disturbances in adolescence, or psychiatric disorders in adulthood, and what relevance has loss of various cognitive functions or early dementia in the elderly? To what extent are sensorimotor deficits or psychiatric disorders relevant? More importantly, how well does a single short-term interim measure performed in early childhood or adolescence adequately predict outcome later in life, and what are the long-term consequences of that? Currently, we do not have the answers.

Learning disabilities is a very crude outcome influenced by many underlying factors, for example, chronic diseases and environmental factors. More importantly, LD is not a specific neuropsychological outcome measure, but rather a categorical determination arising from differences between a child's educational outlook (e.g., IQ) and his or her actual achievement. Focusing on the cumulative incidence of LD implies that follow-up is ceased when an LD is identified, and a priori it is then thought that the LD will persist and never disappear. This impedes estimation of the true prevalence of this outcome measure. Further, a child labelled with LD may at some point in life have a change in achievement placing him or her back in the normal range. Such an incident will not be detected by the current used study designs. Assessment of academic performances has a pragmatic advantage over, for example, IQ testing or similar in that parents are likely to be more interested in how their child will do in school. A recent study employing extensive and repeated neurodevelopmental testing suggested that group testing such as academic performance may lack sufficient sensitivity to detect smaller, minor, or more subtle neurocognitive impairment between children exposed and children not exposed to anesthesia compared with individually administered cognitive tests [26]. It has been claimed that studies using individually administered tests of cognition may be more likely to be positive into any potential phenotype (e.g., abnormalities in speech and language). However, at this point, we do not know under what circumstances individual cognitive testing are actually also meaningful human outcome measures. Many of the outcomes used in these studies are interrelated. One question quickly arises: exactly how different are individually tests of speech and language and school tests? Certainly, good academic achievements require good speech and language skills [27].

Attention-deficit hyperactivity disorder (ADHD) has also been tested as a primary outcome measure to assess for anesthesia-related neurotoxicity [13]. However, the diagnosis and treatment of ADHD are highly disputed. The diagnosis of ADHD is afflicted by ascertainment bias as demonstrated by the large variation in its prevalence across countries, states, races, genders, and ethnicities. Further, in 2011, two million more children were diagnosed with ADHD in the USA compared with 2003, and overall one out of five US teenage boys was labelled with an ADHD diagnosis (more than two-third of these were taking long-term medication such as dexamphetamine). Thus and because ADHD is associated with an array of psychiatric disorders and learning disabilities, its value as an outcome measure in studies on anesthesia-related neurotoxicity is questionable [28, 29]. Recently, autism spectrum disorder has also been used as outcome measure in these types of studies [30]. Similar arguments as just mentioned in relation to ADHD can been applied regarding this outcome measure [31].

24.6   Migration

The degree of migration of study subjects is of major concern in many of the human cohort studies published thus far. As high a proportion as one-third of the original cohort has been reported in some series to move such that information from these individuals could not be retrieved [13, 14]. This is an important issue because significant differences between migrants and nonmigrants are well noted in some of these cohort studies increasing the likelihood for selection biases [32]. Families with a significantly ill child living in close proximity to a major pediatric center are less likely to migrate. Furthermore, children with significant comorbidities are more likely to suffer neurobehavioral problems and require multiple anesthetics.

24.7   Sample Size Issue

The problem surrounding the "sample size issue" was addressed in one of the first human studies on this topic [23]. Since then it has become increasingly apparent that sufficiently large sample sizes are needed to detect modest associations among the multitude of perioperative factors that impact neurocognitive outcomes (see later). In fact, very few of the current available human cohort studies have large sample sizes [21, 22]. The introduction of multiple (individual) testings has been employed to compensate for this fact [19]. However, such an approach carries a high-risk Type I statistical error, which (as mentioned earlier) may be a particular risk in the present context in that many of the tests use are interrelated [27]. Similar problems have been encountered in studies on postoperative dysfunction (POCD) in the elderly [33, 34]. The reality is that to date, there are no reliable tools available to test for the presence of POCD, and simply increasing the number of tests to assess and classify POCD also increases the rate of false-positive classifications.

24.8   Duration and Number of Exposures

Preclinical data suggests that larger anesthetic doses and longer duration may be associated with greater effects (i.e., poorer outcome) [1–9]. Similarly, human studies suggest that one single and short-term anesthetic (and surgical) exposure seems harmless, whereas multiple exposures are associated with poorer outcome (i.e., increased hazard ratios) [14–26]. However, such an association is not necessarily causal, because children who require multiple surgeries are far more likely to suffer serious underlying conditions that – as mentioned above – may independently impact neurodevelopment. Additionally, the effects from surgeries (e.g., stress responses, pain, and neuroinflammation) cannot be disentangled from that of the anesthetic itself in these studies [11, 12]. Very few studies have focused on longer exposures/procedures [35, 36]. In these studies, it appears that many other confounding factors are by far more important than merely exposure to anesthetics.

24.9   Age at Exposure

In preclinical studies, timing of exposure to anesthetic drugs seems to play a pivotal role in mediating the degree of injury as the brain may have periods of increased vulnerability during different stages of development [37]. In young rodents, the period of greatest vulnerability appears to be between postnatal 4 and 10 days (~PD7) and corresponds to the period of the peak synaptogenesis. In guinea pigs, this corresponds to mid-gestation, whereas in rhesus monkeys, it corresponds to up to 35 days of age [3, 4]. In humans, the period of greatest synaptogenesis is thought to occur during the last trimester and up to 2 to 3 to 4 years postnatally. However, there is no evidence to support this contention. Additionally, all brain regions may not develop uniformly, and different regions may be differentially susceptible during different stages of development [3, 4, 38, 39]. A free available website was launched almost 10 years ago to improve accuracy in extrapolating vulnerable periods between different animal species. This website used more modern models and the newest brain developmental data (www.translatingtime.net) [38, 39]. Unfortunately, this new bioinformatics method has not yet been implemented in animal studies on anesthesia-related neurotoxicity. By integrating data from core developmental stages and events from many mammalians into a statistical model, these animal models suggest that the developmental stage of, for example, a rodent cerebral cortex at PD-7 may actually correspond to the maturational stage of the human brain at the very beginning of third trimester [39]. This may well mean that animal experiments using 7-day-old rodents may correlate with providing anesthetics to extremely premature babies.

More recent animal studies have shown that neuronal cell death also occurs in isoflurane- or propofol-exposed adult mice. Two recent studies have demonstrated that different brain regions are vulnerable at different ages, as neurogenesis peaks at different ages among brain regions, and that brain regions with ongoing adult neurogenesis (e.g., dentate gyrus and olfactory bulb) seem to be vulnerable far beyond the previously suggested window of vulnerability, potentially far into adulthood [40, 41]. Thus, in animals, there may be no such thing as a "safe anesthetic period."

Still, it is the general belief that the youngest and most immature infants are at greatest risk. This is unfortunately not reflected in the current human studies published so far on this topic as these usually comprise very few neonates and infants. The few studies that do comprise infants show no differences in outcome following minor surgeries compared to controls but major differences following major surgeries, for example, neurosurgery [21, 22, 35].

24.10   Impact of Surgery

Very few of the available human cohort studies have focused on a single and well-defined surgery [21, 22]. Rather, most studies have pooled data from multiple surgeries (and diagnosis). This is very unfortunate because both surgery and underlying pathology independently influence subsequent neurocognitive outcome. In infants undergoing inguinal and pyloric stenosis repair, academic achievements in adolescence are comparable to the background population [21, 22] and much better compared to infants undergoing, for example, neurosurgical procedures [35].

24.11 Gender Issue

Another important confounding factor is gender. Gender (male) can influence the need for surgery, for example, inguinal hernia and pyloric stenosis repair [21, 22]. Interestingly, it is widely recognized that gender independently impact neurobehavioral outcome (and mortality) in later life. Additionally, gender may also influence an individuals' susceptibility to toxicity – which is an issue also observed in preclinical studies [3].

24.12 Other Important Factors

The single most important cofactor is the effects of surgery itself. The impact of stress responses, nociception, and neuroinflammation need much more clarification.

Higher socioeconomic status and particularly parental (maternal) education are strongly associated with better neurobehavioral outcome and with enhanced capacity to recover from any injury. Interestingly, parental education is more valid than parental occupation and socioeconomic status as these later are subject to changes over time, whereas after the age 30 years, parental educational length rarely changes [42]. Noteworthy, in several of the available human studies, known confounding factors (e.g., gender, age (birth weight), congenital malformations, maternal age, and parental level of education) more strongly affect outcome than exposure to anesthesia and surgery [21, 22].

Many other perioperative factors have the possibility to impact later neurodevelopment possibly to a much larger extents than a brief anesthetic exposure in young life [43]. These include a number of physiological, metabolic, and biochemical factors induced by general anesthetics and surgery, but also the more important questions: who, where, when, and how should small children be anesthetized? For more information about all these issues, the readers are referred to www.safetots.org.

24.13 Ongoing and Future Studies

Currently (i.e., primo 2015), there are at least three ongoing prospective studies. In the Pediatric Anesthesia and Neuro-Development Assessment (PANDA) study, about 500 ASA 1 and 2 children scheduled for inguinal hernia repair before 3 years of age will be compared with an unexposed sibling from a retrospective database. At the age between 8 and 15 years, children will be extensively assessed neurodevelopmentally. Initial results from this study are pending.

The GAS study is a multisite, randomized controlled trial (RCT) in which infants undergoing inguinal hernia repair before 60 weeks postconceptual age are randomized to either general anesthesia or regional anesthesia (spinal or caudal) comparing neurodevelopmental outcome. The follow-up time is 5 years. Enrollment has been completed, but final analysis results are not expected before 2017.

Using an extensive battery of neurocognitive tests (including the operant test battery used in relation to nonhuman primates), the Mayo Safety in Kids study intends to compare the performance of children previously exposed to anesthesia before the age of 3 years with children never exposed. Enrollment is ongoing, but the first results will not be available before 2016.

24.14 Conclusion

Fortunately, it has proven difficult to demonstrate a human equivalent to the animal data demonstrating anesthesia-related neurotoxicity in the developing brain. This fact indicates that the problem most likely is less significant than previously feared. However, that does not mean that the problem is not important. At this point, we know that one single and brief anesthetic exposure seems "safe" and that repeated anesthetic (and surgical) exposures have consistently been associated with poorer outcomes (LD, ADHD, etc.). Importantly, these associations are not necessarily causal, as children who require multiple surgeries are far more likely to suffer serious underlying medical disorders that can impact neurodevelopment. Furthermore, many other perioperative factors influence neurocognitive outcome, and each and every one of them more significantly do so than anesthetic/surgical exposures [40]. Very few neonates, infants, and young children undergo unnecessary anesthesia and surgery. It is ethically unacceptable to subject infants to invasive procedures without the benefit of anesthesia and analgesia. The decision to delay surgery or a diagnostic procedure should be made with a clear understanding that any real added risk of delay is being balanced against a still ambiguous and unknown risk of toxicity. Other than taking sensible precautions (e.g., briefest possible exposures to anesthetics, usage of regional techniques and possibly more opioids, and ensuring as much parental contact as possible), there is no need to change current anesthetic clinical practice and no need to postpone or cancel truly urgent surgeries.

24.15 Author's Comment

In this author's mind, it is highly possible that any definite link between anesthetic drugs or techniques and subsequent neurobehavioral impairment in children will never be established. Hopefully, in this search for any such potential causality in perioperative young children exposed to anesthetics, anesthetists, surgery and surgeons, their overall outcomes will be improved.

References

1. Ikonomidou C, Bosch F, Miksa M et al (1999) Blockade of NMDA receptors and apoptotic neurodegeneration in the developing brain. Science 283:70–74

2. Lunardi N, Ori C, Erisir A et al (2010) General anesthesia causes long-lasting disturbances in ultrastructural properties of developing synapses in young rats. Neurotox Res 17:179–188
3. Vutskits L, Davis PJ, Hansen TG (2012) Anesthetics and the developing brain: time for a change in practice? A pro/con debate. Paediatr Anaesth 22:973–980
4. Vutskits L (2012) General anesthesia: a gateway to modulate synapse formation and neural plasticity? Anesth Analg 115:1174–1182
5. Jevtovic-Todorovic V, Hartman RE, Izumi Y et al (2003) Early exposure to common anesthetic agents causes widespread neurodegeneration the developing rat brain and persistent learning deficits. J Neurosci 23:876–882
6. Paule MG, Li M, Allen RR et al (2011) Ketamine anesthesia during the first week of life can cause long lasting cognitive deficits in rhesus monkeys. Neurotoxicol Teratol 33:220–230
7. Slikker W Jr, Zou X, Hotchkiss CE et al (2007) Ketamine anesthesia during neuronal cell death in the perinatal rhesus monkey. Toxicol Sci 98:145–158
8. Zou X, Liu F, Zhang X et al (2011) Inhalational anesthetic-induced neuronal damage in the developing rhesus monkey. Neurotoxicol Teratol 33:592–599
9. Wu B, You S, Zhenq Y et al (2014) Physiological disturbance may contribute to neurodegeneration induced by isoflurane or sevoflurane in 14 day old rats. PLoS One 9, e84622
10. Pound P, Bracken MB (2014) Is animal research sufficiently evidence based to be a cornerstone of biomedical research? BMJ 348:g3387
11. Hansen TG (2013) Neurotoxicity, general anesthesia and the developing brain: what have we learned from the human studies so far? Curr Anesthesiol Rep 3:175–183
12. Hansen TG (2015) Anesthesia-related neurotoxicity and the developing animal brain is not a significant problem in children. Paediatr Anaesth 25:65–72
13. Sprung J, Flick RF, Katusic SK et al (2012) Attention-deficit/hyperactivity disorder after early exposure to procedures requiring general anesthesia. Mayo Clin Proc 87:120–129
14. Wilder RT, Flick RP, Sprung J et al (2009) Early exposure to anesthesia and learning disabilities in a population-based birth cohort. Anesthesiology 110:796–804
15. DiMaggio C, Sun LS, Kakavouli A et al (2009) A retrospective cohort study of the association of anesthesia and hernia repair surgery with behavioral and developmental disorders in young children. J Neurosurg Anesthesiol 21:286–291
16. Flick RP, Katusic SK, Colligan RC et al (2011) Cognitive and behavioral outcomes after early exposure to anesthesia and surgery. Pediatrics 128:e1053–e1061
17. Sprung J, Flick RP, Wilder RT et al (2009) Anesthesia for cesarean delivery and learning disability in a population-based birth cohort. Anesthesiology 111:302–310
18. DiMaggio C, Sun LS, Li G (2011) Early childhood exposure to anesthesia and risk of developmental and behavioral disorders in a sibling birth cohort. Anesth Analg 113:1143–1151
19. Ing C, DiMaggio C, Whitehouse A et al (2012) Long-term differences in language and cognitive function after childhood exposure to anesthesia. Pediatrics 130:e476–e485
20. Bartels M, Althoff RR, Boomsma DI (2009) Anesthesia and cognitive performance in children no evidence for a causal relationship. Twin Res Hum Genet 12:246–253
21. Hansen TG, Pedersen JK, Henneberg SW et al (2011) Academic performance in adolescence after inguinal hernia repair in infancy: a nationwide cohort study. Anesthesiology 114:1076–1085
22. Hansen TG, Pedersen JK, Henneberg SW et al (2013) Educational outcome in adolescence following pyloric stenosis repair before 3 months of age: a nationwide cohort study. Paediatr Anaesth 23:883–890
23. Kalkman CJ, Peelen L, Moons KG et al (2009) Behavior and development in children and age at the time of first anesthetic exposure. Anesthesiology 110:805–812
24. Stratman G, Lee J, Sall JW et al (2014) Effect of general anesthesia in infancy on long- term recognition memory in humans and rats. Neuropsychopharmacology 39:2275–2287
25. Block RI, Thomas JJ, Bayman EO et al (2012) Are anesthesia and surgery during infancy associated with altered academic performance during childhood. Anesthesiology 117:494–503
26. Ing CH, DiMaggio C, Malacova E et al (2014) Comparative analysis of outcome measures used in examining neurodevelopmental effects of early childhood anesthesia exposure. Anesthesiology 120:1319–1332

27. Flick RF, Nemergut ME, Christensen K, Hansen TG (2014) Anesthetic-related neurotoxicity in the young and outcome measures. The devil is in the details. Anesthesiology 120:1303–1305

28. Visser SN, Blumberg SJ, Danielson ML et al (2013) State-based and demographic in parentre-ported medication rates for attention deficit/hyperactivity disorder, 2007–2008. Prev Chronic Dis 10:20073

29. Visser SN, Danielson ML, Bitsko RH et al (2014) Trends in parent-report of health care provider-diagnosed and medicated attention deficit/hyperactivity disorder: United States, 2003–2011. J Am Acad Child Adolesc Psychiatry 53

30. Ko WR, Huang JY, Chiang YC et al (2015) Risk of autistic disorder after exposure to general anaesthesia and surgery: a nationwide retrospective matched cohort study. Eur J Anaesthesiol 32(5):303–310

31. Loepke AW, Hansen TG (2015) Is this our (paediatric patient's) brain on anaesthetic drugs? The search for a potential neurological phenotype of anaesthesia-related neurotoxicity in humans. Eur J Anaesthesiol 32(5):298–300

32. Katusic SK, Colligan RC, Barbaresi WJ et al (1998) Potential influence on migration bias in birth cohort studies. Mayo Clin Proc 73:1053–1061

33. Lewis MS, Maruff P, Silbert BS et al (2006) Detection of postoperative decline after coronary bypass graft surgery is affected by the number of neuropsychological tests in the assessment battery. Ann Thorac Surg 81:2097–2104

34. Selnes OA, Gottesman RF, Grega MA et al (2012) Cognitive and neurologic outcome after coronary-bypass surgery. N Engl J Med 366:250–257

35. Hansen TG, Pedersen JK, Henneberg SW et al (2015) Neurosurgical conditions and proce-dures in infancy significantly impact mortality and academic performances in adolescence: a nation-wide cohort study. Paediatr Anaesth 25:186–192

36. Andropoulos DB, Ahmad AH, Haq T et al (2014) The association between brain injury, peri-operative anesthetic exposure, and twelve months neurodevelopmental outcomes after neona-tal cardiac surgery: a retrospective cohort study. Paediatr Anaesth 24:266–274

37. Rizzi S, Ori C, Jevtovic-Todorovic V (2010) Timing versus duration: determinants of anesthe-siainduced developmental apoptosis in young mammalian brain. Ann N Y Acad Sci 1199:43–51

38. Clancy B, Darlington RB, Finlay BL (2001) Translating developmental brain development across mammalian species. Neuroscience 105:7–17

39. Clancy B, Finlay BL, Darlington RB et al (2007) Extrapolating brain development from exper-imental species to humans. Neurotoxicology 28:931–937

40. Hofacer RD, Deng M, Ward CG et al (2013) Cell-age specific vulnerability of neurons to anesthetic toxicity. Ann Neurol 73:695–704

41. Deng M, Hofacer RD, Jiang C et al (2014) Brain regional vulnerability to anaesthesia-induced neuroapoptosis shifts with age at exposure and extends into adulthood for some regions. Br J Anaesth 113:443–451

42. Jaeger MM, Holm A (2007) Does parents economic, cultural, and social capital explain the social class effect on educational attainment in the Scandinavian mobility regime? Soc Sci Res 36:719–744

43. Weiss M, Bissonnette B, Engelhardt T et al (2013) Anesthetists rather than anesthetics are the threat to the baby brains. Paediatr Anaesth 23:881–882

Prevention of Chronic Postsurgical Pain

25

Gonzalo Rivera

25.1 Background

Chronic postsurgical pain (CPSP) is conceptualized as pain that extends beyond the period of normal tissue healing, and it is not explained by the initial pathology or surgical complications [1]. In practice, a time frame of pain for more than 2–3 months has gained acceptance as operative definition. The reported prevalence rates range from 5 to more than 50 % in adult surgical population, depending mainly on the type of surgery [2]. CPSP can occur after surgeries such as thoracotomy, extremity amputation, and hysterectomy. However, all procedures including relatively "minor" surgeries (e.g., appendectomy or inguinal hernia repair) have been associated with this condition [3, 4].

Even though CPSP is a well-known entity in the adult literature, this is a relatively unstudied complication in the pediatric population [5]. Considering the growing number of children who undergo surgery every year, there is a necessity to understand the population at risk, possible predisposing risk factors involved, and the eventual long-term effects in functionality and development [6].

25.2 Magnitude of the Problem

The prevalence varies with the nature of the surgical insult and time since surgery but also with the definition criteria used to classify patients with CPSP. Higher prevalence rates are reported in studies that include any report of pain regardless of

G. Rivera, MD
Department of Anesthesia, Clinica Las Condes, Santiago, Chile

Chronic Pain Service, Department of Anesthesia, The Montreal Children's Hospital, McGill University, 2300 Tupper Street, Room C1117, Montreal, QC H3H 1P3, Canada
e-mail: gonzalo.rivera@mail.mcgill.ca; gon.rivera@gmail.com

© Springer International Publishing Switzerland 2016
M. Astuto, P.M. Ingelmo (eds.), *Perioperative Medicine in Pediatric Anesthesia*,
Anesthesia, Intensive Care and Pain in Neonates and Children,
DOI 10.1007/978-3-319-21960-8_25

intensity. Lower rates are typically seen when other criteria than pain (e.g., disability) are also included in the classification [7]. Overall, studies on different pediatric settings suggest that young age at the time of surgery is associated with lower risk of developing CPSP [8].

It has been reported that 1 year after surgery, 22 % of children developed moderate to severe (NRS, $\geq$4) CPSP. This study included children aged 8–18 years who underwent major orthopedic or general surgery, including thoracotomies and laparoscopies. The relative risk of having moderate to severe pain 1 year after surgery was 2.5 (CI 0.9–7.5) if patients experience pain $\geq$3 out of 10 two weeks after discharge [7].

In a retrospective study, 113 children and their parents were enrolled to answer telephone interviews regarding persistence and characteristic of pain after surgery in the preceding 3–10 months. Children between ages of 2 and 17 years who had undergone general, orthopedic, and urologic surgeries were included. Thirteen percent of patients reported the existence of CPSP (average pain level of 4.2 ± 1.5 on a 0–10 NRS) with a median duration of 4.1 months [9].

More specifically, groin pain after inguinal hernia repair is reported to be present in 3.2–13.5 % (severe pain in 2 %) of patients after 3.2–49 years follow-up [10–12]. The prevalence of CPSP after inguinal hernia repair seems to be lower when surgery is performed in childhood since adult reported a 10 % incidence of CPSP [6].

Similarly, results from studies of CPSP after sternotomy and thoracotomy have shown that surgeries during childhood have promising results compared with same procedures in adults in terms of chronic pain. A recent report on CPSP after sternotomy during childhood has shown that pain is present in 21 % of patients (10 % $\geq$4 on the NRS) after a mean follow-up period of 4 years. In adults, sternotomy is followed by CPSP in 20–50 % of patients [8]. Comparably, very young age at the time of surgery was associated with shorter duration of postoperative pain after thoracotomy due to coarctation of the aorta. The prevalence of postsurgical pain (>3 months) after thoracotomy was 3.2 % in the youngest group (0–6 years at the time of surgery), 19.4 % in children aged 7–12 years at the time of surgery, and 28.5 % among those aged 13–25 years at the time of surgery [13].

Spine surgery is associated with variable rates of pain before and after surgery and has been reported with prevalence rates of CPSP ranging from 11 to 68 %, 1–6 years after surgery [6, 14]. Interestingly, Siebert and colleagues have shown that adolescents who experienced no pain before and after spine surgery ("no pain trajectory") were significantly younger than other groups of patients who experienced pain either before or after surgery [15].

25.3   General Mechanisms and Clinical Presentation

The pivotal factor seems to be the nerve damage during the procedure. However, the development of CPSP involves biological, psychological, surgical, and genetic factors interacting in a specific moment [16].

Inflammatory mediators are released by damaged tissue and an inflammatory cascade is triggered after surgery. Several molecules and compounds act directly on the primary afferent terminals, decreasing their excitation threshold (peripheral sensitization) [3]. This response is normal and produces the major part of the acute postsurgical pain. However, one of the triggers of pain chronicity is thought to be the peripheral nerve damage. When nerves are transected or stretched during surgical manipulation, they discharge trains of impulses using glutamatergic neurotransmission via NMDA receptors to sensitize nociceptive pathways in the CNS [16]. This effect produces excitotoxic neuronal destruction and neuroimmune inflammation causing central macrophage activation [17]. All the process of central sensitization is also accompanied by alterations in gene expression resulting in changes in function and synaptic connections in the spinal cord [18].

Interestingly, changes derived by this phenomenon are not limited to the spinal cord. Important alterations in the cortex gray matter and descending systems have also been documented [17].

While mechanisms of peripheral and central sensitization are initially physiologic and protective, under unknown conditions, they become maladaptive and deleterious. The transition is complex and not completely understood. From clinical and epidemiological studies, it is possible to observe that psychosocial and genetic factors have relevant roles in the occurrence of CPSP in an individual.

Clinically, CPSP can have both inflammatory and neuropathic characteristics. Usually, inflammatory symptoms (e.g., swelling, redness) decay over time and respond satisfactorily to NSAIDs. However, neuropathic component may persist for longer periods and is commonly refractory to regular analgesics [19].

Neuropathic pain is usually continuous, like a superficial burning sensation or painful cold. It is also described like paroxystic electric shock or very brief stabbing pain. The neuropathic pain could be spontaneous or elicited by light mechanical (friction, pressure) or thermal stimulation [20]. One of the cardinal manifestations of neuropathic pain is allodynia, in which a non-painful stimulus (e.g., touch) produces pain. A second manifestation is known as secondary hyperalgesia, in which an increase in pain sensitivity occurs in non-injured areas beyond the area of initial injury [21]. In the clinical setting in a patient who is suspected to suffer from CPSP, all these clinical features should be related with the surgical area or scar.

25.4 Factors Associated with CPSP in Children

It is obvious that only a fraction of patients develop CPSP after surgery. However, there is no clear way to know what patient in what situation will evolve with CPSP. In this regard, available literature has highlighted some risk factors for developing CPSP. Since the majority of the information is provided from studies performed in adults, the interpretation of these data in the context of child care should be done carefully.

Arbitrarily, it is possible to group the associated factors for developing CPSP into three main groups: surgical, psychosocial, and patient-related factors.

25.4.1 Surgical Factors

The following surgical factors are linked with an increased likelihood of developing CPSP: type of surgery (e.g., spine surgery, thoracotomy, amputation, etc.), increased duration of surgery, low surgical load in a specific surgery center, open surgeries (vs. video-assisted procedures), pericostal stitches, and evidence of nerve damage. Whether these factors are causally related to the development of CPSP is not completely known [16]. Nevertheless, it seems evident that there is a relation between the magnitude of injured tissues, the probability of nerve damage, and the occurrence of CPSP. As a result, adequate training in less invasive surgical techniques appears warranted. Avoiding an unnecessary surgery is always advisable.

25.4.2 Psychosocial Factors

Preoperative anxiety, post-traumatic stress disorder, introverted personality, pain catastrophizing, poor social support, and emotional numbness have been associated with CPSP or with chronic postsurgical disability in adults [22]. There are no clues to know whether these factors may have the same effect in children. However, it has been reported that anxiety 6 months after surgery is associated with the maintenance of pain after 12 months [7]. It is also interesting that parental catastrophizing scores 48–72 h after surgery can predict pain intensity in their children 12 months later [23]. Adolescents with idiopathic scoliosis who have greater expectations about changes in self-appearance before spine surgery report more pain and experienced less reduction in preoperative pain after surgery [14]. Those findings stand out the intimate relationship between the effect of the psychological "environment" during perioperative period and the occurrence of persistent pain after surgery. The role of eventual psychological interventions or therapies in modifying CPSP remains to be elucidated.

25.4.3 Patient-Related Factors

Experience of pain either before or after surgery is one of the most robust predictors of chronic pain after surgery in adults [6]. No other patient factor is as consistently related to the development of future pain problems as pain: "pain predicts pain" [16]. In a prospective study involving 83 children aged 8–18 years who underwent major orthopedic and general surgery, patients who reported an NRS pain-intensity score ≥ 3 out of 10 2 weeks after discharge were more than three times more likely to develop moderate/severe CPSP at 6 months (RR 3.3) and more than twice as likely to develop moderate/severe CPSP at 12 months (RR 2.5) than those who reported NRS pain score <3 [7]. In this study, the presence of moderate/severe CPSP was not accompanied by high levels of functional disability for the majority of children. Approximately 5–15 % of children with chronic pain report pain-disability of a severity requiring professional attention [24].

As mentioned above, young age at the moment of surgery appears to be a protective factor for developing CPSP. An immature peripheral and central nervous system combined with an enhanced neuronal plastic capacity in the child's brain may contribute to a lower risk for developing chronic painful conditions. Tissues are more indulgent and flexible in children, and therefore many procedures may be less harmful in children than in adults [8].

Contrary to other pain conditions, in the setting of CPSP, the gender difference did not appear to influence the occurrence of persistence of pain after surgery [6, 7].

25.5   Prevention Strategies

Once established, CPSP is very difficult to reverse and complicated to treat. Therefore, a logical answer seems to be its prevention.

25.5.1 Surgical Technique

The primary focus for prevention needs to be an increased awareness among surgeons of ways to avoid intraoperative nerve injury, including careful dissection, reduction of inflammatory response, and the use of minimally invasive techniques [17]. Video-assisted procedures can decrease the damage inflicted to nerves commonly produced by conventional open surgery.

25.5.2 Pharmacological Therapy

A growing number of studies of preoperative systemic drug interventions have been conducted. Those trials included adult population who underwent different surgical procedures such as cardiac surgery, spine surgery, knee arthroplasty, thyroidectomy, breast surgery, and thoracotomy to mention a few. A wide variety of drug classes (NMDA antagonists, lidocaine, alpha-agonists, NSAIDs, steroids, anticonvulsants, antidepressants, opioids, etc.) administered at a variety of therapeutic schemes have been documented [25]. Even if many pharmacological interventions have some positive effect in reducing postoperative pain, they have failed to modify consistently the occurrence of CPSP [22]. Exceptions to this are the use of perioperative ketamine infusions (>24 h) that appear to reduce the incidence of pain at 3 and 6 months after surgery (mainly abdominal and pelvic surgery) and the administration of oral pregabalin which resulted in superiority over placebo (mainly in cardiac surgery and total knee replacement) for pain incidence at 3 months after surgery [26].

Currently, there is no information available concerning the effect of pharmacological interventions on the incidence of CPSP in children.

25.5.3 Regional Blocks

Although regional techniques are effective in controlling acute postoperative pain in different surgical settings, their effectiveness in improving long-term outcomes has been more elusive. In adult population, thoracic epidural anesthesia and paravertebral block, respectively, may prevent CPSP after thoracotomy and breast cancer surgery in about one out every four to five patients treated [27]. Less consistent data is available concerning the role of regional blocks in preventing CPSP after limb amputation. Nevertheless, it has been reported that prolonged postoperative infusion (median duration of 30 days) of local anesthetics via peripheral nerve catheters could be useful for reducing the incidence of phantom limb pain 1 year after surgery [28].

Unfortunately, despite the extensive use of regional blocks in children, including continuous ambulatory techniques [29], the effect of these procedures for the prevention of CPSP has not been studied.

25.5.4 Other Potential Strategies

Different strategies for CPSP prevention have been implemented in adults. Althaus et al. have developed a risk index for predicting CPSP considering different perioperative factors, such as preoperative pain (same and/or other place than the surgical site), acute postoperative pain, recent psychological "capacity overload," and the presence of stress indicators (sleep disorder, trembling hands, tachycardia, etc.) [2]. They found a strong correlation between the number of positive factors in each category and the risk of CPSP (e.g., scoring 4≥ the risk is >70 % of CPSP). Naturally, it is not possible to directly extrapolate these data to children. Nevertheless, this tool highlights the importance of psychological aspects in predicting CPSP. In this regard, it is well known that various forms of cognitive behavioral therapies constitute an essential part of the multidisciplinary treatment of many chronic pain conditions in adults and children [30, 31]. Therefore, it can be anticipated that further psychological research may contribute to improving the prevention and the treatment of chronic pain in children undergoing surgery.

25.5.5 Summary of the Preventing Strategies

The results of studies on preventive multimodal analgesia are equivocal and oriented to adult population. Although sufficient analgesia during the perioperative period is important for the prevention of CPSP, mere short-term blockage of nociception and control of symptoms have not been shown to eliminate the long-term problem [22]. The wide variety of treatment protocols used, even in the same surgical scenario, reflects a current lack of understanding of the critical mechanisms and temporal aspects of development of CPSP [26]. However, this does not exclude the possibility that many interventions may be beneficial in pediatric cases. Since the intensity of acute postoperative pain is the strongest predictor of pain chronicity, standardized pain evaluation and treatment protocols are recommended. Psychological questionnaires and interventions that predict the psychosocial factors in patients that make them susceptible to develop persistent pain should be designed and implemented [32]. Finally, it is essential to ensure patients and parents are adequately prepared and educated for the surgical event and its consequences.

25.6 Concluding Remarks

In conclusion, the available evidence suggests that the prevalence of CPSP is lower if surgery is performed in childhood. When pain is intense and persists, it is likely to have a neuropathic component. At this moment, the refinement in surgical techniques and an adequate acute postoperative pain management constitute the most widely accepted prevention strategies in children. Despite advances in the understanding of the mechanisms involved and the interplay of risk factors in the adult population, the management and prevention of persistent postsurgical pain remain inadequate and poorly studied in children. Further research on the role of presurgical preparation and postoperative care should be conducted for preventing potential disabling consequences.

References

1. Macrae WA (2008) Chronic post-surgical pain: 10 years on. Br J Anaesth 101:77–86
2. Althaus A, Hinrichs-Rocker A, Chapman R et al (2012) Development of a risk index for the prediction of chronic post-surgical pain. Eur J Pain 16:901–910
3. Shipton EA (2014) The transition of acute postoperative pain to chronic pain: part 1 – risk factors for the development of postoperative acute persistent pain. Trends Anaesth Crit Care 4:67–70
4. Gerbershagen HJ, Aduckathil S, van Wijck AJ et al (2013) Pain intensity on the first day after surgery: a prospective cohort study comparing 179 surgical procedures. Anesthesiology 118:934–944
5. Ahn JC, Fortier MA, Kain ZN (2012) Acute to chronic postoperative pain in children: does it exist? Pain Manag 2:421–423
6. Nikolajsen L, Brix L (2014) Chronic pain after surgery in children. Curr Opin Anesthesiol. doi:10.1097/ACO0000000000000110
7. Pagé GM, Stinson J, Campbell F et al (2013) Identification of pain-related psychological risk factors for the development and maintenance of pediatric chronic postsurgical pain. J Pain Res 6:167–180
8. Lauridsen MH, Kristensen AD, Hjortdal VE et al (2014) Chronic pain in children after cardiac surgery via sternotomy. Cardiol Young 24:893–899
9. Fortier MA, Chou J, Maurer EL et al (2011) Acute to chronic postoperative pain in children: preliminary findings. J Pediatr Surg 46:1700–1705
10. Zendejas B, Zarroug AE, Erben YM et al (2010) Impact of childhood inguinal hernia repair in adulthood: 50 years of follow-up. J Am Coll Surg 211:762–768
11. Kristensen AD, Ahlburg P, Lauridsen MC et al (2012) Chronic pain after inguinal hernia repair in children. Br J Anaesth 109:603–608

12. Aasvang EK, Kehlet H (2007) Chronic pain after childhood groin hernia repair. J Pediatr Surg 42:1403–1408
13. Kristensen AD, Pedersen TA, Hjortdal VE et al (2010) Chronic pain in adults after thoracotomy in childhood or youth. Br J Anaesth 104:75–79
14. Landman Z, Oswald T, Sanders J et al (2011) Prevalence and predictors of pain in surgical treatment of adolescent idiopathic scoliosis. Spine 36:825–829
15. Sieberg CB, Simons LE, Edelstein MR et al (2013) Pain trajectories following pediatric spinal fusion surgery. J Pain 14:1694–1702
16. Katz J, Seltzer Z (2009) Transition from acute to chronic postsurgical pain: risk factors and protective factors. Expert Rev Neurother 9:723–744
17. Kehlet H, Jensen TS, Woolf CJ (2006) Persistent postsurgical pain: risk factors and prevention. Lancet 367:1618–1625
18. Ferrari LF, Bogen O, Chu C et al (2013) Peripheral administration inhibitors reverses increased hyperalgesia in a model of chronic pain in the rat. J Pain 14:731–738
19. Fletcher D (2013) Epidemiology of chronic postsurgical pain. In: Mick G, Guastella V (eds) Chronic postsurgical pain. Springer, Paris, pp 13–20
20. Dubray C (2013) How to study chronic postsurgical pain: the example of neuropathic pain. In: Mick G, Guastella V (eds) Chronic postsurgical pain. Springer, Paris, pp 3–12
21. Kyranou M, Puntillo K (2012) The transition from acute to chronic pain: might intensive care unit patients be at risk? Ann Intensive Care 16:36
22. Van de Ven T, John Hsia HL (2012) Causes and prevention of chronic postsurgical pain. Curr Opin Crit Care 18:366–371
23. Pagé MG, Campbell F, Isaac L et al (2013) Parental risk factors for the development of pediatric acute and chronic postsurgical pain: a longitudinal study. J Pain Res 30:727–741
24. von Baeyer CL (2011) Interpreting high prevalence of pediatric chronic pain revealed in community surveys. Pain 152:2683–2684
25. Rashiq S, Dick BD (2014) Post-surgical pain syndromes: a review for the non-pain specialist. Can J Anaesth 61:123–130
26. Caparro L, Smith SA, Moore RA et al (2013) Pharmacotherapy for the prevention of chronic pain after surgery in adults. Cochrane Database Syst Rev 7:CD008307. doi:10.1002/14651858.CD008307.pub2
27. Andreae MH, Andreae DA (2013) Regional anaesthesia to prevent chronic pain after surgery: a Cochrane systematic review and meta-analysis. Br J Anaesth 111:711–720
28. Borghi B, D'Addabbo M, White PF (2010) The use of prolonged peripheral neural blockade after lower extremity amputation: the effect on symptoms associated with phantom limb syndrome. Anesth Analg 111:1308–1315
29. Tsui B, Suresh S (2010) Ultrasound imaging for regional anesthesia in infants, children, and adolescents: a review of current literature and its application in the practice of neuraxial blocks. Anesthesiology 112:719–728
30. Flor H (2012) New developments in the understanding and management of persistent pain. Curr Opin Psychiatry 25:109–113
31. Palermo TM, Eccleston C, Lewandowski AS et al (2010) Randomized controlled trials of psychological therapies for management of chronic pain in children and adolescents: an updated meta-analytic review. Pain 148:387–397
32. Shipton EA (2013) Postoperative pain and preoperative education. In: Schmidt RF, Willis WD (eds) Encyclopedic reference of pain. Springer, Berlin/Heilderburg, pp 3093–3099

Index

A

ABCDEF sequence, 216
ABD. *See* Autologous blood donation (ABD)
Abdominal and pelvic procedures
  common preoperative considerations,
    137–139
  intraoperative management, 139–142
  postoperative management, 142–143
Acoustic impedance monitoring, 387
Acute pain management
  ambulatory regime, 430
  assessment tools, 418–419
  cutaneous sensory receptors, 417
  hemodynamic parameters, 419
  multimodal analgesia, 419
  non-opioid analgesics (*see* Non-opioid
    analgesics)
  non-pharmacological (*see* Non-
    pharmacological management, pain)
  opioids (*see* Opioid analgesics)
  procedure-specific guidelines, 430
  regional anaesthesia (*see* Regional
    anaesthesia)
Acute pain service (APS) team, 431
ADARPEF. *See* Anesthésistes Réanimateurs
    Pédiatriques d'Expression Française
    (ADARPEF)
Adjuvant therapy
  adult pain management, 253
  anticonvulsants, 254
  benefits, medications, 253
  benzodiazepines and baclofen, 254
  gabapentin, 254
  ketamine, 254
  selective serotonin reuptake inhibitors, 254
  tricyclic antidepressants, 254

ADVANCE
  preparation for surgery project, 24
  strategy, 410
Adverse events following immunization
    (AEFI), 48
AEFI. *See* Adverse events following
    immunization (AEFI)
Age at exposure, anesthetic drugs, 442
α_2 Agonists, 31
Airway assessment, 139–140, 217
Airway management
  endotracheal intubation, 263
  intermittent airway obstruction, 263
Airway obstruction
  diagnostic and therapeutic procedures,
    279–280
  emergency airway rescue, 278–279
  mucositis and xerostomia, 240
  neck irradiation, 241
  newborn, evaluation and treatment, 273
  postoperative period, 280
  subglottic and tracheal pathologies,
    277–278
  supraglottic and laryngeal pathologies,
    275–277
  symptoms and signs, 273–274
  TBAO, 274–275
  ulcerative lesions, 240
Aldrete scoring system, 69, 70*t*
Alert, verbal, pain, unresponsive (AVPU)
    acronym, 221
Allergies
  atopy, 44, 45
  causes, 44
  latex allergy, 44, 45
  latex-safe strategies, 46

© Springer International Publishing Switzerland 2016
M. Astuto, P.M. Ingelmo (eds.), *Perioperative Medicine in Pediatric Anesthesia,*
Anesthesia, Intensive Care and Pain in Neonates and Children,
DOI 10.1007/978-3-319-21960-8

Allergies (*cont.*)
    to local anesthetics, 45
    prophylaxis, 46
    radioallergosorbent test (RAST), 46
    skin prick test (SPT), 45
American Academy of Otolaryngology,
        201–202
American Academy of Pediatrics (AAP), 202
American Society of Anesthesiologists (ASA)
        guidelines, 200
Analgesia at home, 430
Anatomical, physiological, and psychological
        peculiarities, trauma, 214
Anesthesia, NMDs
    cardiovascular failure, 161
    hyperkalemic cardiac arrest, 164
    MH, 162–163
    respiratory failure, 160–161
    rhabdomyolysis, 163
Anesthésistes Réanimateurs Pédiatriques
        d'Expression Française
        (ADARPEF), 56
Anterior mediastinal mass (AMM)
    capnogram, 240
    chemotherapy access, 240
    chest X-ray, 239
    general anesthesia, 239, 240
    local anesthesia and sedation, 239
    preoperative echocardiogram, 239
    respiration and avoiding paralysis, 240
    sedation, 239
    tissue types, children, 239
    tumor biopsy, 240
Antifibrinolytics, 95
Anxiety
    components of, 21
    development factors, 22
    high levels of, 22
    low levels of, 22
    transient state, 21
ARDS. *See* Aute respiratory distress syndrome
        (ARDS)
Arteriovenous malformations (AVMs), 127
Asthma. *See also* Upper respiratory infections
        (URI)
    bronchodilators, 43
    bronchospasm, 41
    chest radiograph, 42
    computed tomography (CT scan), 42
    corticosteroids, 43
    day-surgery, 60
    diagnosis of, 42
    flow expiratory volume (FEV$_1$), 42
    medication, children, 43

poorly controlled, 42–43
    regular medication, children, 43
    stepwise management, children, 42
    steroid medication, children, 43
Atopy, 40, 44, 45
Aute respiratory distress syndrome (ARDS), 99
Autologous blood donation (ABD), 94
AVMs. *See* Arteriovenous malformations
        (AVMs)

B
Beckwith–Wiedemann syndrome, 138–140
BIS. *See* Bispectral index (BIS)
Bispectral index (BIS), 78
Bladder detrusor hyperactivity, 262
Blood pressure (BP) monitoring
    arterial cannula, 392, 393
    arterial tonometry, 393
    fluctuations, hemodynamics, 392
    invasive arterial tracing, 393
    pulse transit time, 393–394
    vascular unloading, 393
Botulinum toxin (Botox), 262
BPD. *See* Bronchopulmonary dysplasia (BPD)
Brachial plexus, 428
Brain edema, 124
Brain tumors, 124–125
Breathing
    analgesia, 296
    primary survey, trauma
        destabilization/respiratory
            parameters, 218
        nasotracheal intubation, 218
        tension pneumothorax, 219
    in sleep and airway collapsibility, 193–195
Bronchopulmonary dysplasia (BPD), 43–44
Bronchospasm, 39–41, 44–46

C
Capnography. *See* End-tidal carbon dioxide
        (ETCO$_2$) monitoring
Cardiac dysfunction, neuromuscular
        disorders, 161
Cardiac output (CO) monitoring
    bioreactance, 389
    Doppler techniques, 388
    pulse contour analysis technique, 389
    TEB, 389
    thermodilution method, 388, 390
    transpulmonary thermodilution (TPTD), 388
CBF. *See* Cerebral blood flow (CBF)
Central hypoventilation syndromes, 197–198

Central venous catheter (CVC)
   access, SVC (*see* Superior vena cava (SVC))
   classification, complications
      catheter occlusion, 306–307
      immediate complications, 306
      intermediary complications, 306
      late complications, 306
      risk factors, 307
      rupture, 307
      treatment, 307
   equipment and technique of insertion,
      303–305
   indications, 302
   IVC access (*see* Inferior vena cava (IVC))
Cerebral blood flow (CBF), 115
Cerebral palsy (CP)
   anesthetic management, 260
   blood loss, 266
   cognitive function, 259
   epidural catheter techniques, 267
   fundoplication, 266–267
   gastrostomy, 267
   hemodynamic monitoring, 267
   hip reconstruction, 266
   latex allergy, 266
   lesions/anomalies, 259
   motor defects, 259
   orthopedic surgery, 266
   perioperative management
      airway management (*see* Airway
         management)
      analgesia, 266
      meticulous padding, 262
      pharmacodynamics and
         pharmacokinetics, 264, 265
      positioning, 262–263
      thermal homeostasis, 263
      uncooperative behavior at induction, 265
      venous access, 263
   pneumoperitoneum, 267
   pneumothorax, 267
   preoperative evaluation
      baclofen, 261
      botulinum toxin (Botox), 262
      contractures and deformities, 261
      developmental delay, 260
      epilepsy, 262
      flexion, toes, 260
      gastroesophageal reflux, 260
      laparoscopic fundoplication, 261
      neurolytic blocks, 262
      sarcopenia, 261
      spasticity, 261
      vigabatrin, 261

Cervical collar, 217
CHARGE syndrome, 275
Chemodenervation, 262
Chemotherapy
   awareness, side effects, 255
   cancer treatment, 230
   cardiotoxicity
      chronic anthracycline, 231
      complications, 231
      constrictive cardiomyopathy, 232
      cyclophosphamide, 232
      intraoperative monitors, 232
   hematological effects
      anemia, 235
      dysfunctional coagulation, 235
      meticulous aseptic techniques, 235
      myelosuppression, 235
   hepatorenal toxicity
      cisplatin, 234
      coagulation necrosis, 234
      hepatic injury, 235
      non-cisplatinum chemotherapeutic
         agents, 234, 235
      renal injury, 234
      renal system, 234
   hormone and enzyme production
      alkylating agents, 236
      SIADH, 235
      steroid-induced adrenal
         suppression, 235
      stress response, 235
   neurotoxicity
      cisplatin treatment, 235
      local motor neuropraxia, 235–236
      neurologic consequences, 235
      non-vincristine chemotherapy
         agents, 236
   pulmonary toxicity
      adverse cardiac effects, 232
      bleomycin-induced, 233
      chest X-ray, 234
      complications, 232
      non-anthracycline chemotherapeutic
         agents, 232
      non-bleomycin chemotherapy
         agents, 234
      perioperative inspired oxygen
         concentration, 233, 234
      primary chemotherapeutic
         agents, 233
      pulmonary function tests, 234
Childhood Adenotonsillectomy
      Trial (CHAT), 199
Choanal atresia, 275

Chronic postsurgical pain (CPSP)
  in children
    patient-related factors,
      450–451
    psychosocial factors, 450
    surgical factors, 450
  definition criteria, 447
  glutamatergic neurotransmission, 449
  inflammatory mediators, 448
  inguinal hernia repair, 448
  laparoscopies., 448
  nerve damage, 448
  normal tissue healing, 447
  paroxystic electric shock, 449
  patient classification, 447
  peripheral and central sensitization, 449
  predisposing risk factors, 447
  prevention strategies
    pain management, 453
    pharmacological therapy, 451
    preventive multimodal
      analgesia, 452
    regional techniques, 452
    surgical technique, 451
    treatment protocols, 452–453
  secondary hyperalgesia, 449
  spine surgery, 448
  superficial burning sensation, 449
  thoracotomies, 448
Circulation, 124, 163, 219–220, 240,
      298, 331, 334
Clonidine, 411
Cobb method, 106
Compartment syndrome, 98–99
Congenital chest wall deformities
  pectus carinatum
    analgesic considerations, 134
    background, 134
    Ravitch procedure, 134
    surgical technique, 134
  pectus excavatum
    analgesic considerations, 133
    preoperative assessment of, 131
    reverse Nuss procedure, 134
    surgical technique, 132
Congenital spinal lesions, 126–127
Continuous peripheral nerve blocks
      (CPNBs), 97–98, 427
CPSP. See Chronic postsurgical
      pain (CPSP)
Craniosynostosis repair, 125–126
Cri-du-chat syndrome, 101
Crystalloids, 141
CS. See Intraoperative red cell
      salvage (CS)

D
Damage control strategy (DCS), 224, 225
Day-surgery (DS)
  analgesia
    locoregional, 67–68
    NSAIDs, 67
    pain control, 67
  anesthesia
    airway management, 66
    caudal block, 65
    drugs, 63–64
    fluid therapy, 66
    ilioinguinal/iliohypogastric nerve
      block, 65
    locoregional, 64
    lower and upper extremity nerve
      blocks, 65
    opioids as adjuvants in locoregional, 66
    paravertebral block, 65
    penile block, 66
    spinal block, 64
    temperature, 67
  discharge
    aldrete scoring system, 69, 70t
    clinical criteria for, 69
    modalities for, 69
    observation period, postoperative, 70
    pain therapy prescriptions, 71
    postanesthetic discharge scoring system
      (PADSS), 69–71, 71t
    postoperative management, 70
    recovery from anesthesia, 69
    telephone follow-up after, 71
    tonsillectomy, 71–72
    vital parameters evaluation, 69
  epidemiology, 56
  organizational aspect, 56–57
  patient preparation
    fasting, 62
    information for parents, 62
    pharmacological premedication, 63
    premedication, 62–63
    preoperative evaluation, 61
    written and understandable brochure, 61
  patient selection
    age, 58–59
    ASA physical status, 57–58
    asthma, 60
    incidental heart murmurs, 59
    malignant hyperthermia, 59
    sickle cell disease, 59
    sudden infant death syndrome
      (SIDS), 59
    upper respiratory tract infection (URI),
      59–60

post-discharge nausea and vomiting
        (PDNV), 69
postoperative nausea and vomiting
        (PONV), 68–69
postoperative vomiting (POV), 68
procedure, 60–61
social factor, 61
Developmental delay, 260
Dexmetomidine, 411
Diabetes insipidus, 123
Disability
        chronic pain, 450
        chronic postsurgical, 450
        cognitive function, 238
        compartment syndrome, 98
        neurologic function, 221
        pain evaluation, 418
        trauma injury, 213
Distal tracheal stenosis, 278
DOPES sequence, 218–219
Doppler techniques, 388
Down syndromes, 139–140
Dystrophinopathies, 169

E
Early postoperative negative behaviour
        (e-PONB)
        children, 404
        prevention and treatment
                non-pharmacologic approach, 410
                pharmacologic approach, 411–412
        risk factors
                age and gender, 405
                inhalation anaesthesia, 406–407
                parents and culture, 405
                preoperative anxiety, 406
                propofol, 407–408
                surgery, 406
        tools, 408–410
        treatment, 412
Electrocardiogram (ECG) monitoring
        anesthesia care, 390
        applications, 390
        intravascular/systemic injection, 390–391
Emergence agitation (EA)
        diagnostic criteria, 404
        inadequate pain relief, 404
        restlessness and mental distress, 404
        scales, 408
Emergence delirium (ED)
        definition, 404
        risk factors
                age and gender, 405
                inhalation anaesthesia, 406–407

parents and culture, 405
preoperative anxiety, 406
propofol, 407–408
surgery, 406
End-tidal carbon dioxide (ETCO$_2$) monitoring
        chest compression, 384
        infrared technology, 382
        partial pressure of CO2 (PaCO2), 382–383
        ventilation techniques, 383
Enhanced recovery after surgery (ERAS)
        program, 2–3
Epidural blocks, 427
Epilepsy
        surgery, 125
        valproic acid, 262
ERAS program. See Enhanced recoy after
        surgery (ERAS) program
Esmarch's bandage, 92
ETCO$_2$. See End-tidal carbon dioxide (ETCO$_2$)
        monitoring
Exposure
        allergic reaction, 45
        anesthetic/surgical, 444
        direct external heat sources, 252
        in neonates, 124
        OSA, 188
        passive smoking, 40
        primary survey, trauma, 221
        to secondhand smoke, 41, 45
        "sleep-awake-asleep" technique, 125
Extubation, 66, 111, 155, 171, 172, 225, 279

F
Face, legs, activity, cry, consolability
        (FLACC) scale, 409
Face-mask ventilation, 149
Family
        adverse respiratory events, 40
        anesthesia and surgery, 21, 90
        asthma, 41
        genetically transmitted diseases, 14
        non-pharmacological techniques, 429
        pain, 245
        preoperative anxiety, 21, 23
        preoperative evaluation, 14
Fasting, preoperative, 34
Fat embolism (FES), 99
Femoral nerve approach
        high-frequency linear probe, 360
        hyperechoic, 359
        surgical anesthesia and analgesia, 358
        ultrasound guidance, 360–361
FES. See Fat embolism (FES)
Fundoplication, 266–267

G

Gastrostomy, 267
General anesthesia, infant brain
  age, 442
  anesthesia-related neurotoxicity, 444
  animal studies, anesthesia-related
      neurotoxicity, 438
  brain development, 437
  degree of migration, 441
  duration and number
      of exposures, 441
  gender issue, 443
  human brain, normal development,
      438–439
  human outcome measure, 439–440
  human studies, 439
  impact of surgery, 442–443
  morphological abnormalities, 437
  neuroprotective properties, 437
  nociception and neuroinflammation, 443
  perioperative factors, 443
  sample size issue, 441
  stress responses, 443
  synaptogenesis, 437
Glasgow Coma Score, 221
Glycogenosis, 180
Glycogenosis type II (GSDII), 170–171
Goldenhar syndromes, 101, 274
Guillain–Barrè syndrome (GBS), 169

H

Halogenated agents, 163, 167
HCM. *See* Hypertrophic cardiomyopathy
      (HCM)
Heart murmurs
  brachial and radial pulses, 46
  chest X-rays, 47
  clinical effects, 46, 47
  ECG, 47
  echocardiography, 47
  hypertrophic cardiomyopathy
      (HCM), 46
  innocent and pathological, 46, 47
Heat loss, 263
Hip reconstruction, 266
Hydrocephalus and stunt procedures, 124
Hyperglycemia, 123
Hyperkalemic cardiac arrest, 164
Hypertrophic cardiomyopathy (HCM), 46
Hypnosis, 430
Hyponatremia, 123
Hypothermia, 263

I

Ibuprofen, 425
ICP. *See* Intracranial pressure (ICP)
Iliohypogastric (IH) and ilioinguinal (II) nerves
  in-plane approach, 367, 369
  linear probe, 367
  local anesthetic, 367, 369
  nerve localization, 368
  pharmacodynamic studies, 369
  pharmacokinetic study, 370
  ultrasound technique, 367
Immunomodulatory effects, cancer
  airway lesions, 240–241
  AMMs (*see* Anterior mediastinal
      mass (AMM))
  cancer cell augmentation, 229
  immunosuppression, 229
  neoplasia (*see* Neoplasia/cancer)
  retinoic acid syndrome, 245
  TLS, 243–244
  toxicity, oncological therapies
      (*see* Oncological therapy)
Infantile hemangiomas, 277
Infants
  brain, anesthesia
    age, 442
    anesthesia-related neurotoxicity, 444
    animal studies, anesthesia-related
        neurotoxicity, 438
    brain development, 437
    degree of migration, 441
    duration and number of exposures, 441
    gender issue, 443
    human outcome measure, 439–440
    human studies, 439
    morphological abnormalities, 437
    neuroprotective properties, 437
    nociception and neuroinflammation, 443
    normal development, human brain,
        438–439
    perioperative factors, 443
    sample size issue, 441
    stress responses, 443
    surgery impact, 442–443
    synaptogenesis, 437
  CPSP
    patient-related factors, 450–451
    psychosocial factors, 450
    surgical factors, 450
Inferior vena cava (IVC)
  complications
    catheter migration, 323
    fluid extravasation, 323

lower limb ischemia, 324
portal vein thrombosis, 324
femoral vein
    anatomy, 322–323
    femoral vein catheterization, 323, 324
    reverse Trendelenburg position, 323
    US-guided femoral vein puncture,
        323, 324
Infraclavicular approach
    arterial pulse, 351
    "blind" techniques, 355
    catheter technique, 354
    Color Doppler, 353, 354
    indications, 351
    local anesthetic spread, 353, 355
    ultrasound imaging, 355
Inhalation anaesthesia, 406–407
Interfascial spread of local anaesthetics
        (LAs), 427
Internal jugular vein (IJV)
    anatomy and sonoanatomy, 308–310
    anterior approach, 310
    "blind"/"landmark-guided" approaches,
        310
    posterior approach, 310
    ultrasound-guided anterior approach,
        310–311
Interscalene approach
    carotid artery, 348
    internal jugular (anechoic), 349
    IP, 349, 350
    pneumothorax, 350
    ultrasound imaging, 348
    US-guided nerve stimulating technique,
        349
Intracranial pressure (ICP), 118
Intraoperative bronchospasm, 41
Intraoperative fluid management
    abdominal and pelvic procedures, 141
    trauma, 223–224
Intraoperative management
    abdominal and pelvic procedures, 139–142
    NMDs, 167–171
    OSA, 202–203
    trauma, 223
Intraoperative red cell salvage (CS), 94–95
Intraosseous (IO) access
    complications, 333
    contraindication, 333
    description, 331–332
    devices, 332–333
    perioperative indications, 332
    technique, 332–333

Italian National Program Guidelines, 201
Italian Society of Pediatric and Neonatal
        Anesthesia and Intensive Care
        (SARNePI), 16

J
Jaw thrust, 150, 217, 263
JHSRCS. *See* Johns Hopkins surgery risk
        classification system (JHSRCS)
Johns Hopkins surgery risk classification
        system (JHSRCS), 12

K
Ketamine, 30–31
Ketorolac, 425, 426

L
Laryngeal cleft (LC), 275
Laryngeal mask airway (LMA), 66
    adverse respiratory events, 40
    dexmedetomidine, 33
    gastric access, 263
    general anesthesia, 44
    sizing, 218
    surgical pharyngeal visualization, 202
Laryngeal webs, 276
Laryngomalacia, 275
Laryngospasm, 149
Larynx, 193
Lateral femoral cutaneous nerve (LFCN), 105
Latex allergy, 44, 45, 266
Latex-safe strategies, 46
Lethal triad, 224
LFCN. *See* Lateral femoral cutaneous nerve
        (LFCN)
Limb occlusion pressure (LOP), 92
LMA. *See* Laryngeal mask airway (LMA)
Long QT syndrome (LQTS), 16
LOP. *See* Limb occlusion pressure (LOP)
Lower limb blocks, USG techniques
    femoral nerve approach, 358–361
    saphenous nerve block, 363–364, 366
    sciatic nerve block, 361–363
LQTS. *See* Long QT syndrome (LQTS)
Lumbar plexus, 428

M
Macroglossia, 274
MAC values of halothane, 264

Malignant hyperthermia (MH)
   acute crisis management, 162–163
   patients at risk, 162
   prevention, 162
McGill Oximetry Score (MOS), 191
Mental retardation, 259
MEPs. *See* Motor evoked potentials (MEPs)
Metabolic diseases
   biological signs, 184
   glycogenosis, 180
   Guthrie's test, 183
   mitochondrial cytopathy, 180–183
   perioperative care, 176
   reflex, 183–184
   sources, 176–177
   synthesis of, 177–178
   systematic screening, 183
   urea cycle disorder, 178–179, 183
Midazolam, 30
Mitochondrial cytopathy, 180–183
Mitochondrial myopathies, 166–167, 170
Modified Maintenance of Wakefulness Test
      (MMWT), 82
Modified Yale preoperative anxiety scale
      (m-YPAS), 21, 406
Mortality
   airway problems, 147
   cancer, 229
   gastroschisis, 138
   gender, 443
   general anesthesia, 39
   inflammatory processes, 118
   perioperative hypoxia, 147
   perioperative medicine, 3, 6
   pheochromocytoma, 141
   postoperative phase, 4
   pulmonary toxicity, 232
   retinoic acid syndrome, 245
   subglottic hemangiomas, 277
   trauma, 228
   for traumatic injury, 213
Motor evoked potentials (MEPs), 120
Mouth, 193
Multimodal analgesia, 419
Music therapy, 24
Myasthenia gravis (MG), 166, 169
Myotonic dystrophy, 169–170
mYPAS. *See* Modified Yale preoperative
      anxiety scale (m-YPAS)

N
N-acetyl glutamate synthetase (NAGS),
      178–179
NARCO memory tool, 177

Nasal administration
   α_2-agonists, 32–33
   ketamine, 32
   midazolam, 32
Nasopharynx, 192–193
National Institute for Health and Clinical
      Excellence (NICE-UK), 16
Near-infrared spectroscopy (NIRS)
   brain tissue oxygenation, 391
   cerebral hypoxemia, 392
   cerebral oxygenation monitoring, 391, 392
   neurologic damage, 392
Negative behaviour after surgery
   EA (*see* Emergence agitation (EA))
   ED (*see* Emergence delirium (ED))
   e-PONB (*see* Early postoperative negative
         behaviour (e-PONB))
   postoperative pain (*see* Postoperative pain,
         child's behaviour)
Neonatal larynx, 148
Neonates
   brain, anesthesia (*see* Infants)
   hypotension, 117
   Microstream Sensor, 78
   stress response, 81
Neoplasia/cancer
   cardiovascular effects and considerations, 241
   CNS effects and considerations, 242
   endocrine effects and considerations,
         242–243
   hematological effects and considerations, 243
   hepatic effects and considerations, 242
   myelosuppression, 243
   primary GI tumors, 242
   psychiatric considerations, 243
   pulmonary neoplasms, 241
   renal tumors, children, 241–242
Neurodevelopment
   academic performance, 440
   humans and animals, 438
   perioperative factors, 443
Neuro-endoscopy and anesthesia, 127
Neurolytic blocks, 262
Neuromuscular blocking agents (NMB),
      168, 264
Neuromuscular disorders (NMDs)
   anesthesia, life-threatening complications
      cardiovascular failure, 161
      hyperkalemic cardiac arrest, 164
      MH, 162–163
      respiratory failure, 160–161
      rhabdomyolysis, 163
   intraoperative management
      dystrophinopathies, 169
      GBS, 169

GSDII, 170–171
MG, 169
mitochondrial myopathies, 170
myotonic dystrophy, 169–170
NMB, 168
regional anesthesia, 168
succinylcholine and halogenated
     agents, 167
TIVA, 167–168
postoperative management
pain control, 171
respiratory management, 171–172
preoperative assessment and management
cardiac assessment, 165
chronic treatment, steroids, 166
intravenous line, 166
mitochondrial myopathies, 166–167
myasthenia gravis, 166
neurological assessment, 164
PICU, 166
premedication drugs, 166
pulmonary assessment, 164–165
Neuromuscular scoliosis (NMS), 107, 108
Neurophysiology, pediatric brain
anesthesia and neurotoxicity, 119
arterial carbon dioxide/oxygen tension
     (Pa_{co2}/Pa_{o2}), 116–117
blood pressure, 117–118
brain and inflammation, 118
brain energy metabolism, 116
cerebral autoregulation, 117–118
cerebral blood flow (CBF), 115
cerebral oxygen metabolism, 117
intracranial pressure (ICP), 118
Neurosurgical patient
brain tumors, 124–125
congenital spinal lesions, 126–127
craniosynostosis repair, 125–126
epilepsy surgery, 125
hydrocephalus and stunt procedures, 124
neuro-endoscopy and anesthesia, 127
neurophysiology, pediatric brain
     anesthesia and neurotoxicity, 119
     arterial carbon dioxide/oxygen tension
          (Pa_{co2}/Pa_{o2}), 116–117
     blood pressure, 117–118
     brain and inflammation, 118
     brain energy metabolism, 116
     cerebral autoregulation, 117–118
     cerebral blood flow (CBF), 115
     cerebral oxygen metabolism, 117
     intracranial pressure (ICP), 118
perioperative management
body tempearture, 122
fluid management, 121–122

induction, 120
maintenance of anesthesia, 121
monitoring, 120
positioning, 121
postoperative care, 122–123
preoperative assessment, 119–120
venous air embolism (VAE), 122
postoperative complications
brain edema, 124
diabetes insipidus, 123
hyperglycemia, 123
hyponatremia, 123
perioperative prophylaxis, 124
vascular malformations, 127
NICE-UK. See National Institute for Health
     and Clinical Excellence (NICE-UK)
NIRS. See Near-infrared spectroscopy (NIRS)
NMS. See Neuromuscular scoliosis (NMS)
Noninvasive hemodynamic monitoring
applications, 380
blood pressure (BP) monitoring, 387,
     392–394
cardiac output (CO), 388–390
electrocardiogram (ECG), 390–391
intraoperative monitoring, 380
medications, 379
NIRS, 391–392
Noninvasive respiratory monitoring
acoustic impedance monitoring, 387
applications, 380
$ETCO_2$, 382–384
intraoperative monitoring, 380
medications, 379
pulse oximetry, 380–382
$TC-CO_2$, 384–386
Nonoperating room anesthesia (NORA),
     75–82
Non-opioid analgesics
acetaminophen (paracetamol), 424
clonidine and dexmedetomidine, 426
dexamethasone, 426
dosing, 424, 425
gabapentinoids (gabapentin and
     pregabalin), 426
ketamine, 426
lidocaine infusion, 426
NSAIDs, 425–426
sucrose, 426
Non-pharmacological management, pain
child life specialists, 429
clown doctors, 429
context-induced placebo analgesia, 429
family-based preparation, 429
psychological factors, 429
tablet-based distraction, 429

Non-pharmacological preparation
  parental presence during induction of
      anesthesia (PPIA), 25, 27
  preoperative anxiety
    components of, 21
    development factors, 22
    high levels of, 22
    low levels of, 22
    preoperative visit, 22
    "receptivity" of the patient and the
        parents, 22
    transient state, 21
  for surgery
    ADVANCE project, 24
    age, children, 23–24
    coping techniques, 23
    fasting, 27
    informative approach, 23
    modeling techniques, 23
    MRI, 24
    music therapy, 24
    parents' anxiety, 24
    play and games, 23–24, 26
    play specialist, 24
    success of, 24
    tablet-based interactive distraction
        (TBID), 24
NORA. See Nonoperating room anesthesia
    (NORA)
Nuss procedure, 132–134

O
Obstructive sleep apnea (OSA)
  adenotonsillectomy, guidelines
    AAP, 202
    American Academy of Otolaryngology,
        201–202
    intraoperative management, 202–203
    Italian National Program Guidelines,
        201
    postoperative management, 203
  anesthesia management
    ASA guidelines, 200
    options, 200–201
  central hypoventilation syndromes,
      197–198
  clinical presentation, 188
  consequences, 188–189
  diagnosis
    biomarkers, 192
    cardiorespiratory studies, 191
    diagnostics test, 190–191
    Nap studies, 192
    oximetry, 191

    physical exam and medical history,
        189–190
    radiologic studies, 192
  epidemiology, 187
  infants and premature infants, 195
  medical treatment, 198
  neuronal control
    anatomical balance model, 193–194
    anatomic factors, 194–195
    loop gain, 194
    neural balance model, 194
    pharyngeal dilator muscles, regulation,
        194
  obese child, 195–196
  respiratory control
    larynx, 193
    mouth and pharynx, 193
    nasopharynx, 192–193
    upper airway anatomy
        and relationship, 192
  risk factors, 188
  surgical treatments, 198–200
  syndromes, 196, 197
Obstructive sleep apnea syndrome
    (OSA), 58
Oncological therapy
  chemotherapy (see Chemotherapy)
  radiation toxicity, 238–239
"One-stop anesthesia" modality, 13
"One-stop surgery", 13, 15
Opioid analgesics
  adverse effects, 419
  dosing, 419, 420
  fentanyl, 421
  hydromorphone, 422
  methadone, 422
  morphine, 420–421
  nalbuphine, 422
  oral administration, 419
  oxycodone, 421
  PCA/NCA/PARCA, 423–424
  remifentanil, 421
  sufentanil, 421
  tramadol, 422–423
Oral administration
  α_2-agonists, 31
  intramuscular administration, 63
  ketamine, 30–31
  midazolam, 30
Orthopaedic surgery
  ambulatory surgery, 88–89
  blood management
    antifibrinolytics, 95
    intraoperative blood recovery and
        reinfusion, 94–95

preoperative donation of autologous
blood, 94
transfusion trigger, 95
fasting, 89
intraoperative positioning
and warming, 91
peripheral paediatric
general anaesthesia, 100, 101
lower limb, 103–106
MAC, 100, 101
regional anaesthesia, 100, 101
supraglottic devices, 101
trachea, intubated, 101
upper limb, 102–103
wound infiltration, 101
postoperative care
compartment syndrome, 98–99
pain treatment, 96–98
premedication, 89
preoperative evaluation, 87
procedural sedation, 89–90
tourniquets, 91–93
OSA. See Obstructive sleep apnea
syndrome (OSA)
Outcome human measure, anesthetic drugs,
439–440
Oximetry, 191
Oxygen toxicity, 140

P
Paediatric airway
anatomical considerations, 148
classification
approaches, 151–152
expected difficult airway, 151
impaired normal, 150–151
normal, 150
management
equipment, 155–157
expected difficult airway, 154–155
suspected difficult, 154
unexpected difficult airway, 152–154
obstruction, clinical consequences,
149–150
Paediatric anaesthesia behaviour
(PAB) score, 406
Pain
adjuvants (see Adjuvant therapy)
assessment
parental postoperative, 418
perioperative care of children, 246–247
tools, children, 226, 227
definition, 245–246
measurement, 418

nonpharmacological pain
management, 254
optimal pain management, 246–247
pharmacological treatment, 247–253
post-op pain in cancer patient, 254
sedation techniques, 255
treatment, 247
Paravertebral thorax, 428
Parental presence during induction of
anesthesia (PPIA), 25, 27
Parents' postoperative pain measure
(PPPM), 418
PDNV. See Post-discharge nausea and
vomiting (PDNV)
Pectoralis (PEC) blocks, 428
Pectus carinatum
analgesic considerations, 134
Ravitch procedure, 134
reverse Nuss procedure, 134
surgical technique, 134
Pectus excavatum
analgesic considerations
paravertebral nerve block (PVNB), 133
patient-controlled analgesia
(PCA), 133
thoracic epidural (TE), 133
Nuss procedure, 132, 133
preoperative assessment of, 131
surgical technique, 132
Pediatric airway features, 215, 277
Pediatric anesthesia emergence delirium
(PAED) scale, 408
Pediatric early warning score (PEWS), 15
Pediatric intensive care unit (PICU), 123
Pediatric regional anesthesia network
(PRAN), 103
Periclavicular approaches
advantages and disadvantages, 312
cervicothoracic veins, 313, 315
CVC placement, children, 312, 314
infraclavicular access, subclavian vein
(SCV)
brachial plexus injury, 316
ipsilateral IJV, 317
puncture site, 316
puncture techniques, age category, 317
US-guided approach, 317
panoramic view, major veins, 312, 314
supraclavicular access, brachiocephalic
vein (BCV)
brachial plexus damage, 315–316
cervicothoracic veins, 315
in hypovolemic patients, 314
transpectoral access, axillary vein (AxV),
318–320

Perioperative care
  with cancer
    anesthesia care, 255
    immunomodulatory effects (see
      Immunomodulatory effects, cancer)
    pediatric cancer by age, 229, 230
    pediatric cancer pain (see Pain)
    pediatric cancer stats, 229
    preoperative evaluation and testing, 245
  metabolic diseases
    glycogenosis, 180
    mitochondrial cytopathy, 180–183
    reflex, 183–184
    sources, 176–177
    synthesis of, 177–178
    urea cycle defect, 178–179
  NMD (see Neuromuscular disorders
    (NMDs))
  OSA (see Obstructive sleep apnea (OSA))
  trauma
    anatomical and functional aspects, 215
    anatomical and physiological
      features, 228
    blunt injury in children, 214
    capillary refill time detection, 215
    clinical assessment, 223
    coagulopathy, 223
    DCS, 224, 225
    diagnosis and treatment, primary
      injuries, 213
    history and clinical examination, 222
    imaging and laboratory testing, 223
    intraoperative fluid management,
      223–224
    intraoperative management, 223
    mortality for traumatic injury, 213
    motor vehicle collisions, 213
    pain assessment, 226–227
    pedestrian and bicycle accidents, 213
    pediatric management, 214, 216
    postoperative period, 224–225
    post-traumatic stress disorder, 215
    primary survey, 216–221
    routine laboratory tests, 223
    sedation and analgesia, 225–226
    trauma injury, 213
    trauma management, 213
Perioperative medicine
  anesthesiology and, 5–6
  areas of, 5
  definition, 1
  enhanced recovery after surgery (ERAS)
    program, 2–3
  patient, surgery and complications, 1–2
  postoperative phase

    acute pain management, 4
    chronic postsurgical pain (CPSP), 5
    echocardiography, 4
    hemodynamic management, 4
    intensity of, 4
    noncardiac ultrasound, 4–5
  preoperative phase
    intraoperative phase, 3–4
    pre-habilitation, 3
    risk assessment and optimization, 3
Perioperative prophylaxis, 124
Peripherally inserted central catheters (PICCs)
  catheter placement
    catheter selection, 327
    catheter tip positioning, 329
    insertion technique, 328, 329
    palpation, 326–327
    prevention and detection, 327–328
    sedation, 327
    vein selection, 327
  central vein damage, 326
  complications
    infection rate, 331
    mechanical problems, 330–331
    thrombosis, 331
  decision-making tree, 325
  definition, 325
  fixation and maintenance
    fluoroscopy, 329, 330
    suture-free securing device, 329
  hamper catheter advancement, 326
  indications, 325–326
  local skin damage, 326
  peripheral vein damage, 326
  technical insertion difficulties, 326
Peripheral venous access (PVA)
  arterial circulation, 298
  extravasation, 301
  hematoma, 302
  hypnosis techniques, 296
  indications, 293–294, 296
  near-infrared technology, 299, 300
  phlebitis, 301
  puncture sites
    foot, 298
    forearm and antecubital fossa, 297
    hand, 297
    neck, 298
    scalp, 298
    wrist, 298
  residual anesthetic medication, 302
  transillumination, 299
  USG, 299–301
PEWS. See Pediatric early warning score
  (PEWS)

Pharmacodynamics and pharmacokinetics
  hypnotics, 264
  neuromuscular blocking agents, 264, 265
  opioids, 264
Pharmacological premedication
  ketamine, 63
  midazolam, 63
  oral administration, 63
Pharmacological preparation
  close monitoring after premedication, 28
  drugs and doses, 28, 29
  enteral/transmucosal premedication, 29
  indications for premedication, 28
  nasal route (see Nasal administration)
  oral route (see Oral administration)
  premedication goal, 28
  rectal route (see Rectal administration)
Pharmacological treatment
  acetaminophen, 247
  equianalgesic opioid doses, 251
  fentanyl, 251–252
  hydromorphone, 252
  ibuprofen, 247–248
  methadone, 252–253
  morphine, 250–251
  naloxone, 253
  opioids, opioid-naive neonates, 248, 249
  oxycodone, 253
  parenteral and oral dose formulations,
    248, 250
  patient-controlled analgesia in
    children, 250
Pharmacologic approach, e-PONB
  alpha2-adrenergic agonists, 411
  fentanyl, 412
  intravenous anaesthesia with propofol, 411
  midazolam, 411
  pain management, 411–412
Pharynx, 193
Phenol, 262
PICU. See Pediatric intensive care unit (PICU)
Pierre Robin sequence, 274
Platinum 30 min, 214
Play specialists, 24
Plexus or psoas compartment block
  (PSCB), 104
Polysomnography, 190
PONV. See Postoperative nausea and vomiting
  (PONV)
Postanesthetic discharge scoring system
  (PADSS), 69–71, 71t
Post-discharge nausea and vomiting (PDNV), 69
Postoperative analgesia, 266
Postoperative nausea and vomiting (PONV),
  68–69

Postoperative pain, child's behaviour, 404
Postoperative period
  airway obstruction, 279
  care of children, trauma, 224–225
Postoperative vomiting (POV), 68
POV. See Postoperative vomiting (POV)
PPIA. See Parental presence during induction
  of anesthesia (PPIA)
Prader-Willi syndrome, 196
PRAN. See Pediatric Regional Anesthesia
  Network (PRAN)
Preoperative anxiolysis, 411
Preoperative evaluation
  children care, cancer, 245
  CP
    baclofen, 261
    botulinum toxin (Botox), 262
    contractures and deformities, 261
    developmental delay, 260
    epilepsy, 262
    flexion, toes, 260
    gastroesophageal reflux, 260
    laparoscopic fundoplication, 261
    neurolytic blocks, 262
    sarcopenia, 261
    spasticity, 261
    vigabatrin, 261
  family history, 14
  operating risk stratification
    American Society of Anesthesiologist
      Physical Status (ASA-PS), 12
    Johns Hopkins surgery risk
      classification system (JHSRCS), 12
    NARCO-SS score, 12
  physical examination
    body weight and length, 15
    pediatric early warning score (PEWS), 15
    preschool children, 14
    school-age children, 14
    teenagers, 14
    toddlers, 14
  preoperative assessment, 13
  preoperative test
    anemia, 15
    blood glucose, 16
    chest radiography, 16
    ECG, 16
    guidelines and recommendations, 15
    laboratory tests, 15
    nonselective coagulation screening, 16
    plasma electrolytes, 16
  timing and organization
    "one-stop anesthesia" modality, 13, 15
    "one-stop surgery", 13
    preoperative visit, 13, 14

Preparation, preoperative
  fasting, 34
  non-pharmacological preparation (*See*
      Non-pharmacological preparation)
  pharmacological preparation (*See*
      Pharmacological preparation)
Preventive analgesia, 419
Primary injuries, 213, 214
Primary survey, trauma
  airway, 217
  bleeding/hypertensive pneumothorax, 216
  breathing, 217–219
  circulation, 219–220
  disability, 221
  exposure, 221
  family, 222
  tension pneumothorax, 219
  verbal/slight painful stimulus, 216
Prophylaxis, 46
Propofol anaesthesia, 407–408
Propofol infusion, 411
PROSPECT project, 430
PSCB. *See* Plexus or psoas compartment block
      (PSCB)
Pudendal, 429
Pulse contour analysis technique, 389
Pulse oximetry
  description, 380–381
  external and patient-related factors, 382
  hypoxemia, 381
  oxygenated hemoglobin, 381
  patient-controlled analgesia, 381
  therapeutic decision-making tool, 381
Puncture techniques
  needle tip, 291, 292
  patent vessels, 290
  sites
    foot, 298
    forearm and antecubital fossa, 297
    hand, 297
    neck, 298
    scalp, 298
    wrist, 298
  sliding movements, 291
  US needle guidance, 291

Q
Quadratus lumborum, 429

R
Radiation toxicity, 238–239
Radioallergosorbent test (RAST), 46

Rapid-onset obesity with hypothalamic
      dysfunction (ROHHAD), 198
Rapid sequence induction (RSI)
  technique, 139
Ravitch procedure, 133, 134
Rectal administration
  α_2-agonists, 33–34
  ketamine, 33
  midazolam, 33
Regional anaesthesia
  block techniques and dosing regimens,
      428–429
  continuous infusion, 427
  CPNBs, 427
  epidural blocks, 427
  infusion guidelines, 427, 429
  nerve blocks and dosing regimens,
      427, 430
  peri-and postsurgical stress, 427
  ultrasound guidance, 427
Regional anesthesia, 168
Remote locations
  anesthesiological management
    cerebral activity monitoring, 78
    depth of sedation, definitions, 79
    $EtCO_2$ monitoring, 78
    flexibility, 77
    hemodynamic monitoring (EKG,
        NiBP), 78
    multiple routes of administration, 79
    respiratory monitoring, 78
  complementary techniques, 81–82
  discharge, 82
  inhalation techniques, 79–80
  intravenous techniques
    alfentanil, 81
    dexmedetomidine, 81
    ketamine, 81
    Ketofol, 81
    propofol, 81
    remifentanil, 81
    target-controlled infusion (TCI), 80
  nonoperating room anesthesia (NORA),
      75–82
  pre-procedural assessment
    failed sedations, 77
    fasting status, 77
    LEMON (Look at him, Evaluation,
        Mallampati, Obstruction, Neck), 76
    SOAPME (Suction, Oxygen, Airway,
        Pharmacy, Monitors, Equipment), 76
Retinoic acid syndrome, 245
Reverse Nuss, 134
Rhabdomyolysis, 163

S
Sacral plexus, 428
Salivation, 262
Salt-wasting brain syndrome (SWS), 123
Sciatic nerve block
    biceps femoris muscle, 361
    catheter, 363, 365
    IP midfemoral approach, 363, 364
    IP subgluteous approach, 361, 362
    local anesthetic spread, 361, 363
Scoliosis surgery
    apical vertebra, 106–107
    cerebral palsy, 108
    Cobb method, 106–107
    estimated blood loss (EBL), 109
    extubation criteria, 111
    intraoperative spinal cord monitoring, 110
    motor evoked potentials (MEPs), 110
    neuromuscular scoliosis (NMS), 107, 108
    neurophysiologic monitoring, 110
    preoperative variables, 109
    prone position for posterior approach, 109
    scoliosis, defined, 106
    scoliosis surgery correction, 109
    scoliotic curve, 106
    somatosensorial evoked potentials
        (SSEPs), 110
    spinal fusion surgery, 111
    spinal instrumentation, 108
    surgical procedures, 106
    vertebral rotation and rib cage
        deformity, 108
Secondary injuries, 214
Sedation and analgesia, 78, 81, 127,
        225–226, 255
SFAR. *See* Société Française d'Anesthésie et
        de Réanimation (SFAR)
Shock, 44, 138, 219–220, 449
SIADH. *See* Syndrome of inappropriate
        antidiuretic hormone secretion
        (SIADH)
Sickle cell disease, 59
SIDS. *See* Sudden infant death syndrome
        (SIDS)
Skin prick test (SPT), 45
"Sleep-awake-asleep" technique, 125
Sleep-disordered breathing (SDB), 187
Société Française d'Anesthésie et de
        Réanimation (SFAR), 69, 70
Somatosensory evoked potentials (SSEPs), 120
Spasticity
    baclofen, 261
    intrathecal injections, 261
    vigabatrin, 261

Spontaneous ventilation, 279
SSEPs. *See* Somatosensory evoked potentials
        (SSEPs)
Subglottic stenosis (SGS)
    congenital distal tracheal stenosis, 278
    diagnostic bronchoscopy, 278
    endotracheal intubation, 277
    and laryngeal pathologies
        Benjamin's and Inglis' classification,
            275, 276
        Cohen's and Benjamin's classification,
            276, 277
        vocal cord paralysis, 276
    laryngomalacia, 275
    and tracheal pathologies, 277–278
    tracheomalacia, 278
Succinylcholine, 163, 164, 167
Sudden infant death syndrome (SIDS), 59
Sugammadex, 264
Superior vena cava (SVC)
    catheter malposition, 321
    cavo-atrial junction, 307
    ECG guidance, 308
    fluoroscopy, 308
    immediate complications, 320–321
    internal jugular vein (IJV) (*see* Internal
        jugular vein (IJV))
    late complications, 321
    periclavicular approaches (*see*
        Periclavicular approaches)
    pleural puncture, 307
    spontaneous breathing, 307
    ultrasonography, 308
Surgery
    infants brain, anesthesia, 442–443
    preparation for
        ADVANCE, project, 24
        age, children, 23–24
        coping techniques, 23
        fasting, 27
        informative approach, 23
        modeling techniques, 23
        MRI, 24
        music therapy, 24
        parents' anxiety, 24
        play and games, 23–24, 26
        play specialist, 24
        success of, 24
        tablet-based interactive distraction
            (TBID), 24
SWS. *See* Salt-wasting brain
        syndrome (SWS)
Syndrome of inappropriate antidiuretic
        hormone secretion (SIADH), 123

T
Tablet-based interactive distraction (TBID), 24
TAP. *See* Transversus abdominis plane
    (TAP) block
Target-controlled infusion (TCI), 80
TBID. *See* Tablet-based interactive distraction
    (TBID)
TC-CO$_2$. *See* Transcutaneous CO$_2$ (TC-CO$_2$)
    devices
TCD. *See* Transcranial Doppler (TCD)
TCI. *See* Target-controlled infusion (TCI)
Temperature, 263
Tension pneumothorax, 219
Thermal homeostasis
    forced air systems, 263
    hypothermia, 263
Thermodilution method, 388, 390
Thoracic electrical bioimpedance (TEB), 389
TIVA. *See* Total intravenous anesthesia (TIVA)
Tizanidine, 262
Tonsillectomy, 71–72
Total intravenous anesthesia (TIVA), 121,
    167–168
Tracheal intubation, 41, 102, 150, 153–155,
    218, 240
Tracheomalacia, 278
Tranexamic acid, 266
Transcranial Doppler (TCD), 120
Transcutaneous CO$_2$ (TC-CO$_2$) devices
    advantages and disadvantages, 386
    cutaneous vasoconstriction, 385
    diabetic ketoacidosis (DKA), 385
    neonatal population, 384
    pulmonary ventilation-perfusion
        matching, 385
    ventilation techniques, 384
Transpulmonary thermodilution (TPTD), 388
Transversus abdominis plane (TAP) block
    IP TAP block, 372, 373
    local anesthetic dispersion, 374
    needle insertion, 371
    neuraxial blockade, 372
    oblique fascia, 372
    subcostal/lateral, 429
Treacher-Collins syndrome, 101, 274
Trisomy 21, 138
Tumor lysis syndrome (TLS), 243–244

U
Ultrasound (US) equipment
    adult and pediatric, young children, 290
    block technique, 343

cart-based echographs, 342
curvilinear probes, 289
Doppler and Zoom functions, 288–289
high-frequency probes, 289
linear probes, 289
needle handling skills, 346–347
probes
    linear transducers, 343
    nerve block, 345
    sector, 343
    types, children, 343, 344
small-footprint probes, 289
sterile probe covers and sterile gel, 290
ultrasonography, 345, 346
Ultrasound guidance (USG)
    advantages, 286–287
    applications, 285
    equipment
        adult and pediatric, young children, 290
        curvilinear probes, 289
        Doppler and Zoom functions, 288–289
        high-frequency probes, 289
        linear probes, 289
        small-footprint probes, 289
        sterile probe covers and sterile gel, 290
    gel models, 293, 295
    learning curve, 293, 295
    limitations, 287
    post-procedural screening, 287, 288
    puncture techniques, 290–293
    sterile setting and ergonomics, 293, 295
    sterility and ergonomy, 293, 295
    during vascular access, 288, 289
Umbilical, 429
UMSS. *See* University of Michigan Sedation
    Scale (UMSS)
Uncooperative behavior management, 265
University of Michigan Sedation Scale
    (UMSS), 82
Upper limb blocks, US-guided techniques
    axillary approach
        anechoic structure, 356
        brachial plexus block, 356
        catheter, 357, 359
        compression, 356, 357
        high-frequency linear probe, 357, 358
        in-plane technique, 357
        local anesthetic, 357, 359
        vascularization, 356
    brachial plexus, 347
    infraclavicular approach, 351–355
    interscalene block approach, 348–350
    supraclavicular approach, 351–353

Upper respiratory infections (URI). *See also*
    Asthma
    day-surgery, 59–60
    endotracheal tube or LMA, 40
    laryngospasm, 40, 41
    propofol anesthesia, 40
    risk factors, 40, 41
    salbutamol, 41
    symptoms of, 40
Urea cycle defect, 178–179
USG regional anesthetic techniques
    axillary approach, 356–359
    cart-based echographs, 342
    continuous peripheral nerve blocks,
        374, 375
    lower limb blocks (*see* Lower limb blocks,
        USG techniques)
    truncal blocks
        iliohypogastric (IH) and ilioinguinal
            (II) nerves, 367–370
        rectus sheath block, 370–372
        TAP, 371–374
    ultrasound equipment (*see* Ultrasound
        (US) equipment)
    upper limb blocks (*see* Upper limb blocks,
        US-guided techniques)
    USG, 341

V
Vaccination, 48
VACTERL association, 138
VAE. *See* Venous air embolism (VAE)
Valproic acid, 262
Vascular access, perioperative period
    arterial access
        axillary artery, 336
        brachial artery, 336
        complications, 336–337
        dorsalis pedis artery, 336
        femoral artery, 334–336

indications and equipment, 333–334
ischemia, 336, 337
local infection, 337
posterior tibial artery, 336
radial artery, 334, 335
temporal artery, 336
ulnar artery, 336
vasospasm, 336–337
bedside ultrasound examination, 285
CVC (*see* Central venous catheter (CVC))
IO route
    complications, 333
    contraindication, 333
    description, 331–332
    devices, 332–333
    perioperative indications, 332
    technique, 332–333
PICCs (*see* Peripherally inserted central
    catheters (PICCs))
portal vein thrombosis, 338
PVA (*see* Peripheral venous
    access (PVA))
real-time needle guidance, 285
ultrasound guidance (*see* Ultrasound
    guidance (USG))
umbilical arteries, 338
umbilical vein, 337–338
Vascular malformations, 127
Venipuncture, 27
Venous air embolism (VAE), 120, 122
Venous thromboembolism (VTE), 99–100
Ventilation techniques, 279
Vocal cord paralysis, 276
von Willebrand factor type I, 262
VTE. *See* Venous thromboembolism (VTE)

W
Wolff-Parkinson-White one (WPW), 16
WPW. *See* Wolff-Parkinson-White one
    (WPW)

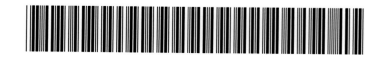